NURSING ADMINISTRATION HANDBOOK

Fourth Edition

Edited by
Howard S. Rowland
&
Beatrice L. Rowland

AN ASPEN PUBLICATION®
Aspen Publishers, Inc.
Gaithersburg, Maryland
1997

This publication is designed to provide accurate and authoritative information in regard to the Subject Matter covered. It is sold with the understanding
that the publisher is not engaged in rendering legal, accounting, or other
professional service. If legal advice or other expert assistance is required, the
service of a competent professional person should be sought. (From a
Declaration of Principles jointly adopted by a Committee of the American Bar
Association and a committee of publishers and associations.

Library of Congress Cataloging-in-Publication Data

Nursing administration handbook / edited by Howard S. Rowland &
Beatrice L. Rowland — 4th ed.
p.   cm.
Includes bibliographical references and index.
ISBN 0-8342-0926-8
1. Nursing services—Administration. I. Rowland, Howard S.
II. Rowland, Beatrice L.
[DNLM: 1. Nursing, Supervisory. 2. Nurse Administration. WY 105 N9734 1997]
RT89.N765   1997
362.1'73'068—dc21
DNLM/DLC
for Library of Congress
96-39566
CIP

Orders: (800) 638-8437
Customer Service: (800) 234-1660

About Aspen Publishers • For more than 35 years, Aspen has been a leading professional
publisher in a variety of disciplines. Aspen's vast information resources are available in both
print and electronic formats. We are committed to providing the highest quality information
available in the most appropriate format for our customers. Visit Aspen's Internet site for more
information resources, directories, articles, and a searchable version of Aspen's full catalog,
including the most recent publications: **http://www/aspenpub.com**
Aspen Publishers, Inc. • The hallmark of quality in publishing
Members of the worldwide Wolters Kluwer group.

Editorial Resources: Ruth Bloom

Library of Congress Catalog Card Number: 96-39566
ISBN: 0-8342-0926-8

Printed in the United States of America

1 2 3 4 5

Table of Contents

Preface

Throughout the 1990s, new and radical developments in the health care field have been introduced at a breathless pace. Today the key note being struck repeatedly is "change," to accommodate new realities: from reactive health care to illness prevention, from costly procedures to cost-conscious efficiencies, from one-stop hospital stays to an array of care delivery options, from segmentation of treatment to a continuum of care, from curing illness to caring for clients, from a broad focus on process to a fixed one on outcome, from nursing staff to interdisciplinary providers, from individual to team accountability, from problem solutions to process/system improvements, and so on.

The most competent and experienced nurse administrators have to hustle to keep up with new developments that daily affect their nursing departments both directly and indirectly. And administrators in training are confronted by major transitions in management theory, practice, and even vocabulary, in addition to the structural changes taking place in the field.

The times are both exhilarating and daunting, providing new opportunities while offering few reliable precedents for guidance. Individuals just starting in this field need a road map to negotiate their way through an increasingly complex and rapidly evolving field. The *Nursing Admin-*

istration Handbook has a long track record, both as a textbook and as a hands-on tool for nurse executives seeking insight and step-by-step guidance in all aspects of administration. We are determined that it remain the leading text in the field. That is why this fourth edition of the *Nursing Administration Handbook* freshly surveys the entire field of nursing administration and incorporates the most significant new developments and current practices.

This edition includes completely new chapters, major enhancements in most other chapters, and a host of updates and revisions throughout. No chapter has been left untouched. The new materials and expert insights are supplemented by a wealth of guidance from prominent nurse educators and nurse administrators working in the field. Our goal has been to provide the vital information required by the nurse administrator who wants to stay ahead of—not just in step with—the pack.

Major additions and updates in the extensive new material introduced in this edition are outlined below.

The executive challenges of today are freshly dealt with in three new chapters: Chapter 6, "Change and Transformation," discriminates among reengineering, restructuring, and redesign, which are all reconfiguration techniques currently used to improve health care systems and departments. Chapter 37, "New Realities," reviews the transitional measures and the new structures being put into place in the delivery of health care services in the managed care environment. Chapter 8, "Teamwork," provides practical guidance for coping with the new team-based workplace.

New perspectives on management style and methods are covered in a widely altered and expanded Part I of the book. Chapter 1 emphasizes the significance and reliance on leadership skills. Chapter 2 provides information on the transformation of the nurse manager's role. Explanations of newly developed administration methods—facilitating, collaborating, participative decision making, systematic problem solving—are some of the issues reviewed in Chapters 3 through 5. And new appendixes provide an extensive guide to the sophisticated tools managers are now expected to use in the increasingly significant disciplines of strategic planning and quality evaluation.

New mandates, technical developments, and critical concepts in the health care field are discussed in several totally revamped chapters. These include Chapter 22, "Quality Concepts," and Chapter 16, "Information Management and Technology," two areas of overwhelming importance in health care. Administrative responsibilities in patient care are newly presented in two chapters: Chapter 14 offers an updated view of nursing delivery systems and the documentation of care; Chapter 15 focuses on the patient as customer and on patient-centered relations. Communication has become increasingly important as nursing staff work in closer coordination with other departments to improve patient care or administrative procedures. Chapter 28 provides fresh and valuable approaches for hand-

ling conflict, dealing with staff diversity and cultural congruence, and developing negotiating skills.

In addition, there are major revisions in most chapters to bring readers abreast of other current practices. Some of the topics discussed include the legal and regulatory environment affecting nursing personnel, additional concerns regarding nurse liability, current union issues, worker safety, computer software to support scheduling and the budget decision-making process, financial delegation, the nurse administrator's ethical stewardship, the application of management principles to encourage a learning environment, and the educational needs of new-style leaders.

Finally, although much has been added, replaced, updated, and revised in this new book, we want to assure users of earlier editions that the features that many have found critical to successful nursing management—which may explain why the *Nursing Administration Handbook* is called a classic—are still very much in place. Our intention is to preserve these essential elements along with the most recent developments to make this book an up-to-date and comprehensive single-volume resource on nursing administration. To that end, much of the organization and the internal headings of the earlier edition have been maintained to facilitate the use of this handbook as a thoroughly updated, though still familiar, reference.

Our goal is to provide the users of this edition of the *Nursing Administration Handbook* with dependable administrative knowledge, effective practices, and the specific tools necessary so that they can deal confidently with the new developments now impacting the field of nursing administration and will be fully ready for those developments that are still emerging.

Part I

Management

Chapter 1

Leadership

LEADERSHIP IN A RADICALLY CHANGING HEALTH CARE ENVIRONMENT

In health care, the structures and mechanisms for delivering services are being modified daily. The new configurations are having a significant impact on managers and organizational leaders, whose ability to understand and cope with the processes at work is being severely challenged.

New Requirements*

Using the principles of partnership, equity, accountability, and ownership, leaders are beginning to create a more interactive milieu that balances the roles of providers with the expectations of communities within an environment of fixed resources. Leaders must now be fluid and flexible in style and approach and create the kind of situation that will allow those who do the work of health care to connect in new ways and to interact as necessary to build a truly comprehensive continuum of services. (See Table 1–1.)

New structures, principles, relationships, and behaviors require new approaches and skill foundations for leaders. Leading and managing without relying on the traditional superior-subordinate relationship demands different skills from those most managers now have. It means seeing the world of health care work from within the new paradigm and helping others develop new ways of working and relating. It means being able to assess individual strengths, skills, and needs and doing what is necessary to learn to be effective. It calls for support, integration, linkage, and risk-taking. It means leaving disciplinary, departmental, compartmental, segregated, and polarized structures and behaviors behind and constructing a framework in which new equity-based values, structures, relationships, and behaviors converge around the communities served by health care providers.

ELEMENTS OF LEADERSHIP IN HEALTH CARE

Establishing and Reinforcing Values*

People who work in health care organizations are guided more by vision, goals, and values than by production targets and output payments. Lead-

---

*Source: Adapted from Tim Porter-O'Grady and Cathleen Krueger Wilson, *The Leadership Revolution in Health Care: Altering Systems, Changing Behaviors*, Aspen Publishers, Inc., © 1995.

*Source: David B. Starkweather and Donald G. Shropshire, "Management Effectiveness," in *Manual of Health Services Management*, Robert J. Taylor, ed., Aspen Publishers, Inc., © 1994.

Table 1–1 Current Viewpoints on Leadership

Tasks of Leadership*

- Envisioning goals
- Affirming values
- Motivating people
- Managing resources and circumstances
- Achieving a workable level of unity
- Explaining mission, goals, policies, and issues
- Serving as a symbol of the work group's identity
- Representing the group externally
- Renewing tangible and intangible resources, particularly people

Leadership Behaviors**

- Challenging the process
  - –Search for opportunities.
  - –Experiment and take risks.
- Inspiring a shared vision
  - –Envision the future.
  - –Enlist others.
- Enabling others to act
  - –Foster collaboration.
  - –Strengthen others.
- Modeling the way
  - –Set the examples.
  - –Plan small wins.
- Encouraging the heart
  - –Recognize individual contributions.
  - –Celebrate accomplishments.

Formalized Role for Leadership***

- Establishing and promulgating the organization's mission, renewing and revising it as necessary
- Building on the mission, defining and establishing a clear vision for what the organization can and resolves to become, encouraging staff participation in its development
- Developing other leaders at every level of the organization who help fulfill the organization's mission and vision
- Accurately assessing the needs of the organization's patients (and other uses of the organization's services) and developing an organizational culture that focuses on improving performance to meet these needs
- Defining a strategic plan that is consistent with the organization's mission and vision
- Clearly communicating the mission, vision, and plan throughout the organization
- Fulfilling the organization's vision by providing the framework to accomplish the goals of the strategic plan
- Developing this framework through the proper direction, implementation, coordination, and, ultimately, improvement of services throughout the organization

*Source: Gardner, J.W. *The Tasks of Leadership*. Paper prepared for the Leadership Studies Program. Washington, DC: Independent Sector, March 1986.

**Source: Adapted from Kouzes, J.M. and Posner, B.Z. *The Leadership Challenges*. San Francisco: Jossey-Bass, 1987, p. 14.

***Source: Adapted from © *1994 Accreditation Manual for Hospitals* (Volume I—Standards). Oakbrook Terrace, IL: Joint Commission on Accreditation of Healthcare Organizations, 1993. Reprinted with permission.

---

ership in health care therefore involves establishing and reinforcing a service-oriented ethic.

Health care enterprises also do not possess tight corporate hierarchies where things get done because managers order them to be done. To a great extent, commands in health care enterprises will be followed only if they are accepted as legitimate and reasonable by those expected to respond. But what is reasonable and legitimate? This is what leadership establishes.

Many health care enterprises (including most hospitals) are tax-exempt community benefit organizations and, as such, must accept the main responsibility for setting community service goals and strategies.

In short, health care organizations are value driven, and their leaders establish and nurture the appropriate values. Below is a description of seven ways in which they can do this.

Possess Vision

The effective manager must be able to articulate a clear vision for the organization or his or her unit and do it in such a way that others come to believe in that vision. Subordinates must buy into what the unit must do to advance the vision. They must become excited by the vision and develop a "can do" attitude. Whatever the source, the manager has to personally own the vision; otherwise, the manager will fail to inspire others.

Commit to the Development of Others

The manager must encourage and support the efforts of individuals within the organization to maximize their understanding and skills and must create a working environment that motivates them to commit their personal energy and talents to the pursuit of organizational objectives. In this role, the manager is more a mentor, educator, and coach than a boss.

Commitment to the development of others is an expression of trust in subordinates and in their initiative and creativity. This trust even encompasses permission to take risks and make mistakes, present alternative views, and offer dissent. This is leadership by empowerment. Subordinates will rise to the occasion when they feel trusted and empowered.

Establish Values

It is the leader's job to discover and declare what his or her organization stands for, to establish a morality that becomes the standard for others, and to declare this in clear and inspiring terms. Organizations are strongly guided by culture; managing the evolution of organizational culture is the process of establishing values. It is important for subordinates' self-esteem and respect that they know their actions are being evaluated in the context of a value system. They also are sensitive to these values and can be relied upon to reflect them in their behavior. The effective manager reinforces this system of values by personal example. This is "principled leadership."

Look for and Learn about New Methods and Techniques

The health care environment is rapidly changing, and organizational managers must be open to new knowledge. Managers at all levels need to go beyond organizational boundaries to look, learn, and bring back new concepts and techniques.

New methods are of tremendous assistance in learning what to do and how to do it better; they are frequently employed by the top managers responsible for the well-being of the entire organization.

"Looking beyond" is a strategy other managers need to use as well. Department managers, for example, need to communicate with other department managers to determine whether the fit, integration, and contributions of their departments are proper and effective and whether changes, new directions, and new priorities are in order. Leadership requires looking beyond; looking beyond leads to learning; and a learning organization is a more effective organization.

Establish Priorities and Direction

Establishing priorities adds focus. Setting the direction of the organization shows people what priorities are highest, how the organization's vision and values can be put into action, and where they should place their energies. Leadership establishes the strategic direction, and this focuses the organization's efforts on addressing its priorities and problems and how to translate a plan into action. Problem solving is less difficult if the manager creates an atmosphere in which others feel empowered to solve problems. Problem solving is a shirt-sleeve management task.

Balance the Interests of All Affected Customers

Health care organizations are composed of and associated with myriad interest groups: employees, physicians, nurses, the community, patients, suppliers, insurers, leaders, politicians, the media, and so on. Often they do not have a specific group of owners (stockholders) whose interests clearly should be given the highest priority. The effective health care manager works to balance the interests of all the stakeholders, usually to the benefit of the largest good. This balancing often calls for skills in facilitation, negotiation, and conflict resolution. It also requires consideration of ethical issues.

Demonstrate a Commitment for the Public Benefit

Obviously, organizational benefit is a goal of each manager. However, health care managers typically place community benefit and patient benefit at the top. This is the major difference between these executives and their business counterparts. The latter must "do no harm" and must "do well"; the former must "do good" for the public and patients they serve. Of course, the commitment to doing good must become a major element of the enterprise's value system. The effective leader must not only have and demonstrate a commitment to the public benefit but know how and when organizational objectives and actions should be modified in order to meet broad community needs.

Attributes Associated with Excellence in Nursing Leadership*

Excellent executive nursing leadership is vital to the survival of health care agencies in the current turbulent environment. Nurse executives play a critical role in determining the vision for health care facility departments and in setting the climate for changing practice. It is thus crucial to identify and define the leadership role of the nurse executive. One long-range study, completed between 1986 and 1989, examined excellent nurse executives' leadership styles. Nurse administrators with a reputation for excellence were selected for in-depth interviews on the characteristics of leadership in nursing. The following discussion identifies the primary themes that

emerged from the ideas and concepts and practices of the executives interviewed.

Nurse executives identify excellent nursing *leadership* with universal leadership skills. Nurse executives deviate from the general leadership description when they emphasize nursing's responsibility to influence the practice environment. They stress the importance of creating an environment in which the professional nurse can participate at both the organizational and the professional level. This emphasis on nursing practice exists because people come to the health care facility for patient care. As one executive stated, "The primary role of any nursing administrator is to facilitate clinical practice at the bedside level."

Another aspect of excellent nursing leadership is the integration of nursing into the overall organizational effort. The effective nurse executive is a *team player* who receives interdisciplinary respect and cooperation. Team players contribute to and ultimately determine the success or failure of the organization.

Negotiation skills are another must for the excellent nurse leader. The leader appreciates the difference between negotiation and compromise. The idea becomes "give some to get some," because "winning a battle might mean losing the war." Such executives are not afraid of losing or withdrawing from a battle. They prefer to reframe "battles" as team efforts aimed at a mutually agreed-upon outcome.

Excellent nurse executives serve as *ambassadors* representing nursing in its relations with the medical staff, the board, administrators, and the public. They have the ability to "translate the patient care needs into a language that the people of the power tables understand and appreciate."

Excellent leaders have *strong value systems*. The following qualities were identified: honesty, fairness, integrity, trust, and caring, accompanied by a drive for quality and excellence. These leaders are willing to take a stand on issues and remain true to their convictions. Nurse executives consistently *model* these values with the expectation that staff will emulate these values when caring for patients.

Excellent nursing leaders are *creative*, have a *vision* of what can be accomplished, and are

Source: Janne Dunham and Elaine Fisher, "Nurse Executive Profile of Excellent Nursing Leadership," *Nursing Administration Quarterly*, Vol. 13:2, Aspen Publishers, Inc., © 1989.

risk takers. Their vision is dynamic. They have good ideas and are open to new ideas from others.

Excellent nursing leaders are *charismatic*. They challenge, interest, and excite people about the vision, so that staff members also become committed to accomplishing the vision. The executives' vision surpasses that shared with staff members. The part of the vision shared with staff members stretches them, yet not so much that they think the vision is not possible.

Executive leadership involves *constant communication*, both written and oral, combined with strong interpersonal skills. Part of the effectiveness of top nurse executives' communication stems from a commitment to being direct as well as from an ability to ask the right questions. Knowing when to say, or not to say, something and knowing when to listen are considered very important. Executives use their vision to structure *goals* and set the direction.

Empowerment occurs when the vision and direction are clear. The leaders empower staff members by motivating them to make the vision a reality.

Empowerment requires recognizing staff potential and unleashing that potential to accomplish the vision. It involves turning "control over to nursing staff leaders while at the same time helping to guide the direction and create the environment." "Excellent nursing leadership is orchestrating your professional practice climate in such a way that the system moves effectively in the caring of patients and is cost-effective, yet your hand is hardly noticed."

Executives agree on the importance of recognizing excellence in others. Leadership "is not always being in front and having a whole army of followers." Although there is a place for leaders, leaders without an army of excellent people to support their efforts are not going to achieve what they are employed to achieve. There was agreement that power comes from below, not above.

Selection of *excellent staff* is a key factor. Excellent leaders teach and train staff, often serving as role models, *mentors*, and facilitators. Excellent leadership is being visible to staff and establishing relationships with them.

Excellent nurse leaders are decision makers. They have a well-developed sense of timing in addition to the ability and confidence to make immediate decisions, wait for outcomes, and persevere when necessary. They know when to make decisions, when to delay them, and when to let others make them.

Excellent nurse leaders *constantly grow and learn*. They learn by listening to those around them, staying current, challenging themselves continuously, and learning from their own mistakes and the mistakes of others.

There was consensus that excellent nursing leaders have well-developed *business skills*, including an understanding of finance and budgeting (i.e., knowing the bottom line), resource management, long- and short-range planning, systems analysis, and human resource management.

Excellent nurse leaders are involved outside the health care facility in professional organizations or in influencing governmental policy. This involvement is intraorganizational and broad based.

LEADERSHIP STYLE

Factors Affecting Leadership Style*

The leadership style adopted by the manager depends a great deal on factors such as (1) the importance of the results, (2) the nature of the work, (3) the characteristics of the workers, and (4) the personal characteristics of the manager. If work activity must be performed immediately, perhaps under disaster or crisis conditions, the health care manager may have to adopt a style from the autocratic end of the continuum. At other times, when work need not be done immediately, another style, perhaps consultative or participative, may be used.

----

*Source: Copyright © 1977, Jonathan S. Rakich.

The type of work being performed by subordinates can influence which style is most appropriate. If it is routine clerical work and must have a specific sequence flow, the manager may be more consultative than democratic in determining how and when the work activity will be performed. However, if the work is creative and flexible and other departments do not rely on its timely completion, the manager may be able to adopt a participative or democratic style. Certainly, the manager of the billing or accounts receivable department will adopt a different leadership style than the manager of a medical research department.

The subordinates' characteristics—their training, education, motivation, and experience—can influence the leadership style adopted by the manager. This factor is closely related to the type of work, since staff skills tend to correspond closely with the work required. If the subordinates are skilled professionals, the manager may seek their opinions more readily (consultative or participative style) in determining how and when the work is to be performed. If they are unskilled, not necessarily dependable, or inexperienced, the manager may have to make most of the decisions. Further, there are some employees who, because of their value systems or previous experiences, will not accept decision-making responsibility if it is offered.

Finally, the personal characteristics of the manager can affect the leader authority style adopted. Some individuals, by reason of their personality traits, previous experiences, values, and cultural background, function better under one style or another and may find it difficult to change with the situation. No one style is appropriate at all times. Which style is correct can only be answered after an evaluation of the situation, including the work environment, what is to be done, the nature of the employees, the personality of the manager, and the organizational climate.

Styles*

Various terms such as *autocratic* and *democratic* have been attached to the decision-mak-

---

Source: Jonathan S. Rakich, Beaufort B. Longest, and Thomas R. O'Donovan, *Managing Health Care Organizations*, W.B. Saunders Co., © 1977. Reprinted by permission of CBS College Publishing.

ing behavior vis-à-vis the manager and the subordinates. These labels are traditionally called "styles of leader decision authority" and can be displayed on a continuum. In addition, terms such as *employee-centered* and *work-centered* have been used to describe various supervisory styles used by managers in overseeing work activity. Rather than nodes on a continuum, they represent opposite ways in which managers interact with subordinates.

Autocratic

In the continuum of leader authority presented in Figure 1–1, the "autocratic" end represents the manager who makes decisions and announces them to the group. The use of the autocratic style means that the manager has made a decision pertaining to what the purpose of the group activity is, how the group activity is to be structured, and who is to be assigned to what specific tasks. The total interacting relationship and the work setting have been decided by the manager. The role of subordinates is to carry out orders without having any opportunity to materially alter the decisions that have been made. The manager provides little opportunity for a subordinate to participate in making decisions.

In health care settings, the pure form of the autocratic leader decision authority style is seldom exercised by administrators. It is often the physician who adopts this style as the individual responsible for the activities required for patient care. Out of necessity, the physician must make decisions that no one else can. Consequently, he or she will make decisions and announce them to other personnel, such as nurses and technicians, who will be expected to carry out the activities without deviation.

Consultative

The "consultative" style appears to the right of "autocratic." In this situation, the manager "sells" the decision or presents ideas and invites questions from subordinates, or both. Specifically, the manager makes decisions concerning the work activity to be carried out, its purpose, how it is to be done, when, and by whom and attempts to sell the subordinates on the decisions. The manager may recognize the possibility of some resistance and invite questions; however, unless overwhelming reasons cause a change in the decisions made, they stand.

Participative

If the manager presents a tentative decision that is subject to change or presents the problem to the subordinates, gets suggestions, and then makes the decision, he or she uses a "participative" style. The manager identifies the purposes, the problems, and the means by which the activities should be carried out; presents a tentative decision already made or seeks subordinate opinion; and then makes the decision. In this instance, the "area of decision freedom for subordinates" is much greater and the "use of authority by the manager" is much smaller than with the autocratic and consultative styles.

Participative management is a very powerful motivator in enabling employees to have some measure of influence and control over work-related activities. The work group can influence the decisions made concerning work activities and their purpose.

Democratic

Within a "democratic" style, the manager defines the limits of the situation and the problem to be solved and asks the group to make decisions. The subordinates have a relatively large "area of decision freedom," as indicated in Figure 1–1. The boundaries of activity are set by the manager, who permits the group to make decisions within those limits. For example, a nurse manager might allow only registered nurses to give medication but might permit them to decide among themselves who will give the medication and who will perform other tasks that must be done.

Laissez Faire

The term *laissez faire* was originally coined for the doctrine that government should not interfere with commerce. It is sometimes called "free rein." Under such leadership, subordinates are permitted to function within the limits set by the manager's own superior. There is no interference within the group by the manager, who, although participating in the decision making, attempts to do so with no more influence than any other member of the group. The subordinates basically have complete freedom in making decisions, with minimum participation by the manager. The manager is merely a figurehead. This style of leader decision authority is rarely found in health care organizations.

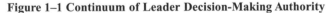

Figure 1–1 Continuum of Leader Decision-Making Authority

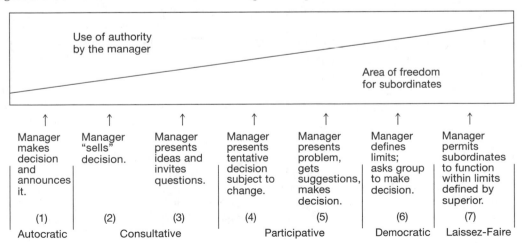

Source: Reprinted by permission of *Harvard Business Review.* Exhibit from "How To Choose a Leadership Pattern" by R. Tannenbaum and W. Schmidt (May/June 1973). Copyright © 1973 by the President and Fellows of Harvard College; all rights reserved.

NEGOTIATING A NEW ADMINISTRATIVE POSITION*

The following strategies could help a newly appointed chief nursing officer.

First, establish your agenda. While the expectations are high, establish a philosophy that can be narrowed down to a phrase or two that you can use over and over and to which you can return when the time comes to be firm. A phrase that succinctly captures what is important to you helps your staff have something about which to get excited.

Decide on your objectives and share them symbolically. Using a few well-chosen strategies is better than diffusing your agenda in many different directions. Using a new logo to announce a nursing model or offering a special class at the facility helps you send a serious message in time-efficient ways.

Develop positive coalitions quickly. As much as is possible, begin to network with your staff, professional colleagues, and other executives. An easy method is to determine the areas of conflict that a predecessor may have had and target those as opportunities. Be clear about your objectives in developing the coalitions; you still do not know enough about the culture to make good decisions this early in the game.

Maintain the old symbols as much as possible. Even apparently innocuous systems can be symbolic, and care should be taken not to disassemble any structure whose purpose or history makes it important.

Maximize the use of personal charisma to reach your constituents, but do not rely on it. It is possible to use charisma in nursing, but you must demonstrate regard and respect for the established layers. Allowing staff access to you via conferences and regular bulletins helps to underpin your philosophy. Allowing staff nurse access via an open door is fraught with difficulty no matter how attractive the prospect may appear, and, initially, open-door access should be reserved for formal structures like exit interviews.

Use your supporters to get your message out. You will need all the support you can get in the opening days of your tenure, and you should use every opportunity for good publicity and every photo opportunity. Making rounds on the weekends and assisting in minor ways on the units are all means by which "institutional legends" are born. You should be careful to be consistent with your general philosophy; otherwise the mixed messages you will send can confuse your agenda and disgruntle your budding cheerleaders.

Know the institutional legacy. A new incumbent needs to know that there often is a legacy of bad feeling—the only variables may be the degree of intensity and the significance. Interviewing, asking questions, and seeking feedback may help ferret out the problem and help you begin to incorporate the appropriate people into your network. These techniques also help you to develop information about opposition to your plans and assist you in planning a response.

Optimism and an upbeat attitude are winners. An air of enthusiasm and interest and exploration is satisfying to staff who have undergone the loss of leadership and are looking to be included in a meaningful future.

Use the theory of small wins to consolidate your agenda. Publicize the gains that you and your staff have made. Pay attention to the impact of recognizing the hard work that contributed to your success. Acknowledging staff who have published or earned a degree or have been selected for office says a lot about what you value and helps your staff understand that the future is created with small steps and successes. Keep reminding them that their actions directly reflect your agenda, and reward them consistently and often.

PREPARING FOR THE FUTURE— NETWORKS*

It is essential that nurse executives thoroughly prepare themselves for the fast-approaching

*Source: Judeth N. Javorek, "What Ronald Reagan Has To Do with Making It in a New Position," *Nursing Management*, Vol. 21, No. 9, September 1990. Reprinted with permission.

*Source: Rhonda Anderson, "Nursing Leadership and Healthcare Reform, Part III, Nurse Executive Role in a Reformed Healthcare System," *Journal of Nursing Administration*, Vol. 23:12, December 1993. J.B. Lippincott.

health care system changes. The individuals ready for the future are those who have ensured that their leadership skills are ready. These include the following skills (as identified in a recent *Healthcare Leadership Forum* on "Bridging the Gap in Healthcare"): mastering change, systems thinking, ability to develop and share a vision, and supporting continuous quality improvement.

Other primary areas of expertise must be ensured in strategic planning, finance, and the status of current and proposed relevant public policy.

In addition, it is critical that nurse executives take an early, informed, and proactive role in the development of integrated health care networks and delineate the nurse executive role in that network. In general, all effective executive leadership in an integrated network will need to be able to:

- Create and realize a network-wide strategic vision and mission.
- Develop a continuum of care that helps individuals manage their health care.

- Assess community needs and develop strategies and systems to meet those needs.
- Promote learning environments that are flexible, responsive, cost-effective, and outcome oriented.
- Create and assess the data to quantify patient care clinical and financial outcomes and community/population needs.
- Function as a strategic operations expert.
- Lead change and help constituencies with new ways of thinking and operating.
- Work interdependently with physicians, payers, consumers, governments, and others to meet common goals.
- Analyze and respond to legislative, payment, and public policy initiatives.

Essentially, each executive's role should result in cost-effective, quality patient care delivery across the integrated network. Those who can clearly articulate their unique contribution to the integrated network will emerge in a challenging new position.

Chapter 2

The Role and Characteristics of Management

DIFFERENTIATING MANAGERS FROM EXECUTIVES*

As the layers of nursing administration have proliferated with the changing structure of health care facilities, a distinction has evolved between the concepts of managers and executives. This contrast is largely the result of basic entrepreneurial activities, the growth of large-scale hospital chains, the separation of ownership and control, the development of strategic management theory, and the differentiation of operational responsibilities from key leadership responsibilities.

Management implies a dynamic and proactive approach to running operations. It suggests that managers are concerned not only with achieving efficient operations but also with ensuring that effective performance is attained. The manager will react to resource allocations in an organization by negotiating, arguing, politicking, or using other means to acquire a larger allotment. Pressures on the organization are resolved by adjusting the current process and structure of service delivery for immediate resolutions. The manager may also be actively involved in de-

fining a vision of which goals and objectives of the program, department, or organization will pursue.

The primary feature that differentiates managers from executives is the extent of their authority to formulate organizational vision. Managers hold limited strategic vision for their program, department, or organization because they are extremely involved in controlling current operations. They have restricted time, freedom, and prerogative to determine where an organization is headed over the long run. On the other hand, executives are more interested in forming a strategic vision of where a program, department, division, or organization is headed and in elucidating the conceptual steps that are required to arrive at that point. As a result, executives have an expanded vision for the organization.

Managers are oriented toward current operations. Consequently, their effort is directed to operations management or fine-tuning of operations. This is generally reflected in a short-run outlook in planning. Goals and objectives are primarily set for a period that is consistent with the current budgeting cycle. The culmination of this operations orientation is a limited vision of where an organization is headed. Less effort is devoted to conceptualizing which direction the organization should pursue because so much effort is given to how the organization is currently performing.

*Source: Judith F. Garner, Howard L. Smith, and Neill F. Piland, *Strategic Nursing Management: Power and Responsibility in a New Era*, Aspen Publishers, Inc., © 1990.

Executives are normally oriented toward both current operations and long-run strategy. They attend to operations to make certain that efficiency and effectiveness goals are achieved. They do not dwell on current operations, however; that is a responsibility for managers.

Executives maintain an outlook of the long run. Their planning horizon is seldom less than one year. They concern themselves with events outside the organization and the manner in which those events might be detrimental to operations. The result is an expanded vision of the direction in which the organization is headed. Executives temper this vision with a healthy awareness of internal operations. The abilities and limitations of the organization are well analyzed. Therefore, executives avoid moving too quickly or ambitiously and thereby endangering fiscal solvency, competitive posture, and the general essence of the organization. Executives define the organization and determine what the organization will become many years hence.

FUNCTIONS OF MANAGEMENT

Overview of Traditional Functions*

The duties common to all managers are most often referred to as functions of management. They include planning, organizing, directing, coordinating, and controlling. (See also Table 2–1.)

Planning

The planning process is largely one of forecasting and decision making. Forecasting provides the manager with information and messages about the future. By combining the forecast with other data related to the past and present, a manager can then select those courses that appear to be most appropriate in terms of forecasting conditions. Yet, while a manager can be assisted in the planning process by various staff groups, it should be noted by each manager that the ultimate responsibility for planning rests with him or her alone.

Since planning is always future oriented, it can be further characterized as the process whereby the management of an organization bridges the time span between where it is at present and where it wants to be at some point in the future. In doing so, planning involves the choice of objectives along with the policies, strategies, programs, procedures, and rules that are necessary for their accomplishment. In this sense, planning directs managers' thinking toward *what* they expect to do, *why* it will be done, *where* it will be done, *when* they expect to do it, *how* it will be done, and *who* is going to do it.

Organizing

Basically, the purpose of organizing is to establish a chain of command and a division of labor. To accomplish these ends, organizing involves the identification of duties to be performed; a grouping of these duties to indicate division, unit, section, or departmental arrangements; and an assignment of authority according to the line, staff, or functional relationships that will exist between individual jobs and total organizational units.

The steps outlined above can, of course, be applied either to the initial design of an organizational structure or to the maintenance of the structure once it has been established. In each case, the process is indispensable, since it combines human and material resources into an orderly and systematic arrangement that provides the basic ingredients necessary for a coordination of effort.

Directing

Planning can determine what will be done, organizing can combine the necessary resources for doing the job, coordinating can maintain harmony among the resources, and controlling can monitor performance, but it is direction that initiates and maintains action toward desired objectives. Direction is, therefore, closely interrelated with leadership, in that a manager's style of leadership is determined by the manner in which he or she exercises authority in the direction of subordinates.

Source: Gene Newport, *Tools of Managing,* © 1972. Addison-Wesley, Reading, Massachusetts. Pp. 7–9. Reprinted with permission.

Table 2–1 Summary of Managerial Roles

Role	Description	Identifiable Activities
Interpersonal		
Figurehead	Symbolic head; obliged to perform a number of routine duties of a legal or social nature	Ceremony, status requests, solicitations
Leader	Responsible for the motivation and activation of subordinates; responsible for staffing, training, and associated duties	Virtually all managerial activities involving subordinates
Liaison	Maintains self-development network of outside contacts and informers who provide favors and information	Interdepartmental relations and other activities involving outsiders
Informational		
Monitor	Seeks and receives wide variety of special information (much of it current) to develop thorough understanding of organization and environment; emerges as nerve center of internal and external information on the organization	Handling all contacts categorized as concerned primarily with receiving information (e.g., periodical news, observational tours)
Disseminator	Transmits information received from outsiders or from other subordinates to members of the organization; some information factual, some involving interpretation and integration of diverse value positions of organizational influencers	Forwarding mail into organization for information purposes, verbal contacts involving information flow to subordinates (e.g., review sessions, instant communication flows)
Spokesperson	Transmits information to outsiders on organization's plans, policies, actions, results, etc.; serves as expert on organization's industry	Department meetings; handling contacts involving transmission of information to outsiders
Decisional		
Entrepreneur	Searches organization and its environment for opportunities and initiates "improvement projects" to bring about change; supervises design of certain projects as well	Strategy and review sessions involving initiation or design of improvement projects
Disturbance Handler	Responsible for corrective action when organization faces important, unexpected disturbances	Strategy and review sessions involving disturbances and crises
Resource Allocator	Responsible for the allocation of organizational resources of all kinds—in effect the making or approval of all significant organizational decisions	Scheduling; requests for authorization; any activity involving budgeting and the programming of subordinates' work
Negotiator	Responsible for representing the organization at major negotiations	Negotiation

Source: From *The Nature of Managerial Work* by Henry Mintzberg (pp. 92–93). Copyright © 1973 by Henry Mintzberg. Reprinted with permission of Harper & Row Publishers, Inc.

Success in carrying out this function depends on many factors. Among the most important are delegation, communication, training, and motivation. Through delegation, subordinates receive the authority required for the fulfillment of their responsibilities. Communication provides individuals with the information needed in performing their jobs and allows for feedback of results related to their performance. Training is involved with the initial orientation of employees in addition to the continued direction of learning once they are on the job. Finally, motivation is concerned with assisting individuals in satisfying their needs in such a way that they continue to exhibit behavior that is consistent with their potential.

Coordinating

A coordination of effort involves the synchronization of activities toward established goals. If all employees are given the right to do a job in their own way, each is usually guided by his or her own ideas of what should be done. And even though these individuals may be quite willing to cooperate, the end result could well be a waste of time, effort, and money, since there is no meaningful direction to guide their efforts. Consequently, coordination is required and becomes a major responsibility of all managers.

To reiterate, coordination is different from cooperation. While the latter may arise spontaneously among the members of a group, coordination occurs only through effective leadership.

As with a tug of war, the manager can make a great contribution by learning when and how to let go of the rope, so to speak, in order to call the cadence that causes the team to pull together. In this sense, coordination is the means of concentrating and applying cooperative effort to accomplish a task with economy and effectiveness. Therefore, it becomes the very essence of management and results from good planning, organizing, directing, and controlling.

Controlling

The purpose of control is to see that actual performance corresponds to that which is called for in various plans. All managers exercise control by (1) knowing or establishing the standards that relate to a particular course of action, (2) measuring actual performance against the standards, and (3) correcting deviations from standards, when necessary.

Leadership is also essential to control, since inanimate objects are really not controlled in the strict sense. People operate machines, use equipment, follow procedures, and, in fact, bring an organization to life. Thus control focuses on the direction of human behavior, but leadership is needed to cause persons to perform in a desired manner.

Each of the functions and activities identified here is performed by every *professional* manager at every level. The differences are ones of magnitude and frequency. Figure 2–1 shows the variation in the percentage of effort devoted to

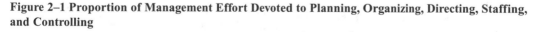

Figure 2–1 Proportion of Management Effort Devoted to Planning, Organizing, Directing, Staffing, and Controlling

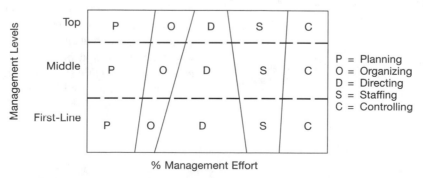

each of the five functions at three levels of management.

As is readily apparent from the illustration, the biggest variation in proportionate effort is in the directing function. The closer the manager is to production activity, the larger is the proportion of effort likely to be devoted to the directing function. Conversely, the farther away from production the manager gets, the less time and effort should be devoted to directing and the more attention should be given to the other functions. Obviously, the actual mix of the various functions will not be as smooth as in the illustration, and it will be influenced by other factors as well. Nevertheless, the marked change in the mix as a manager proceeds up the management ladder is inescapable. Therefore, a highly successful first-line manager will not necessarily make a good middle manager. Nor, on the other hand, will a middle manager who possesses the necessary skills to perform effectively at that level be a guaranteed success as a first-line manager. Note: For a self-evaluation tool measuring managerial qualities see Appendix 2–A.

The Transformed Nursing Manager*

Transformational leadership is less like directing and controlling than it is like coordinating, integrating, and facilitating. The manager does not envision, create, direct, or produce. These are the unilateral realities of the Industrial Age. The more dynamic, interactive, and synergistic requirements of the emerging age call for a new set of skills and insights on the part of the leader.

The transformational leader facilitates the development of changed relationships and moderates the dialogue necessary to create newer understanding in the workplace. Most of the creativity and content of change will come from the service providers of the organization and take place in the clinical service units. It is there that most of the change in service and relationships will unfold. In order to accomplish this, much dialogue, mediation, and integration will have to occur. Many of the groups necessary to the change in service design and relationship have not and do not have the relationship necessary to work out the character of newer work arrangements, let alone define their content.

The new leader must be able to work beyond the parameters of a single discipline or department and must apply skills that facilitate communication, dialogue, group management, consensus building, conflict resolution, and issue mediation. The ability to bring groups together, create a safe working environment, and challenge and lead others into a context that helps work and relates in concert is central to the emerging leadership role. This person must be able to explore carefully yet specifically the discomforts, uncertainties, misconceptions, and fears of disparate groups and then lead them into new definitions of relationship and service.

Bringing groups together to plan strategies and build newer work relationships and designs is simply the first step for the leader. Work and human enterprise are full of the potential for conflict and uncertainties. Add a dose of economics and the relational challenges can become intense. Newer models for problem identification and solution seeking must emerge from out of the workplace between the involved parties. The transformational leader does not see himself or herself as the moderator or mediator of this conflict. Rather, the leader seeks to develop mechanisms and processes where problem solving, dialogue, solution seeking, and opportunity building occur between and among the invested players independent of the leader's role. Indeed, the leader teaches and builds self-sufficiency and interdependence and provides models for the parties to use, which assures problem solving and relationship building without creating the need for the leader's intervention.

*Source: Tim Porter-O'Grady, "Transformational Leadership in an Age of Chaos," *Nursing Administration Quarterly*, Vol. 17, No. 1, pp. 17–24, Aspen Publishers, Inc., © 1992.

The transformational leader creates a context that encourages the development of "self-leadership" in the work environment. In this way the transformational leader models leadership characteristics rather than simply expressing leadership behaviors he or she wants others to use. Instead, the leader seeks to create those same skills in others so that they may be self-directed, solution based, and creative in unfolding their own group process and clinical work. Dependency relationships are untenable in the role of the transformational leader and all effort is undertaken to extinguish such characteristics and replace them with equitable, constructive, and self-managed behaviors.

The effort to create equity and to establish new kinds of relationships takes precedence in the newer organizational configurations. Multidisciplinary and collaborative structures are essential to effective service provision. Artificial role and departmental differentiations are no longer viable strategies for building patient-based and outcome-focused service arrangements. The notions of "fault" and unilateral ownership of problems or blame generation simply do not reflect a structure out of which collaborative relationships and mutuality can arise. As the disciplines are forced to relate at increasing levels of intensity, the ability to confront, focus, find common ground, and move to solution finding and relationship building will be essential. Indeed, new work models are building on interdisciplinary and cross-referenced designs that are patient based and reflect a level of collaboration never previously experienced. Instead of simply talking to each other in a language only they can understand, a new level of conversation is required, creating a way of talking and relating that all can comprehend. The leader's ability to bring these diverse forces together to work in concert with each other is the challenge of the time. Successful care models will depend upon effective coalitions that include the whole spectrum of health care disciplines. See Table 2–2 for an overview of transforming a nurse-manager's role.

Table 2–2 The Transformation of the Nurse Manager's Role

The shifted emphasis and upheaval in organizational theory demand that managers revise their roles as follows:

manager → leader
director → coach
boss → mentor
quality assurance → continuous quality improvement
department perspective → organizational perspective
clinical audits → research
participatory management → self-governance
coordinator → project manager
turf protection → collaboration
control → partnership
planning → strategic vision
vertical management → horizontal management
budgeting → fiscal accountability
status quo → innovation
department focus → product-line focus

Recommended Reference Reading: Contemporary Competence Clusters

- Cluster I—Manager who needs to function as a coach, a technologist, a visionary, a facilitator: See Peter Drucker, *The New Realities* (New York: Harper & Row, 1989).
- Cluster II—Manager who needs to function as an egalitarian "associate," a communicator, a mobilizer: See J. Champy, *Reengineering Management* (New York: Harper Business Publishing, 1995).
- Cluster III—Manager who needs to acquire competence in personal mastery (through self-examination), systems thinking, mental modeling, shared visioning, team-linked learning: See P.M. Senge et al., *The Fifth Discipline Fieldbook* (New York: Doubleday/ Currency).

MANAGERIAL SKILLS*

It has been suggested that there are three skill areas with which managerial competence is likely to increase.[1] An individual can harness and develop these managerial skills through experience and formal learning. It is unlikely that the individual is born with these skills. The term *skill* itself conveys an idea that the ability to perform a task can be learned and developed. Technical, human, and conceptual skills all contribute to managerial success.

In this context, *technical skill* refers to managers having an understanding and proficiency in a specialized activity that requires knowledge and ability in the use of tools, processes, and procedures.

In this context, *human skill* refers to the manager's ability to function as a work-group member and his or her success in developing cooperative behavior among the employees. Two components make up this human skill: the perceptual aspect and the subsequent behavior that stems from human perception. The manager must strive to develop an awareness and understanding of the employees' and his or her own attitudes, beliefs, and values regarding human relations. The manager needs to recognize how and where these attitudes, beliefs, and values (such as prejudices and feelings) are apt to hinder or enhance appropriate work behavior.

Conceptual skill refers to the individual manager's ability to see the organization systematically. An organization reflects complex interactions among its properties, the whole being greater than the sum of its parts. The manager should understand how organizational functions and recurring problem areas interact and are interdependent. By being cognizant of these interdependencies and their relationships, managers are more apt to enhance the organization as a whole. Efforts at change and decision making do not occur in a vacuum; they have systemic implications.

These domains of skills—technical, human, and conceptual—can be applied to nurse manager tasks to construct a competence skill list for developing and evaluating nurse managers (see Tables 2–3 through 2–5).

MANAGERIAL ACCOUNTABILITIES*

General Accountability

Five basic areas of accountability—human, fiscal, material, support, and systems resources—fall squarely within the manager's scope of accountability. They are resource driven and focus on context, not content. Each entails specific role obligations that provide the content

---

*Source: Eduardo S. Rodela, "Managerial Work Behavior and Hierarchical Level: Implications for the Managerial Training of First-Line Supervisors," *Health Care Supervisor*, Vol. 9:3, Aspen Publishers, Inc., © April 1991.

[1]Katz, R.L. "Skills of an Effective Administrator," *Harvard Business Review* 52, no. 5 (1974): 90–112.

*Source: Tim Porter-O'Grady and Cathleen Krueger Wilson, *The Leadership Revolution in Health Care: Altering Systems, Changing Behaviors*, Aspen Publishers, Inc., © 1995.

Table 2–3 Competencies Reflecting Technical Skills

Nursing Practice Technology

- Maintain professional-technical competence in an area of nursing practice.
- Achieve goals of direct patient care.
- Act as a patient advocate.
- Support family members.
- Support the goals of biomedical research.
- Demonstrate knowledge of purposes, procedures, and processes of biomedical research.

Management Technology

- Organize, direct, and control operations essential to goal achievement.
  - Assume responsibility for decision making within one's scope of control.
  - Exert authority.
  - Perform effectively in ambiguous situations.
  - Plan and implement political strategies to achieve both short-term and long-term goals.
  - Influence the acceptance of one's decisions.
  - Take calculated risks.
  - Assume accountability for one's decisions.
- Select a leadership style appropriate to the work, the workers, and the situation.
- Obtain, process, and disseminate information essential to job performance.
  - Systematically scan relevant information resources.
  - Select relevant information.
  - Use appropriate information resources in planning.
  - Identify priorities.
  - Organize information meaningfully.
  - Present information effectively using oral and/or written communication processes.
- Solve or mitigate problems.
  - Assess the nature of a problem.
  - Identify appropriate means for solving a problem.
  - Involve others in the use of problem-solving processes.
  - Persevere in the search for a solution.
- Initiate, stimulate, and facilitate change.
  - Effect a planned change.
  - Anticipate change.
  - Support the change initiatives of others.
  - Respond flexibly to a changing environment.
- Develop systems for the conduct of work.

- Coordinate the optimal use of organizational resources.
  - Delegate appropriately.
  - Manage time effectively.
  - Use available technologies.
- Manage resources.
  - Consider time, space, materials, equipment, finances, and people as potential resources.
  - Document the need for resources.
  - Conduct interviews with prospective personnel.
  - Obtain necessary resources.
  - Function with limited resources.
  - Allocate resources.
  - Account for resource utilization.
  - Use budgetary processes.
  - Use fiscal systems for financial analysis, forecasting, and monitoring.
- Provide learning opportunities to enhance employees' personal and professional growth.
  - Identify present and potential learning needs of staff.
  - Identify and mobilize educational resources.
  - Use role modeling to teach others.
  - Control the physical and interpersonal climate for learning.
- Evaluate the performance of employees.
  - Base expectations for performance on knowledge of competent patient care.
  - Base expectations for performance on knowledge of the demands of research on patient care requirements.
  - Clarify expectations for performance and the rationale for expected behaviors.
  - Base evaluation on objective analysis of relevant behaviors.
  - Communicate evaluation of performance and related decisions in an objective and supportive manner.
  - Use praise and constructive criticism appropriately.
  - Document performance evaluation in writing.
  - Apply civil service and public health service procedures and criteria in rating performance.
  - Develop mutual plans for improving performance, including a mechanism to evaluate progress toward goals.
  - Use appropriate formal and informal rewards.
  - Stimulate improved performance.
  - Maintain confidentiality.

Source: Maryann F. Fralic and Andrea O'Connor, "A Management Progression System for Nurse Administrators, Part I," *The Journal of Nursing Administration*, April 1983. Reprinted with permission of J.B. Lippincott Company.

Table 2–4 Competencies Reflecting Human Skills

- Communicate clearly and dispassionately with peers, colleagues, subordinates, and superiors.

    –Foster open communication through clear expression and receptive listening.
    –Explain the rationale for one's decisions and requests.
    –Explore reasons for another's position on an issue.
    –Deal with anger and frustration in a direct and constructive manner.
    –Demonstrate sensitivity and insight regarding the perceptions and reactions of others.

- Facilitate communication between staff and others in the organization.

    –Obtain, process, and disseminate information essential to job performance.
    –Represent staff in contexts external to the unit.
    –Build networks by establishing relationships with appropriate people inside and outside the organization.

- Establish a climate of mutual trust and respect.

    –Maintain a predictable leadership style.
    –Maintain credibility.
    –Maintain confidentiality.
    –Maintain integrity.
    –Deal with staff in a fair and just manner.
    –Act as advocate for staff.

- Work harmoniously with peers, colleagues, subordinates, and superiors.

    –Collaborate with others to achieve goals.
    –Act interdependently as necessary.

- Foster an innovative and motivating work environment.

    –Initiate, stimulate, and facilitate change.
    –Provide meaningful, productive work.
    –Provide learning opportunities to enhance employees' personal and professional growth.

- Act assertively to achieve goals.

- Use power, status, and influence appropriately to achieve goals.

- Promote group work to solve problems and achieve goals.

    –Promote the participation of others in group processes.
    –Participate in group processes.
    –Promote the solidarity and growth of groups over time.

- Facilitate the management of an employee's personal or professional crisis.

- Manage conflict.

    –Assess the characteristics of conflicting parties and situations.
    –Structure the environment in which the conflict is addressed.
    –Intervene to ameliorate or eliminate the cause of a conflict.
    –Mediate a conflict using appropriate strategies.

- Perform under varying degrees of stress.

- Objectively analyze and respond to others' critique of one's performance.

- Assume responsibility for one's personal and professional growth.

- Act as a patient advocate.

Source: Maryann F. Fralic and Andrea O'Connor, "A Management Progression System for Nurse Administrators, Part I," *The Journal of Nursing Administration*, April 1983. Reprinted with permission of J.B. Lippincott Company.

Table 2–5 Competencies Reflecting Conceptual Skills

- Analyze the work to be done.

  –Identify discrete elements of the work.
  –Identify optimal sequences for work processes.
  –Establish priorities.
  –Assess the degree of uncertainty inherent in the work and surrounding the work.

- Formulate goals.

  –Define the unit's purpose and objectives.
  –Define mutual expectations of staff and manager regarding unit goals.
  –Establish directions for the unit through priority setting.

- Assess resources.

  –Consider time, space, materials, equipment, finances, and people as available resources.
  –Evaluate available resources in terms of strengths, weaknesses, and limitations in a systematic, businesslike manner.
  –Maintain objectivity.

- Predict outcomes.

  –Identify and interpret recurrent patterns of organizational events, considering both people and systems.
  –Make rough correlations regarding the probable impact of variables on organizational events.

- Plan for the future.

  –Formulate a vision for the future of the unit, service, and/or organization.
  –Develop and communicate a long-range plan against which results can be measured.
  –Develop short-term strategies to achieve the long-range plan.

  –Effect a marketing plan designed to facilitate the long-range plan.
  –Retain a practical view of possible means of shaping and responding to future eventualities.

- Clarify relationships of the unit to the larger organization's parts and whole.

  –Articulate goals and functions of the organization, the service, and their units.
  –Retain a perspective on organizational goals and functions.
  –Achieve congruence between unit, service, and organizational purposes and objectives.

- Maintain a professional identity.

  –Identify standards of professional nursing practice.
  –Foster the growth and development of the profession.
  –Recognize the social responsibilities imposed by one's professional identity.
  –Facilitate the education of nursing students.

- Maintain an awareness of societal trends.

  –Recognize the social climate in which health care is delivered.
  –Recognize the political constraints within which the health care delivery system operates.
  –Recognize trends in health and illness that may impact health care delivery.
  –Recognize existing and emerging technologies that may impact health care delivery.
  –Recognize the nature of the contemporary worker.
  –Recognize the nature of the contemporary health care professional.

Source: Maryann F. Fralic and Andrea O'Connor, "A Management Progression System for Nurse Administrators, Part I," *The Journal of Nursing Administration*, April 1983. Reprinted with permission of J.B. Lippincott Company.

of the manager's role in various functional levels of the organization.

Human Resources

Managers have traditionally had the task of providing the right people for the right work in the right place at the right numbers and at the right time. They still have this task. They are accountable for ensuring that staff are available in a balance that is appropriate given the demands and the material resources. Self-scheduling, computer-based programs, and unit checks can be used to coordinate resources and service demands. The role of the manager is to see that a system is in place, that it works effectively, and that the human resources are appropriate given cost parameters and service demands.

Fiscal Resources

The creation, management, and evaluation of the use of an organization's fiscal resources are a central function of managers. The object is to match service operations and goals with the fiscal resources dedicated to achieving the organization's purposes. However, it is important to make sure fiscal resources are used effectively. The system that addresses this issue and applies and evaluates the use of fiscal resources falls within the accountability of the manager. Here again the manager may work with mechanisms that depend on staff involvement such as cost-center budgeting, staff-driven financial plans, staff fiscal control mechanisms, point-of-service cost evaluation, and per subscriber cost parameters. The role of the manager is to ensure that whatever methods are used work well and facilitate the effective use and stewardship of the fiscal resources.

Material Resources

Many of the same principles apply to both material resource and fiscal resource management. Material resource allocation and use techniques can also be staff driven. Capital planning and acquisition processes can be team based and team evaluated. The role of the manager is to ensure that there are appropriate mechanisms to handle material resource issues effectively and without exceeding the parameters provided for the sources.

Support Resources

Creating a milieu that makes it possible for the staff to be self-directed and deal with clinical and service issues and that empowers the teams to control their relationships and work is part of the support role of the manager. Primary tasks include resolving development issues, enhancing the learning context, providing the tools to problem solve, and providing access to the expert resources of the organization. The manager must be concerned with the competence of the staff in managing their work and the environment of empowerment that pervades the organization. Offering opportunities for empowerment and ensuring a proper and sustainable milieu are of critical importance.

Systems Resources

Linking all the parts of the system together to facilitate the work is a fundamental task of the manager. Systems resources such as experts, service supports, organizational structure, quality measurement, data collection and generation, outcome measurement, and competence enhancement provide the kind of support necessary to sustain a team's efforts.

The manager must make certain the systems data are presented in such a way that they can be understood and are useful. Indeed, the manager's role centers on the generation and interpretation of the information necessary to support the work of the providers. Information from budget data to clinical outcome data can have significant implications for service or care delivery. Accurate and meaningful systems data assist the providers in making the right decisions and validating their work.

Nurse Manager Accountabilities

The general managerial accountabilities have been reformulated and added to by the American Organization of Nurse Executives to create a nurse manager–specific list of accountabilities that takes into consideration the special aspects of applying general accountabilities in a patient-oriented organization (see Table 2–6).

THE CREATIVE EXECUTIVE*

There is and always will be a need for effective leadership. However, the leadership role must

---

*Source: Adapted from A. Bennett, "The Innovative Supervisor," *Health Care Supervisor,* Vol. 4, No. 2, pp. 183–184, © 1986, Aspen Publishers, Inc. and T. Porter-O'Grady and C.K. Wilson, *The Leadership Revolution in Health Care: Altering Systems, Changing Behaviors,* pp. 108–110, © 1993, Aspen Publishers, Inc.

change with the times. Before individuals can move to outcome-based, resource-oriented, and service-driven leadership, they must abandon out-of-date mental maps and create new alternatives to getting the job done.

Creative leaders approach new role demands with an attitude of self-design or improvisation. They see this time of transformation in health care as a period to play with career possibilities— to revisit their reason for choosing management as a field of endeavor and their vision for their lives. The creative reworking of leadership roles requires of the individual a certain learning resourcefulness, a preponderance of free-style actions and outcome-driven actions, and a tendency to reject stereotypical answers. By applying these

---

Table 2–6 Accountabilities of the Contemporary Unit Manager

Accountability

The **unit manager** in many settings may be considered a middle management role and may in fact coordinate the activities of several nursing units with a broad overall perspective and related strategies. The unit manager has 24-hour accountability and is primarily responsible for production of the desired product, which in nursing is positive patient health outcomes and conditions during illness and adjustment. The unit manager manages staff, materials, and systems and is accountable for:

- providing staff resources necessary to do the work of the unit(s)
- providing materials, through budgetary management, to ensure that equipment, supplies, educational materials, and so forth are available
- managing systems (e.g., staffing patterns, staff numbers needed, application of goals and objectives to the unit, interfacing with others to produce positive work flows)
- supporting shared governance models (in many hospital settings)

The overall accountability of the unit manager remains to the patients and the organization; the specific aspects often are charted by the management method in place, whether a traditional or a staff empowerment model. In shared governance, the manager moves from a narrowly defined, fixed role to a much broader role. The manager's role also changes from a controlling role to a supporting and facilitating role as the staff take an active role in nursing practice decisions.

Role Responsibilities

Regardless of the management model in practice, the unit manager uses some form of manager influence—motivation, power, leadership, or behavior modification—in achieving organizational objectives. In staff empowerment models, the nurse manager involves staff in the management process and key skills of planning, organizing, staffing, leading, communicating, and decision making. From a patient care management perspective, the unit manager oversees budgetary issues, staffing and scheduling, and hiring and retention practices and communicates with multiple disciplines to promote most effectively the care, cure, and comfort provided by the nursing staff to the patients.

Source: Catherine E. Loveridge and Susan H. Cummings, *Nursing Management in the New Paradigm*, Aspen Publishers, Inc., © 1996.

skills and strategies in the process of improvisation, managers will find it less burdensome to make sense out of their experience and achieve a fit with new role definitions. The real question for each individual is whether or not improvisation is a last resort or a purposeful way of working into the future. Can the individual, in other words, switch from the discipline of a self-managed career to the art of self-design?

What are some of the areas of supervisory skills and ability central to innovation?

First, there is the idea of viewing the organization as a total system that operates as a part of a larger system. Innovative supervisors are capable of doing new things because creativity and ingenuity are nurtured through a concern and commitment that go beyond the narrow limits of the functional boundaries of the work unit for which they are responsible. Second, innovative supervisors have the skill and ability to establish and achieve innovative goals that evolve from foresight with respect to advancing organizational performance. Third, these supervisors possess the ability to maximize performance of available human resources. The innovative supervisor knows that fulfilling the role of manager rather than "part-time worker" allows worthwhile extensions to helping employees not only to handle problems, but also to participate in all parts of the problem-solving and innovative process. Fourth, supervisors who are innovative handle and impart information that is not only essential when considering that employees change their attitudes and their expectations, but that is also essential when creating an environment in which newness and novelty can flourish. Fifth, this innovative leader effectively manages human affairs at work, counteracting such barriers to change as the absence of a unity of purpose, threats to harmonious relationships, resistance and resentment, incompetence, or workers' unwillingness to produce.

Underlying these basic requirements for innovation in supervision is the need for problem-solving ability—being able to take a problem and develop its issues and dimensions, generate alternative ideas for solution, and derive feasible initiatives from the alternatives. To make this change process work well, the effective, innovative supervisor does eight things. This innovator

1. recognizes when the problem in question is *really* the problem;
2. opens the mind to ideas;
3. provides sight, insight, and excitement;
4. focuses on the unusual, seeing what others have ignored;
5. tempers innovativeness with practicality;
6. engenders cooperation and coordination;
7. thinks through the work needed to turn an idea into meaningful action; and
8. asks the right kinds of questions in different ways.

The list of questions is as follows:

- Do I believe in the old saying, "Problems have a way of working themselves out if you leave them alone"?
- Have I ever caught myself saying "We tried that, but it did not work"?
- Do I prefer waiting for someone else to try a new idea first, rather than take a calculated risk on it myself?
- Do my people show any fear of being threatened by new ways of doing things?
- What is the degree of my discomfort about the anticipated complexity and uncertainty that lie ahead? What has been the degree of pleasure associated with my past problem-solving opportunities?
- Do I perceive problem solving as a discrete activity or as an integral element of the management process?
- Do I really hold to the belief that "the best is yet to be"?
- What level of value do I place on my current skills in identifying problems requiring solution? My skills in devising successful methods to solve these problems? My skills in gaining acceptance and support from people affected by, and involved in, change?
- In my past problem-solving efforts, how well have I applied the principle of systematization?

- Have I ever chosen a solution, yet realized I still had a problem?
- How active and successful have I been this past year in producing new ideas?
- How good am I at noticing details ignored by others?
- Am I functioning as a manager or as a "part-time worker"?
- When solving problems, do I approach the need for change with confidence, hope, and enthusiasm?
- Do I approach problems with an open mind, with an absence of any preconceived notions, and with an organized plan of questioning? Did I, in fact, ask any good questions today?

NURSE POWER

Overview*

Power has multiple meanings and frequently negative connotations. It is used here to mean the ability to get and use whatever resources are needed to achieve nursing goals.

Organizational power refers to the power that exists within hospitals and other health care institutions. This kind of power is in the decision-making process of organizations. It is organizational power that nurses need to influence the conditions of nursing work.

In addition, individuals have *personal power* derived from the decisions they make on a daily basis about how they are going to organize their lives. Political scientists refer to an individual's sense of political efficacy—that is, the individual's feeling that he or she can influence events through personal effort. A sense of political efficacy becomes a self-fulfilling prophecy. If individuals believe that they make a difference and can influence events in their lives, they are likely to participate actively in trying to get what

they want. This participation will make them feel more powerful even if it is not all that successful. However, the opposite is equally true. If individuals believe themselves powerless to influence events and therefore do not even try, they are going to feel even more powerless.

Sources of Power and Influence

Where does power come from? Writers and researchers seem to agree that the major sources of power and influence are as follows:

- *reward power*—power to reward behavior, give positive opportunities, or remove negative effects
- *coercive power*—the ability to impose penalties for nonconformity
- *legitimate power*—power based on the internalized norms, beliefs, roles, and values of those being influenced
- *referent power*—power based on identifying with other people who have power
- *expert power*—power that derives from the knowledge, abilities, and credibility of the person exerting influence
- *informational power*—power arising from the ability and opportunities of an individual to gain and share valuable information (e.g., access to and influence on organizational gossip can be a valuable resource)

Power holders usually have a combination of these sources of power. But having power is not in itself sufficient to make an individual powerful—his or her sources of power must be used as resources to achieve desired goals. Nursing has and always has had power; the problem lies in the use, nonuse, or misuse of this power.

Powerful Leaders

One factor that clearly distinguishes good leaders from bad, effective leaders from ineffective, and liked leaders from disliked ones is the ability to mobilize organizational resources to make things happen.

Source: Jennie Larsen, "Nurse Power for the 1980s," *Nursing Administration Quarterly*, Vol. 6:4, Aspen Publishers, Inc., © 1982.

The assignment of formal organizational authority does not necessarily ensure access to power in the organization. For example, how much power does a nurse manager really have in the typical hospital? How much power does he or she have to hire and fire, make budget decisions, grant staff development opportunities, or redesign nursing jobs?

Nurse managers need organizational power to back up nursing demands and decisions and ensure the confidence and loyalty of staff nurses.

Organizational power is derived from having influence at the decision-making levels of the organization, from having informal connections with sponsors and peers, and from having a visible high-status position. People are quite knowledgeable about who has power in the organization and who does not. When asked, organizational members will often state they prefer to work with managers who can get things done.

Powerful nursing leaders tend to generate high group morale, primarily because of their ability to get things done. Powerful nursing leaders are mobile and aid in the advancement of their staff nurses. These leaders tend to adopt participatory management styles in which they share information with the staff nurses, delegate responsibility, and are flexible about organizational rules.

Understanding How To Make an Impact*

Opportunities for health care managers to participate in strategy-level issues are increasing. Such involvement implies that fresh perspectives may be incorporated in developing organizational strategies and that more avenues may exist for coordinating strategy with implementation. However, integration depends on how well operating-level managers work with strategic-level movers and shakers.

Movers and shakers are those who alter the strategic direction of an organization or program. They can also significantly affect service deliv-

ery. Movers and shakers include leaders on the board of trustees, articulate and motivated providers who are formally or informally associated with an organization, capable or powerful top management staff members, and community leaders.

Movers and shakers are effective agents of change within organizations because they possess certain characteristics. Health care managers should understand these characteristics so that they can build productive relationships with movers and shakers (see Figure 2–2).

First, the *charisma* associated with outstanding leaders is reflected in superior *expertise* based on expertise based on effective communication skills and presence. Next, expertise based on a broad experiential base coupled with penetrating analytical skills allows movers and shakers to earn exceptional authority and power. Third, movers and shakers are able to focus on strategic visions and *policy-level decisions*.

Movers and shakers work through other team members to select and implement solutions that are consistent with organizational mission statements. Fourth, their *entrepreneurial* mindset enables them to take calculated risks and design creative solutions in response to formidable challenges. Finally, movers and shakers are not reticent to *face facts* and make tough decisions.

Not all movers and shakers possess all of these characteristics equally. Nor are they all concerned about the same issues. As individuals, they bring differing interests and capabilities to health care organizations. Health care managers may strive to cultivate some of these characteristics themselves, or they may seek to establish productive relationships with the movers and shakers themselves.

Managers have numerous opportunities to interact with powerful movers and shakers who influence the direction of health care organizations. By constructively using the ideas, insights, and power of movers and shakers, health care managers should be able to discharge their responsibilities more effectively.

At least three methods exist for enlisting the cooperation and support or the indirect benefit of power and influence of movers and shakers: (1) developing a trusting relationship, (2) using

*Source: Howard L. Smith, Richard A. Reid, and Neill F. Piland, "Building Productive Relationships with Movers and Shakers," *Health Care Supervisor,* Vol. 9:3, Aspen Publishers, Inc., © 1991.

Figure 2–2 Reflected Power: Developing Relationships with Movers and Shakers

Identification of Movers and Shakers	Strategies for Building Productive Relationships

Strategies for Building Productive Relationships

1. Develop trusting relationships.
   - Demonstrate dependability.
   - Provide periodic feedback.
   - Maintain consistent management behaviors.
2. Use borrowed power judiciously.
   - Facilitate information analysis.
   - Defer actions until trust is formed.
3. Maintain visible alliances.
   - Invest in the relationship.
   - Devise innovative strategies to continue the relationship.

borrowed power judiciously, and (3) maintaining viable alliances. Depending on their situation, health care managers may be able to adopt one or more of these approaches to increase their personal and professional effectiveness.

Fitting into the Executive Team*

The chief nurse officer (CNO) position has evolved from the traditional director of nursing position responsible for maintaining the functioning of a more simply defined single department to a nurse executive position responsible for managing many facets of patient services. More than any other member of the executive management team, the CNO must be acutely aware of both clinical and managerial demands, acutely aware of the politics of power in the institution, and acutely wary of getting caught in power struggles.

The CNO's broad scope of responsibility and interface with all areas of health care facility operations makes the CNO the prime resource of the chief executive officer (CEO). At first appraisal, the CNO seems to occupy a paradoxi-

cal position, maintaining independence and integrity while at the same time representing the CEO and personifying the CEO's goals and philosophy. Clearly, acknowledgment of a shared philosophy eliminates the paradox. The foundation of the relationship of the CEO and the CNO is, however, more than shared goals; it is the ability of two personalities to connect in a way that feels balanced and brings about positive results.

The mutually supportive relationship between the CEO and the CNO can be enhanced by keeping in mind these practical suggestions.

- Detect potential problems and resolve them yourself whenever possible, while always keeping the CEO informed. Be aware that your decisions and actions reflect directly on the CEO.
- Be conscious of your visibility. In your interface with the facility's many departments and in leading your own, you are under the scrutiny of the entire institution and are representing the CEO.
- Maintain professional networks in nursing, in other health care–related organizations, and in the community. You serve as a vital link and may be the first to know about both current and future issues, trends, and problems.

***Source:* Lenore M. Appenzeller, "The CNO-CEO Relationship," *Aspen's Advisor for Nurse Executives*, Vol. 3: 6, Aspen Publishers, Inc., © 1988.

- Foster and maintain a positive and active relationship with the medical staff. In addition to being a liaison between physicians and administration, you must establish a collegial working relationship with the medical staff leadership. Without this, the CEO will be thrust into the peacekeeper role, which will not be appreciated.

- When presenting a proposal or suggestion, give the CEO the opportunity to review material in advance. Keep in mind that the CEO is everyone's boss and must consider the impact on the entire institution. Put yourself in the CEO's position.

- Offer the CEO options; no one likes being boxed in. Particularly when presenting alternatives for resolving a problem or conflict, stubbornness, ultimatums, and lack of flexibility are counterproductive.

- Give the CEO the opportunity to change his or her mind. Allow for graceful adaptation, changes of opinion, and room to negotiate.

- Do not avoid responsibility. You may have to "take the heat" for others' decisions as well as your own. You are a member of a management team and must support its decisions.

Strategies for Influencing Staff*

Among the influence strategies that effectively channel the elements of the leader's power into productive results are the following.

Obtain and share accurate information. In many situations, a leader is able to influence oth-

*Source: Claudette G. Varricchio, "The Process of Influencing Decisions," Nursing Administration Quarterly, Vol. 6:2, Aspen Publishers, Inc., © 1982.

ers primarily because of access to accurate information and the ability to communicate it effectively to followers.

Demonstrate expertise. The degree to which a leader is perceived as having special knowledge or skill is an important factor in influencing others. An expert's opinion is more influential than that of a majority of the group.

Use legitimate authority in effective ways. Legitimacy is based on norms and expectations held by group members.

Encourage subordinates to identify with the leader. A subordinate either has or wants a feeling of oneness with the leader. Such identification comes from a feeling of knowing the leader, sharing common goals and values, and being able to talk with him or her. The leader's communication skills are an important aspect of this strategy.

Use rewards and punishments effectively. Basic to coercion is the perception by one or more persons that another person is able to mediate rewards for them. If both "sides" do not agree about what constitutes a reward, however, the strategy is weak. If what the manager thinks of as a reward is not perceived by the staff as such, the reward will not be an effective means of influence.

Understand how to manipulate cues affecting a decision. This can involve the manipulation (withholding) of information to promote ignorance, for example. This strategy restricts the number and range of perceived alternatives, affects the quality of a decision, and affects the values and abilities of the decision maker.

Effectively control the work environment. Agendas are an important type of environmental control. The agenda for a meeting or a listing of decision priorities provides an important control on the influence of others.

Appendix 2–A

A Set of Self-Evaluation Tools

Try the quizzes that follow, sticking reasonably close to your own experience. Mark each item Yes or No.

Leading

Of all management skills, leadership is most highly valued—and most difficult to define. Nevertheless, while leadership has many unknowns, some insightful checkpoints can provide a rough rule-of-thumb measure of this crucial skill.

___Do you do a good job of getting staff to cooperate in achieving goals?

___Do staff bring their really tough work problems to you?

___When the heat's on, can you get staff to go "full steam" without any gripes from them?

___When you are not around to supervise personally, do your subordinates go on working pretty much as usual?

___Do you have a good record of helping individuals improve their job performance?

___Is your record free from any justified complaint about showing favoritism?

___Can you usually get people to accept changes, even if they have to make a big adjustment?

___In an argument or a controversy involving other departments, do you back up your staff when you know they are right?

___Do you have relatively little trouble in getting staff to level with you?

___Do you often use encouragement?

___Do staff seem to take criticism from you and respond constructively?

___Do you find it easy to get volunteers?

___Do you make special efforts to be fair in assigning tasks?

___Are you proud of your staff? Do you show it?

Planning

The ability to study cause and effect, to see short-range difficulties in the light of long-range goals, is a key to overall executive accomplishment.

___Do you review objectives periodically so that your planning can be updated?

___Do you take advantage of group brainpower by permitting subordinates to participate in planning procedures?

Source: From *The Executive Deskbook,* 2nd edition, by Auren Uris, © 1970, 1979, by Litton Educational Publishing Inc. Reprinted by permission of Van Nostrand Reinhold Company.

____Would you benefit by formalizing your planning procedures, that is, allocating specific time periods to planning activities?

____Do you use the basic tools of planning—calendar, pencil, paper, charts, graphs, pertinent records of past performance, and so on?

____Is your planning flexible enough to meet changing conditions—higher standards, shorter deadlines, and so on?

____Are your planning methods organized well enough for you to be able to explain them to someone else?

____Do you try to develop the skills of your subordinates as an aid to achieving your most ambitious plans?

____Do you devote training time to helping your subordinates plan their activities?

____Do you refrain from planning the activity of any subordinate who should be on his or her own?

____Do you not allow your subordinates to perform planning functions that you should be doing?

____Do you ask your superior for enough information to make your planing sufficiently long range?

____Do you consult your superior to get suggestions on your planning activities, including suggestions on objectives, resources, methods, and evaluation of results?

Order-Giving Review (Directing)

How good is your command of the order-giving process?

____Before giving orders, do you
  −clarify the end results you're after?
  −prethink the moves required to meet objectives?
  −decide on the right people to do the job?
  −help make needed resources available to them?

____In giving orders or instructions, do you
  −suit the type of order to the individual: a direct order for the beginner, "result-wanted" order for the veteran, and so on?
  −indicate, wherever necessary, the addi-

tional information (data, reference material) the staff will need to finish the job?
  −try to put into your instructions the challenge that will create the strongest motivation for the individual?
  −provide written instructions and other support material, as needed?

____In setting goals for subordinates' activities, do you
  −let them join in a discussion of the relevance and importance of goals?
  −permit those with initiative enough leeway to exercise it?
  −give those who lack self-confidence the opportunity to check back with you as often as will be helpful?

____To aim at better teamwork, do you
  −give your group the opportunity, where possible, to share in planning operations?
  −keep group goals clearly in view at all times?

Your Decision-Making Practices

Your decision-making success depends on how well you can evaluate or compare alternative solutions to your problems, despite time pressure and insufficient data.

____Do you avoid leaving yourself high and dry because of failure to decide on a course of action *in time*?

____Similarly, do you avoid making decisions *before* you have to, and later receive information that would have changed your actions?

____In developing alternative courses of action to given problems, do you make use of the experience and knowledge of
  −your superior?
  −colleagues?
  −professional sources of know-how?
  −your subordinates?

____In evaluating the advantages and disadvantages of alternatives do you
  −list the pros and cons of each possibility in writing (at least for critical decisions)?
  −check the opinions of experts or people with relevant experience?

—try to quantify as many factors as possible, to make comparisons easier and more meaningful?

____In your final selection of a course of action, do you consider the possibility of combining the favorable aspects of two or more alternatives?

____In analyzing decisions that misfired, was the reason

—a misunderstanding of the objectives you were trying to achieve?

—a miscalculation of the difficulties of the situation?

—an overestimation of the abilities of your subordinates?

—an underestimation of their abilities?

—a failure to keep up with new developments affecting your decision?

Problem Solving

Unsolved problems are stones in the road of progress. The executive administrator is confronted by an unending parade of problems day in, day out. Are you able to keep the stones out of the road?

____Do you go looking for problems in order to account for

—plans that have not jelled?

—unanticipated developments?

—unexpected behavior on the part of your staff?

____Do you agree that a problem generally holds the clue to its solution?

____When you are faced with a problem, do you automatically

—start digging out the relevant facts?

—mentally line up the people who can help solve the problem?

—try to approach the situation on a logical, systematic basis?

____Do you motivate the problem-solving activities of your subordinates by communicating to them the excitement and challenge of facing up to a tough problem?

____Do you give your unconscious a chance to work on your problems by generating mental input—focusing on the circumstances and facts of the difficulty, thinking about the problem, and not trying to think through to a solution, leaving that to your unconscious mind?

____As a starter for creative problem solving, do you examine and challenge the assumptions you may have about the circumstances of the problem as well as the possible solution?

Scoring for each category: If the nos outweigh the yeses, you should be dissatisfied with your score. Go back over all the questions. Each one highlights a major opportunity for leadership performance. Questions you answered no are prime areas for improvement.

Chapter 3

Planning, Directing, and Controlling

PLANNING

The Nature of Planning*

The function of planning incorporates both strategic and tactical planning. *Strategic planning* involves determining the direction in which an organization should be headed. *Tactical planning* involves allocating resources that enable an organization to reach strategic objectives.

Second, plans are primarily mechanisms for guiding organizational efforts. The real test of planning is the ability to direct efforts on a daily basis, that is, to move from the abstract to the implemented. It is not enough just to create plans. They must be articulated and then put into action. Once the action occurs, control should be implemented to ascertain whether performance targets have actually been achieved. For a comprehensive plan to work effectively, each step must receive equal attention, and the cycle must be completed (i.e., from planning to implementation and then to control) before returning to planning. It should also be remembered that plan-

ning, to be effective, should not occur just at the top echelons. It should be implemented throughout an organization (see Figure 3–1).

Third, planning is a continual process that moves from setting the mission to setting operational objectives.

Fourth, values and expectations often determine what missions and strategies are adopted. Finally, reviewing and evaluating plans support control. Planning does not occur in a vacuum. Accomplishments or failures are ultimately analyzed, and the information gained thereby is used to revise plans where necessary.

Figure 3–1 Prerequisite for Effective Planning

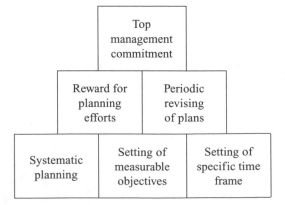

---

*Source: Judith F. Garner, Howard L. Smith, and Neill F. Piland, *Strategic Nursing Management: Power and Responsibility in a New Era*, Aspen Publishers, Inc., © 1990.

In many health care organizations, the short run is the immediate fiscal period. Intermediate plans cover one to two years. Long-term plans fall in the three- to five-year range. Variances in health care markets, the general economy, public regulation, patient preferences, industry structure, social climate, societal values, competition, and related factors tend to shorten the time frame of planning. Nonetheless, it is useful for health care organizations to extrapolate their efforts to five to ten years in the future.

Strategic Planning*

Strategic planning requires an assessment of organizational or departmental strengths and weaknesses before identifying opportunities and external threats. This means there is a cooperative effort between nursing services and overall organizational services. Thus, strategic planning for the health care facility constrains, and is constrained by, planning at the nursing department level. This synergy implies that nursing services and nursing directors can significantly influence the types of strategies a health care facility pursues in delivering patient care, and the end results occurring for organizational performance.

The Relationship of Strategic Planning and Performance

Nursing directors are responsible for developing strategies that enhance nursing department performance and that thereby affect overall health care facility performance. This relationship is explained below and demonstrated in Figure 3–2.

Strategic planning, as presented in Figure 3–2, may range from no planning to structured strategic planning. Planning can lead to a harmonious fit between an organization and its context. The result of such congruence is a

greater capacity to achieve performance. When a nursing director invests in strategic planning efforts, the anticipated outcomes are higher quality of care, greater staff satisfaction, lower patient care costs, and higher contribution to the profit margin of the health care facility.

Strategic planning articulates specific objectives and a map for reaching those objectives. If a nursing director failed to expend effort on planning, departmental performance would suffer, and, because of the cost contribution of nursing care, the facility's performance would also be negatively affected.

Nursing directors may emphasize several strategies to reach the performance targets established in a planning process. Management strategies and cost-control strategies are discussed below because they would have an immediate impact on financial outcomes, which are an important factor in health care facility performance.

Management Strategies. There are three primary management strategies: operations control, performance monitoring, and staff development strategies. In terms of operations control, nursing directors can improve documentation to ensure that nursing care costs are accurately accounted for, adjust nurse and support staffing to reflect patient census trends, and act to ensure that health care facility charges reflect nursing costs. Performance monitoring strategies may involve upgrading utilization review efforts, improving staff performance reviews, and upgrading quality assurance. Finally, in the staff development area, nursing directors can (1) attempt to enhance continuing education (for nurses in methods of cost control and for nurse managers in managerial topics); (2) institute participative management to promote group ownership of objectives; (3) implement clinical ladders as a means to motivate staff; (4) increase registered nurse salaries to minimize turnover costs and to enhance personal productivity; and (5) recruit capable staff, which should lead to higher performance levels.

Cost Control Strategies. Cost control strategies are categorized as either staffing or operations control strategies (Figure 3–2). Cost control through staffing may involve

Source: Howard L. Smith, Sat Ananda Mahon, Neill F. Piland, "Nursing Department Strategy, Planning and Performance in Rural Hospitals," *Journal of Nursing Administration*, Vol. 23:4, April 1993, J.B. Lippincott Company.

Figure 3–2 Model of Strategy and Planning for Performance

Management Strategies

Range of Strategic Planning Options		Operations Control	Staff Development	Performance Results
• Structured strategic plans • Structured operational plans • Informal plans • No planning	+	• Improved documentation • Census-based staffing • Adjusted charges for nursing costs **Performance Monitoring** • Upgraded utilization • Improved performance reviews • Upgraded quality assurance	• Continuing education in cost control • Continuing education for nurse managers • Participative management • Implemented clinical ladders • Increased salaries • Recruited capable staff	Affect → • Net income per patient day • Cost per patient day • Operating margin

Cost Control Strategies

Staffing	Operations Control
• Decreased staffing level • Eliminated overtime • Decreased RN to patient ratio • Decreased agency utilization • Reduced continuing education • Reduced staff benefits	• Changed structure of nursing department • Improved supplies management • Involved staff in budgeting process • Decreased administrative overhead

• decreasing staffing levels over the long run in view of utilization trends
• eliminating overtime paid to nurses
• decreasing the ratio of registered nurses to patients
• reducing use of nursing agency personnel
• reducing continuing education expenses
• reducing staff benefits

These strategies accomplish specific cost objectives. Cost control may also involve attention to specific operations control strategies, including

• reducing administrative overhead (i.e., by running the department with fewer nurse managers)

• improving supplies management to reduce inventory and ordering costs and to better manage waste
• involving staff in the budgeting process to promote group ownership of objectives and to educate staff about fiscal constraints
• changing the structure of the nursing department to enhance responsibility for specific operating objectives

Phases*

The different phases of the planning process are interdependent and continuous; they fre-

---

Source: Planning for Nursing Needs and Resources, National Institutes of Health, DHHS, 1972.

quently overlap in time and are often not discrete. Several of these phases are separated and discussed below as though a plan is totally developed and then implemented. This is not meant to convey the idea that planning always takes place in rigid and sequential steps. Viewed in phases, the planning process consists of

1. seeking common purposes and objectives
2. identifying issues and concerns
3. determining organizational structure for planning
4. selecting participants (and hiring staff if necessary)
5. collecting and analyzing data
6. assessing needs and resources
7. developing recommendations
8. developing the plan of action
9. implementing the plan of action
10. evaluating and reviewing progress in implementing and in continuous planning.

No one phase of planning is more important than another. Each has significance for bringing about the actions needed to solve nursing problems.

Framework for Organizing

To design and create a planning mechanism adapted to the department's conditions and needs, the nurse manager must do the following:

- Assess planning experience and readiness for planning.
- Outline the perimeters of nursing concerns and required actions and set the objectives of planning.
- Pinpoint data and information needs and availability.
- Determine what special studies or surveys may be required.
- Consider and understand the so-called power structure in the area affected.
- Decide what tasks must be undertaken to assess needs and resources and to reach planning objectives.
- Identify leaders and select participants for functional tasks.

- Determine staff requirements.
- Set a tentative timetable.
- Estimate budgetary requirements.

Determining Objectives

The nursing concerns requiring assessment by planning groups should first be identified. Then a study outline should be completed for each concern. The outline should list influential factors, information needed for assessment, sources for data, and any required special studies.

The completed study outline provides a basis for determining planning procedures and the course to be followed. The planning techniques, data requirements, and need for special surveys and studies will, in turn, influence staff and budgetary requirements.

Other concerns or aspects of issues and problems requiring analysis and study will emerge as planners begin to seek solutions to particular nursing problems.

Collecting Data

Using Existing Data. The use of data from existing sources presents few problems and precludes elaborate, time-consuming data collection. Use of these data involves the following: (1) identifying their sources; (2) assessing their relevance, timeliness, and accuracy; (3) abstracting the data from the original sources for use in the planning documents in a way that would be most meaningful to the planning group; and (4) analyzing the meaning and implications of the data in terms of the planning objectives.

Methods of Collecting Original Data. Questionnaires, interviews, and observation are used to collect original data. Any one or all of these methods may be employed to gather data on the same subject.

Administering a questionnaire, perhaps the most widely used method for original data collection, is the simplest type of data-collecting method. It is also less expensive and time-consuming than other methods. Questionnaires are used to elicit data on the following: (1) *objective facts*, such as the number of facilities and services available and the number of personnel employed; (2) *behavioral variables* that may be of interest to planning groups, such as kinds of nursing activities performed; (3) *evaluations*, such as feelings about the quality of patient care; and (4) *specified events*, such as the time spent by nurses on clerical activities.

Interviews are used when questionnaires cannot provide the depth of response required. The unstructured interview permits probing into the responses solicited to verify meaning and to obtain in-depth data. The highly structured interview allows for the collection of standardized data and information and for probing to clarify and broaden responses.

Observation is used for studies in which evaluation is the primary objective or where the data required are complex, are difficult to obtain, and need considerable interpretation. Such studies would include, for example, evaluating the activities of staff or the quality of their performance. Data are recorded in the form of an evaluative rating of what is being observed, a narrative description of what was seen, or entries on a checklist. The use of this method requires considerable control over the observation to ensure reliability.

Developing the Plan of Action

When recommendations have been formulated and priorities have been determined, they are then incorporated into a definitive plan for meeting nursing needs. In developing the plan, attention is given to the following:

- specifying goals, objectives, and policies for carrying out recommendations and suggested programs
- phasing activities so that resolution of problems requiring immediate action leads to actions and measures for attaining long-range goals
- indicating the individuals to carry out each recommendation
- specifying a time span for achieving specific objectives or steps in the plan
- providing methods for evaluating progress in meeting objectives

The plan of action should build on existing services and staff resources. The diversity of needs, resources, and existing patterns of education and service must be dealt with.

In developing the plan, problems likely to be encountered in its phasing must be considered (e.g., resistance to the introduction of new concepts). Measures to surmount potential obstacles must be worked out in advance and integrated into the plan. Criteria for a good plan are outlined in Table 3–1.

CREATIVITY AND INNOVATION

To navigate the chaos of the 1990s successfully, the health care organization must be able to tap into the creative potential of its employees. Health care organizations today face a critical choice: Innovate and change, or expect to be replaced by organizations that do. It is the choice between chaos and transformation.

Creativity and innovation are hallmarks of the most successful health care organizations in the country today. Successful innovation is not magic or something that just happens when the synergy is right. Organizations with a track record

---

Table 3–1 Evaluation Criteria

A plan is good or generally acceptable if it

- is in line with a clearly stated objective
- indicates the procedural method for putting the plan into action
- can be communicated effectively (allowing for appropriate dissemination methods)
- is operational, professionally sound, and economically feasible
- represents an integrated whole and not an isolated entity
- allows for alternate courses of action as changes occur and opportunities for new approaches arise
- wisely uses human talents, abilities, and skills to their maximum potential and makes judicious use of material resources in order to improve patient care and educate the nursing staff

Source: Planning for Nursing Needs and Resources, National Institutes of Health, DHHS, 1972.

of successful innovation have discovered that innovation must be managed. Innovation management is a developmental process, a process of becoming that does not happen overnight. These organizations have established an internal climate that supports entrepreneurial activity and goes beyond paying lip service to the idea of innovation and employee entrepreneurship. They recognize that innovation must be systematic, organized, and managed rather than sporadic, incidental, and accidental. Innovation is expected and encouraged in the organization and seen as part of the work to be done rather than something that happens in addition to the "real work" of the staff.*

A Process for Managing Innovation*

A five-phase process can help the leader manage the process of innovation. The primary issues of each phase are identified below, and although it is recommended that they be considered sequentially, the issues of one phase can also appear and are appropriate to consider throughout the entire cycle.

Phase 1: Preparation

In the first phase, preparation, the two major issues of purpose and allocation of resources must be considered and managed. This phase is the foundation of the process. It is primarily leader-driven and the responsibility of the nurse executive and the team of internal leaders. Clear lines of responsibility should be identified and decisions made about appropriate levels of authority.

Simply put, innovation must be an important element of the department's mission and a part of the everyday language before it will be accepted as a value. Adequate resources also must be available if innovation is an expected part of the work of the organization. This includes time,

access to other people, funding, and personal development time.

Managers should be prepared for their roles as innovation managers. Individual innovators need programs or opportunities that focus on innovation and the skill development needed by a successful innovator. All members of the department benefit from general programs focusing on the need for innovation, essential skills, and their role in supporting fellow staff members who are innovators.

Phase 2: Movement

During the second phase, the structural elements supporting innovation throughout the department need to be established. If the vision is clear, the structure needed to support that vision will follow. The two aspects of this phase are planning and decision making.

Planning for a structure that will support innovation in the department is critical. The nurse executive facilitates this planning with participation and input from all levels within the department. A process for evaluating new ideas, gaining approval, and obtaining funding must be established. Two separate structures may be needed, one for large projects that involve integral changes in the department and actual funding, and a simpler process for ideas with less impact and a lesser need for resource allocation. Once innovation-supporting structural changes are determined, assignment of responsibility is necessary. How will the process be initiated? Who will be responsible? How will levels of authority be decided?

Phase 3: Team Creativity

This phase is described as team creativity, or maturation, as the innovators within the department actually begin using the structure that has been established. The issues of priority setting, climate developing, coordination, cooperation, team building and networking, and internal communications must be considered. Each of these issues is an important key, and lack of attention to any one will result in a system out of balance.

Source: Jo Manion, "Chaos or Transformation? Managing Innovation," *Journal of Nursing Administration*, Vol. 23:5, May 1993, J.B. Lippincott Company.

Phase 4: New Reality

The fourth phase is the new reality. The key issues relate to stabilizing the environment, maintaining the direction that has been set, and actually producing results from the innovative projects and changes that have occurred. A common error made in innovation management is expecting productivity improvements or gains too early in the cycle.

Stabilizing the innovation is an important step and should be considered carefully. Ways to anchor the change must be sought.

Phase 5: Integration

The final phase of the developmental cycle is integration or closure. The key issues in this stage relate to evaluative functions and quality. Although evaluation is an important process throughout this developmental cycle, at this phase it is a key issue. The innovation should be measured for its beneficence and effectiveness. In anticipation of later evaluation, key indicators of success are established during the planning phase. The process used to develop or implement the innovation is evaluated. Key questions should include: what did we learn; what would we do differently; and is there anything we can stop doing? Cultivate an attitude within the department that these questions are a normal part of the process. Never let the evaluation process be construed as placing blame.

Creating a climate and structure within an organization that empower clinical staff and managers alike takes a strong commitment and consistent effort on the part of the executive and leadership team. To make the leap from creative ideas to a new reality requires a process for managing innovation. It requires establishment of a supportive climate and individuals who have advanced skills in creativity, developing new ideas and plans, and the implementation of change. Transformation of the organization is the potential result.

*Guidelines for Implementing Innovations**

Identification of strengths and areas needing improvement provides a database around which changes can be made. The plan of systematic evaluation should provide direction and valuable information. Avoid the attitude of "change for change's sake (see box)."

Develop a master plan with target dates for time of accomplishment of different aspects. This is your blueprint. The job, when looked at as a whole, may appear overwhelming. Break it down into small pieces that can be handled. Recognize that the timetable may have to be revised.

Ensure staff involvement. People tend to support what they help plan. The size of your staff will cause your approach to vary. If you have a staff of 20, you can use approaches that would not work with a staff of 200.

Define the constraints under which you must operate. These may be in terms of money, time, skill of staff, equipment, and clinical facilities.

Identify and analyze the choices, for there is more than one way to get to an objective.

Consider all the ramifications of the change. Innovations that are helpful in one area may have undesirable side effects in other areas.

Plan for evaluation. Have you ever noticed that in most books evaluation is often the last chapter? It is even listed as the last step in the nursing process. It should start at the beginning of your process and continue throughout.

Perhaps the most important point is to make failure acceptable. Risk taking is associated with change, and this can be anxiety producing. Not succeeding should not become degrading to individuals.

When working with staff, bring out hidden agendas so that real issues can be handled. Remember, one of the factors for promoting change is not threatening the autonomy and security of individuals.

Source: D. Shumaker, "Change Theory and Instructional Innovation," *Instructional Innovations*, National League for Nursing, Pub. No. 16-1687, 1977. Reprinted with permission.

Five Strategies for Moving from Fear to Earning

The following five strategies can help employees move from a position of fear to one of earning:

1. **Make leadership visible.** Leadership has to project certainty and confidence because people desperately need to believe that leaders know what they are doing. When anxiety is high, so are dependency needs; people need help in having faith that the future will be better. When a major change is instituted, a kind of corporate vacuum is created during which employees wait to see what will happen.

   The best strategy is to fill the vacuum with positive ideas before others fill it with negative ones. This means telling people what is happening and what the leader is going to do. It is important to use any opportunity available to informally discuss plans, using both personal and organizational forms of communication.

2. **Communicate concern for the individual.** Employees need to believe that leadership understands how they feel because they are working under difficult circumstances. Leadership needs to communicate a true understanding of how stress affects subordinates.

   In its weekly newsletter, one organization gave a list of departments and phone numbers available for emotional support and counseling that included an em-ployee assistance program, pastoral care, employee relations, and the name of a behavioral psychologist known to the organization. When possible, try to retain employees by retraining or relocating them. Out-placement services are an important way to acknowledge the employee's contribution to the organization.

3. **Provide information on the process of the change, including both the good news and the bad news.** This strategy will help reduce the rumors that seem to develop a life cycle of their own when no real information is available. It is important to remember that in high anxiety, very little appears logical and rational.

   Employee forums need to be made available on an around-the-clock basis so that employees can continually express concerns and ask questions. Bulletin boards must be strategically placed to provide updates on available positions along with diagrams depicting planned changes. It is important to publicize progress, as well as to acknowledge people who have accomplished the goals.

4. **Make it possible for people to earn security and experience belonging.** It is all right to make security conditional, if the real terms of the contract are made overt and clear. Individuals who are effective role models should be pointed out as examples. Providing educational tools and specific training sends a message to the employees that retraining will follow expectations. Whenever possible, avoid layoffs. However, when layoffs are necessary, base them on merit, not seniority, or one is merely regressing to the entitlement phase.

5. **Reduce the emphasis on the hierarchy.** When people feel powerless, they become preoccupied with issues of power and they never feel safe. The role of the manager is changing from that of director to one of a facilitator of teams. In so doing, the manager must learn to ask smart questions, not give smart answers.

Source: Vicki Lachman, "The New Employee Contract: From Entitlement to Achievement," *Aspen's Advisor for Nurse Executives*, Vol. 11:7, Aspen Publishers, Inc., © 1996.

Transition Tactics

Resisters should become "targets" of the administrator's strategy for making the effective change. The administrator should take the following steps:

- Allow targets to ventilate their fears, concerns, insecurities, and grief in an environment that treats these feelings as legitimate.
- Focus targets' attention on the future, not the past.
- Reward those who are supportive of the change and apply pressure to those who are resistant.
- Assign roles, tasks, and responsibilities so targets feel they are involved and exercising influence.
- Provide targets with the logistic, economic, and political resources needed to achieve what you asked of them.
- Identify anchors who targets can trust and who will remain constant and provide stability.
- Provide targets with training in how to understand their own reactions, as well as the reactions of others, to the change process.

Source: Donna Richards Sheridan, "In the Business Literature," *Aspen's Advisor for Nurse Executives*, Vol. 6:2, Aspen Publishers, Inc., © 1990.

When deadlocks occur, brainstorm and try to identify alternatives. Try not to vote in this kind of situation.

Try not to have a final or "set" decision in a small group that will result in defensiveness when recommendations are presented to the total group and suggestions are offered, for it is likely they will be. Label materials "Draft 1, 2, 3" or "Working Copy." This helps develop the mental set that decisions can be changed. They are not carved in stone.

The final guideline is to maintain a perspective. Remember, there is nothing like a little experience to upset a theory.

CONTROLLING

Overview*

Controlling is the management function in which performance is measured and corrective action is taken to ensure the accomplishment of organizational goals. It is the policing operation in management, although the manager seeks to create a positive climate so that the process of control is accepted as part of routine activity. Controlling is also a forward-looking process in that the manager seeks to anticipate deviation and prevent it.

The manager initiates the control function during the planning phase, when possible deviation is anticipated and policies are developed to help ensure uniformity of practice.

Close supervision and a tight leadership style reflect an aspect of control. Through rewards and positive sanctions, the manager seeks to motivate workers to conform, thus limiting the amount of control that must be imposed. Finally, the manager develops specific control tools, such as inspections, visible control charts, work counts, special reports, and audits.

The Basic Control Process

The control process involves three phases that are cyclic: establishing standards, measuring performance, and correcting deviation. In the first step, the specific units of measure that delineate acceptable work are determined. Basic standards may be stated as staff hours allowed per activity, speed and time limits, quantity that must be produced, and number of errors or rejects permitted. The second step in the control process, measuring performance, involves comparing the work (i.e., the service provided)

Source: Joan G. Liebler, Ruth E. Levine, and Hyman L. Dervitz, *Management Principles for Health Professionals*, Aspen Publishers, Inc., © 1983.

against the standard. Employee evaluation is one aspect of this measurement.

Studies of consumer/client satisfaction are key elements when services are involved. Finally, if necessary, remedial action is taken, including retraining employees.

Note: For further discussions of control methods, see Chapters 13, 21, and 35.

Characteristics of Adequate Controls

Several features are necessary to ensure the adequacy of control processes and tools.

Timeliness. The control device should reflect deviations from the standard promptly and at an early stage, so there is only a small time lag between detection and the beginning of corrective action.

Economy. If possible, control devices should involve routine, normal processes rather than the special inspection routines at additional cost. The control devices must be worth their cost

Comprehensiveness. The controls should be directed at the basic phases of the work rather than the later levels or steps in the process.

Specificity and Appropriateness. The control process should reflect the nature of the activity. Proper quality-of-care inspection methods, for example, differ from a financial audit.

Objectivity. The processes should be grounded in fact, and standards should be known and verifiable.

Responsibility. Controls should reflect the authority-responsibility pattern. As far as possible, the worker and the immediate supervisor should be involved in the monitoring and correction process.

Understandability. Control devices, charts, graphs, and reports that are complicated or cumbersome will not be used readily.

Tools of Control

Certain tools of control may be combined with the planning process. Management by objectives, the budget, the Gantt chart, and the Program Evaluation Review Technique (PERT) network are examples of tools used both for planning and controlling. The flowchart, the flow process chart, the work distribution chart, and work sampling (see Chapter 21) all may be used in planning workflow or assessing a proposed change in plan or procedure. They also may be adapted for specific control use, such as when the flowchart is employed to audit the way in which work is done, as compared to the original plan.

Specific, quantifiable output measures may be recorded and monitored through a variety of visible control charts. In addition to these specific tools, the manager exercises control through the assessment and limitation of conflict, through the communication process, and through active monitoring of employees.

How To Control*

Money, Material, and People

Essentially, a manager controls three entities or a combination of them: money, material, and people. Each, however, is handled differently; each takes a separate skill. Money and material are usually more constant and easier to budget. Money will buy just so much, and the manager has only so much money and must decide what to do with what is available.

But people are not that easy to budget (control); no two are alike and each person may show different qualities from one time to the next. That is what makes a person an individual. When budgeting (controlling) people, the manager must consider that they work at a different speed in the morning than in the afternoon, and with a different attitude on Monday than on Friday, or on evenings than on nights.

Often, people may try to control without a plan, which means they are doing some guesswork with their controlling. For example, when someone decides in the middle of a project that it is taking too many supplies and too much time,

---

Source: Copyright © 1977, Martin Broadwell.

and *then* starts to "control," very likely there was no preset plan to begin with.

A rule of thumb—really more of a guide—is that when the manager needs to take drastic action with people, materials, or money, either the planning or the controlling stage broke down. In general, controlling consists of (1) determining standards, (2) measuring results against standards, and (3) taking remedial action as necessary.

Determining Standards

In determining standards, look for answers to some basic questions: Who sets the standards, and how will you know they are the standards? Your plan may or may not specify how far you can stray from the standards without courting trouble. You must have this information; you cannot hope to control without it.

You also need to know who will measure the results of your work and who will see the results of those measurements. Is there a quality control person (such as a systems engineer or an infection control officer) who reports to higher management? Or has someone on your own staff been given partial responsibility for watching quality?

Of utmost importance is what will be measured and why it in particular is being measured. Are you getting valid information or just watching a meaningless figure?

It is also important not to overreact to situations. For example, your superior tells you to watch out for certain problems or expenditures, and you set up a control system much more complicated than you need. Long after the crisis is past, you are still filling out forms and sending reports up the line. Once forms and reports come into being, getting rid of them is next to impossible. Start them only under extreme need.

What are some items that can be measured? Obviously, you want to measure output of services. How long did it take? How much did it cost? What was the final quality?

Then you need to look closely at expenses. When you measure them, you must measure all of them. Are you taking into account everything that is being charged to the particular job? Are

you including staff help and hidden costs that eventually will need to be shown?

Using Resources

You must also account for the use of resources. Again, this means people, time, and money—but here you measure efficient use. Are you doing a good job of matching people and jobs? Remember, a job done well is not necessarily proof of good supervision. You must consider who is doing the job. If your staff are capable of doing much more because of experience, education, training, or talent, you cannot be too proud that they have done the job well. Your goal is to match ability with job requirements as closely as possible, then let the people grow out of their jobs as they develop. As a manager, you must constantly measure—at least in your mind—both how well the employee matches the job and whether he or she has outgrown it.

This is also true for other resources. Are you really getting the most out of overtime? Are you doing jobs that could be left undone or eliminated altogether, then using overtime for essential things? Sometimes managers can trap themselves this way, spending valuable time on unimportant chores, forcing themselves into overtime. Or staff may be used on nonessential assignments when they could be working on more worthwhile projects. You can have everyone pitch in and help when admissions are very heavy. But if this means you neglect other work that will put you behind schedule or cost you time and money later on, you have made a bad decision.

Using the Budget

The budget is perhaps the oldest and best control device you have. It gives you something to measure your progress by and something at which to aim. As you compare yourself constantly with the budget, you also get feedback on where you can expect to be at the end of the budget period.

Here are a few basic points of reference on budgets. First, a budget is put together to let the administration know just how much money is needed and where it can best be spent. Good budget planning takes local needs into account, and good budget designers solicit help from all levels in determining the best use of funds.

The trouble starts when each level becomes unrealistic about its needs. With each unit adding just a little extra, a little cushion here or there, the total budget becomes bloated. Either the demand is too big or the health care facility must look for more money than it really needs. When this happens, someone at the top usually starts to whittle the figure, and everyone gets hurt.

Do not include in your budget anything you cannot substantiate; sooner or later, you will have to account for what you requested. If your figures will not stand the test, not only will the budget be cut, but your reputation as a manager will suffer.

Measuring Results

Once you have determined the standards by which you are to control, you must measure the results against those standards. Sometimes this is routine—a simple matter of seeing how many patients were treated, and so forth, then reporting the obvious results by whatever method is provided.

All evaluating is not that obvious or that easy, however. In some situations, so many contributing factors are involved that it is unclear just what the results mean.

One of the best evaluation methods is the process known as sampling. There is nothing complicated about it. It is simply a means of looking at large or complicated services and obtaining reliable results without taking a measurement on *every* detail and *every* person involved in that effort. Instead, a small, average sample is taken and its results are used to represent the entire operation. Or one complete case or instance out of several can be taken, assuming that the rest are like this one.

You can look for ways of getting true samples regularly: Check the employee absentee list occasionally and notice if certain persons or a constant number are absent regularly. Spot-check three or four days in a row and notice how much time the employees are taking for break or when they are coming back from lunch. Look at patient complaints once a week for several weeks and find out what is causing trouble. These are good indicators of how well you are doing and a good means of controlling.

When sampling will not help in measuring results, and the measuring seems too difficult to do on the whole operation, you may choose to look for a substitute measurement. Thus, you can examine something like absenteeism or tardiness and get a good idea of the group's morale. High turnover may be a good substitute measurement of the extent of available job enrichment and training. A look at previous records may be a good measure of motivation or employee morale in the work unit, providing other things are equal. The substitute measurement may be a tangible means of measuring intangibles such as attitudes, job satisfaction, morale, and so forth.

Taking Remedial Action

Controlling would be useless if it did not include the final facet of control: taking remedial action when required. When measuring processes show that things are running smoothly, you should be a good enough manager to recognize it and leave things alone. But when results show that a situation is getting out of hand or that you should be doing better, you should step in and take action.

You may not be the one to take the action, but you might instigate it by reporting to the right person. If you have found a problem on the unit, ask yourself who should know about it. The obvious answer is: Someone who can do something about it. Whether the problem is overtime, a union grievance, or whatever, telling the right person as soon as possible may ward off a much more serious problem later on.

However, it is better to solve the problem yourself than to pass it on to someone else. This means you must have the authority to take the necessary remedial action. It also means you may need to repeat the entire planning, organizing, and directing functions. If that is what the remedial action requires, that is what you, the good manager, should do.

Systems Engineering

Activities*

Health systems engineers (frequently referred to as industrial or management engineers) are employed by hospitals and other health care institutions to study facility design and utilization, information flow, human resource utilization, and the degree to which performance objectives are being met, in the expectation that they will be of aid in reducing costs and improving the quality of and access to care.

The following activities summarize the majority of services provided by systems engineers:

- the analysis, design, and improvement of work systems, work centers, and work methods
- the establishment of work standards for determining staffing patterns, human resource utilization, and costs
- the development of job descriptions, job evaluation plans, merit rating procedures, and employee motivation plans
- the design of physical facilities, layout and arrangement, floor space utilization, material flow, and traffic patterns
- the installation of systems for production control, inventory control, and quality control in the storing, handling, processing, and using of materials and supplies
- the economic analysis of alternative combinations of human resources, materials, and equipment, and the development of models to optimize such combinations
- the simplification of paperwork and the design of forms
- the improvement of organizational structure, authority-responsibility relationships, and patterns of communications
- the development of data processing procedures and management reports in order to establish information systems for managerial control on a continuing basis
- the generation of technical information, the forecasting of future needs and demands, and the conversion of relevant information into a form useful in managerial and administrative decision making
- the performance of general staff work for the administrator for his or her use in policy determination, fiscal budgeting, building plans, and public relations[1]

Analysis*

Operations Analysis. This function is described as making a thorough analysis of an operation by dissecting it into its component parts or elements. Each part or element then is considered separately, and the study of an operation becomes a series of fairly simple problems. Systems engineers have found from experience that few established methods cannot be improved if examined sufficiently.

Process Analysis. Another term for a similar evaluation is *process analysis.* It is described as "the act of studying the process used for producing a product for the purpose of developing the lowest-cost, most efficient process which will yield products of acceptable quality." Applied to health care, the end result of a process should result in better health, although objective measurement may be difficult. When a current process is evaluated to find ways of improving it, the analysis usually is made with the aid of one or more types of process charts. The process chart is a convenient way to show the relations among operations, the steps of a process, and factors such as distance moved, working and idle time, cost, operations performed, and time standards. It permits the quick perception of a problem so that improvement can be undertaken in a logical sequence.

---

[1]Harold E. Smalley, *Hospital Management Engineering,* Prentice-Hall, Inc., Englewood Cliffs, N.J., © 1982, p. 397. Copyright © Harold E. Smalley. Reprinted by permission of the author.

*Source: David F. Johannides, *Cost Containment through Systems Engineering,* Aspen Publishers, Inc., © 1979.

---

*Source: David F. Johannides, *Cost Containment through Systems Engineering,* Aspen Publishers, Inc., © 1979.

Systems Analysis. Another evaluation term is *systems analysis*. A system is defined as a network of interrelated operations joined together to perform an activity. In a sense, it is a broader application of the operation analysis definition, with key elements reviewed for their negative or positive impact on the decision points of the system.

Systems analysis requires 10 steps of the systems engineer:

1. Define the problem.
2. Prepare an outline of the systems study.
3. Obtain general background information on the areas to be studied.
4. Understand the interactions between the areas being studied.
5. Understand the existing system.
6. Define the system requirements.
7. Design the new system.
8. Prepare economic cost comparisons.
9. Sell the new system to management.
10. Provide implementation, follow up, and reevaluation.[1]

In addition to this process, an effective system should produce the following important results:

• the right information furnished to the right people, at the right time, and at the right cost
• a decrease in uncertainty and improvement of decision quality

---

• an increased capacity to process present and future volumes of work
• an ability to perform profitable work that was previously impossible
• increased productivity of employees and capital, and reduced costs[1]

To achieve these results, one step is all-important—the design of the new system. Here the information developed earlier is combined into a synchronized approach to desired goals. It requires the recognition that alternative configurations may offer success in varying degrees, which must be assessed. It is a practical process that is limited by the availability of such resources as time, money, and human resources. It remains a key instrument for implementing decisions.

Systems Theory*

The systems model is made up of four basic components: inputs, throughputs or processes, outputs, and feedback (Figure 3–3). The overall environment also must be considered.

Inputs. A systematic review of inputs for a health care organization or one of its departments could include

• characteristics of clients: average length of stay, diagnostic categories, payment status
• federal and state laws concerning employers: collective bargaining legislation, the

---

[1]John M. Fitzgerald and Ardra F. Fitzgerald, *Fundamentals of Systems Analysis*, John Wiley & Sons, © 1973. Reprinted with permission.

[1]Ibid.
Source: Joan G. Liebler, Ruth E. Levine, and Hyman L. Dervitz, *Management Principles for Health Professionals*, Aspen Publishers, Inc., © 1983.

Figure 3–3 Basic Systems Model

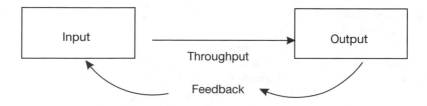

Occupational Safety and Health Act, workers' compensation, Civil Rights Act

- multiple goals: patient care, teaching, research

Throughputs (Withinputs). Throughputs are the structures or processes by which inputs are converted to outputs. Physical plant, workflow, methods and procedures, and hours of work are throughputs. Throughputs are analyzed by work sampling, work simplification, methods improvement, staffing patterns, and physical layout analysis. For example, a chief of service cannot control patient arrivals for walk-in service in a clinic; this input is imposed on the system. The policies and procedures for processing walk-in patients, however, constitute a cluster of throughputs that can be determined by the manager.

Outputs. Outputs are the goods and services that the organization (or subdivision or unit) must produce. These outputs may be routine, frequent, predictable, and somewhat easy to identify.

Some outputs for health care institutions are

- processing of specified laboratory tests within 10 hours of receipt of specimen
- retrieval of patient medical record from permanent file within 7 minutes of receipt of request
- 100 percent follow up on all patients who fail to keep appointments

Feedback. Changes in the input mix must be anticipated. To respond to these changes, managers need feedback on the acceptability and adequacy of the outputs. It is through the feedback process that inputs, and even throughputs, are adjusted to produce new outputs. The communication network and control processes are the usual sources of organized feedback. The management by objectives process, short interval scheduling, and PERT networks constitute specific management tools of planning and controlling that include structured, factual feedback.

If there is an absence of planned feedback, if the communication process is not sufficiently developed to permit safe and acceptable avenues for feedback, or if the feedback is ignored, feedback will occur spontaneously. In this case, it tends to take a negative form, such as a client outburst of anger, a precipitous lawsuit, a wildcat strike, a consumer boycott, or an epidemic.

Closed Versus Open Systems. Systems may be classified as either closed or open. An ideal closed system is complete within itself. No new inputs are received, and there is no change in the components; there is no output of energy in any of its forms (e.g., information or material). Few, if any, response or adaptation systems are needed because such a system is isolated from external forces in its environment and internal change is self-adjusting.

Organizations have been viewed as closed systems; that is, the emphasis has been placed on the study of functions and structure within the organization without consideration of its environment and the consequent effect of environmental change on its processes.

An open system is in a constant state of flux. Inputs are received and outputs produced. There is input and output of both matter and energy, continual adaptation to the environment, and, usually, an increase of order and complexity with differentiation of parts over time.

Classic functions of a manager, which are carried out in the distinct, unique environment of a given organization, are reflected in the systems approach. Table 3–2 summarizes this interrelationship.

Management by Objectives*

There are three distinct phases in the management by objectives (MBO) cycle: the planning phase, the performance review phase, and the feedback phase leading to a new planning phase. Table 3–3 summarizes the MBO cycle in terms of each phase, key activities for the phase, and the participants involved in each phase.

*Source: Joan G. Liebler, Ruth E. Levine, and Hyman L. Dervitz, *Management Principles for Health Professionals,* Aspen Publishers, Inc., © 1983.

Table 3–2 Relationship of Classic Management Functions and Systems Concepts

Systems Concept	Predominant Management Function
Input analysis Identification of constraints Assessment of client characteristics Assessment of physical space Budget allocation analysis	Planning
Throughput determination Development of policies, procedures, methods Development of detailed departmental layout	Planning and controlling
Specification of staffing pattern	Staffing
Methods of worker productivity enhancement	Controlling, leadership, and motivation
Output analysis Goal formulation Statement of objectives	Planning
Development of management by objectives plan	Planning and controlling
Feedback mechanisms Development of feedback processes	Controlling, communicating, and resolving conflict
Adjustment of inputs and outputs in light of feedback Adjustment of internal throughputs	Renewing planning cycle

Planning

Selection of objectives is the basic activity on which the MBO process is built, and it must be given careful attention. A guiding principle for the choice of objectives is the rule of the critical few, also referred to as the Pareto principle. In essence, this concept reflects the probability that most of the key results will be generated by only a few of the activities, while most of the activities will generate only a few of the key results.

Performance Objectives. In the MBO process, the performance objectives developed are essentially operational goals or objectives. The objectives that are determined for an MBO sequence should be distinguished by three characteristics.

- *Specificity.* Each objective should include a plan that shows the work to be done, the

time frame within which it is to be accomplished, and a clear designation of the individual who is to accomplish the work.

- *Measurability.* Each objective, as far as possible, should have quantifiable indicators for the measurement of work accomplished. If an activity cannot be quantified, qualitative factors should be developed.

- *Attainability.* Each objective should be realistic; it should be possible to carry out the activity within the time frame established.

Performance objectives have much in common with operational goals, which will be discussed here briefly in conjunction with their use in management by objectives.

Operational Goals. In addition to the formal statements of objectives and desired functional statements of performance, a manager may wish

Table 3–3 Summary of MBO Cycle

Phase	Key Activities	Participants
Planning	Identify and define key organizational goals. Identify and define key departmental goals that stem from overall goals. Identify and define performance measures (operational goals) for employees.	Manager
	Formulate and propose goals for specific job. Formulate and propose measures for specific job.	Subordinate
	Participate in management conferences. Achieve joint agreement on individual objectives and individual performance. Set up timetable for periodic meetings for performance review.	Manager and subordinates
Performance review	Continue to participate in periodic management conferences. Adjust and refine objectives based on feedback, new constraints, and new inputs. Eliminate inappropriate goals. Readjust timetable as needed. Maintain ongoing comparison of proposed timetable and actual performance through use of control monitoring devices, such as visible control charts.	Manager and subordinates
Feedback to new planning stage	Review overall organizational and departmental goals for the next planning period, such as the next fiscal year.	Manager

to develop operational, or working, goals for internal department use only. Operational goals are also highly specific, measurable, and attainable; they must be sufficiently concrete to relate the overall goals and objectives to specific actions.

Operational goals may be seen as temporary measures that take into account the reality of changing, usually difficult, work situations. They reflect the impact of a high turnover rate, absenteeism, employees in a trainee status, physical renovation of the work area, or temporary emergency situations. Operational goals may become progressively more refined as progress is achieved in certain areas.

Performance Review

The performance objectives determined in the MBO conference must be fair, based on all known relevant conditions, adjusted to the in-

dividual's capability, and adjusted to the specific constraints of the work situation. The objectives themselves do not vary from one performance meeting to another, but the points to be measured are subject to change because of variations in conditions during work cycles.

The purpose of performance review is not only to monitor the performance, but also to make adjustments as indicated by the situation. Successful use of management by objectives includes the allowance for a margin of error, that is, planning for mistakes and accepting the human factor. This planning for contingencies gives realism to the objectives and is helpful in enhancing employee acceptance of the process.

Feedback

There are several, even many, management conferences to formulate the original plans, to adjust these plans during the performance review phase, and to obtain the necessary feedback. During the management conferences between workers and managers, specific planning takes place, as follows:

- Appropriate objectives are identified through mutual agreement.
- Time periods for achieving the objectives are established.
- Responsibility in terms of results is defined.
- Revision and adjustments are made periodically.

Formats for MBO Plan

The format for writing a detailed MBO plan varies; managers develop a format to suit their own needs unless a specific format is imposed by a higher authority in the organization. Regardless of what format is used, certain information should be included routinely in the MBO plan.

- department
- unit or subdivision
- overall objectives and the derived operational objectives
- the period covered in the MBO cycle
- key participants
- workflow factors and special constraints
- identification of training needs
- methods of evaluation to be used
- detailed time plan

DIRECTING/FACILITATING

Directing*

Directing is the management function that initiates action. It obviously includes giving directions, assignments, and instructions. But it also includes building an effective group of subordinates who are motivated to perform. The amount of directing done by each manager varies a good deal; first-line managers do a great deal of detailed directing, whereas top managers spend more time in other managerial functions.

Some managers see a need for strong controls and detailed directions. The behavior of subordinates is to be regulated through coercion and punishment if they do not perform properly and through monetary rewards if they perform well. This type of manager believes in close supervision, detailed instructions, and exact deadlines. The manager is doing the planning of work and making the decisions. Some employees like this style and respond well to it, especially those with skill deficiencies, lack of experience, or personalities that want firm and structured direction.

Other managers, who are more in step with current management attitudes, believe that most people will work hard and assume responsibility provided they can satisfy personal needs and organizational goals at the same time. Therefore, these managers do not see the sharp division between leaders and followers. They feel that performance is better regulated by internal controls (within the person) than external controls. In this human resource approach, employees participate in setting the goals for work to be done, thus becoming committed and enthusiastic about its accomplishment. The manager assumes that untapped talents will become evident and maximize the contributions the employees can make toward the goals of the enterprise.

The contemporary manager's role has reinforced this image of the worker. The manager's directing function is changing to an empowering/guiding/facilitating role.

Facilitating*

Facilitation involves easing a group through a logical and satisfying process. A process is sat-

Source: David B. Starkweather and Donald G. Shropshire, "Management Effectiveness," in *Manual of Health Services Management*, Robert J. Taylor, ed., Aspen Publishers, Inc., © 1994.

Source: Tim Porter-O'Grady and Cathleen Krueger Wilson, *The Leadership Revolution in Health Care: Altering Systems, Changing Behaviors*, Aspen Publishers, Inc., © 1995.

isfying when it follows a sensible set of steps and when it feels psychologically agreeable. The right people are in the right place, and the environment is conducive to the success of participative processes and teams.

Facilitators need to understand how people operate in groups and how to use group dynamics to help teams accomplish their work. Using group dynamics is no easy task, as most groups are made up of people who have varying levels of cognitive complexity and are at different stages of development. The dynamics of most groups thus tend to reflect degrees of comfort with uncertainty stemming from unlike judgments and reasoning.

To function in a facultative role, a leader must be a masterful communicator. In the new health care organization, leader communication can no longer be dominated by task-oriented and position power messages. Leader communication that emphasizes receptivity, similarity, immediacy, and equality is crucial for encouraging high levels of participation among workers.

Receptivity is evidenced when leaders communicate in words and action an openness to exploring work issues, even if they are personally uncomfortable with exploration of such issues. *Equality* messages are intended to communicate that everyone's point of view is equally valuable to explore as input into a decision.

Facilitating leaders are flexible. They understand the development of teams and recognize that at varying stages of development different things are needed from the leader. (See Chapter 8.) Novices to the work of groups may unknowingly encourage groups to avoid conflict or cause them to become paralyzed by discussion in order to find the "perfect solution." In fact, many group decisions require challenging discussions and/or conflict resolution prior to implementation. The key is to find the best balance between those task activities that move a group through its agenda and the maintenance processes that address positive and negative group dynamics. It is the quality of the interaction that is the focus of facilitation skills rather than the persons doing the interacting.

COLLABORATION

Collaboration is an increasingly important component of restructured delivery systems. Consistency in approach, in communication, and in care planning is vital because of the many interactions among patient care teams, multiple managerial levels, departmental coordinators, and external care providers. Yesterday's turf holder mentality is being relinquished slowly but surely as the health care process becomes an interdisciplinary, interdepartmental system with the patient as its focus point. Interaction requires the skill of collaboration and a framework for collaborative practice. If collaborative practices are underdeveloped in these times of dynamic change, health care providers will not be able to respond in the manner needed.

The Collaborative Condition or the Collaborative Partnership

In a collaborative relationship, there is an agreement to pursue a common purpose and a sharing of knowledge to resolve problems, decide issues, and set goals within a structure of collegiality. The partners decide together the kinds of activities and functions that each will contribute. Issues of power and control are discussed, along with other issues that could affect the nature of the relationship. Although a collaborative relationship is typically intense, it does allow for the separateness of each partner. Indeed, the recognition of separateness is an essential feature of collaboration. Each partner agrees to contribute special talents and skills to the pursuit of a common purpose in return for the benefits the partners hope to achieve as a result of the other partner's contribution of any special talents and skills.

It is to be expected that the levels of contribution will differ depending on the skills required and the resources available. Each partner will have a different mix of those elements upon which the relationship is to be built. The interests of each of the parties to the collaborative venture must be enumerated for all so that they can be properly attended to in building the relationship. It is the combination of the various interests that defines the collaboration and gives it a purpose. Knowing each party's reason for being present helps keep group members focused and aware of the factors that bring them together.

Generally the first step toward collaboration occurs when an individual recognizes the potential mutual benefits in a specific set of circumstances. The next step occurs when that individual communicates the insight regarding collaboration to another. All collaboration begins with a vision of what could be and moves from vision to actuality through a series of steps that result in the effective operational process (see Table 3–4).*

Establishing a Platform for Collaboration between Managers**

The goal of a collaborative relationship is to achieve mutual benefit through partnership. It is a strategic alliance that may vary in structure and focus. As applied in the organizational context, alliances may range from simple selected exchanges of information to the joint production of a product or service to achieve a common goal. There is generally an expectation on the part of each member of the alliance that the result of joint efforts will add value to the achieved outcome.

Outcomes of effective alliances are often judged by how well the following takes place: goals are achieved, resources are secured and retained, key stakeholders are satisfied, and each alliance member increases in organizational value.

---

*Source: Tim Porter-O'Grady and Cathleen Krueger Wilson, *The Leadership Revolution in Health Care: Altering Systems, Changing Behaviors*, Aspen Publishers, Inc., © 1995.
**Source: Mary Etta Mills and Mary S. Tilbury, "Collaboration: The CNE-CFO Connection," *Nursing Administration Quarterly*, Vol. 17:4, Aspen Publishers, Inc., © Summer 1993.

Table 3–4 Elements of Collaboration Along the Continuum

Individual
- Knowledge of the parameters
- Willingness to negotiate roles
- Commitment to the work
- Investment in the outcomes
- Discovery of a quid pro quo
- In it for the long term

Partners
- Mutually agreed relationship
- Continuous dialogue about the issues
- Flexibility in work relationships
- A process for conflict resolution
- A strategy for role clarification
- A mechanism for integrating with others

The development of a collaborative relationship occurs in several stages. Generally, there is a recognition on the part of each individual that the person with whom he or she would collaborate has the ability to influence an existing situation in a way that could be favorable.

Collaboration then entails mutual work to develop a plan and a targeted approach to accomplish the desired outcome. The active implementation of the plan, regular discussion, modification, and evaluation of action can set the stage for this type of interaction to become normative.

While the creation of a collaborative relationship might initially focus on leadership or management style, it may later focus on issues of control and substantive direction. A solid collaborative approach on the part of senior managers is based on an ongoing dialogue of formal and informal communication that defines working agreements regarding the identification and management of resources. Ultimately, critical elements of collaboration include communication, competence, trust, commitment to goals, and consistency of purpose.

*Role of the Nurse Manager in Fostering Collaborative Practice**

The nurse manager is pivotal in achieving successful collaborative relationships among physicians, nurses, and other health care providers. First, the nurse manager needs to ensure that organizational structure not only overcomes barriers to effective collaborative practice but facilitates its success. The second task of the nurse manager relates to the facilitation of professional growth and development and maturity among clinical care providers. Nurse managers can increase the likelihood of successful outcomes by ensuring that the following work environment variables are monitored.

Coordination components vital to collaborative practice include structural elements such as support systems, decision-making opportunities and specificity of work protocols.

Collegiality in the work setting refers to relationships among individuals who occupy positions of equal and unequal status. Collaborative practice cannot exist except in a culture characterized by collegiality that offers mutual respect for professional knowledge and contributions.

Communication is the most critical component of collaborative practice: Setting up a communication structure and using it are critical to the success of the relationship.

Competency of each nurse participant is mandatory in order to achieve respect in the professional relationship. A high regard for one's competence related to clinical care is also essential for development of a sense of independence, which is a cornerstone for successful collaboration. It is the nurse manager who creates a practice environment in which each worker is able to achieve personal maximum potential.

Education is the most fundamental of all nurse manager behaviors related to creating an environment where collaborative practice can function. The nurse manager must articulate a clear definition of collaborative practice, a vision for achieving the goal of collaborative practice, and the desired outcomes of collaborative practice. In addition, nurse managers must be attuned to the clinical readiness of staff members to assume active roles in collaboration. Each participant in a collaborative model must develop a high level of clinical knowledge and expertise in order to enter the relationship as a partner. The role of the nurse manager is to facilitate nurse clinicians in their pursuit of clinical excellence, with the desired outcome being a high level of self-efficacy.

MEETINGS*

Meetings are an essential aspect of consultative and participative leadership styles. Joint decisions and actions take longer to arrive at than do unilateral decisions and edicts, since true two-way communication including discussion and feedback requires more time than so-called one-way communication. However, the extra time spent in meetings represents the best available technique for arriving at joint conclusions and determining joint actions.

Types of Meetings

Information Meetings

The *information meeting* is held simply for the transfer of information. The group leader has something to pass along to employees or others and you choose to do this with a meeting rather than by some other means. The basic purpose of any information meeting is to transfer information to the group, and in this setting the leader may do most or all of the talking. Although there are usually questions and discussion for the sake of clarification, the transfer of information is essentially one-way communication.

Source: Adapted from Judith A. Evans, "The Role of the Nurse Manager in Creating an Environment for Collaborative Practice," *Holistic Nursing Practice*, Vol. 8:3, Aspen Publishers, Inc., © April 1994.

Source: Charles R. McConnell, *The Effective Health Care Supervisor*, ed 3, Aspen Publishers, Inc., © 1993.

Discussion Meetings

The objective of a *discussion meeting* is to gain agreement on something through the exchange of information, ideas, and opinions. The essence of the discussion meeting is interchange; the exchange of information must be established between and among all participants.

- A *directed* discussion meeting may be appropriate when a conclusion, solution, or decision is evident. The conclusion has already been determined; yet it is not simply being relayed to the group as straight information. It is the leader's objective to gain the participants' acceptance of the solution. In effect, a directed discussion is a "sales pitch."
- A *problem-solving* discussion meeting is held when a problem exists and a solution or decision must be determined by the group. Although the answer determined by joint action may well turn out to be based on the ideas of a single participant, at the outset it is apparent only that there is a problem with which several parties could reasonably be concerned.
- The purpose of an *exploratory* discussion meeting is to gain information on which the manager or others may eventually base a decision. The objective is not to develop a specific solution or recommendation but rather to generate and develop ideas and information for others (perhaps for the group leader but possibly for the nurse executive or some other manager) who must make the decision.

The Staff Meeting

The *staff meeting* may be an information meeting, a discussion meeting, or both. A staff meeting is usually held for the purpose of communication among the members of a group. Staff members may report on the status of their activities, and thus each may be required to effect the one-way transfer of information to others. This meeting form is also used to solve problems, sell ideas, and explore issues, and depending on the business at hand, it may take on any or all of the three forms of the discussion meeting.

Determining the Need for a Meeting

Having defined the problem, the nurse manager should not automatically assume that a meeting is inevitable. Other means of organizational communication are available, and all are valid and may be preferred under certain circumstances. In determining the need for a meeting, the nurse manager should consider the following:

- How many people are involved? If very few, perhaps the telephone, letters, or memos can be used.
- Will a meeting save time? Often a problem can be solved by a memorandum or report, but if an exchange of ideas is needed, then a meeting may avoid a seemingly endless series of other contacts.
- Should everyone get the same story? Perhaps the issue is complex or technically involved, calling for different levels of participation by both medical and nonmedical personnel. Perhaps there are policy issues to be considered, suggesting that certain matters be taken up at a policy-making level before they can be dealt with generally.

Most important, it is necessary to clarify the nature of the situation to enable a group to begin dealing with that situation. Before the invited participants attend the meeting, they must understand the "need"—what they are going to discuss when they get there.

COMMITTEE SYSTEMS

Committee organization is one mechanism by which the nurse executive distributes the necessary activities of the nursing division and contributes to the larger organization. Care is needed in selecting a system of committee work. The executive needs to keep committees productive and on target.

Setting up a Committee Structure*

In designing a committee structure for the nursing division, the nurse executive first examines the objectives and functions of the division to decide which objectives and functions can be best met through committees and which can be best handled by other means.

Committee structures are preferable for two kinds of situations: those requiring multiple input for goal attainment and those in which diverse representation facilitates implementation of proposed activities. Multiple input is required when the combined knowledge of various specialists is needed for completing the committee charge. Still other committees simply need multiple input for brainstorming and for reaching the most satisfactory solution. Diverse representation on a committee also may help in project implementation, lending legitimacy to projects and encouraging acceptance of solutions because of the democratic appeal.

Some questions the executive may use as guidelines in evaluating committee structure and function are the following:

- Are there adequate committee structures to enable the division to reach its goals? Are there any obvious omissions?
- Does each committee fill a vital need that is not within the scope of any other committee?
- Does each committee have a clear reason for existing?
- Are the purposes of the nursing committees consistent with the avowed divisional definition of and philosophy of nursing?
- Is the total number of committees logical for the size of the nursing division and the thrust of its objectives?

Types of Committees*

There are several different kinds of committees formed to serve specific functions.

*Source: Adapted from Barbara Stevens Barnum and Karlene M. Kerfoot, *The Nurse as Executive*, ed 4, Aspen Publishers, Inc., © 1995.

Standing committees reveal the nurse executive's operational definition of nursing since these committees represent the focal point of action in providing nursing services.

For example, Executive A divides operations into products, procedures, and patients. In each case, the committee has a specific output that clearly belongs to it (e.g., a new product, a new procedure, a new care plan). The committee structure gives a view of nursing as being composed of a series of separate parts that, when added together, form the totality of nursing.

Executive B has a different concept and tends to view nursing as a process rather than as consisting of parts. The committees seem to flow from each other; work of a care evaluation committee naturally leads to the work of the care improvement committee. Similarly, improving patient care will call for changes by the nursing systems improvement committee. All three of these committees may involve things, actions, and people. All three focus on processes. Some of the items that were *ends* for Executive A (products and procedures) here become *means* to the goals of Executive B.

No one division of standing committees is right or wrong. There can be as many possible organizations of standing committees as there are different executives to think of them. The real question is whether the selected committee structure accurately mirrors the philosophy of nursing of the organization and provides for effective management.

The design group, sometimes called the task force or project team, is a temporary committee, brought into existence to investigate and to propose solutions for a specific problem. The design group is a problem-solving, problem-oriented unit that ceases to exist once its problem is satisfactorily solved. Design groups tackle many different kinds of problems: administrative, procedural, interdepartmental, and patient oriented. Indeed, they may be used for any problem that best can be solved by a select, informed group. The composition of the design group is dictated by the problem or goal itself. Those persons who have the most knowledge and experience to bring to bear on the subject are appointed to the committee.

Groups based on organizational position and function exist in most nursing divisions. A head nurse group and a steering committee of nurse managers are examples. In determining whether such groups should be formally designated, the nurse executive needs to evaluate the desirability of providing a vehicle for group cohesion and power. Most nurse executives find it useful to create an administrative council to provide a source of communication and participative management.

The functions of groups based on organizational position differ from the functions of regular committees. These ongoing groups typically monitor and respond to the changing work environment. They tend to be responsive to immediate administrative problems of diverse kinds and function to grease the wheels of the day-to-day operations. The content with which they deal varies greatly over time.

Interdivisional committees have assumed significant importance in the restructured environment, and nursing presence at such meetings has become critical. Usually interdivisional committees result when the following conditions arise:

- when coordination of goals and activities is necessary, such as between service and education or among divisions working toward a common strategic plan
- when recurrent problems occur because of conflicting goals or systems, as may occur between nursing and human resource departments

In addition to the assigning of appropriate-level personnel to interdivisional committees, the nurse executive must always consider that the division needs to put its best foot forward in interdivisional work. A committee member must be one who will impressively contribute and represent the best nursing has to offer.

The institutional or corporate-level committee must include a representative of the nursing division. The nurse executive must be assertive in claiming that space, for sometimes there will be resistance to suggestions that nursing join such committees. In some instances, membership may

be won by proving that nursing (and its informational input) is essential to the effective performance of the committee in question.

Sometimes, achievement of full committee rights is won step by step. It is better to have attending rights than no rights at all. Once nursing's presence is taken for granted, the executive is in a better position to press for more committee power. Attendance at medical committees and major administrative committees is essential, as is access to the institution's board. At the worst case, the nurse executive can expect to make several presentations to the board yearly. At best, the nurse executive may be a voting board member. Often, the reality falls between—with attendance without vote as a satisfactory compromise.

What Makes Committees Work?

Committees work when they are formally organized, have assigned jobs to do, have a leader, keep written records of their deliberations for future reference, and know results are expected. Committees fail when they are not wisely constituted, when their purpose is vague or is lost sight of, when members are not well oriented and are not convinced that the results will be worth the effort, when they meet only for the sake of meeting, or when the preparation for their meetings is inadequate.

Elements To Consider

1. Purpose. The charge to the committee should be clearly defined, and its responsibilities, duties, and objectives should be spelled out. The choice of chairperson and members and the willingness of individuals to serve largely depend on the committee's purpose.

2. Need. Is the committee the best technique for accomplishing the purpose that has been defined? If so, should a new committee be formed or can an existing committee do the job? Or would a conference of one or two sessions do it just as well?

3. Functions. What kind of committee is this going to be? Is it to be administrative, assigned a definite action responsibility such as that for the development of policies and procedures? Or is it to be advisory, set up to explore, to communicate, and to coordinate?

4. Organization. How many members will it have, and how will they and the chairperson be selected and appointed? Will there be ex officio members and will they have votes? To whom will the committee report? How often will it meet? Who will call special meetings? Who should receive copies of the minutes? Will the committee spend money, and how much? Who will be responsible for arrangements, agenda, and call notices?

*5. Selecting the Leader.** First, would the prospective leader be optimistic about the committee's task? The leader's attitudes have a very definite influence on the group.

Second, would the prospective leader be able to organize the committee into a tightly knit task-oriented group? A clue as to whether a potential leader would be able to organize the group efficiently might be found by looking at the employee's daily work patterns. An employee who is conscientious, organized, and efficient would probably bring those same patterns to the committee.

Third, would the prospective leader be able to ask pertinent questions and to listen to and comprehend the answers that are received?

6. Committee Members. A sensitive administrator will carefully select individuals who can comfortably work with other individuals. The following questions might be asked of potential committee members. If the answer is yes to most of these questions, the chances are good that he or she will be a productive member of the group.

- Has this individual worked on committees before? If yes, was his or her input constructive?

- In general, does the individual relate well to his or her peers within the organization?
- When there is conflict, can this individual look at the underlying causes of the problem?
- Does this individual think critically?
- Can this individual look past his or her interests in order to examine all sides of an issue?

7. Feedback. When an administrator lets committee members know that he or she is pleased with the work they are doing, gives suggestions on how they could do their work better, and is available as a resource person, he or she is providing a healthy impetus for the committee.

An administrator cannot afford to set up committees and let them flounder. He or she must keep track of what is going on within the committees and give encouragement and support.

8. Committee Recommendations. Taking the suggestions of the committee seriously does not necessarily mean always agreeing to what a committee has recommended. It does mean, however, that the administrator will carefully look at the suggestions, meet with the committee to understand the logic behind the recommendations, and then respond to the output of the committee.

Making a Committee Effective*

To have effective committees, managers need to deal with the committee itself and any inherent problems.

One common problem in committees is failure of members to acquire the necessary commitment. Committees are seen by some as add-on functions, not as critical as their day-to-day work. Leaders of committees must be given clear charges so that they understand their responsibility. Further, they must be able to communicate this sense of purpose to members. Reviewing committee achievements and requiring that

---

Source: Items 5 through 8 are adapted from Robert Veninga, "Applying Hospital Control to Hospital Committees," *Hospital Topics*, June 1974. Adapted with permission.

Source: Adapted from Barbara Stevens Barnum and Karlene M. Kerfoot, *The Nurse as Executive*, ed 4, Aspen Publishers, Inc., © 1995.

the chairperson submits reports of progress in addition to mere minutes is one administrative tool to keep a committee on target. But a group needs to be given enough authority to fulfill its objective and the ability to implement its decisions. The executive may give a committee power to recommend or power to decide. Committee members must clearly understand their powers in each case.

Sometimes, in attempting to give equal consideration to various factions, a dual leadership is created with cochairpersons. But a committee that is the responsibility of more than one person may not be perceived as the responsibility of anyone in the long run. Usually, it is better to alternate chairpersons than to split the responsibility.

In addition to placing responsibility and holding leaders accountable, the executive needs to provide for effectiveness in the committee process. Simply put, leaders should be taught how to run an effective meeting. In the best of all situations, the leader and all the members will be familiar with how groups work. Further, chronically unproductive committees must be closely examined.

Often a committee is unproductive because it does not really need to exist (e.g., when its objectives are either not attainable or not important at the particular time). When the objectives are judged valid but the committee is still unproductive, it is trying to do the job with the wrong people. A committee leader without appropriate skills also may be the problem. Another possibility is an incompatible mix of members, incompatible in regard to the objectives of the committee, not necessarily incompatible in their interpersonal relations with one another.

*Leading Committee Meetings**

Start on Time. Executives may want to allow some flexibility in how closely to adhere to a rigid starting time. If the meeting is a one-time

---

Source: Charles R. McConnell, *The Effective Health Care Supervisor,* ed 3, pp. 300–303. Aspen Publishers, Inc., © 1993.

affair involving a number of people who are organizationally scattered, perhaps including some who are superior in the management structure, it may be advisable to bend a few minutes on starting time. (In a practical sense, it is likely to wait more than a few minutes for a tardy person to show.) Also, a one-shot meeting is not a regular part of someone's schedule or pattern of behavior. It is perhaps best to allow some slack in scheduling; for instance, a session may be scheduled for 1:30 P.M. although it is probable it will not start until 1:45 P.M. Try not to overdo this practice; it suggests disrespect for those who do show up on time and deference to the latecomers.

In the case of a regularly scheduled meeting (for instance, a monthly staff meeting held at 3:00 P.M. on the third Thursday of each month), begin precisely on time. The more deference paid to chronic latecomers, the more likely these people are to remain chronic latecomers. Also, chronic tardiness can often be an indication of other problems, such as hostility, disrespect, lack of interest, or perhaps inflated ego.

Making it a habit of starting on time can go a long way toward curing chronic tardiness. If it is 3:00 P.M. and only half the staff are present, start the meeting even though the remainder will be trickling in over the next several minutes. Out of respect for those who show up on time, do not repeat what has already been said for the sake of the latecomers. Rather, let the late arrivers know they have to wait until after the meeting to find out what they missed from those who were present. Make it plain, also, that the content of the early part of the meeting is not always filler or "warm up" material that people can afford to miss. Make it a habit to start regularly scheduled meetings precisely on time, and most chronic latecomers will change their ways as they get the message and become accustomed to this pattern of behavior.

State the Purpose of the Meeting. First tell the group why they are there and what they need to accomplish. Also, give them the best estimate of the amount of time the meeting should require. *Ending* time can be fully as troublesome as *starting* time in some situations. A meeting can be a form of escape for some people who lead busy, hectic working lives, and some people may tend to prolong the session with irrelevancies if progress is not well controlled. (It has been suggested that an effective way to get a one-hour meeting concluded in one hour is to schedule it to start an hour before lunch or an hour before quitting time.) In short, the first item of business should be to advise those attending why they are there, what they are expected to accomplish, and approximately how long it should take.

Encourage Discussion. Do not allow the meeting to move in such narrow lines that valuable input is lost. Ask for clarification of comments that are offered. Consider requesting opinions and asking direct questions, particularly of the few "silent ones" who frequently populate meetings. Remember, if the meeting has been structured wisely then everyone who is there is there

for a good reason. It is part of the job of meeting leader to do everything possible to get those people talking who ordinarily tend to remain quiet.

Summarize Periodically. Agreement in a discussion meeting is usually not reached in a single, progressive series of exchanges. Rather, agreement accrues as discussion points are sifted, sorted, and merged, and a solution or recommendation begins to take form. Capture this by periodically summarizing what has been said, giving the group a recounting of where they are and where they seem to be headed. If they can agree with the summary of progress—essentially, their thoughts encapsulated and restated—then the meeting is on the right track.

End with a Specific Plan. When the meeting is over the leader should be able to deliver a final summary stating what has been decided and

---

Exercise Control: A List of Don'ts

Of Yourself

- Don't let your ego get in the way simply because you are the meeting leader and thus automatically "in control" of the proceedings.

- Don't lecture or otherwise dominate the proceedings. Remember, the setting is a meeting, not a speech or a class.

- Don't direct the others by telling them what to do or what they should say or conclude. This would amount to one-way communication, which is only marginally appropriate even when the purpose of the meeting is purely informational.

- Don't argue with participants. Discuss, yes—argue, never.

- Don't attempt to be funny. What may be funny to one person may not be to another. The best laughs generated at a meeting are those that arise naturally from the discussion.

Of the Group

- Don't allow lengthy tangential digressions to pull you away from the subject of the meeting. Granted many legitimate problems are identified through tangential discussions, but, legitimate or not, if they do not relate to the problem at hand they are diluting the effectiveness of the meeting. Should a legitimate problem arise, make note of it but sideline it for action at another time or at another meeting and proceed with the subject at hand.

- Don't allow monopolizers and ego-trippers to take over. Although certain talkative people may have significant contributions to make, their constant presence center stage serves to narrow the discussion and discourage marginally vocal contributors from opening up at all. Overall, your effectiveness as a meeting leader will largely be determined by how effectively you control the discussion of the group.

who is going to do what and by when. Far too many meetings are frustrating affairs that may feel productive while under way but afterward leave participants hanging with a sense of incompleteness.

No one should leave a meeting without full understanding of the decisions made, the actions to be taken, the people responsible for implementation, and the timetable for implementation. If the subject is sufficiently complex, it may be to the leader's advantage to call for understanding by going "around the table," asking everyone for their interpretations of what has been decided and how they see their roles, if any, in the implementation of the decision. In any event, do not let the group leave without a clear understanding of what has been decided and what happens next.

Follow Up. As far as a leader's authority over the problem extends, it is up to him or her to follow up to determine that what has been decided gets accomplished. He or she should also see that minutes of the meeting, should they be necessary, are prepared and distributed; provide later assurance to all participants that what they decided has in fact been accomplished; and schedule a follow-up meeting should one be necessary.

USING CONSULTATION SERVICES

Management consulting services include identifying and investigating problems involving organizational structure, policies, and procedures; program design and implementation; interpersonal relationships; and continuous quality improvement methods.

Types of Consultation*

There are two types of consultation services: *expert* and *process.* The primary difference between them is the way in which the consultant implements the process.

In *expert consultation* the consultant generally identifies problems, makes decisions, and implements strategies without involving the members of the organization in the process. The expert consultant is hired to "fix" the identified problem.

In *process consultation* members of the organization are an integral part of the process consultant's approach. Process consultants act as resources, using their expertise to advise and guide. The process consultant is hired to help the members of the organization fix the problem.

The manager must give special attention to the selection of a consultant and ongoing management of the process (see Table 3–5). The following phases are valid for both types of consultancy:

- preparation, in which the organization identifies a need and existing resources within the organization to meet that need
- initial contact and selection, involving selection of the consultant and establishing the parameters of the consultation
- implementation, during which the agreed-on project is undertaken
- completion, which includes evaluating and terminating the consultation

In both types of consultation, the consultant is an advisor who is providing a service based on some special knowledge and skill. However, neither type of consultant has any magic cure for what ails the organization. Further, neither has any direct authority, and both are dependent on organization members for the information needed.

Finding a Consultant*

Some consultants are employed by firms specializing in consultation to nursing or offering a broader range of services. Some are self-

*Source: Marie C. Berger, Leslie N. Ray, and Virginia Del Togno-Armanasco, "The Effective Use of Consultants," *Journal of Nursing Administration*, Vol. 23:7/8, July/August 1993, J.B. Lippincott Company.

*Source: "JONA's Semiannual Directory of Consultants to Nursing Administration," *Journal of Nursing Administration*, February 1984. Reprinted with permission.

Table 3–5 Guidelines to Relations with Consultants

Paid Consultants	Volunteer Consultants
• Define the problem clearly. • Consider cost. • Interview prospects; look for skill, objectivity, responsibility. • Get references from persons whose judgment you trust. • Do not be unnecessarily impressed by credentials. • Review any published work. • Spell out responsibilities of both the agency and the consultant. • Inform staff and board. • Retain your authority in working with consultants. • Listen to, monitor, and analyze consultant findings. • Be prepared to make decisions throughout the process. • Terminate if work is unsatisfactory.	• Recruit experts with talents appropriate to need: managers in private industry, university faculty, health professionals. • Be aware of political climate in your choice of expert. • Call upon those that you know have done a good job. • Approach formally through organization channels to allow the expert more ease in making commitment. • Allow the expert sufficient time within his or her busy schedule. • Offer some form of recognition for help received. • Keep in mind that your responsibility and judgment must prevail.

Source: Health Manpower Planning Process, DHHS, Pub. No. (HRA) 76-14013, 1976.

employed, either full or part time, and may hold other jobs as well. There are few practical opportunities for these consultants and firms to publicize their services widely to the specific persons who might use them. Thus, when a nursing administrator needs advice from outside his or her agency to assist with a problem or project, it is often difficult to find the consultant best suited for the job.

The *Journal of Nursing Administration* publishes each year in the August issue a directory of consultants to nursing administration. Information regarding size of the organization, time in operation, areas of expertise, and fee structure is provided. The directory includes the names of over 350 independent consultants and consulting firms. The listings are grouped according to 37 areas of expertise.

Chapter 4

Problem Solving and Decision Making

PROBLEM SOLVING

Problem-Solving Styles*

It has been proposed that individuals have a favored problem-solving style. A manager's problem-solving style is important, because it is the manager's behavior that defines what is acceptable in the work group. A mismatch between problem-solving styles of managers and subordinates influences subordinates' job satisfaction and job performance.

Style is a marked preference, a character difference, a pattern that is relatively stable over time and incident. Individuals with different styles acquire, store, retrieve, and transform information differently. From time to time, circumstances may force individuals to operate outside their preferred style. They can do this, but it is stressful, and as soon as possible individuals return to their preferred style. Excessive demands to use other than the preferred style result in a desire to leave the situation.

Two problem-solving styles are suggested: the adaptive style and the innovative style.

- *Adaptors* accept the customary viewpoints and paradigms in which the problem is embedded. They generate ideas to solve problems based on existing definitions of the problem.
- The habitual *innovator* detaches the problem from its cocoon of accepted thought, reconstructing both the problem and its attendant paradigm in the search for a solution.

Adaptors and innovators have very different personality characteristics. Adaptors are prudent, safe, cautious, and dependable. When criticized, adaptors respond by becoming more conforming and compliant.

In contrast, innovators have little self-doubt, enjoy unstructured situations, and are capable of system maintenance work for only short periods of time. Because of these characteristics, adaptors and innovators frequently clash when working together in organizations.

Neither the adaptive nor the innovative problem-solving style is better. Different styles are needed at different times in an organization or in different types of organizations. Many long-established organizations are settled and have a large investment in staff, systems, and other resources. These organizations value continuity and want change to occur at a manageable pace.

*Source: Carolyn E. Adams, "The Impact of Problem-Solving Styles of Nurse Executives and Executive Officers on Tenure," *Journal of Nursing Administration*, Vol. 23:12, December 1993. J.B. Lippincott Company.

In these stable organizations, adaptors are hired, trained, and promoted. In contrast, in new organizations or organizations characterized by chaotic, turbulent, or rapidly changing environments, there is a preponderance of innovators. Innovators take control in unstructured situations and operate well in times of crisis.

Selecting a Problem for Study*

As a first step in the process of selecting a problem for study, managers should attempt to develop a complete list of all work situations in which there are indications of problems (see box). This listing should be kept current by adding to it any newly identified problem situations as they come to mind.

The next step is to establish an order of study priority with respect to the various work problems that have been identified. In ranking the relative importance of each of the listed problems, certain factors should be considered in making a decision. Some of these relevant factors are listed below in the form of questions, which should, of course, be adapted to the needs of the specific problem situation involved.

Which problem situation is causing the most difficulty?

How soon must a solution be found to the problem situation?

Is the problem situation in question really the one to be solved, or is it simply a part of a still larger problem that requires study?

What is the status of the job in question? Is it temporary in nature? If not, what will be the future demands?

Is the timing for study appropriate from the standpoint of employee turnover, absenteeism, work demands, and personalities presently involved in the job situation?

Is there a good chance of achieving success in the way of improvement?

> ### Problem Indicators
>
> - *Backlog* of unfinished work in any operation
> - *Delays and interruptions* in the performance of a function or service
> - *Overtime* that is needed repeatedly in the carrying out of an activity
> - *Waste* of effort, equipment, material, human resources, time, or space
> - *Complaints* from patients, staff, or visitors
> - *Costs* of the function that seem to be unduly high
> - *Absenteeism* or *turnover* occurring continually in any health care facility area
> - *Loss* or *damage* of supplies or equipment; also injury to employees and others
> - *Congestion* or *disorderliness* of a work area involving one or more individuals
> - *Excessive time* being devoted to an activity in proportion to the actual end result
> - *Location* of an object in an out-of-the-way place
> - *Fatigue* due to walking, bending, reaching, or other nonproductive or tiresome work motions

How soon can discernible results be attained? What may be the extent and the nature of the benefits to be achieved?

How long has it been since any changes were introduced on the job in question? What were the experiences with these changes?

What are the staff's attitudes toward the existing process or procedure? How much employee resistance or resentment may be anticipated?

Are there any management policies or professional requirements that might limit changes in the existing situation?

Are there any management plans presently under way that might either eliminate the problem situation or have some effect on the nature of the problem?

---

*Source: Addison C. Bennett, *Methods Improvement in Hospitals*, J.B. Lippincott, © 1964. Reprinted with permission.

Analyzing and Solving Problems

Nursing administration is faced with a comprehensive array of managerial problems and other specific problems.

*Problem Analysis and Strategy Planning**

1. Identify the difficulty, the concern, the problem.
   - Who sees it as a problem?
   - Who is affected by it?
   - How are they affected?
   - What significant events or typical incidents illustrate the problem?
   - To what extent are there differences in goals toward which individuals or groups are working in this situation?
2. Identify the various values (assumptions, beliefs, or feelings that serve as criteria by which goals are determined) of the total organization, any groups, and the individual persons involved.
3. Identify the various norms (i.e., behavior patterns highly valued or discouraged) of the total organization and any groups.
4. Identify the various individuals and groups that influence (i.e., have power and/or status) the decisions and behavior of the total organization, groups, and individuals.
5. Identify the various sanctions (i.e., punishments and rewards) by which norms are maintained in groups or the total organization.
6. Identify your roles (i.e., positions and functions) in the situation. What other roles seem important in the situation? As you refer to other people, explain the relationships between you and them.
7. Identify the various patterns of communication (i.e., who talks to whom, formally and informally). You may wish to diagram this.

Figure 4–1 Problem Analysis and Strategy Planning

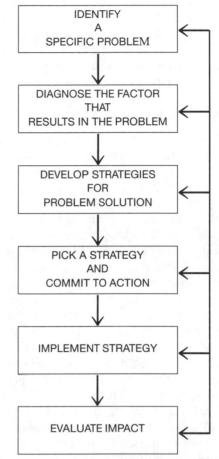

Source: Reprinted with permission from *Power: Use It or Lose It,* © 1977, National League for Nursing.

8. Identify the various steps (i.e., defining, clarifying, developing alternatives, etc.) and categories by which the group makes decisions.
9. Identify the various actions that relevant groups take that help the organization maintain its identity and separateness.
10. Identify the means by which groups maintain linkage (communication) with other groups.
11. Review the diagnosis and decide what the underlying problems seem to be now.
12. Determine which elements or processes seem to be most critical to the problem.
13. List what you have tried to do about the problem within the past six months. (In-

Source: Reprinted with permission from *Power: Use It or Lose It,* © 1977, National League for Nursing.

clude as specifically as possible the goals and strategy that informed your actions, as well as the effects of the actions.)

14. Decide what you might try to do about the problem within the next six months. List as many specific actions as you can and their anticipated effect on relevant organizational elements and processes.

Identification of Process Problems*

Often, the root cause of a problem is hidden deep within the procedures and processes used to create a service or system. Typically, people try to compensate for a problem by trying to fix the obvious rather than by developing a systematic plan to get to the original source. They try to solve one piece by adding or rearranging steps, not realizing that they are distorting other parts of the process. As problems arise from the distortions, additional steps are added to compensate. The process then becomes more complicated or complex and adds extra work without adding value to the service. This unnecessary work is called *complexity*. Almost all processes include work that would not be necessary if systems worked flawlessly. The types of complexity can be described as follows.

Mistakes and defects cause work to be repeated, or extra work is required to remedy the error. They are reflected in infections and other complications, as well as in administrative delays and higher costs.

Breakdowns and delays require waiting or rework. They are reflected in longer stays for patients, uneven workloads for staff, and administrative backlogs.

Inefficiencies consume more material, time, and movement than are essential. They are reflected in lack of productivity, poor record-keeping, and higher costs.

Inconsistency results in erratic or unreliable performance. It may result from lack of a plan or systematic method for dealing with a task, for example, so that performance varies in consis-

tent ways. Or it may be due to a special cause or be the result of specific circumstances (an equipment breakdown or a temporary staff shortage that disrupts the normal routine).

There is a high probability that a process or system will have at least one of the problems listed above; many will have several problems. The team (those who work within the process) should examine the process to identify areas, tasks, and jobs that fall into one of these categories and then work to track down the root causes. Team members should keep in mind the Pareto principle, or 80/20 rule; 80 percent of the trouble usually comes from 20 percent of the problems.

PARTICIPATORY PROBLEM SOLVING: QUALITY CIRCLES*

> This viable approach has the capacity to tap into both the leadership abilities of the manager and the potential problem-solving abilities and creativity of the total health care staff. The process itself, as a participatory technique, and the skills developed to work the process are highly acceptable in quality management philosophy.

A quality circle is generally defined as a group of people (usually between 4 and 15) who work in the same or a similar area who voluntarily meet on a regular basis to identify, assess, and solve problems in their area of work.

The three most often mentioned management objectives of quality circles are (1) to improve patient care quality in the health care facility, (2) to improve productivity, and (3) to improve employee motivation and morale. Other objectives may include the following: to instill cost-containment awareness in employees, to encourage and use employee creativity, to help employees develop into managers, and to help employees grow professionally and personally.

---

*Source: James E. Orlikoff, "Quality Circles in the Hospital Setting," *Topics in Health Record Management*, Vol. 3:4, Aspen Publishers, Inc., © 1983.

The objectives that top management will have for quality circles will differ from the objectives of the employees who choose to participate in the circles. Management and employee objectives should be complementary but not necessarily identical for a quality circle program to succeed.

Characteristics

For a quality circle program to succeed, the following characteristics must be present:

- Participation in the circles must be voluntary.
- Management must be supportive of the program (by allowing circles to meet on company time, by officially recognizing the activities and results of circles, and by allocating resources to support the program). Training in problem-solving methods, group process techniques, data gathering, and data analysis must be a fundamental component of the program.
- Quality circle members must work together as a team.
- The program must have a people-building, not a people-exploiting, orientation.
- Circle members must work to *solve* problems, not just to identify them.
- Each circle must have the right to select its own problem for study and resolution.

Quality Circle Program Organization

A quality circle program should not be imposed on employees by being presented as a new organizational structure. Rather, such a program should be integrated into the existing organizational structure of the organization. The quality circle program will, however, have an independent organizational infrastructure consisting of a steering committee, a facilitator, a leader, circle members, a problem-solving process, and management presentation.

The Quality Circle Steering Committee. The steering committee is the body that directs the overall quality circle program. The members of the committee should include representatives of the medical staff and of the major departments of the organization. The committee

- develops the overall objectives of the quality circle program
- develops a plan to implement the program (beginning with a pilot program)
- develops an informational and promotional campaign for the program
- develops a description of the job and qualifications of the facilitator
- chooses a facilitator
- determines the person to whom the facilitator reports
- determines how quality circles will interface with other health care facility systems (such as suggestion and reward programs, employee development programs, and facility functions such as quality assurance)
- determines the financial support for the program
- identifies areas where quality circles can be pilot tested
- establishes implementation dates for the pilot circles
- establishes some type of measures for the pilot and the entire program
- determines how often and for how long the circles will meet
- establishes a reward and recognition program for circles

The Facilitator. The facilitator will be the person directly responsible for guiding and coordinating the activities of the circles throughout the organization. The facilitator will, at a minimum, perform two general functions: (1) train all circle leaders and (2) act as process observer and technical assistant to the circles. The facilitator acts as the bridge between all the circles and coordinates the circle activities with the rest of the health care facility.

Specifically, the facilitator trains circle leaders and acts as a resource in the areas of group process techniques; group problem-solving techniques; data gathering, statistical analysis, and data display techniques; and management presentations.

The Leader. Generally, the leader for each quality circle is the first-line manager of the employees who are the circle members. In this way, the circle fits into the existing organizational structure of the institution and will therefore be more likely to be accepted by all involved in the quality circle program.

The Members. The members of any given circle are employees in the same area or department who volunteer to participate in the circle. They may drop out of the circle if they desire, and other employees who did not choose to volunteer at first may do so later. Eight is the optimum number of members per circle. There should be no more than 14 members.

The Problem-Solving Process. Each circle should follow these steps.

1. The members identify a list of problems in their area.
2. The members select one problem for study.
3. The circle analyzes the problem (the circle may call in internal experts to give them technical assistance in analyzing the problem).
4. The circle presents its findings and recommended solutions to management.
5. Management reviews the circle's presentation and decides whether or not to implement the circle's suggestion.
6. Based on management's decision, the circle implements the action designed to correct the problem.

Management Presentation. Using charts, graphs, and other visual aids, the circle members present their analysis to management. This procedure is viewed as being intrinsically rewarding to circle members and is an opportunity for management to communicate enthusiasm and support to the members for their activities and accomplishments.

THE NATURE OF DECISION MAKING

Decision making is choosing options that are directed toward the resolution of organizational problems and the achievement of organizational goals.

The purpose of decision making within the health care organization is the coordination of goals and objectives of its members to deliver optimal patient care while controlling cost. The nurse manager, as a decision maker, has a vital role to play in bringing to fruition the achievement of these organizational goals and objectives.

Certain attributes are essential for the decision maker to make effective and efficient decisions. First, the nurse manager must have the freedom to make the decision in question. This requires the necessary power and knowledge to select the decision. Second, the manager must have the capacity and ability to make a wise decision. This requires sound judgment, deliberation, objectivity, and experience. Finally, the manager must have the will, motivation, and commitment to choose. This requires volition, a conscious activity of the will to make a decision. These qualifications are essential for the nurse manager, since decisions affect others and may encompass life-and-death situations.

Some subtle obstacles to rational and objective decision making include biases or prejudices, ignorance, time and financial constraints, resistance to change, unclear goals and objectives, and the fear of risk taking. The nurse manager must make a conscious effort to be constantly attuned to these influences in order to make intelligent and objective decisions. There are a series of steps to guide the decision-making process.*

Risk, Uncertainty, and Judgment**

Some decision-making theorists speak of something called "perfect information." This is a state that exists only when one knows all there is to know about all aspects of every available alternative. If there truly were such a thing

Source: Kathleen Kerrigan, "Decision Making in Today's Complex Environment," *Nursing Administration Quarterly,* Vol. 15:4, Aspen Publishers, Inc., © 1991.
**Source:* Charles R. McConnell, *The Effective Health Care Supervisor,* ed 3, pp. 265–268. Aspen Publishers, Inc., © 1993.

as perfect information there would be no decision at all: the "decision" would have made itself because the only true alternative would be self-evident.

Because there is no such thing as perfect information, there are always elements of risk and uncertainty in a decision-making situation. Risk is there because something may be lost— be it time, money, effectiveness, or perhaps life itself—if the wrong decision is made. Uncertainty also exists; since one does not know everything about all aspects of the situation and has no guarantees that things will come out right, it is not known whether the choice is the right one.

One of the major objectives in the decision-making process is to minimize risk and uncertainty by learning as much as practical about each decision-making situation. Since risk and uncertainty are always present, there is always the need for judgment in decision making. Decisions do not make themselves: people make decisions. All of the efforts at gathering and analyzing information, as well as all sophisticated quantitative decision-making techniques, are no more than efforts to reduce the extent of pure judgment required in decision making.

In the last analysis many decisions will be right or wrong because of human judgment regardless of the amount of quantitative information involved. The objective is not to try to eliminate judgment from decision making. This cannot be done. Rather that judgment must be refined by learning as much as it is practical to learn about the alternatives.

The No-Decision Option

In even the simplest of decision-making situations there are always at least two choices: to decide or not to decide. The no-decision option is the case in which one selects the latter choice. In effect what one does is "decide not to decide." This does not have to be a consciously made decision, but it can, and very often does, occur by default through procrastination. Taking no action on a problem amounts to the exercise of the no-decision option.

Appreciate that whether the no-decision option is exercised by choice or through procrastination it is still a decision. Frequently it is the decision with the most potentially far-reaching consequences. All too often we adopt an attitude, either consciously or unconsciously, that suggests: "If I'm really quiet maybe it'll go away." Sometimes it does indeed go away and things get better. However, things usually do not get better. To cite one of the corollaries of the well-known Murphy's Law: "Left unto themselves, things invariably go from bad to worse."

The Range of Decisions

Decision-making situations may range from the highly, but rarely totally, objective, with plenty of factual information on which to decide, to the purely subjective or totally judgmental decision. The decision-making process described in this chapter essentially applies to all decisions; the differences lie in the kinds of information with which we must deal in developing alternatives.

We can usually be more comfortable with so-called objective decisions. We have facts, figures, and other data to work with. We compare prices, statistics, hours, pieces, or some other specific indicators and make our choices. Orderly approaches to decision making are possible, and improved facility at making such decisions comes with practice in conscientiously following the steps of the process through decision after decision.

The highly subjective decision is another matter. Little or no data are available. We must make our choices based on rules and regulations, policies, procedures, and precedents, and very often on our basic sense of what is right or wrong, fair or unfair, or logical or illogical. Many personnel-related decisions fall in the area of the subjective, and while the basic decision-making process does not apply nearly as specifically as with most objective decisions, improved decision-making ability again comes largely through experience.

Although decisions may range from the mostly objective to the wholly subjective, the character of any particular decision may be greatly influenced by the conditions under which it must be made. The single circumstance that probably has the greatest effect on the character of any particular decision is the imposition of pressure.

Decision-making pressure is often felt as a limitation of the time available in which to investigate properly and render a decision. It is one thing to face a situation in which you have more than adequate time to develop and assess all workable alternatives; it is another matter entirely to realize that undesirable consequences will result if a decision is not rendered by a deadline—and that this deadline does not leave time enough for reasonable investigation. Unfortunately many supervisory decisions are pressure decisions, and we have to accept the fact that limited time will squeeze us into a less-than-desirable pattern of analysis and action. In this regard, time may constrain not only the alternatives but also the entire decision-making process.

Responsibility and Leadership

An anonymous quotation goes, "It's all right to pull decisions out of a hat as long as you're wearing it." While this statement is only partially true (it is *not* usually all right to pull decisions out of a hat) the point about responsibility is well made. If we assume the authority to make a decision, we should be charged with equivalent responsibility. In making decisions for a department they should be consistent with supervisory charge. It is the supervisor's responsibility for the output and actions of employees. However, one should not make a decision with which other employees or the supervisors of other departments must comply. In accepting a given amount of responsibility one ordinarily acquires decision-making authority consistent with that responsibility. No supervisor's decisions should exceed the limits of designated authority.

Also on the subject of authority, when delegating certain decision-making powers to employees, be sure to extend authority and responsibility in equivalent amounts. Authority and responsibility are each weakened, if not negated entirely, by the absence of the other. How much decision-making authority is delegated to employees will be a direct reflection of leadership style. Generally the autocratic or authoritarian leader will prefer to retain all such authority while the participative leader will involve the employees in shaping and choosing decision alternatives.

No Magic Formula

It is possible to create valid guidelines for making many decisions. It is done all the time: rules, regulations, policies, and procedures are generated to guide decisions. However, in spite of what a few determined bureaucratic leaders may believe, it is not possible to anticipate all contingencies and premake all decisions. It is not possible to cover everything with rules that say, in effect, "When this situation arises, apply this remedy." Good supervisory decisions will remain a matter of arriving at a proper emphasis on all decision elements through judgment based on facts and figures, knowledge, experience, advice, intuition, and insight.

Process*

The basic method for making a decision involves a sequence of six steps.

Step 1: Analyze and Identify the Situation. As a manager, you first clarify the situation you are trying to resolve. Sometimes this step is simple. For example, there may be a vacancy on your staff. You want to promote one of several possible subordinates into the spot. You have to make a decision and choose among them.

However, some situations may not be clear-cut: A department in your jurisdiction is doing poorly. Before you can make a remedial decision, you have to take into consideration the circumstances, find out *what* is wrong and *why* it is wrong, in order to proceed.

Source: The Executive Deskbook, 2nd edition, by Auren Uris, © 1970, 1979, by Litton Educational Publishing Inc. Reprinted by permission of Van Nostrand Reinhold Company.

Step 2: Develop Alternatives. In every decision-requiring circumstances, there are at least two possible actions, for example, taking action or not taking action. In most cases there are more. For instance, in filling a vacancy on a leadership level one might choose among the following:

- Leave it unfilled.
- Hire from the outside.
- Promote the person who is most familiar with the duties of the open job.
- Set up some kind of test that will make it possible to grade the qualifications of applicants for the job.
- Ask for volunteers.

Step 3: Compare Alternatives. There are few cases where the nurse executive is lucky enough to have one alternative that represents the likelihood of 100 percent satisfaction. Usually each alternative has advantages and disadvantages. An alternative that you might prefer may be too costly, or you may lack the staff to carry it out. Where the decision is crucial, take the time to actually write out the advantages and disadvantages of each alternative.

Step 4: Rate the Risk. One of the differences between decision making and problem solving is that a proper solution to a problem is sure-fire, if it is indeed the right solution. The results are practically ensured.

But in decision making, the usual situation is one in which every alternative being considered includes an uncertainty factor. Since managers seldom have total information about the situation they are dealing with, they can never be sure that the decision they make will be completely satisfactory.

Accordingly, in considering alternatives, it is important to rate the degree of risk each one involves. Obviously, this must be an estimate. Yet this approximation should be a part of the considerations that lead you to select the most desirable alternative.

In rating the risk, you may use percentages or any other rating system you prefer: grading from 1 to 10, using the academic A–F rating, and so on.

Step 5: Select the Best Alternative. If the previous steps have been done carefully, it is possible that the most likely alternative will be self-evident. But there are other possibilities.

- No alternative is desirable. The riskiness of all alternatives, for example, may properly persuade you not to take any action, because no move you can think of at the time promises to be successful.
- Merge two or more alternatives. In some cases you may find that while no single alternative provides the averages you want, combining elements of two or more provides you with the most likely plan.
- The "resources factor" may swing your decision. Alternative A may have more advantages than Alternative B. However, in carrying out Alternative B, you may have a piece of equipment that promises to save the day. Or, and this element is often crucial, you may have a subordinate of outstanding skill that will make Alternative B a much better bet because of his or her availability for this move.

While it is wise to gather information and check facts, be sure to get expert opinions and project the possibilities into the future. There will still remain some uncertainty in your attempt to pinpoint the best move. This uncertainty element can never be completely eliminated, and the usual practice is for the nurse executive to select between two otherwise "even" alternatives by hunch or intuition. Do not underestimate the importance of your feeling. Veteran nurse executives consider intuition a standard part of decision making and use it when facts, logic, or systematic considerations are unavailable.

Step 6: Get into Gear. After a decision has been made, it must be made operative. You, or a subordinate, must take on the assignment of getting the people, resources, and so on, involved in putting the decision to work.

It may seem like an unnecessary emphasis to make this final point at all. But the fact is that many a decision, made even after days or weeks of effort, fails to produce results; or the decision is followed up in such a weak fashion that despite its many excellences only mediocre results are achieved.

In short, a decision implemented with energy and conviction can make a sizable difference in the outcome. For example, the manner in which a decision is communicated to the people who will be affected by it is, in itself, an important factor. And the manner in which the assignments represented by the decision are given to the people that are to carry out the plan is a major aspect of its effectiveness.

SUPPORTING NURSE EXECUTIVES' DECISION MAKING

Nurse executives need to be aware of the impact that technology can have on their decision-making processes. A computerized decision support system (DDS) can make their jobs considerably easier.

Decision support systems offer methods for refining the decision-making process. Although computers provide historic financial information, as well as payroll and patient billing information, computers also perform many more functions that can help nurse executives and their staffs identify and gather decision-making data and, in some cases, identify the preferred alternative. Nurse executives need to be aware of the latest technology that their institution has and request the programming assistance that will enable them to harness the power that comes with the information.*

Assistance with Managerial Decisions*

At different levels, nurse executives participate in managerial activities in several catego-

*Source: Adapted from Sheila M. Jacobs and Sandra Pelfrey, "Decision Support Systems," *Journal of Nursing Administration*, Vol. 25:2, February 1995. J.B. Lippincott.

ries. For example, strategic planning involves top-level management in the task of setting long-range goals for the organization. It concentrates on determining which new services to offer, given the anticipated needs of the community and the support resources that would need to be amassed.

Tactical control involves monitoring and controlling operations and allocating resources effectively. An example of tactical control would be determining the mix of professional nurses and paramedical staff members needed to staff specific units. Operational control deals with supervising daily operations. Managers look at current patients and their levels of acuity to determine the level of nursing care required on individual units.

When considering the possibility of computerized assistance for decision making, consider the types of decisions that will be made. There are three basic types of decisions: structured decisions, unstructured decisions, and semistructured decisions.

Structured decisions use defined rules and relationships to arrive at answers. The decisions often are made by traditional computer programs, with the decision-making procedures specified in advance.

Unstructured decisions involve complex situations and usually are one-time or ad hoc decisions. There are no clear procedures for making these decisions, and human judgment and intuition are needed.

The semistructured decision-making process cannot be defined completely in advance. The decision is not entirely unstructured, nor is it entirely structured; therefore, both human intuition and computer modeling methods can be used.

The decision type directly relates to the categories of managerial activities described above. Strategic planning activities generally involve unstructured decisions, whereas tactical control decisions generally are semistructured, and operational control decisions usually are structured.

Managers dealing with tactical and strategic planning activities, or semistructured and unstructured decisions, need computerized support that has ad hoc inquiry and analysis capabilities, thus, the emergence of decision support systems.

Decision support systems are computer-based systems that provide interactive information support to managers during the decision-making process. Decision support systems use (1) analytical models, (2) specialized databases, (3) a decision maker's own insights and judgment, and (4) an interactive, computer-based modeling process to support the making of semistructured and unstructured decisions by individual managers.

Decision Support System Components*

In addition to the human user (whose judgment, intelligence, and intuition are critical) a decision support system has the following computer-based components: (1) the dialogue/user interface, (2) the database, and (3) the analytical model base. These components make a decision support system easy for nontechnical users to operate, allow access to a wide variety of data, and provide a variety of analysis and modeling capabilities.

The *dialogue component*, or user interface, enables the decision maker to interact or converse with the system.

A decision support system must have a *specialized database* that contains the data needed to support specific types of decisions. These data are used by the system's analytical models and also may be used for responses to queries by the decision maker. Some of the data for a decision support system database comes from the organization's internal, operational database—the database that is used for traditional data processing. Other decision support system data come from external sources, such as the government, professional organizations, suppliers, and

competitors. The remaining data are personal data entered by the decision support system user.

The *model base component* gives a decision support system its analytical capabilities, through a collection of mathematical models and analytical techniques. A simple example is:

$$Revenue - Expenses = Profit$$

A decision support system may contain general purpose models as well as customized models for specific decisions. The models may be fairly simple, such as determining the optimal quantity of a specific product that should be ordered, or more complex, such as forecasting the number of patients needed to support construction of a new surgical suite.

The analytic modeling techniques available with a decision support system can be extremely useful and cost-effective to a decision maker.

"What if" analysis highlights the impact that changing the value of one or more variables has on other variables. For example, the impact of using overtime in some areas instead of hiring new employees can be assessed.

Sensitivity analysis is used to find the impact of changing the value of one variable repeatedly to see how this affects other variables, for example, increasing overtime pay in increments to determine the level at which a new hire is preferable.

Goal-seeking analysis sets a target value for a variable to see what level of another variable is needed to reach the target value. An example of this might determine the staffing complement that will provide the necessary coverage while remaining within certain dollar constraints.

Optimization analysis involves finding an optimum value for a variable, for example, the best employee health care option given the nature and needs of the staff and the budget.

The model base, like the database, is managed by a software system. The model base management system interacts with the dialogue component so that the user can create, modify, store, and run models and view the output. The model base management system also interacts with the

Source: Sheila M. Jacobs and Sandra Pelfrey, "Decision Support Systems," *Journal of Nursing Administration,* Vol. 25:2, February 1995. J.B. Lippincott.

database component to obtain the data needed by the models.

Decision-Making Tools and Techniques*

Managers may test alternatives through the use of decision-making tools and techniques.

Alternative Opinion Method

A manager may obtain the *considered opinion* of experts to sharpen the arguments for and against an alternative. The resulting comparative assessment helps the decision maker to select a course of action.

When the *devil's advocate* technique is used, the decision maker assigns an individual or group the duty of developing statements of all the negative aspects or weaknesses of each alternative. Each alternative is then tested through frank discussion of weaknesses and error before the final decision is made.

Source: Joan Gratto Liebler, Ruth Ellen Levine, and Jeffrey Rothman, *Management Principles for Health Professionals*, ed 2, Aspen Publishers, Inc., © 1992.

Factor Analysis Matrix

The factor analysis matrix is an effective comparative analysis tool for the decision maker who must overcome personal preference to make an impartial decision. As a first step, the decision maker develops the criteria under two major categories: essential elements (musts) and desired elements (wants).

The choices available are compared through the development of a table or matrix. The factors can be assigned relative weight, as in a point scale, and the alternative with the highest point value becomes the best option. Even without the weighting factors, the matrix remains useful as a technique of factual comparison (see Figure 4–2).

Decision Tree

A managerial tool used to depict the possible directions that actions might take from various decision points, the decision tree forces the manager to ask the "what then" questions (i.e., to anticipate outcomes). A simplified, nongraphic version is demonstrated in Table 4–1. Possible events are included, with a notation about the probabilities associated with each. The basic decisions are stated, with all the unfolding, prob-

---

Figure 4–2 The Payoff Table

Results

Alternatives	180 (.6)	200 (.4)
180	1 $9	2 $24
200	3 $10	4 $10

Expected costs if 180 are ordered:
$9 (.6) + $24 (.4) =
$5.40 + $9.60 = $15.00

Expected costs if 200 are ordered:
$10 (.6) + $10 (.4) =
$6.00 + $4.00 = $10.00

Explanation: The chart above depicts data from an outpatient department of a large hospital where paper gowns are used. It is determined that on a weekly basis, there is a 60 percent probability that 180 gowns will be used and a 40 percent probability that 200 gowns will be used. Costs are assigned to each of these alternatives. The cost of 180 gowns is $9.00. The cost of 200 gowns is $10.00. If there were a shortage of gowns, a special order would entail an extra cost of $15.00. Thus, if 180 gowns are available and the amount used during the week is 180 the cost is $9. If 180 gowns are available but 200 gowns are needed, the cost will be $24 ($9 for available gowns plus $15 for the special order). If 200 gowns are available and 180 are used the cost is $10. If 200 gowns are available and used the cost is $10.

Decision: Alternative 4 appears to be the least costly option while providing a sufficient number of gowns.

Source: Kathleen Kerrigan, "Decision Making in Today's Complex Environment," *Nursing Administration Quarterly*, Vol. 15:4, Aspen Publishers, Inc., © 1991.

Table 4–1 The Decision Tree

Objective of Decision	Alternative/Action	Probability	Expected Outcome
Adequate staffing with wisest expenditure of money	1. Hire FT RN $16/hr	a. Increased patient load (.7) (will have to pay) $16 × .7 = $11.20 b. same patient load (.3) $16 × .3 = $4.80	$16.00 Adequate staffing
	2. Pay OT $24/hr	a. Increased patient load (.7) (will have to pay) $24 × .7 = $16.80 b. same patient load (.3) (will not have to pay)	$16.80 Adequate staffing
	3. Hire per diem RN $20/hr	a. Increased patient load (.7) (will have to pay) $20 × .7 = $14.00 b. same patient load (.3) (will not have to pay)	$14.00 Adequate staffing, least cost

Explanation: This chart shows data from an intensive care nursery in which it is predicted that during the fiscal year, patient census will increase. There is a 70 percent probability that the patient load will grow and a 30 percent probability that it will remain the same. The goal of the unit is to provide adequate staffing of nurses while controlling cost. Salary for a full-time (FT) registered nurse (RN) is $33,280 or $16 per hour. Overtime (OT) cost is $24 per hour, while per diem RN cost is $20 per hour.
Decision: Alternative 3 appears to be the least costly option while providing adequate staffing.

Source: Kathleen Kerrigan, "Decision Making in Today's Complex Environment," *Nursing Administration Quarterly*, Vol. 15, No. 4, © 1991, Aspen Publishers, Inc.

---

able events branching out from them. Decision trees enable managers to undertake disciplined speculation about the consequences, including the unpleasant or negative ones, of actions. Through the use of decision trees, managers are forced to delineate their reasoning, and the constraints imposed by probable future events on subsequent decisions become evident. Each decision tree reveals the probable new situation that results from a decision.

Operations Research

By definition, operations research is an applied science in which the scientific method is brought to bear on a problem, process, or operation. It is a technique for quantitative problem solving and decision making in which mathematical models are applied to management problems.

Simulation is the representation of a process or system by means of a model. Through the development of models, managers attempt to gain additional information about the uncertainties in a situation; those elements are brought into focus and assessments are made concerning the degree of chance associated with them. The underlying premise is that delays are costly, yet too little activity on another occasion is also costly.

Gaming is the simulation of competitive situations in which the element of uncertainty is introduced as a result of some other, often competing, decision maker's action. In the management field, games give reality to training situations and to the decision-making process. Unlike other forms of simulation, gaming uses human decisions, although they may be computer assisted.

AFTER THE DECISION*

Recognizing Uncertainty

The nurse executive has two resources after making a decision.

Test Run

In some cases it is possible to try out the decision short of full implementation. For example, a nursing director has decided to adopt a new scheduling procedure throughout the department. He or she makes a trial run of the procedure and tests it out in a single unit. If satisfied with the results, the director goes all out. If not, he or she can rethink the decision.

Flexibility

It is possible to develop a decision with "branching" steps. For example, an executive says, "Let's use training method A with a group of 10 people, and training method B with another 10. Then we can compare results, and adopt the method that works best for all our new aides."

Implementation

Not *what* you do, but the *way* you do it holds the secret of a successful outcome in decision making. This is the opinion of a veteran executive decision maker who has seen in both her own experience and that of colleagues the crucial role played by implementation in determining the outcome of decisions.

There are several basic considerations to be made in implementing a decision.

Commitment. Once a course of action has been decided, others involved must be willing to put aside all hesitations, partial commitments to other courses of action, and so on. You have made a decision. You must move ahead on the decided course without further hesitations or doubts.

Announcement. In some cases, this element is minor. But in others, the way in which a decision is revealed to staff can make a difference in its acceptance and its viability. When a decision is stated with resolution, confidence, and optimism, its chances of success are considerably increased, as compared to a reaction of doubt, hesitation, gloom, and pessimism.

Staff. Who gets to do what in putting a decision to work is often a crucial factor. Some alternatives simply cannot be adopted because the people to develop them are not available.

In considering the human resources aspect of implementing a decision, think of it not only in terms of quantity but in terms of quality. You may have enough people to do a job, but ascertain that they have the skills, experience, initiative, and so on, to achieve assigned objectives.

Increasingly, nurse executives are learning to use small groups rather than individuals in staff assignment in some situations. Would a team of two or three be better for a given assignment than a single individual?

Time. Exactly when to start a plan, what deadlines to set, what pace to adopt, must be clearly spelled out. An undertaking started prematurely may suffer just as much as one started too late. On the question of pace, you must consider whether a particular project should get "crash" treatment or may be spaced over time. Considerations may involve the state of mind of a work group. For example, you may want to announce an exciting new program in the fall, when people are psychologically "ready to buckle down," rather than during the summer doldrums.

Responsibility. You may want to stand at the helm to make sure that the implementation of the decision remains on course. Or you may want to delegate this responsibility. If you make the latter move, the individual you select and the manner in which you hand out the assignment may be crucial.

There is a big difference in the motivating effect of "Jan, there's a little project I'd like you to take over for a few weeks," and "Jan, there's an important responsibility I've decided to turn over to you, and the outcome of it is so important that

*Source: The Executive Deskbook, 2nd edition, by Auren Uris, © 1970, 1979, by Litton Educational Publishing Inc. Reprinted by permission of Van Nostrand Reinhold Company.

it can make a considerable difference in our future."

When Decisions Go Sour

Nurse executives—using one method or another—somehow manage to make decisions. But only a small percentage of decision makers know how to proceed when a decision goes wrong. And even the most carefully considered, well-planned decision can turn sour. Five positive moves may save the day.

Recognizing. This move is a "must" prelude to all the others, involving clear-headed, honest recognition of the fact that, on this particular decision, you have come up with a clinker. It may not be your fault at all. Other people, other forces, other events may be wholly or partially responsible. But whatever the cause, there is nothing to be gained by clinging to a losing situation. Executives who do not—or will not—recognize the inevitable, who are determined to make a decision work, to stick it out come what may, are only compounding wrong. The best response is to accept the losses, analyze the causes, and try to recoup what you can.

Reversing. Many a decision is the result of a multistep process. From step A to step B to step C and so on until the final stage is reached. Somewhere along the line you may have tripped. Can you, after thinking things out, retrace your steps to the point where the misstep occurred? Backtrack from E to B, for instance? Then revising B, begin a subsequent series of steps, this time

in the right direction? If so, you are halfway home.

Replacing. There will be times when you have a decision that looks great—on paper. You have followed all the proper procedures, made all the right moves, said all the right things. Then, in execution, up pops a weak link—and trouble. Does this mean that your idea is not workable? Not at all.

The weak link should be replaced, the decision can look good again—on paper and in execution.

Revising. In some instances, of course, a decision turned bad cannot be remedied by simply replacing or retracing. Accordingly, major surgery is called for, a complete revision of the original plan. Now is the time to ask yourself, "Do I have an alternative? Is there a workable plan B that I can substitute for unworkable plan A?" Undoubtedly, in arriving at plan A you had considered other ways, other means of achieving your objective. Can one, or a combination of these—with additions, subtractions, or amendments, successfully serve your purpose? Possibly it can.

This stage, incidentally, may call for consultations up, down, and along the line.

Reviewing. Results are the proof of the decision-making pudding. When they go wrong, analyzing when, why, and how can teach you a great deal: about your own decision-making ability, about techniques that need sharpening, about pitfalls to be avoided, about planning, performance, and people. Failure often triggers more knowledge than success.

Chapter 5

Delegation and Time Management

THE NATURE OF DELEGATION

Delegation is both a process and a condition. It is, in part, the process of assigning work to an employee. The *process* is generally well understood, but much consideration of delegation stops at this point. The *condition* of delegation, which must be achieved by going well beyond the process itself, exists when there is thorough, mutual understanding by supervisor and employee of what specific results are expected and how these results may be achieved. Too often, delegation is treated as a simple process and no steps are taken to attain the true condition of delegation.

Actually, there is no difference between empowerment and *proper* delegation. Even in a standard thesaurus *empowerment* and *delegation* are synonyms for each other along with *commission, assignment, deputation*, and a number of other words.*

Proper Use of Subordinate Leaders**

How your subordinate leaders perform is a reflection of your own leadership.

Source: Charles R. McConnell, *The Effective Health Care Supervisor*, ed 3, Aspen Publishers, Inc., © 1993.

**Source:* Fred Fiedler et al., *Improving Leadership Effectiveness*, John Wiley & Sons, Inc., © 1976. Reprinted with permission.

Matching Abilities. You may find it relatively easier to modify your subordinates' leadership situations than your own, once you determine the types of situations in which they perform best. You are in an excellent position to counsel them on the types of leadership situations in which they appear to perform well. You are able to give them not only guidance, but also tangible assistance by modifying their leadership situation. If you desire, you can work with them to analyze their situation and determine what is best for them.

There are many different ways in which you can help match your subordinate leaders' job situation with their abilities. You can assign the leader to harmonious or to more conflicting groups, and gradually change the composition of the group to make it more harmonious or more challenging as a problem in human resources administration. You can assign to one leader highly structured tasks, or give highly detailed and specific instructions on how the task is accomplished. You can assign to another leader the problems and tasks that are naturally more vague and nebulous, or you can give your instructions in a less specific manner and imply that the leader and his or her group are to develop their own procedures in dealing with the problem.

Providing Support. You can shore up the leader's authority by providing a great deal of support and backing, by ensuring that all the organizational information is channeled through the leader, and by extending greater authority to reward and punish or by letting everyone know that you will almost certainly accept the leader's recommendations.

You can give leaders close emotional support by making yourself available to them for guidance and advice, by being as nonthreatening as possible, and by giving them assurance that you stand behind them. Alternatively, you can take a more aloof evaluative stance, implying that subordinate leaders are on their own and that it is up to them to find the right methods and to develop the appropriate policies to deal with their problems. While this latter way of dealing with your subordinate leaders might appear cold, certain types of leaders are better able to perform in this type of climate than in a warmer, more accepting atmosphere. There are also leaders who prefer this type of relationship with their boss. Different types of people perform better under different sorts of control, and you should not automatically assume that your preference is shared by all.

Assigning Appropriately. You can also modify the leadership situation of your subordinate managers by selection and placement, that is, the proper assignment of your subordinates to a leadership situation in which they are most likely to perform well.

Knowing the personality of your subordinates and the nature of the task, you can select the leader who will excel at the beginning or the type of leader who will gradually mature into a great performer.

You may require that certain leaders obtain intensive training, knowing that others may perform just as well with little or no training (remembering that all leaders must have minimum qualifications to be considered for a leadership position).

You should ensure that leaders are either placed in a position in which they can perform well or that the situation is modified so that their leadership potential is used to the fullest.

Consider the options that are open to you in selecting subordinate leaders for maximum performance. If you opt for long-range performance,

see Table 5–1 for recommendations that might guide your procedures. The general rule is that you wish to keep task-motivated leaders in high-control and low-control situations or get them there as soon as possible, and relationship-motivated leaders in moderate-control situations or get them there as soon as possible.

THE NUTS AND BOLTS OF DELEGATION

Supervisory work can be separated into two general categories: technical tasks and managerial tasks. Most technical tasks are likely to be subjects for delegation, although there may be a few that continue to be controlled by the nurse manager because they are of sufficient importance to warrant his or her personal attention or because they occur so infrequently that time invested in training would be wasted.

Most pure managerial tasks cannot be delegated; they require supervisory authority. For instance, staff input and assistance can be obtained in planning, scheduling, budgeting, purchasing, and other such activities, but the tasks of approving, recommending, or implementing still call for the exercise of supervisory authority.

How to Delegate*

Select and Organize the Task

Take the time to make a list of duties you perform that could reasonably be delegated to an employee; concentrate on ongoing functions, on jobs that regularly recur. The following should be done automatically: preparing routine reports, answering routine correspondence, preparing service schedules, ordering supplies, serving on certain committees, performing actual patient care or other technical tasks. Many other activities may present themselves as candidates for delegation. List them all, and rank them accord-

---

Source: Adapted from Charles R. McConnell, *The Effective Health Care Supervisor*, ed 3, Aspen Publishers, Inc., © 1993.

Table 5–1 Guide for Assigning Subordinate Leaders

> *Explanation: Leadership Style Terms*
>
> 1. *Relationship motivated:* concerned with maintaining good interpersonal relations, sometimes even to the point of letting the task suffer.
> 2. *Task motivated:* emphasis on task performance. These leaders are the no-nonsense people who tend to work best from guidelines and specific directions.
>
> *Explanation: Leadership Situation Terms*
>
> 1. *High-control* situations allow the leader a great deal of control and influence and a predictable environment in which to direct the work of others.
> 2. *Moderate-control* situations present mixed problems—either good relations with subordinates but an unstructured task and low position power, or the reverse.
> 3. *Low-control* situations offer the leader relatively low control and influence, where the group does not support the leader and neither the task nor position power gives him or her much influence.

If the situation for the experienced leader is:	The situation for the inexperienced leader is:	If the leader is:	To obtain best long-range performance, proceed as follows:	To obtain best short-run performance, proceed as follows:
High control	Moderate control	Task motivated	Train leader Structure task Increase position power Support leader	If possible, do not select If selected, train Structure task Provide position power
		Relationship motivated	Do not increase leader control Rotate eventually	Select if possible Do not train Keep task structure low
Moderate control	Low control	Task motivated	Do not increase leader control	Select if possible Do not train or structure task more than necessary
		Relationship motivated	Train leader Structure task Support leader Increase position power to move situation to moderate as quickly as possible	If possible, do not select If selected, train intensively, support, structure task
Low control	Very low control	Task motivated	Support leader Structure task	Select if possible
		Relationship motivated	Increase position power Train leader	Do not select

ing to two criteria: the amount of your time they require and their importance to the institution. In short, establish a priority order of tasks for delegation.

Do not, however, attempt to delegate all these nonmanagerial duties at once. Pick *one* task to begin with, preferably that which is either of most importance to the institution or takes the largest part of your time or both. Plan on delegating a single function, or as much of one as possible, to a single person and thus avoid the situation in which a function is so broken up that no one person is able to develop a sense of the whole job.

Determine the specific authority you will have to provide the person to whom you delegate an activity. Plan also on defining the limits of that authority.

Select the Appropriate Person

Pick the employee you will delegate to by matching the qualifications of available employees with the requirements of the task to be delegated. How well you can do this will depend to a great extent on how well you know your employees' strengths and weaknesses and attitudes and capabilities.

Beware of either overdelegating or underdelegating. When you overdelegate, the employee to whom you give a task is clearly not ready to handle it. While a modest amount of challenge is certainly desirable, too much challenge can be overwhelming to the employee. Overdelegation frequently leads to an employee's failure in a first attempt at handling increased responsibility, a harsh beginning that is not easily overcome. On the other hand, underdelegation—assigning a task to an employee who is overqualified and can obviously handle it with the greatest of ease—can be fully as damaging. Underdelegation is a waste of an employee's capabilities and often results in that employee's boredom and stagnation.

Instruct and Motivate the Person

One of the most common errors in delegation is turning an employee loose on a task with inadequate preparation. In gathering the information you need to turn over a job, it may be necessary for you to put those instructions in writing as well as to teach the employee how to do the job personally. When you are completely ready to turn a task over to an employee, you should be able to provide satisfactory answers to the following questions on instruction and motivation.

- Am I prepared to give the reasons for the task, fully explaining why it is important and why it must be done?
- Are all the details of the assignment completely clear in my mind? Should they be conveyed in writing?
- If necessary, can I adapt all the instructions and procedural details to the level of the employee's knowledge and understanding?
- Does the assignment include sufficient growth opportunity to motivate the employee appropriately?
- Does the employee have the training, experience, and skills necessary to accomplish the task?

Turning a task over to an employee then becomes a critical exercise in two-way communication. When meeting to make the actual assignment, encourage the employee to ask questions. If questions are not readily forthcoming, ask the employee to restate your instructions. Whenever possible, demonstrate those parts of the activity that lend themselves to demonstration and have the employee perform those operations to your satisfaction.

Keep in mind that if delegation is to serve its proper purpose, the nurse manager must be willing to accept the employee's decisions. In addition, the employee must be able to see the importance of the delegated task. The employee also must have the time to perform the delegated task.

Last in the process of turning over a task, but extremely important, is the necessity for you and the employee to achieve agreement on the results you expect.

Maintain Reasonable Control

Know your employees well enough to be able to judge who needs what degree of control and assistance. Since the degree of control necessary will vary from employee to employee, the hazards of overcontrol or undercontrol are always present. *Overcontrol* can destroy the effects of delegation. The employee will not develop a sense of responsibility, and you may remain as actively concerned with the task as though you had never delegated it at all. *Undercontrol* is also hazardous in that the employee may drift significantly in unproductive directions or perhaps make costly or time-consuming errors that you could have helped to avoid.

Having decided the approximate extent of control the individual needs, set reasonable deadlines for task completion, or for the completion of portions of the task, and prepare to follow up as those deadlines arrive. Give the employee plenty of time to do the job, including, if possible, extra time for contingencies. Then, if you make it a habit always to follow up on deadlines, your employees will pick up on this pattern and expect you to look for timely results.

Throughout the entire delegation process, try to avoid being a crutch for the employee. Regardless of how much guidance and assistance you are called on to provide, try to avoid solving problems for your employees. Rather, focus on showing your employees how to solve their own problems. To keep failures to a minimum, regularly assess your performance with the questions listed in the following box.

Where and When To Delegate*

The following situations should be areas to consider for delegation.

Routine Tasks. Screening mail, preliminary interviewing of job applicants, handling minor scheduling problems—activities like these may be parceled out to subordinates when you are not inclined to do them yourself.

---

*Source: From *The Executive Deskbook*, 2nd edition, by Auren Uris, © 1970, 1979, by Litton Educational Publishing, Inc. Reprinted by permission of Van Nostrand Reinhold Company.

> ### Assessing the Quality of Your Delegation
>
> - Did I assign a task only to take it away before the employee could truly demonstrate any competence at the task?
> - Did I maintain too much or too little control?
> - Did I split up an activity such that no single person with some authority could develop a sense for the whole?
> - Was I overly severe with an employee who made a mistake?
> - Am I giving proper credit to the employee for getting the job done?
> - Am I keeping the more interesting tasks for myself, delegating only the mundane or unchallenging activities?
> - Have I slacked off in my own work as I delegated certain activities, or have I used the time saved to increase my emphasis on managerial activities?

Tasks for Which You Do Not Have Time. There is another group of activities, not necessarily routine, but of comparatively low priority. When you have time for these, you prefer to do them yourself. But when more urgent matters occupy your attention, these may be passed along to a capable subordinate.

Problem Solving. Some executives properly turn over a problem situation to a subordinate. This is usually of a low or medium priority area; and actually there may be one (or more) of your subordinates with a particular knowledge or skill in the area that qualifies him or her to take on the task. In addition, he or she will be motivated to give it special attention, since it will represent a challenge.

Change in Your Own Job Emphasis. For the average executive, job content changes over the years, slowly in some cases, rapidly in others. As executives become aware of these changes in emphasis, they understand that new elements in their activity require more of their time. To make the time, the executive must, as a practical matter, delegate "old" aspects of his or her responsibility to subordinates.

Capability Building. Last but not least, delegation may be used to increase the capability of individual subordinates and your staff as a group. Properly managed, delegation becomes the means by which you train and develop the skills of subordinates.

When Not To Delegate

Just as there are situations for which delegation is a solution, there are circumstances that make it inadvisable.

Delegation can cause trouble if the wrong duties are handed over. Some of your responsibilities are yours for keeps.

- *The power to discipline.* This is the backbone of executive authority.
- *Responsibility for maintaining morale.* You may call on others to help carry out assignments that will improve morale. You cannot ask anybody else to maintain it.
- *Overall control.* No matter how extensive are the delegations, ultimate responsibility for final performance rests on your shoulders.
- *The hot potato.* Do not ever make the mistake of passing one along, just to take yourself off the spot.

Some jobs must be retained. It is best to keep them in certain circumstances.

- *Jobs that are too technical.* Staff scheduling or annual budgeting may be routine to you but completely beyond a subordinate's skill.
- *Duties that involve a trust or confidence.* Examples include handling confidential department information and dealing with the personal affairs of one of your staff.

Barriers to Delegation

A variety of obstacles to effective delegation can be found in the delegator, the delegatee, and, possibly, the situation itself.

Accepting the Risks*

One theorist says the most difficult part of learning to delegate is learning to accommodate differences. It is easy to accept the idea that people are not the same; it is much harder to accept its application. There can be immense variations not only in the quality and quantity of work performed but also in the ways it is done. The manager must be prepared to accept and live with the subordinates' methods and decisions. It may be a very big order, but the manager cannot reap the benefits of delegation unless he or she is willing to accept the risks. Delegation is a calculated risk, and managers must expect that over time the gains will offset the losses.

Overcoming Resistance to Delegated Assignments**

Delegation may fail to the extent that employees believe you are "pawning off" your work if all of the steps essential to thorough delegation are not followed. Employees will frequently resist delegated tasks and resent doing them if the tasks are inappropriately organized, the staff have been inadequately instructed (or not instructed), or if staff are left to drift for themselves too much of the time. An employee who is ill prepared to handle a certain task may well resent having to do that task.

Also, much of the employee attitude can be attributable to the nurse manager's failure to address the motivational side of delegation properly. Employees need to understand both why a given task must be done and what they can expect to get out of doing it. An employee who believes in the importance of the task is far more likely to give it an honest effort than one who is led to believe the task is unimportant.

It is always fair for an employee to wonder "What's in it for me?" regarding any assigned

---

Source: Reprinted by permission of the publisher, from *The Time Trap*, by R. Alec Mackenzie, pp. 133–134, © 1972 by AMACOM, a division of American Management Associations, New York. All rights reserved.
**Source:* "A Supervisor Asks: 'Delegation's Downside,'" *Health Care Supervisor*, Vol. 10:2, Aspen Publishers, Inc., © December 1991.

WHY MANAGERS FAIL TO DELEGATE

____They are workaholics or perfectionists.
____They are insecure because:
- they are afraid that the delegate will fail
- they are afraid that the delegate will do it better than they do
- they are afraid that they will be accused of dumping

____They do not like to turn over what they enjoy doing.
____They do not think their staff are ready or willing.
____They have had unpleasant previous experiences with delegation.
____They don't know how to go about it.

WHY DELEGATES RESIST

____They don't think they are qualified.
____Previous efforts have failed.
____Their teammates may not approve.
____They don't think they have the time.
____They don't like what is delegated or see some reward in it.
____They don't think they will have enough authority.
____They lack confidence that the delegator will support them.
____They think they are being manipulated or dumped on.

Source: W. Umiker, *Management Skills for the New Health Care Supervisor,* ed 2, Aspen Publishers, Inc., © 1994.

task. Let any employee know what *is* in it for him or her, that doing the task will provide relief from other tasks (thus introducing some variation into the job), the opportunity to learn new and different tasks and increase his or her scope of familiarity with the department, the chance to expand his or her basic knowledge and in this fashion enhance growth possibilities within the organization, and more capability to interact with other employees as the general level of familiarity grows to include a greater variety of tasks. If an employee's attitude regarding a particular task is, "I'm stuck with this because the boss doesn't want to do it," then the forces of dissatisfaction are present. It is up to the nurse manager to attempt to head off dissatisfaction by looking for a positive side of the task to apply as a motivator.

Assigning Unpleasant Tasks. Of course, there are some tasks that few people will want to take on because they are, by nature, menial or tedious.

A task that is unpleasant but nevertheless recognized as necessary must be accomplished as efficiently as possible in a manner that maintains fairness among the employees of the department.

It is often not the tasks themselves that are resisted—as long as they are indeed accepted as necessary—but more often a sense of unfairness or inequitable distribution of work that employees will resist.

One simple suggestion that might work under some circumstances is simply to take the unpleasant task and split it up so that it is accomplished on an equal basis by all members of the group.

You will accomplish more with your employees in the long run by not openly acknowledging the unpleasant nature of a task but simply stressing the necessity for getting this task done and thus acknowledging its importance.

TIME MANAGEMENT

Most people think their time problems are external, that they are caused by the telephone, meetings, visitors, and delayed information or decisions.

In almost all cases, it is possible to influence, if not control, externally generated time problems. More difficult to identify, as well as to manage, are the internally generated time wasters: procrastination and indecision, lack of self-discipline, the inability to say no, the inability to delegate, or the tendency to fight fires, to act without thinking, and to jump from task to task without finishing any of them.

Time is a constant that cannot be altered. The clock cannot be slowed down or speeded up. Thus we cannot manage time itself. We can only manage our activities with respect to time.

The same skills are needed as those used in managing others—the abilities to plan, organize, delegate, direct, and control. Time management is simply self-management. It is impossible to be effective in any position without controlling one's time effectively.*

Paradoxes in Time Management*

Open-Door Paradox. By leaving a door open in hope of improving communication, managers tend to increase the wrong kind of communication, that of a trivial or socializing nature. This multiplies interruptions and distracts from more important tasks. The "open door" was originally intended to mean "accessible," not physically open.

Planning Paradox. Managers often fail to plan because of the time required, thus failing to recognize that effective planning saves time in the end and achieves better results.

Tyranny-of-the-Urgent Paradox. Managers tend to respond to the urgent rather than the important matters. Thus, long-range priorities are neglected, thereby ensuring future crises.

Crisis Paradox. Managers tend to overrespond to crises, thereby making them worse.

Meeting Paradox. By waiting for latecomers before starting a meeting, managers penalize those who came on time and reward those who came late. So next time those who were on time will come late, and those who were late will come later.

Delegation Paradox. A manager tends not to delegate to inexperienced subordinates due to their lack of confidence. Yet subordinates can win the manager's confidence only by gaining the experience that only comes through delegated authority.

Cluttered-Desk Paradox. Managers leave things on their desks so they will not forget them. Then they either get lost or, as intended, attract attention every time they are seen, thus providing continual distractions from whatever the manager should be doing.

Long-Hours Paradox. The longer hours managers work, the more fatigued they become and the longer they assume they have to complete tasks. For both reasons they slow down, necessitating still longer hours.

Activity-versus-Results Paradox. Managers tend to confuse activity with results, motion with accomplishment. Thus, as they gradually lose sight of their real objectives, they concentrate increasingly on staying busy. Finally, their objective becomes to stay busy, and they have become confirmed "workaholics."

Efficiency versus Effectiveness. Managers tend to confuse efficiency with effectiveness. They will be more concerned about doing the job right than doing the right job. No matter how efficiently a job is done, if it is the wrong job, it will not be effective.

Paradox of Time. No one has enough, yet everyone has all there is.

Structure for Time Management*

It is possible to be busy—very busy—without being very effective. Hard work without accomplishing set goals leads to frustration and stress.

---

*Source: E.B. Schwartz and R.A. Mackenzie, "Time Management Strategy for Women," *Management Review*, September 1977. Reprinted with permission of the author.

*Source: Suzanne Carter, "Working Harder and Getting Nowhere—No Wonder You Are Stressed!" *Nursing Administration Quarterly*, Vol. 18:1, Aspen Publishers, Inc., © Fall 1993.

The first step in eliminating this stress begins with the belief that people have the power to control their work situation and, for that matter, their lives. Next, armed with this belief, individuals can determine their priorities and goals. Only then can they manage time in a way that permits them to achieve these goals.

This approach to reexamining goals and priorities is described by Covey in his book *The 7 Habits of Highly Effective People.* According to Covey, three habits are critical to this examination: being proactive, beginning with the end in mind, and putting first things first. Embracing these habits will provide a new personal road map. Managing time according to priorities or simply "putting first things first" is advocated.

The time management matrix provides a framework for prioritizing daily activities. This grid classifies activities by importance and urgency. Activities may fall into one of four categories: important and urgent, important and nonurgent, nonimportant and urgent, and nonimportant and nonurgent.

The first category, important and urgent, is where many nursing administrators spend most of their time. What could be more urgent and important than the life and death situations of a health care facility? Examples of time spent in this category include patient emergencies, disasters, staffing shortages, lack of resources, and bed shortages. This style of management is typically problem oriented. Some of these crises can be avoided if more time is spent addressing these issues in a nonurgent mode.

The important, nonurgent category includes those activities that are critical to the accomplishment of goals but may not require immediate attention. Examples of these activities include planning activities, coaching and counseling of staff, and monitoring of quality care through rounds and patient interviews. Time spent in this quadrant may reduce the amount of time spent in the urgent mode.

The third category, nonimportant and urgent, fills an administrator's time in many organizations. Reports, proposals, and projects demanded by the organization but not necessary to the accomplishment of the organization's or manager's goals fill the day.

Finally, the fourth category includes nonimportant and nonurgent activities. It consists of many of the great time wasters. These include poorly organized meetings, wandering phone calls, and duplicative paperwork.

It is readily apparent that while spending time in quadrant II is desirable, and time spent in quadrants I and III should be minimized, time spent in quadrant IV should be avoided. Applying this grid to activities and then examining the four quadrants closely will determine which activities lead to the accomplishment of priorities and goals. Daily work routines must then be adjusted to allow time for activities that lead to goal accomplishment.

Associating Management Style by Time Management. Quadrant II leadership is proactive rather than reactive. It emphasizes important, nonurgent activities, focusing on goal accomplishment rather than a problem-oriented approach to management.

Since this management style is proactive and not problem oriented, these nursing leaders have a clear idea of where they are going. They have defined goals and a detailed plan of action. They have work lists broken down weekly or possibly even daily. At the start of each week and perhaps at the start of each day, they schedule time for these important tasks.

Quadrant II leaders delegate effectively. They recognize that delegation takes time and that it involves teaching and coaching. These nursing leaders recognize the importance of staff development and invest time and resources in this activity. Most important, they spend time troubleshooting, counseling, and monitoring progress toward stated goals. Thus, quadrant II leaders are proactive, goal directed, and focused. Since they spend time in activities that they believe are important, they are more satisfied with work and less stressed.

Planning to Manage Time*

As mentioned before, a paradox of time is that if managers take time to plan, they will have more time. An hour of effective planning can save three to four hours in execution and produce better results.

Planning answers basic questions: Where am I now? Where do I want to be? How do I achieve this? The first question calls for an assessment of the present situation, the second involves setting goals, and the last requires an outline for action.

Audit: Where Am I Now? To plan more efficient use of time, you must first determine how you use it now, how it should be used, and how to schedule its proper use.

Most people are unaware of exactly how they spend their time. Practically every serious study of managers' use of time stresses the surprise of most managers when they discover where their time is really going. Yet, unless they know, they cannot choose among alternative ways to use it.

Probably the simplest and most accurate way to find out where your time goes is to keep a *time log*. You must log daily activities against a time segment (e.g., each 15-minute interval) and account for the time used. The object is to locate a trend or pattern in daily activities.

A time log is a "self-help" tool, a way to look closely at the day, as how you really spend your time. It aids both in planning time and in delegating tasks to others.

One week is usually long enough to log your time. Job priorities should then be compared with what you actually do. Can nonessential work be spotted? Unnecessary meetings? People who should not have been seen? Time spent on things that do not relate to goals? Problem areas?

A *time analysis* of the data from the time log often confirms some time wasters and makes managers aware of others they did not suspect they had. It can also help measure progress in solving these time wasters by showing how much time was saved each day and how results have improved. It can be used continuously to signal deviations from plans and therefore encourage immediate correction.

Goal: Where I Want To Be. How can good use of time be made without goals and priorities? Defining goals, an overall direction—professionally and personally—is crucial. Goals for your life, the year, and the day should be set. "What do I expect to accomplish today?" "What are the most important things to get done at home and at the office?" Put them in writing. A goal or plan that is not written down is a dream.

Plan: How To Achieve This. Once goals are established, a plan is needed to reach them. It commits managers to "making it happen" rather than to letting things happen and then reacting to crises. At the end of each workday, prepare a list of what must be done at the office on the following day. Do the same thing in the evening for the home. A list not only ensures against forgetting but also leaves the mind free from important matters. The palest ink is better than the best memory.

Time management experts that most people waste 80 percent of their time on unimportant things. The 80/20 law says that 80 percent of value comes from 20 percent of the things people do. Of 10 tasks, for example, two yield 80 percent of the valued results. For effective time management, the key is to find these two, label them top priority, and *do* them. On a busy day, the remaining eight can probably be postponed without real harm.

Doing the most important things first is valuable when emergencies interrupt the day. If the highest priorities have been accomplished, managers are free to respond to the crises.

In assigning priorities, you must ask: How does that task relate to my goals and objectives?

Source: E.B. Schwartz and R.A. Mackenzie, "Time Management Strategy for Women," *Management Review*, September 1977. Reprinted with permission of the author.

What is the immediacy of the task? Is it really that important? Why am I doing it? What am I doing that should not be done at all? Could others do it? What is the nature of the task (for example, can it be combined with anything else)?

In setting priorities for paperwork, group it into three categories: Priority One (most important, handle at once); Priority Two (less urgent, do when you get to it); and Priority Three (low priority, keep it just in case someone asks; throw away when the drawer is full). By setting priorities, you can distinguish "most important" tasks from the "most urgent," perhaps eliminating a tendency to operate by crisis.

Action

Many people know what they want and how to accomplish it, but they procrastinate. Take your plan for the day and then start with the most important thing you need to do. The first hour sets the style for the rest of the day.

In fact, discretionary time—time you can really control—generally comes only in fragments later on. Most managers have only a half hour to two hours a day of discretionary time. This time should be invested on the most important things. At least what does not get done will be less significant and less important.

Give total attention to each task. If you do not have time to do it right, when will you have time to do it over? Highly successful people concentrate on whomever they are talking to or whatever they are doing. Sincere total attention, as well as being a timesaver, is also great human relations.

Complete each task the first time. Get all needed data before you start writing a report or speech. Arrange to work without interruptions and finish the job in one session if at all possible. Make it a rule to try to handle each piece of paper only once.

Make it a practice, too, to be brief, to the point, and understood. Words saved are time saved. Learn to speak up and shut up. Also, learn to listen skillfully. Studies indicate people lose more than two-thirds of what they hear immediately after they hear it.

Be considerate of other people's time. Organize to cut down on frequency of visits. When you must see someone, phone for an appointment. Efficient people rarely see you unless they have important things to discuss. Usually, several items are saved for a single conversation. This saves time for you and for them.

Minimize meetings. Call a meeting only when it is more efficient than the telephone. Send an agenda before the meeting to each person who will attend and keep the discussion limited to the necessary points. Whenever those involved are not aware of the agenda prior to the meeting, time will be wasted in orientation.

Set a specific time limit for the meeting and keep it. An announced starting and ending time allows for those involved to plan the balance of their day. And do not attend meetings that are not absolutely necessary; instead, ask for a copy of the minutes.

Use telephone timesavers. Prior to important calls, outline the basic points that must be made during the conversation. Then, when you make the call, identify yourself and move immediately into the business of the call.

Eliminate unproductive reading. Read reports and other documents once and act or reply at once. Read less essential material when you need a break, have a break, or are traveling.

Close your door when you have jobs that must be completed. Too many interruptions? Close the door. Do not take telephone calls. Get the work done.

The average manager is interrupted every eight minutes all day long. Successful control on interruptions is essential.

Follow up on the day's work. Control also means follow up, adjusting the plan, time schedule, and performance in terms of objectives and conditions. At the end of the day, analyze what tasks were not completed. Track and eliminate time-killers. Did you spend too much time on the phone? Were tasks left undone because you did not want to do them and therefore managed to postpone them? Give them top priority on the next day's list and do them.

Some people, believing they work better under pressure, procrastinate until forced into action. Do they really work better under pressure or just faster and less effectively?

Timesaver Strategies*

There are numerous suggestions for saving time. The following are brief recommendations on using time to one's own advantage. Although it is not possible to put all of these into effect immediately, *now* is the time to start.

Eliminate paper. Do not allow it to accumulate. The best advice regarding paper control is to pick it up once and dispatch it. Assign it to someone else, make a decision, give it to the secretary, or use the "round file."

Conduct regular communication sessions. Establish a set time, day, and place for regular meetings. Say it once to 20 people rather than 20 times to individuals.

Block your time. Some projects demand uninterrupted time. Plan and prepare for these by setting aside a block of time to complete the task. In some institutions a quiet hour is observed. During this time telephone calls, visits, and interruptions of any kind are not permitted for those people involved. The results have proven to be most rewarding.

Take time to train. The time spent in effectively training one's staff pays great dividends in both time saved and increased productivity. This ties in with proper delegation.

Relinquish ownership. A common time trap indigenous to managers is accepting problems that are not theirs. Determine who owns the problem and graciously return it to its rightful owner. Also, involving employees in the art of problem solving will help them to grow.

Simply say no. The victor of time management does not try to be all things to all people. Persons who attempt to do this end up being nothing to themselves. Learn the fine art of saying no. Refuse to accept those things that are not your responsibility or that you cannot handle at that time.

Plan your emergencies. Despite the apparent contradiction in terms, it is possible to carefully plan one's time so that marginal emergencies are controlled. For the manager who schedules and plans ahead, it is possible to expect the unexpected. Most health care managers are able to predict the time of day, week, month, or year when their workload increases. Managers can anticipate when budgets are due, when reports need to be submitted, and so on. Many emergencies are somewhat predictable and managers can plan the time to deal with them.

Be complete. A real and insidious time robber occurs without people being aware of it. It is work that is left unfinished: the stopping and getting back into the project again, working at an uneven pace that shifts from slow to frantic, and the missing of deadlines. To combat this time robber, managers must be complete and finish what they initiate. Work should be accomplished at a reasonable and controlled pace. Deadlines should be set and met.

Get away. Minivacations are a strong deterrent to time anxiety. These are selected brief interludes during the course of the day to "get away from it all." Selected means that these minivacations should be scheduled at specific times. What is done during the 5- or 10-minute respite is up to the individual. The only restrictions are that it not be work related and that it be something the person enjoys. It may be a brisk walk around the block, listening to favorite music, reading poetry, or whatever. A minivacation is to be taken daily, perhaps once in the morning and again in the afternoon. It will help to reduce stress and revitalize a person so that he or she may continue to take charge of time.

Source: Victor J. Morano, "Time Management: From Victim to Victor," *The Health Care Supervisor*, Vol. 3:1, Aspen Publishers, Inc., © 1984.

Chapter 6

Change and Transformation

OVERVIEW

Many hospitals have begun laying the groundwork necessary for a major redesign of the basic inpatient care process. As implemented in most U.S. hospitals, total quality management (TQM) and continuous quality improvement (CQI) represent necessary, but not sufficient, conditions for the redesign process to occur.

The modern hospital's departmental and compartmental organizational structures were essentially established early in the twentieth century. Following the lead of medicine, the organization of hospitals has been driven by the specialization of knowledge, skills, and technologies employed to provide individualized patient care services. Over time, individual allied health provider groups laid claim to discrete aspects of the traditional nursing care process and promoted profession-based patient-service differentiation. With each profession-based differentiation, new supervisory and departmental structures came into being. Hospitals came to be organized around the provision of an increasing array of discrete patient care services, rather than around the best methods of meeting patients' health care needs. As a result, hospitals have become highly bureaucratic and inefficient organizations typi-

fied by extensive vertical management hierarchies that support a highly compartmentalized organizational structure.

However, process improvement experiments and research have confirmed that compartmentalization in hospitals limits the industry's ability to enhance clinical and service quality and negatively affects overall operational efficiencies. Many persons in the field are beginning to conclude that the existing organizational structures and patient care processes need to be critically examined and fundamentally redesigned. Common buzzwords related to this notion include *reengineering, restructuring,* and *work and job redesign.*

A critical challenge for health care organizations and departments is the decision to transform, reengineer, restructure, or redesign what is being done today to ensure the organization's long-term viability.*

*Source: Douglas S. Wakefield, Stacey T. Cyphert, James F. Murray, Tanya Uden-Holman, Michael S. Hendryx, Bonnie J. Wakefield, and Charles M. Helms, "Understanding Patient-Centered Care in the Context of Total Quality Management and Continuous Quality Improvement," © Journal on Quality Improvement. Oakbrook Terrace, IL: Joint Commission on Accreditation of Healthcare Organizations, 1994, Vol. 20, No. 3. Reprinted with permission.

Scope of Transformation

Accurate definition and articulation of the scope of the change effort is the first step to success.

- *Reengineering* is used to denote massive and radical change. It means changing an organization in a complete manner, stemming from a re-evaluation of mission, market share, and finance.
- *Restructuring* is changing the table of organization within an institution, division, or unit and reconfiguring the infrastructure.
- *Redesign* is used to describe a situation in which work roles and processes are redesigned as part of an internal systems change.

Source: Sheila Lenkman, "Making Sense of Redesign," *Aspen's Advisor for Nurse Executives*, Vol. 10:10, Aspen Publishers, Inc., © July 1995.

The Change Continuum

All plans to make a change from one situation to another may be considered a project. But, in today's language, the word *project* has been relegated to designate the most simple form of retooling. Moving incrementally along with continuum of change, the next point is improvement. This leads into process redesign before moving on to the more radical change efforts, restructuring and reengineering.

Nurse managers must determine their position on this continuum. It is necessary to differentiate among these approaches even though the initiation of the more radical methods is beyond the power scope of the local nurse manager. (Nurse executives and directors can—and do—influence and participate in structural and reengineering changes on the departmental and overall institutional level.) Just as important for the manager is understanding the concept of change, for whichever transformation path is taken into the future, change is bound to occur.

Leading the Initiative

The Manager's Role in Reengineering*

Inherent in the concept of reengineering is radical change. When a change occurs through process reengineering, change ensues throughout the organization.

To support an environment for organization-wide reengineering, management roles need to be re-created (see Table 6–1). Although changes in various responsibilities will evolve as an outcome of reengineering, the imperative for strong leadership remains constant.

In terms of role structure, reengineering initiatives require an approach different from other, more recent approaches for initiating change, such as total quality management, continuous quality improvement, and quality circles. In those approaches, change is generally initiated from the bottom of the organization, with staff driving the project while receiving support from top management. In reengineering, the initiative must be led by one person or a group at the top level of management; if it is led from the bottom up, it will be blocked by organizational barriers. This phenomenon is due in large part to the radical change inherent in the reengineering project.

The leader's role requires someone who has enough authority over all stakeholders in the process(es) that will undergo reengineering to ensure that reengineering can happen. This requirement is essential because the reengineering process crosses many organizational boundaries. As a consequence, issues of turf protection need to be successfully confronted and resolved. Thus, the leader must possess the inherent authority to make reengineering happen.

---

*Source: Adapted from Dominick L. Flarey and Suzanne Smith Blancett, "Management and Organizational Restructuring: Reforming the Corporate System," in *Reengineering Nursing and Health Care: The Handbook for Organizational Transformation*, Suzanne Smith Blancett and Dominick L. Flarey, eds., Aspen Publishers, Inc., © 1995.

Table 6–1 Managerial Roles in Reengineering Initiatives

There are five major new roles created through and developed by reengineering initiatives.

- *Leader*—A leader must emerge who can oversee the entire project and ensure that it happens. This reengineering leader, in most instances, should be the chief executive officer or the chief operating officer, so that top management will continue to be engaged and committed to the project. This top-level leadership will also solidify the perception by the entire organization that top executive management is truly living out its responsibility to lead the organization through its re-creation.
- *Process owner*—Process owners are generally the managers who are responsible for specific processes. The major imperative for their role is to facilitate process reengineering and to ensure the integration of departments that is necessary to re-create the organization. They must think differently and support the facilitation of an organizationwide change initiative. It is their responsibility to remove the traditional barriers and boundaries that have slowed the organization down in its past attempts to respond swiftly to the changing external environment.
- *Reengineering team*—The reengineering team is the group that actually reengineers processes and systems. Its membership generally consists of multidisciplinary rep-

resentatives throughout the organization. Reengineering team members take on a true leadership role. One of their primary responsibilities is to sell the change concept to everyone in the organization and to be role models for change. These members lead by doing and, as a direct consequence, motivate others to cooperate with the actual reengineering process.
- *Steering committee*—The steering committee is generally made up of senior and middle managers who assume accountability for developing policy and standards related to reengineering efforts. They also serve as the primary body responsible for the ongoing evolution of the project. Their other major responsibility is to evaluate the need for additional resources for reengineering and to ensure that such resources are available to the reengineering team.
- *Reengineering czar*—Every organization that reengineers needs a full-time leader who is an expert in process reengineering and serves as a teacher and mentor to the reengineering team. This new leader must also be well versed in the use of specific tools for process reengineering, as well as in the tools and statistical analyses used to evaluate reengineering projects. In this role, the reengineering czar serves as an internal consultant to the organization for its reengineering initiatives.

Source: Adapted from M. Hammer and James Champy, *Reengineering the Corporation: A Manifesto for Business Revolution*. New York: Harper Business; 1993.

Leading a Successful Work Redesign Change*

Work redesign changes how we work and how we look at work. It changes relationships with coworkers, and it necessitates system changes to support the new work order. It alters roles, often dramatically. It challenges historical truisms and established professional territories.

The successful organization undergoing work redesign will understand that cultural change takes considerable time. To implement a successful work redesign project, an organization should make provision for the following issues.

Support of Projects. The health care facility and nursing administrative staffs must enthusiastically demonstrate that the project is a priority. Administrative staff must also be willing to open up the system to review and revision. If the system does not change, the staff will be very limited in the amount of work redesign they can accomplish.

Source: Jennifer E. Jenkins, "Work Redesign: Ensuring Success," *Aspen's Advisor for Nurse Executives*, Vol. 7:10, Aspen Publishers, Inc., © July 1992.

The nurse manager is a key element in work redesign. The manager must actively encourage and celebrate staff ownership of the process. Once the parameters are defined, the staff must be free to redesign the way work is done on their unit to suit their patient populations and staff expertise and knowledge. Essentially, the nurse manager acts as coach, mentor, and resource.

Empowered Choice. Work redesign involves two or more people working together for an extended period. Staff involved in work redesign need to be empowered to determine how it will be accomplished in their own area (within limits set by the organization). This is best handled by having representatives from the units or departments involved meet to hammer out the plan.

Another empowered choice staff must have is freedom to change the solid lines around job descriptions. That is, job descriptions must be flexible to permit the registered nurse (or others) to delegate work based on the knowledge and skill of the worker and the individualized needs of the patient.

Appropriate Cultural Environment. Making work redesign more than a temporary Band-Aid requires a cultural change. Organizations must do the following:

- Permit workers to systematically examine their work.
- Provide training for those directly and indirectly involved.
- Coach risk takers.
- Ensure adequate time for change to become a part of everyday practice and thinking.

It cannot be stressed enough that adequate time is required for successful work redesign. The period from decision to implementation may be 4 to 12 months. It will take an additional two to three years for the change to become a natural way of doing work.

Encouragement of Continuous Improvement. Successful work redesign is based on the premise that it is a journey and not a destination. Continuous evaluation of goals, expectations, and outcomes will be necessary to update the project to reflect changing resources, patient populations, employee mix, and treatment modalities. When something does not work, a system for examining the cause and effect is vital. Contributing factors are examined and solutions tried. When all is going well, people must ask, "Is this the best we can do?" or "Do we need to be doing this?"

Nurse Manager as Coach

Throughout the process, the nurse manager monitors and fine-tunes. He or she meets regularly with the redesign staff to offer encouragement, support, coaching, structure, and a sense of perspective. The nurse manager ensures that there is a well-thought-out plan, monitoring tools, communication and education plans for all staff; keeps administration informed; and brings information from the health care facility to the staff as needed. When the staff lose perspective, the nurse manager can be very helpful by using humor and getting staff to review their accomplishments. By keeping staff focused on both short- and long-term goals, the manager ensures that there will be small successes on the way to the larger goal.

Purpose of the Redesign*

To decide whether one component or a combination of components is needed in a redesign, the planning team clearly identifies the purposes of the redesign. What are the reasons for redesign? What objectives will be achieved by a redesign? (For a summary of questions to address before attempting a change project, see Table 6-2.) Examples of common purposes for redesign include improved continuity of patient/family care, increased nurse satisfaction, reduced or more efficient resource utilization by patients and their families, more efficient use of human resources, standardization of patient outcomes, a flatter organizational structure, streamlined

---

Source: Doris Milton, "The Evaluation of New Nursing Structures in Single or Multifacility Systems," in *Building New Nursing Organizations, Visions and Realities*, Cathleen Krueger Wilson, ed., Aspen Publishers, Inc., © 1992.

Table 6–2 Questions To Guide Conception of a Change Project

- What specific problems will be addressed through the implementation of a new nursing structure?
  - organizational structure problem
  - delivery system problem
  - nursing role/performance problem
  - coordination problem
  - integration problem
- What needs are being expressed? Is there consensus among the needs being expressed? Will a change in the nursing structure meet these demands?
- How will needs be prioritized? Which needs will be left unaddressed?
  - professional nursing needs
  - physician needs
  - consumer needs
  - support department needs
  - manager needs
  - facility administration needs
- Is the targeted nursing structure performing as it was originally intended to perform? Where are the performance gaps and how are structure performance problems manifested?
  - How many and which types of individuals and groups are affected by the poor performance?
  - How severe is the performance problem of the targeted nursing structure?

- Will the nursing structure need to be modified or replaced?
- Is the problem experienced in the same manner across the nursing organization? If not, how are differences manifested?
- Is the organization open and ready for change?
  - Ad hoc task forces are commonly called upon to solve problems.
  - There is a positive questioning attitude.
  - Reward systems are tied to innovation and excellence.
  - Trust exists.
- Have there been past attempts to remedy the situation?
  - Which groups or individuals were involved?
  - What solutions were attempted?
  - Did the intervention succeed or fail? Why?
- Do the basic resources exist within the organization to support the introduction of change?
  - leadership
  - information systems
  - time and money
  - environment
- Is the rationale for the change accurate and realistic?
  - change for change sake
  - knee-jerk response or quick fix
  - thoughtful project conception

Source: Cathleen Krueger Wilson, *Building New Nursing Organizations, Visions and Realities*, Aspen Publishers, Inc., © 1992.

---

management teams, development of collaborative practice, and increased patient/family satisfaction with care and preparation for discharge.

The planning team then considers whether the component or combination of components selected for redesign will achieve the objectives. Each component or combination of components may be very worthwhile, but may not change what needs to be changed at that facility. It is important to think about what needs to be altered so that the objectives for the redesign will be met.

When one or more structural redesigns are chosen, it is important for all who are involved to achieve consensus on exactly what this structure will look like. If the structural change is being implemented in different patient care areas or on several units, the commonalties that must be present and the differences that are possible need to be addressed.

Decisions concerning the type of restructuring are very difficult and time consuming, since redesign is not the reshuffling of the same old pieces.

Considerations in Change Projects*

Transformation efforts are complex change projects requiring a great deal of thought before they are ever implemented. Take the following steps to avoid unanticipated or negative outcomes from work redesign. (Also see Table 6–3 for examples of practical ways in which leadership can positively influence patient care delivery redesign.)

Determine the amount of dollar savings to be had or the desired outcome of a system change (in plain language, know exactly why you are doing this and what the desired outcome is).

Know your labor pool capabilities, whether nursing or across the house, and *determine the needed skills, cross-training, and support.*

Document the unique needs in management and supervision, orientation, and continuing

---

education of multitask, cross-trained individuals; gather a database on all activities and tasks to be reallocated.

Consistently review the effectiveness and efficiency of the redesigned roles; calculate organizational bottom-line productivity rather than departmental or role productivity.

Know the current level of satisfaction for all parties influenced by the new design. Review the impact on patient and physician satisfaction as implementation proceeds.

Know the scopes of practice within nursing. Review state codes and determine whether some functions that are not permitted to be performed by nursing staff are allowable if performed by nursing personnel allocated to another department.

Document the fiscal impact of change by constructing spreadsheet simulations of proposed work redesign changes using average hourly salaries.

Understand the other changes occurring in the institution that have an impact on the patient unit labor force.

*Source: Sheila Lenkman, "Making Sense of Work Redesign," *Aspen's Advisor for Nurse Executives*," Vol. 10:10, Aspen Publishers, Inc., © July 1995.

Table 6–3 Change and Transition Strategies

Action	*Purpose*
Create a climate that acknowledges the psychological impact associated with change and provide opportunities to openly discuss this dynamic.	This is extremely important because people going through the change zone often feel guilty that they are not coping better.
Establish effective integrating mechanisms that facilitate healthy communication and constructive conflict resolution.	Monitoring the state of the transition keeps it on track, so that nothing falls through the cracks between what was and what is yet to be.
Involve people in the change process to the greatest possible extent, especially when jobs are being redesigned. This can be accomplished through "freeing people up."	Meaningful participation in retreats, work groups, and other exchanges promotes ownership of the change and therefore superior acceptance.

Source: Sister Anne Hayes and James N. Phan, "Mercy Healthcare's CARE 2000: An Evolution in Progress," *Nursing Administration Quarterly*, Vol. 20:1, Aspen Publishers, Inc., © Fall 1995.

THE PROCESS OF CHANGE

The Classic View of Change

If one were to attempt to characterize the nature of change, three types of change could be identified. *Structural change* affects the organizational process, such as alterations in authority charts, budget procedures, or rules and regulations. *Technological change* affects the physical environment and work practices or systems. *People-oriented change* affects the performance and conduct of employees, such as the introduction of different training schemes, appraisal systems, sets of standards, or promotional devices.*

*Phases**

Kurt Lewin identified three phases of change—unfreezing, moving, and refreezing.

Unfreezing is the development of a need to change through problem awareness. Even if a problem has been identified, a person must believe there can be an improvement before he or she is willing to change. Coercion has been used for unfreezing. Removing a person from the source of his or her old attitudes to a new environment, punishment and humiliation for undesirable attitudes, and rewards for desirable attitudes affect change.

Moving is working toward change by identifying the problem or the need to change, exploring the alternatives, defining goals and objectives, planning how to accomplish the goals, and implementing the plan for change.

Refreezing is the integration of the change into one's personality and the consequent stabilization of change. Frequently, staff use old behaviors after change efforts cease. Related changes in neighboring systems, momentum to perpetuate the change, and structural alterations that support the procedural change are stabilizing factors.

Introducing Change*

Change does not simply happen; it is brought about by forces within the organization. There are various organizational approaches used to introduce change. At one extreme is the *unilateral* approach, in which authoritative decisions are made at the top of the power structure and handed downward. At the other extreme is the *delegated* approach, in which subordinate levels hold the responsibility for new solutions to identified problems. In between is the *shared power* approach, the most successful means of arranging change, in which higher level authority interacts with lower level decision groups. Each of these approaches takes several forms.

Unilateral Approach

By Decree. An impersonal announcement handed down by the top echelon, a one-way declaration of intention usually phrased in a memo, policy statement, or lecture. The assumption is that automatic compliance with authority will produce changed behavior and anticipated improvements.

By Replacement. A singling out of strategically located key positions to be filled more effectively by new personnel. This is a device used when the decree approach is insufficient, but it rests on the same assumptions that upper authority control and mandate are necessary to bring about change at the bottom organizational rungs.

By Structure. A relatively formal mechanism for change that relies on a redesign of the organizational pattern, with the assumption that the creation of new or different slots will result in improved performance. If the arrangement is not adjusted to the informal authority lines evident in current practices, it will be ineffective, becoming merely an exercise in logic on paper.

*Source: G. Matsunaga, "Nurse Administrator Must Be Chief Initiator of Change," *TheAmerican Nurse*, April 1975. Reprinted with permission of the American Nurses' Association.

*Source: Larry E. Greiner, "Patterns of Organization Change," *Harvard Business Review* (May–June 1967), pp. 121–122.

Shared Power

By Group Decision Making. A two-phase approach where upper authority identifies the problem, but subordinates debate and select the most appropriate solution for stimulating change. The assumption is that participation in the change decision increases support and commitment.

By Group Problem Solving. The two functions of problem identification and solution are faced by the subordinate discussion group in recognition of the members' practical experience and knowledge of the issue at hand.

Delegated Power

By Case Discussion. A generalized discussion of a situation aimed at developing problem-solving skills that can then be applied by staff to carry out changes.

By Sensitivity Sessions. A psychologically oriented method that does not deal with task-oriented problems or changes but instead places emphasis on social or interpersonal processes. Led by a professional trainer, the members of the group develop self-awareness and insight into the attitudes of others. This increased understanding is expected to lead to informal and self-initiated change. Customarily used for top management, the method has been used in nursing services (e.g., by an entire staff of an individual unit).

Steps To Support a Cultural Change*

The success of innovation—a major change—is determined not by how it was implemented or how it is being carried out but by the effect this innovation has on patient outcomes.

Step 1: Assess the Unit Culture

Each nursing unit has its own distinctive culture. Hence, there is no one right way to implement changes. Rather, each change must be individually adapted to each work group. Indeed, new practice patterns will play out differently on different units, depending on the culture and the needs of that unit. Thus, the same innovation should be implemented differently in each unit so as to fit in with a particular culture.

The change agent must identify the cultural elements of each innovation and compare these elements with the culture of the nursing unit undergoing the change so as to predict which aspects of the unit's culture will encourage or resist the change.

Step 2: Identify Cultural Elements of the Innovation

The next step of the cultural innovation process is to review those elements of the innovation that may effect cultural behaviors, such as

- power relationships within the group
- priority behaviors that the group considers to be the best use of time
- peer relationships and support systems within the group
- the group's preferences for stability versus change

These are the behaviors that the change agent is advised to consider when comparing a work group's current behavior with the behavior that would result from the innovation so as to predict how the group might react to the innovation.

The best places to find the cultural elements associated with an innovation include the following:

- descriptions in the literature of how an innovation has altered a specific work group
- conversations with those who have experienced how an innovation has changed their organization
- reports that indicate how to tell whether or not what has been done is "the real thing" for a given innovation

---

Source: Adapted from Harriet Van Ess Coeling and Lillian M. Simms, "Facilitating Innovation at the Unit Level through Cultural Assessment, Part 2: Adapting Managerial Ideas to the Unit Work Group," *Journal of Nursing Administration*, Vol 23:5, May 1993. J.B. Lippincott Company.

Steps 3–5: Compare the Unit Culture with a Specific Innovation

These steps occur more together than in sequence. Step 3 involves comparing the unit culture with the essential elements of an innovation to determine which cultural behaviors will drive and which will restrain the innovation.

- When the culture is similar to the innovation and thus serves as a driving force, it should be supported.
- When the culture conflicts with the innovation and thus acts as a restraining force, the restraining power can be lifted by reframing the innovation, customizing the innovation, or, if necessary, changing the culture.

In step 4 the manager thus strengthens the unit norms that support the change. Finally, in step 5, the manager works to decrease the cultural forces that resist the new practice pattern by reframing or tailoring the innovation or changing the culture (see box).

- *Reframing* involves changing the conceptual or emotional view of a situation. It is a way of seeing things differently, but in a way that still fits the facts. In reframing, the interpretation of the situation changes, but the facts remain the same.
- *Customizing/tailoring* new strategies to fit with the existing culture involves altering the proposed change to fit the culture of the work group and introducing the idea in such a way that it will mesh with current cultural rules.
- *Changing the culture* means assisting employees to learn new behaviors and give them confidence that they can perform the new behaviors. Continuous reinforcement of one or more teaching sessions will be necessary for permanent change.

Lessons on Changing the Workplace*

Bottom Up and Top Down. It is easier to make change with administrative support. Be sure to clarify what levels of risk taking can be tolerated. It is most important to have the staff who provide the care or service support the need for and create the change. It is essential to have both.

The Quality Advantage. Build the change process on the institution's quality structures and processes. They support the empowerment of the front-line worker and make it clear where the decision-making responsibility lies. Physicians are more willing to change when they perceive the organization is improving systems.

The Right Pace. Too much change too fast is overwhelming, and change that is too slow is stagnating. Recognize the difference between the grumbling noise that accompanies growth and the serious noise that says "fix me." The pace of change depends on staff, unit, and department readiness; administrative support; and leaders who can lead. Build on strength. Do not lose momentum.

Time and Energy. Do not underestimate the work and commitment needed to carry on culture changes when roles change or are created. The web of interpersonal relationships becomes more intricate. The manager's role becomes more complex. More work is created for departments, for example, staffing and recruitment. Plan on ways to support each other and celebrate the small steps forward. Do not add onto already "full plates" without looking at what can come off.

Labor Unrest. Expect staff turnover and labor unrest. Changes in working conditions and expectations may result in turnover. Some staff leave because the hours no longer fit their needs or their practice does not fit the standards. Union organizing activities can result as work roles,

***Source:* Margaret Peruzzi, Denise Ringer, and Karen Tassey, "A Community Hospital Redesigns Care," *Nursing Administration Quarterly*, Vol. 20:1, Aspen Publishers, Inc., © Fall 1995.

conditions, and expectations undergo examination and change.

Flexibility. Be ready with plan B. Change is a series of approximations. Expect that delays in achieving intermediate goals and midcourse changes will occur. Have alternate plans ready that lead toward the same goal to keep the project on track.

Consultants. Use consultants selectively for their knowledge and ability to help chart the course through change. Use internal staff to implement change. A judicial mix of line and staff leaders who have earned the staff's respect and trust and have long-term accountability for project outcomes can engineer change best.

Communication. Do not depend on the grapevine to inform others. Use every means possible and use them frequently to tell the hospital what is happening and how it is going. Write in the health care publications, talk on the health care circuit, and invite other organizations to come and see for themselves. Do it, and do it often. Add more to whatever you may think is enough.

Caring. Value and care for employees as well as patients so that employees can help patients recover at a cost that society can afford. Caring is the bottom line. Make decisions in regard to that core value.

SPECIFIC ATTRIBUTES OF REENGINEERING, RESTRUCTURING, AND REDESIGN

The Reengineering Revolution*

Reengineering is the hottest thing in management today. It is an intense method that focuses on the radical redesign of systems and processes to achieve quantum leaps in performance and defined outcomes. Reengineering is about revising a process or system; it is about starting over from scratch. The proponents of the reengineering concept, M. Hammer and J. Champy (*Reengineering the Corporation: A Manifesto for Business Revolution*, New York: Harper Business, 1992), envisioned a system of reinvention and re-creation: a tossing out of "old thinking" in order to redesign a better way of doing things.

Table 6–4 summarizes the core features and philosophies of reengineering. To reengineer successfully, it is essential that everyone involved in the project have a solid, fundamental under-

---

*Source: Dominick L. Flarey and Suzanne Smith Blancett, "Reengineering: The Road Best Travelled," in *Reengineering Nursing and Health Care: The Handbook for Organizational Transformation*, Suzanne Smith Blancett and Dominick L. Flarey, eds., Aspen Publishers, Inc., © 1995.

Table 6–4 Core Features of Reengineering

- **Radical change**—The focus is on radical change in processes and systems.
- **Discontinuous thinking**—It involves a radical departure from dysfunctional ways of doing and thinking; it means breaking old assumptions and rules.
- **Innovation**—The emphasis on creativity and re-creation, going where no one has gone before.
- **Dramatic improvements**—The major imperative is realization of quantum leaps in defined outcomes, yielding dramatic, not just incremental, improvements in processes and systems.
- **Start-from-scratch initiative**—The focus is on what can be, rather than what is.
- **Genesis effect**—It is a birth, a new beginning, a time of creation.
- **Cross-functional**—This is a synergistic process, crossing multiple functions and boundaries.
- **Futuristic**—The emphasis is not on the present or past but on future operations, which demands visionary thinking and leadership.
- **Driven from the top down**—This effort requires the absolute commitment and continuous support of top-level management to be successful.
- **Organization focused**—All elements of the organization are readily involved and positively affected.

standing of these core elements. These elements also provide guidelines for ongoing assessment of whether or not reengineering is occurring.

The key to successful reengineering is to stay focused on the core features and elements of the process. The greatest mistake is to focus on the peripheral organizational elements. Confusion and frustration will generally result, and the overall objective of making radical changes and quantum leaps in performance will never be realized.

Reengineering and Strategic Planning

Reengineering must be planned well in advance. It needs to be written into the organization's strategic plan and planned for as a major initiative toward organizational transformation. It must become a routine management strategy. One method of incorporating reengineering into the constant, overall operations of the organization is to frequently address the following questions:

- What are our customer's needs, requirements, and expectations?
- What trends and changes are clearly affecting our business?
- What is the current environment of competition like?
- Which elements of our current processes and systems are not adding value?
- What is the future vision for this organization?
- What are the organizational goals and objectives for realizing the vision?
- How can current performance or products be reinvented or re-created?
- What radical changes can be made to ensure our future success?
- How flexible and fluid is the organization?
- How do we envision our future? Where do we want to be five years from now?
- What major paradigm shifts in the world are predicted to occur over the next decade, and how will they affect our business?

In many cases, simply addressing these questions will most certainly lead organizations to many reengineering initiatives.

Suggested Phases for a Reengineering Initiative

Phase 1: Internal and External Assessment. Before reengineering can happen, it is paramount that a comprehensive analysis of the organization's internal and external environment be undertaken. This analysis lays a solid foundation for the overall reengineering effort. Internal assessment means taking a long, hard, critical look at the organization. It means facing the realities of the evolution of the organization and its current status.

The assessment process must be a group effort of the organization's management team. The first task of internal assessment is to thoroughly assess the culture of the organization. The next step in the internal assessment of the organization is a focus on customers. Questions need to be answered about their needs and expectations and the level of their satisfaction. Then the assessment must identify what is dysfunctional in the organization. To complete the internal assessment, the management team must analyze basic questions on current status of quality, leadership, performance, costs, human resources, and the efficiencies of the organization. Once all of the components of the internal assessment have been completed, a clear and compelling picture of the organization will emerge.

A comprehensive assessment of the external environment must also be completed. This evaluation is essential so that the management team can fully understand the nature of the health care business and the need to act quickly to confront the realities of the changing health care system.

Phase 2: Visioning. The first step in the visioning process is to accept the realities of the internal and external assessments. The team needs to thoroughly discuss its dissatisfaction with what currently exists and to make a commitment to change the organization.

The vision must be created by the entire management team, not just a choice few. This strategy will foster a real ownership by the team for the vision. The vision must be realistic, tangible, and not so far-fetched that it cannot come to fruition. Most important, the vision must be constantly and clearly communicated to everyone in the organization and to key players outside the organization, such as the community, vendors, and payers. The vision statement should be posted in easily accessible places throughout the organization.

The vision is the foundation for the transformation of the organization.

Phase 3: Planning. This phase focuses on what needs to be done to realize the vision. Planning must focus on four major imperatives for transformation and realization of the vision statement.

- Increase the quality of all services delivered.
- Dramatically improve the work environment for employees.
- Increase customer satisfaction.
- Develop efficient and effective processes that contribute to care delivery in a cost-effective way.

The planning session must tap the skills and abilities of the management team and must be led by top management. Then the teams need to meet in small planning groups and begin writing the project plan. The goals and objectives of the project must be established. A timetable for the project should also be developed at this point. A project can take from a few months to four years, with the typical project taking 9 to 12 months.

Phase 4: Starting from Scratch. The very core of reengineering is found in the phase of starting from scratch. The previous phases lay the foundation for this critical point in the process. In this phase, actual reengineering of processes occurs. Reengineered processes need to look very different from traditional ones because reengineering is about radical change and dramatic improvements, innovation, and re-creation. To reengineer, the teams go to the drawing board, start with a blank sheet, and totally re-create the process (see Table 6–5).

Phase 5: Testing. Once teams have completed the creation of new processes, the testing phase can begin. In this phase, a performance model of the newly engineered process is developed.

Phase 6: Evaluation. The reengineering team and the employees systematically evaluate the new processes over a defined time frame. To assist in the evaluation process, defined outcomes for the project must be established. These are broad-based outcomes that can be established for any reengineering project in health care.

Phase 7: Revisiting. The last phase of the initiative is to revisit the reengineering process periodically. As change continues in the health care environment, the methodology for reengineering must constantly be revisited. As change occurs,

---

Table 6–5 Guidelines for Recreating (Reengineering) the Process

- Delete everything that does not add value; this is the essence of reengineering.
- Let no organizational facet be immune to change or elimination.
- Be innovative—break all assumptions.
- Focus on the breadth of the process.
- Innovate mental work, and do not replicate physical work.
- Focus on total customer satisfaction.
- Coordinate the management of change into the new process.
- Focus on the objectives of process reengineering.
- Focus on defined outcomes of the new process.
- Re-create processes so that workers make the decisions.
- Remodel the workflow to streamline operations.
- Incorporate automation, which is a key enabler in process reengineering.
- Design work into process teams.
- Focus on keeping the process simple.
- Cut out all redundancy in the new process.
- Implement quality initiatives in the new process.
- Set up the process for ongoing, continual improvements.
- Challenge the process as it is being created, and constantly rethink it.

environments are affected, and the need for more internal change becomes manifest. The health care system will never be static; it will constantly evolve.

Restructuring the Nursing Department*

Restructuring refers to major change initiatives, which might include the reduction of costs by being leaner, the alteration of nursing practices to gain greater focus, the discontinuation of activities unrelated to core competencies, and the creation of new organizational structures that permit participation, stimulate innovation, and flex in response to competing demands.

The restructuring of a nursing organization is clearly a major change initiative. The successful design of new nursing structures will depend on the effectiveness of project planning, management, and evaluation. Table 6–6 presents some outcomes of successful restructuring.

Stages of Restructuring

Project conception is initiated when there begins to be awareness about the limitations of a particular nursing structure. At this stage, the nursing organization moves toward problem definition through the initial assessments of strengths and weaknesses. Faltering nursing structures are examined to better understand the gap between how the structure is actually performing and how it needs to perform to meet current demands. Symptoms of poor performance are noted, along with past attempts to remedy the situation. The needs of various users, the readiness of the organization for change, the identification of potential solutions, and the delineation of general goals for the change project are also examined in great detail. This stage culminates with the production of a realistic assessment of nursing structure per-

---

*Source: Cathleen Krueger Wilson, *Building New Nursing Organizations, Visions and Realities*, Aspen Publishers, Inc., © 1992.

Table 6–6 Outcomes of Successful Restructuring

A thoughtful, well-designed, effectively implemented and evaluated restructuring project will have certain outcomes, beyond those pertinent to the change itself.

____ The structures that remain after restructuring will have added value to patient care activities.

____ Cost-cutting strategies are clearly aligned with improving delegation downward, creating a high-commitment organization.

____ Redeployment is the hallmark of the change process, so that good people are reassigned to other parts of the system. This breeds trust, security, and commitment to the future.

____ Time is no longer spent on costly, labor-intense services that detract from the provision of quality care. Nursing roles reflect only nursing work.

____ The change is seen as long term and one of continuous improvement to ensure quality. Planning and evaluation activities, as well as the allocation of resources, evidence the long-term point of view.

____ There is a clearly identified match between the organization's mission and philosophy and the new structure. Hiring practices, socialization of new employees, rewards/incentives, and administrative decision making exemplify this connection.

---

formance, organizational strengths, and weaknesses and a list of potential solutions.

Next, the organization enters into the *project selection* stage. At this junction in the project cycle, choices must be made among the potential solutions, the needs of multiple users of the nursing structure, and the value of a new structure to the whole organization. If these differing requirements can be linked together in a meaningful way, then a decision to change can be finalized.

Formal planning follows the decision to change. Identification of project timelines and outcomes, selection of a project team, delineation of implementation strategies, and selection of an evaluation methodology are the key activities encompassed in this stage of the project cycle.

Project implementation includes those activities for initiating a change, including reeducation strategies, communication methods, and controlling functions.

Milestone evaluation and project modification phases follow implementation and include the pilot evaluation and ongoing evaluations of a change, which are then used to modify the project design, if such alteration is warranted. The project is terminated with a final evaluation of the overall change.

Work Redesign*

A fundamental goal of work transformation in health care is the redesign of jobs and work processes to support seamless care throughout the organization. (See Table 6-7.)

Nurse executives, as part of the leadership team of a work transformation project, are particularly challenged to evaluate critically the structure of nursing within the organization and traditional practices and beliefs.

Numerous approaches have been created to assist leadership teams with the arduous task of integrating functional structures and practices into a seamless care delivery model without dismantling the intrinsic value of the process components. Approaches to work transformation need to be tailored to the unique attributes of the specific health care organization.

Considerations Critical to Creation of New Roles

Initiate the work transformation project with commitment to a vision that calls specifically for

---

*Source: Carol Boston, "Breaking Down the Walls without Tearing Down the House," *Journal of Nursing Administration*, Vol. 24:3, March 1994. J.B. Lippincott.

Table 6–7 Outcomes of a Redesigned Patient Care Delivery Model

A patient care delivery model that focuses on the seamless integration of health care delivery will include the following:

- Many clinical tasks and activities are assigned to unlicensed ancillary support staff in either existing or newly created roles. Wherever possible, cross-trained caregivers will provide routine care that is protocol driven.
- Clinical activities requiring professional judgment and decisions are allocated to registered nurses, creating registered nurse roles that support scopes of responsibility at the upper limits of licensure.
- High-performance work teams are created to manage the entire care delivery experience for groups of patients. Jobs are designed for all professionals, including nurses, that optimize and maximize professional education, personal expectations, and licensure stipulations.
- The seamless care delivery process for patients can be optimized with a navigator or case manager guiding the patient through the entire experience, from preadmission to postdischarge.

---

a seamless care delivery continuum and elimination of a department/functional focus. A successful work transformation effort starts with a clear vision of the attributes of a seamless continuum of care and measurable outcomes to be achieved in the process. Highly structured, compartmentalized organizations may have difficulty with this philosophical shift in breaking down traditional boundaries; however, this vision is critical to achieving outcomes.

Use a multidisciplinary approach to identify all clinical tasks and activities necessary to support a comprehensive patient care experience within the organization. This team will work collaboratively to identify those activities required to manage the patient care experience across traditional organization boundaries, whether they are at the department or functional level. By focusing on all clinical components and activities of patient care, this analysis will form the framework for discussion of appropriate clinical roles and responsibilities in an integrated approach to the patient care delivery experience.

Use a multidisciplinary approach to reach consensus on clinical activities that require professional licensure or certification. Once all clinical activities have been identified, the team can consider how they can be most appropriately allocated among members of the care delivery team, at all times focusing on the patients' needs versus those of individual departments. Each caregiver on the team will have ownership for the entire patient experience, rather than the individual tasks within it.

Validate the delineation of clinical roles with relevant licensure, regulatory, and accrediting agencies. The roles and accountabilities of the various caregivers agreed to by the team should be compared with state laws and practices, as well as requirements of outside agencies such as the Joint Commission on Accreditation of Healthcare Organizations and state accreditation bodies. Do not depend on acceptable historical practice and organization beliefs to drive the creation of jobs that are compliant with external requirements.

Use designated, specific focus groups to gain feedback on the new clinical roles and to achieve front-line consensus for the delineated clinical accountabilities of various caregivers in the integrated model.

Pilot test the care delivery model and the new clinical roles, ensuring the existence of the infrastructure essential to support these roles. Pilot units should be selected carefully to ensure that all staff members are committed and prepared to support the unit and the new care delivery roles that are patient focused rather than department driven.

Carefully disseminate the care delivery model organizationwide, and provide for role customization, as appropriate. Instill broad competencies for care delivery roles so that essential competencies for all care delivery roles are consistent throughout the organization.

PRACTICAL TIPS ON TRANSFORMATION PROJECTS

Starting Out

Development of a Vision*

Some people advocate tearing down the old system and starting from scratch. Whether or not you concur, you need as fresh an approach as possible; you do not want to be unduly burdened with the paradigms of the past in the design of future improvements. You also need to learn from mistakes and victories of the past. In addition, the powers that be simply may not permit starting from scratch, at least until some credibility has been established for the approach and team.

It is probably best to start with a high-level analysis and then concentrate on a small number of processes. Try using the following design approach.

Make a list of what you like and do not like about the existing system, and what you would like to see. Feel free to consult others—process owners, users, customers, suppliers, auditors, and others. Then lay this aside for awhile.

Look at alternatives, learn about what else is available, benchmark, and so forth. Read books, take seminars and courses, read reports and success stories, and make pilgrimages to hallowed sites of success.

Brainstorm approaches. Agree on mission, vision, and focus. Set some overall improvement targets.

Then construct an *abbreviated* "as-is" process map to determine what is happening now and where the waste and delays are occurring. Use this to better understand the process, generate issues lists, and target more specific improvements than from the previous steps.

Construct a "to-be" model of the proposed process, including flow diagrams, organization, forms, procedures, and so forth.

**Source:* Reprinted with permission of APICS-The Educational Society of Resource Management, Falls Church, VA. 1994 APICS International Conference Proceedings.

Challenge Existing Approach*

Start with an assumption in the back of your mind that the old way can be improved enormously—the odds are with you. Allow yourself to be proved wrong in some areas, but do not count on it. This forces more critical thinking. Compare the results of the current process to your ideal mission statement and note the differences. Then brainstorm how it can be improved significantly.

It is hard to get people to challenge existing approaches, unless you do the following:

- Remove possible threats to them for doing so. This can best be done by demonstrating that staff can do it and survive. Ensure that people are rewarded, not punished, for making improvements. One organization was in the habit of laying off team members after improvements were made—a real motivator.
- Expose teams to alternative models for doing business. This can be accomplished through education, site visits, reading, participation in professional societies, and group discussions.
- Assign leadership or lead the charge yourself. Set the example by challenging the status quo and soliciting better ideas. Encourage others to do this as well.

There is no need to be totally original in your thinking. Find out what "best practices" are in your industry and others with transferable concepts. Possibly even collaborate with other organizations in developing better processes (void where prohibited by law).

Try to disregard the existing organizational structure when developing the ideal process. Look at the objectives that need to be accomplished, the processes that are needed to support them, and, finally, at the resources (including organization) needed to accomplish them.

Plotting the Process*

Service delivery processes need to be evaluated critically at the microlevel so that redundancies and non–value-added steps can be eliminated. This goal can be accomplished through the use of a method called *process steps innovation* (PSI), which identifies opportunities to streamline workflow. The following components are incorporated in the process:

- creation of a general flow map, which provides a snapshot of the whole task
- creation of a detail flow map, which provides a ground-level picture of every step that takes place in each area of the general flow map
- assessment of turnaround time—the time it takes to complete a detail step and the attachment of cost to same

In general, a *process timeline* outlines the general categories and subprocesses required at each phase of the redesign. The value of such a document lies in identifying needed resources as well as the sequence in which key activities should occur so that the redesign proceeds as smoothly as humanly possible.

The timeline allows the redesign team to look at the total process in a snapshot type format. It allows the owner of the process to have control over such things as the budget. It provides a communication tool to all members of the redesign team. It describes who is doing what and when. The timeline also provides information on the cost to the organization from start to end.

An additional advantage of using a process timeline is that it provides a written format for

Source: George Miller, "Reengineering: Forty U$eful Hints," *Hospital Materiel Management Quarterly*, Vol. 17:2, Aspen Publishers, Inc., © November 1995.

Source: Sister Anne Hayes and James N. Phan, "Mercy Healthcare's CARE 2000: An Evolution in Progress," *Nursing Administration Quarterly*, Vol. 20:1, Aspen Publishers, Inc., © Fall 1995.

the redesign. Therefore, when a member of the redesign team vacates a position, someone else can take over with little or no delay in the process.

Project/Planning Team Structure*

The following approach sets up a master project working with multiple planning teams.

*Source: Cathleen Krueger Wilson, *Building New Nursing Organizations, Visions and Realities*, Aspen Publishers, Inc., © 1992.

It enables a maximum number of people to be involved in planning, while a limited number make the final planning recommendations. This approach addresses the inefficiency created by large groups while maximizing participation. The project team has one member from each major group affected by the change, plus top administration. The project team has the authority to request work of the planning teams, accept the work completed, or to return it for more study. In addition, the project team implements and monitors the activities it has approved.

The project team has many planning teams assigned to it, which do the actual staff work needed for the design of implementation activities. These are described in the box below.

- *Planning Team #1: Organizational Preparation*—Planning and scheduling the communications required to assist key groups in understanding the change and the timetable for implementation
- *Planning Team #2: Management Development*—Identifying management skills required for implementation and providing management education if necessary; delineating expectations of managers during implementation, including time frames for manager behavioral changes
- *Planning Team #3: Operations*—Planning for operational needs during implementation, including information systems, accounting department function changes, and communication requirements
- *Planning Team #4: New Structure*—Designing the new delivery system, specifying implementation steps and schedule
- *Planning Team #5: Human Resources*—Developing new job description and performance appraisals along with date of implementation
- *Planning Team #6: Evaluation*—Creating the design and methodology for evaluations; scheduling for baseline, midpoint, and final evaluation points

---

Part II

The Working Environment

Chapter 7

Organization

OVERVIEW

The organization is designed to integrate the efforts of individuals and groups to accomplish the work to be done. Each organization has its own culture, which provides meaning to the decisions made and the directions taken in accomplishing the mission. Several of the organizational structures presented emphasize command and control perspectives, or empowerment perspectives, which reflect beliefs about how systems operate and how people work together.

Elements of Organizational Structure*

Organizational structure is the way in which the component units of the organization are related to one another to accomplish the goals of the organization. It is defined as the formal pattern of relationships among positions, directing the processes and functions of the organization. The components of the structure include standardization, centralization of authority, specialization, coordination, communication, and innovation.

Standardization is defined as a dimension of structure indicating the degree to which the organization relies on rules and procedures to guide the behavior of employees. An example of standardization is a department policy that explains the procedure for an employee to request vacation time.

Centralization of authority is defined as a dimension of structure indicating the degree to which the locus of authority is contained in one or a limited number of positions. An example of centralization of authority is the chain of accountability displayed in the organizational chart.

Specialization is defined as a dimension of structure specifying the extent to which the duties of each role are clearly specified. This may be narrowly defined to specific tasks within an organization (e.g., phlebotomist) or more broadly defined as a specific function (e.g., financial duties).

Coordination is defined as a dimension of structure that identifies the process of combining the efforts of subsystems to achieve the goals of the organization. An example of coordination is the clinical pathway developed for an oncology client.

*Source: Catherine Loveridge, "Organizational Design," in *Nursing Management in the New Paradigm*, Catherine Loveridge and Susan H. Cummings, eds., Aspen Publishers, Inc., © 1996.

Communication is defined as a dimension of structure in which information is transmitted throughout the organization to provide data for decision making, to motivate employees, to exercise control, and to express satisfaction or dissatisfaction with operations.

Innovation is defined as a dimension of structure that describes the extent to which the organization supports and encourages the development of unexpected and creative solutions, for example, an organization's commitment to the implementation of nursing research findings in clinical practice.

Organizational Models*

The elements of organizational structure assume different degrees of prominence in different organizational models. The most common of these models include the functional model, the bureaucratic model, the matrix model, and the shared governance model.

1. Functional Model

The functional model of organizational structure relies on dividing up activities to maximize standardization and routinization of repetitive tasks. An example of this type of organization is found at the nursing unit level by assignment of a medication or treatment nurse who is responsible for administering medication to all clients on the unit. The intent of this type of organization is to improve efficiency by streamlining processes. In this model, *line activities* are those activities directly involved in the principal work of the organization showing a direct line of authority. *Staff activities* are those activities provided to support the work of the line. For example, in nursing, the nurse educator who is responsible for the orientation of new nurses would be considered in a staff position. Usually,

no subordinates report directly to those in staff positions. The *chain of command* describes the flow of authority in an unbroken line from the highest level, usually the executive, to the lowest. The second principle, *unity of command*, specifies that no subordinate should be responsible to more than one superior. In organizations in which professional nurses are employed, these components of a functional organization are of limited usefulness because professionals are responsible not only to the organization as employees hired to provide specific services but also to society in fulfilling a commitment that is the basis of the bond established between society and the profession.

2. Bureaucratic Model

In the bureaucratic model, coordination requires that people responsible for subdivisions of work be placed in authority positions where work is coordinated by orders from superiors to subordinates, reaching from the top to the bottom of the enterprise. The chain of command in a bureaucracy is represented by levels of graded authority in which there is supervision of lower offices by the higher ones.

The bureaucratic model of organization includes many features of the functional model, but it is more complex. The term *bureaucracy* has often been used to indicate difficulties in getting things done. In reality, many features of a bureaucracy are desirable, but the ways in which these elements have been put into practice often cause the problems associated with the term.

Other characteristics include the principle of fixed and official jurisdictional areas, generally ordered by rules or administrative regulations; the fact that management is a primary duty and as such requires specific management expertise and full-time commitment; and the fact that management follows general rules that can be learned and applied equitably, so that no favoritism or special privilege is permitted.

This limited viewpoint has resulted in centralized decision making, in which authority is vested in the department rather than shared with the individual clinician, standardized policies and procedures replace individualized care, manage-

Source: Adapted from Catherine E. Loveridge, "Organizational Design," in *Nursing Management in the New Paradigm*, Catherine E. Loveridge and Susan H. Cummings, eds., Aspen Publishers, Inc., © 1996.

ment replaces leadership, and quality equates to adequate rather than excellent. Reliance on rules that assist in confronting complex rather than simple problems results in confusion when rapid change is required to meet uncertain conditions.

3. Matrix Model

The matrix organizational design was developed to improve the responsiveness and focus of organizations. Characteristics of this design include the distribution of authority and resources to the operational level of the organization, dual reporting and accountability channels, and multidisciplinary membership.

The matrix model of organization provides the expertise needed to provide quality care through the functional leadership dimension. At the same time, cost and efficiency are controlled through the service or product dimension. Although this model is being used more frequently in complex organizations, it still presents challenges for the professional employee. The dual channels of authority can be confusing to both managers and employees and can lead to interpersonal and role conflict.

4. Professional Practice Model

This model is a new organizational structure that evolved in health care facilities where industrial designs have proved inadequate to address professional employee issues. The foundation for these models is the assumption that professionals, those who do the work and are closest to it, need little administrative direction. Their professionalism substantiates their ability to be accountable as individuals and to evaluate and govern themselves through a structure of their peers. These models include *shared governance at the department level* of the organization and *self-directed work teams* at the *unit level of operation*.

Shared governance. In shared governance, the organization formalizes its commitment through a vote of the staff and the development of by-laws designed to direct the way in which authority, responsibility, coordination, and communication will be allocated throughout the new structure. This form of participatory structure is treated at length later in this chapter.

Self-directed work teams. Self-directed work teams offer a unit-level approach to improving accountability by the staff in clinical practice. In this organizational model, staff are represented on committees and councils (e.g., research, education, quality improvement, and clinical practice) that are responsible for developing policies and making decisions regarding their areas of responsibility. These teams may be multidisciplinary in membership and may operate in a process system. The team may also be structured on a hierarchical basis, that is, on many different levels such as in a patient care team. Nontheless, the authority is still participatory or shared. In addition, these self-directed work teams often assume responsibility for aspects of operational management. (Further discussion on this development appears later in this chapter and also in Chapter 8.)

A comparison of the major organizational models along with the components of organizational structure is presented in Table 7–1.

Management Challenge: Coordination and Structure*

Determining the proper structure for health care organizations will be one of the management challenges of the next century. This is because there must be a fit between a health care organization's structure and strategy and the environment in which it operates. In the delivery of health care, coordination and integration across many work groups are required if the institution is to provide each patient with the right thing at the right time in the right place. In a health care facility, almost every part must operate in coordination with the others. This puts a heavy burden on the enterprise: Its managers must ensure that adequate communication occurs between operating units, scheduling, and staffing for those tasks that need to be performed at precise times.

Enterprises that function with operating units in relative isolation and with low requirements

---

*Source: David B. Starkweather and Donald G. Shropshire, "Management Effectiveness," in *Manual of Health Services Management*, Robert J. Taylor, ed., Aspen Publishers, Inc., © 1994.

Table 7–1 Chart —Key Concepts in Organizational Models

	Standardization	Authority Centralization	Specialization	Coordination	Communication	Innovation
Functional Mode	Maximized for uniformity	Authority flows from highest to lowest positions	Development of specialists for repetitive work	Departments report to an administrator who integrates activities	Upward communication from departments and downward directives from administration	Limited to leadership group
Bureaucracy	Written procedures guide practice	Authority flows from highest to lowest positions	Staff positions serve line positions	Span of control in positions arranged in a hierarchy to permit direction from superiors	Formal channels through chain of command	Limited to span of operation
Matrix	Integration of procedures for effective results	Dual authority from functional and service lines	Multidisciplinary use of special expertise	Maximized due to integration of several disciplines	Maximized across organization	Maximized due to synergism
Shared Governance	Policies and procedures developed by those governed by them	Accountability for practice placed with practitioners, organizational responsibilities shared with administration	Roles for expert clinicians designed by staff group	Councils include representatives from all groups	Coordinating council disseminates all decisions to members	Encouraged through council support

for coordination can function fairly well using *vertical communication:* Information passes up and down the hierarchy, and it is sufficient for coordination between units to take place at the top. By contrast, health care organizations, with their high coordination requirements, must have effective *horizontal communication:* Information must pass between parts at the operating level as well as at the top.

Management Structure

Organizational coordination and integration are determined largely by management structure. The management structure of an organization determines not only the authority and account-ability of various persons in the structure but also the pathways of communications and coordination between units—who does what for whom and when. The management structure assigns responsibility for effective coordination to certain points, usually called the points of integration.

Management structures that enhance vertical communication take advantage of specialization. But the grouping together of specialists limits their ability to communicate and coordinate with other personnel in the organization; they are more likely to work with each other to improve their internal functioning. An example is the hospital pharmacy. If a large hospital is structured along vertical lines, all the pharmacists employed by the enterprise are placed in one department and one location, and the official in charge of that department deals with coordination between the pharmacy and other operating units. The point of integration is near the top of the enterprise and not at the operating level. It is usually found in a functional organization.

Restructuring to enhance horizontal coordination results in a relatively flat hierarchy. The organization must abandon the efficient grouping of like specialists and instead establish points of integration at operating levels. For example, each pharmacist might now serve a group of patient care units totaling, for example, 75 beds to improve the integration of the pharmacy function with the rest of the patient care operation.

A number of other health care facility functions and departments can similarly be restruc-tured. The final result is that the health care facility becomes a product organization: The management structure no longer groups like specialists together, the point of integration is at the operating level, and the new "mini-facilities" (75-bed units) each contain a mix of people whose functions need to be coordinated and integrated. The term *product organization* is applicable because the basis of organizing is to provide patient care (a product) effectively rather than to perform certain specialized functions efficiently.

Choosing an Integration Structure

The kind of structure chosen—functional or product—depends on the size and complexity of the enterprise. The general problem with a large functionally structured organization is that its lines of communication and accountability have become overlong, running through numerous vertical layers. Information is distorted and de-layed, yielding either wrong responses to prob-lems or responses that are too late. Further, the specialized units become more isolated and cease to understand or even care about their fit with the rest of the enterprise. Top management in-troduces more and more staff level coordination and control specialists, but without reorganiza-tion, they remain ineffective (and are expensive as well).

A small organization must organize along functional lines because it would be too costly to duplicate all the specialists. But since it is small, the job of integration is done fairly well anyway.

By contrast, a large organization can afford to organize along product lines. In fact, this is a better alternative for it, because a large organi-zation structured functionally does a poor job of integrating around its product.

ORGANIZATIONAL CHARTS

Organizational charts are graphic representa-tions of how organizational systems are arranged. On the surface they primarily appear to define structure by illustrating the titles of departments and the titles of the people in charge. They also depict systems of communication, authority, and decision making, however. In fact, they are the formal representation of how the organization, the largest system, has chosen to arrange those functions and subsystems that must come together for the organization to act as a system to realize its goals. (See Figures 7–1 and 7–2.)

In daily use, organizational charts are looked at most often to determine lines of authority and reporting relationships. They usually take a pyramid shape, with one person at the top and several expanding layers of management between the top and the front line, where the service is provided or the product manufactured. This shape was believed to be best suited for organizations that are experiencing high growth and have an interest in control and planning; however, it may no longer be pertinent in today's organizations.

Organizational charts can also serve a useful purpose for the working nurse manager. They can be a valuable resource in determining the systems that the nursing department affects and in deciding who needs to be included in planning changes because of the possible impact on

Figure 7–1 Standard Nursing Organization

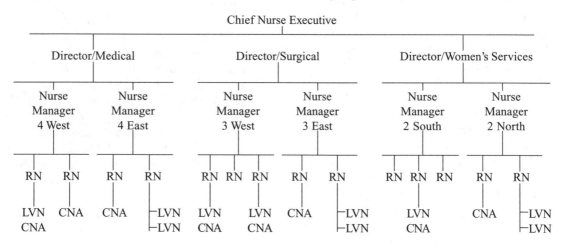

Bureaucratic Model of a Nursing Department

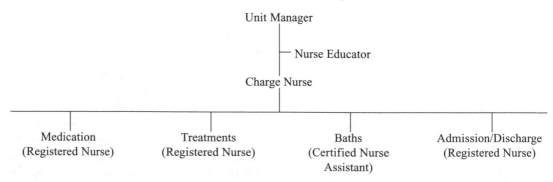

Functional Model of a Nursing Unit

Source: Catherine Loveridge, "Organizational Design," in *Nursing Management in the New Paradigm*, Catherine Loveridge and Susan H. Cummings, eds., Aspen Publishers, Inc., © 1996.

Figure 7–2 Flattening the Organizational Structure

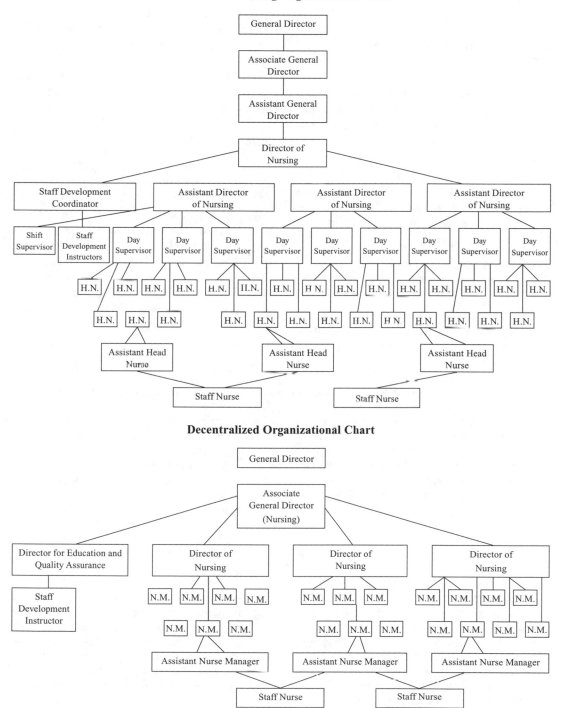

Traditional Nursing Organizational Chart

Decentralized Organizational Chart

Source: Reprinted with permision from *Nursing Economics,* 1993, Volume 11, Number 1, pp. 46–47. Reprinted with permission of the publisher, Jannetti Publications, Inc., East Holly Avenue, Box 56, Pitman, NJ 08071-0056; phone (609) 256-2300, fax (609) 589-7463. (For a sample issue of the journal, contact the publisher.)

their system. Furthermore, they clarify who needs to approve decisions or participate in making them.*

Organizational Status of the Nurse Administrator**

In this era, many new forms of organization in health care are likely to be seen. The corporate models will vary, and the horizontal linkages of similar organizations (e.g., numbers of acute care hospitals) and vertical linkages of different purpose institutions (e.g., acute care plus long-term care facilities) will call for experiments in organizational arrangements. In all cases, the nursing executive's objective is to see that nursing achieves the recognition in organizational design required for it to achieve its necessary goals in the organization.

The two levels of nurse executives in many organizations today include (1) the institutional executive and (2) the corporate nurse officer. There are complexities related to both these positions, but everyone needs a clear understanding of who is accountable to whom for what functions and responsibilities.

Institutional Nurse Executive

Nurse executives in a single institution (freestanding or in a corporation) need to consider their placement on the table of organization. Ideally, they will prefer to report to the chief executive officer (CEO). Whatever that person's title—CEO, president, or other—CEO will be used here to indicate the top hired official with accountability to a board or to a central corporation officer in a multi-institution corporation. It is preferable in most cases that chief nurse executive officer (CNEO) report to this person in the facility. (See Table 7–2.)

*Source: Alice A. Kayuha, "Organizational Systems," in *Nursing Management in the New Paradigm*, Catherine Loveridge and Susan H. Cummings, eds., Aspen Publishers, Inc., © 1996.

**Source: Barbara Stevens Barnum and Karlene M. Kerfoot, *The Nurse as Executive*, ed 4, Aspen Publishers, Inc., © 1995.

Table 7–2 Nurse Executive's Responsibility to the Governing Board and the CEO

- *To demonstrate how accomplishment of the nursing department's mission statement will support the overall organizational achievement of its missions.* The mission statement of the department of nursing does not restate that of the organization but rather describes specifically how the nursing department will support achievement of the organization's mission.
- *To define outcomes of nursing services.* Nurse executives must define outcomes of nursing services, provide a clear picture of contributions by nursing, and define how nursing can be packaged and marketed.
- *To show connections between market positions and level of expert nursing services as a competitive edge.* The nurse executive must be able to articulate what services nurses provide that are unique and cannot be provided by other workers.

- *To interpret specific threats and opportunities in changing environments.*
  - Opportunities are any favorable situations (often a trend or change) that can be exploited by implementation of a strategy.
  - Threats are any unfavorable situations in the nursing department's external environment that are potential barriers or constraints to fulfilling the nursing department's mission, and therefore the organization's mission.

  Factors in the external environment can be listed and prioritized depending on the organization. Nurse executives can analyze these factors, outline the implications for the specific organization, and pose relevant strategic strategies for discussion, debate, modification, and board approval.

Source: Diane E. Nitta and Joan Gygax Spicer, "The Nurse Executive's Responsibility to the Governing Board," *Aspen's Advisor for Nurse Executives*, Vol. 4:11, Aspen Publishers, Inc., © August 1989.

At one stage, the pattern of having the CNEO report to the top executive was almost routine, but with growing complexities in health care industry, some major institutions have redesigned to have the CNEO report to the second administrative officer, here titled chief operating officer (COO), although the titles may vary.

When the institution is very large, there may be some justification for having the CNEO report to the second officer, thus the "inside" role of managing the institution may fall to the COO. If, however, reporting to a COO actually means that nursing is seen as merely one operational center among others, then the candidate should be concerned about the placement. The issue is, What does the organizational placement of the CNEO say about how nursing is perceived by the organization?

Multi-Institution

In the multi-institution corporation, CNEOs may have a dual reporting relationship whereby they report to both an institutional CEO and a corporate nurse executive. A matrix design of this sort is common today, and the important need is for clarity concerning the nurse executive's accountability to each boss. Is the position in a hierarchical line reporting arrangement to both superiors? Or is the relationship to a corporate nurse executive a coordinative (staff) relationship? Or are both relationships that of line authority, with the content of accountability different to each superior?

The answers to these questions may be complex; the issue is whether the nurse executive knows what product is required by each boss. Further, the CNEO will want to be assured that he or she has the authority requisite to deliver on those expectations.

Corporate Level Nursing Officer

If the nurse executive is seeking a corporate position, the question of authority becomes even more important. If the nurse executive is responsible for CNEOs who also report to institutional CEOs, what is his or her power to enforce directives for these nurse executives? Has the organization developed ways to resolve conflicts if, for

example, he or she issues a corporate directive that conflicts with orders given to the institutional CNEOs by their respective CEOs?

Lines of relationship and power are complex today, but when there are no institutional paths for resolution of conflict, there may be difficulties ahead. One mitigating force, of course, is the nurse executive's ability to foster positive interpersonal relationships. But that skill alone will not suffice for the nurse executive in a highly competitive environment with other executives who care more about building kingdoms than fostering cooperation.

NURSING DEPARTMENT ORGANIZATION

Overview*

The nursing services department is organized in a pyramid fashion very much like the health care facility as a whole. The primary responsibility rests with the director of the nursing services department, referred to as the director of nurses (DON) or vice president of nursing.

Directors are usually selected because of their management abilities; they are often registered nurses with advanced degrees (sometimes in the specific discipline of nursing services administration). Often, the director has one or two assistant directors to aid in the management of the department. The title of nurse manager is frequently given to the position held by a registered nurse who supervises or directs the activities of two or more nursing units. The nurse manager may manage and direct the many nursing service activities during the evenings, nights, or weekends; thus, the titles of night manager, weekend manager, or day manager are often applied. If a health care facility has a nursing school, the director of nursing is often responsible for both the nursing services and the nursing school. Or the nursing school may have its own director who reports to the director of nurses. If there is no

---

Source: I. Donald Snook, *Hospitals: What They Are and How They Work,* ed 2, Aspen Publishers, Inc., © 1992.

school of nursing, the training function of the nursing department is usually assigned to an assistant director who is responsible for the education, orientation, and continuing in-service education of all employees in the department of nursing.

The nursing services department is also organized along geographic lines. Each of the nursing service responsibilities for patient care is decentralized to a specific location in the health care facility called a nursing unit or patient care unit. Certain responsibilities and functions to operate a nursing unit are assigned to a head nurse. A head nurse or nurse manager supervises the personnel in a patient care unit. This person is accountable for the quality of the nursing care on the unit, controls the supplies, and schedules the staff. Usually the head nurse has a series of staff nurses. The staff nurses are assigned specific responsibilities for the nursing care of patients on the nursing unit.

The Nursing Unit

The nursing care of the health care facility is organized in a decentralized fashion into patient care units or nursing units. The size of nursing units varies. They can be very small, with 8- to 10-bed units for specialized care, or they can be large, with 60- to 70-bed units. Perhaps the most common size is between 20 and 40 beds per unit.

*Specialized Nursing Units**

In addition to the overall responsibilities and functions of nursing services, the units also carry more specific responsibilities and functions of patient care, varying with each nursing unit. The establishment and execution of educational programs for staff and student nurses may also be functions of these special nursing units.

Medical and Surgical. While medical conditions are not easily divided into distinct categories, medical nursing is considered a specialty in that normal and abnormal reactions or symptoms of diagnosed diseases must be recognized and reported. The patient with a stroke or a cardiac condition requires a much different type of nursing from that given the patient with an ulcer or diabetes. Patients who undergo surgery also require special preoperative and postoperative care.

Pediatrics. This service embraces the care of children. Care of the newborn is usually in a separate unit located in the obstetric unit. The activities of the pediatric unit require understanding of the unique needs, fears, and behavior of children, which is reflected in the type and degree of nursing care given. Where illnesses require protracted convalescence, educational and occupational therapy become concerns of the nursing service. Relationships with parents pose further important responsibilities.

Obstetrics. Prenatal care, observation, and comfort of patients in labor; delivery room assistance; care of mothers after delivery; and nursing care of newborns are important responsibilities of this unit. Obstetric nurses assist in instructing new mothers in postnatal care and care of the newborn. Care of the newborn, particularly the premature, requires special nursing skills dictated by their unique requirements.

Psychiatric. While most emotionally disturbed patients are treated in specialized facilities, the general hospital also recognizes a responsibility and provides care for the mentally ill. Nursing care of patients with mental illness requires a knowledge of their various behavior patterns and how to cope with them. Techniques must be learned for dealing with all types of problem behavior so that skilled, therapeutic care is given to such patients.

Operating Room. This unit has primary responsibility for comforting patients in the operating room, maintaining aseptic techniques, scheduling all operations in cooperation with surgeons, and determining that adequate human resources, space, and equipment are available.

Source: Job Descriptions and Organizational Analysis for Hospitals and Related Health Service, U.S. Training and Employment Service, U.S. Department of Commerce, 1970.

Nursing personnel assist the surgeon during operations and are part of the surgical team. Preparation for operations includes sterilization of instruments and equipment; cleaning up after operations is also part of the unit's responsibility. In many health care facilities, the recovery room unit is an adjunct responsibility of the operating room unit. Special nursing attention must be given to patients after an operation until they have completely recovered from the effects of anesthesia.

Emergency Department. This unit is responsible for emergency care and for arrangements to admit the patient to the health care facility, if necessary. The unit completes required records; makes reports to police and safety and health agencies; handles matters of payment and notification of relatives; and refers patients to other services within the facility or community, as needed.

Special Care Units*

The contemporary health care facility may have a variety of special care units to manage and maintain patients with special illnesses and injuries. These areas may include hemodialysis or renal dialysis centers, inpatient alcoholic and drug addiction units, pediatric units, and skilled nursing facilities for long-term care, as well as the more commonly found units discussed below.

Intensive Care Units. The most common type of special care unit in a hospital is the medical/surgical intensive care unit (ICU). The purpose of ICUs is to manage the critically ill patient who is in a precarious clinical status and requires "eagle eye" supervision. ICU cases could be patients in shock, patients who have had strokes, or persons with heart failures, serious infections, respiratory distress, and so forth.

By marshaling the hospital's resources in one geographic area, it is much easier and efficient to provide high-quality care. Not only are sophisticated equipment and instrumentation avail-able in ICUs, but a highly concentrated nursing staff is also used.

Coronary Care Units. Coronary care units (CCUs) do for cardiac patients what ICUs do for severe medical and surgical patients.

For both ICUs and CCUs, it is usual to have a medical director assigned either full time, part time, or on a rotating basis to manage the units medically. Individual attending physicians manage their own patients.

The nurse's role in these units is critical. The nurses should be intelligent observers, and they must be able to interpret changes in a patient. Under critical circumstances, they might have to diagnose and even treat the patient. One of the prime objectives of the CCU is to detect early signs of impending cardiac disaster so that it can be treated before cardiac arrest takes place.

Neonatal ICU. A special offshoot of the ICU is the neonatal intensive care unit, which specializes in the management of critical health problems in the newborn. Caring for the critically ill newborn requires a specially trained nurse and physician. Neonatal intensive care units have had great success in the handling of premature infants, giving them a new lease on life.

Using a Clinical Nurse Manager Framework*

In one decentralized nursing service system (Figure 7–3), each major clinical nursing specialty has become a division. The individual divisions function with a high degree of autonomy under the direction of a division head and with the coordinated efforts of clinical coordinators and clinical nurse managers.

Just as each major clinical specialty becomes a division, each patient care area becomes a unit under the direction of a clinical nurse manager. The units may vary in patient census and patient

---

Source: I. Donald Snook, *Hospitals: What They Are and How They Work,* ed 2, Aspen Publishers, Inc., © 1992.

Source: D.M. Stitely, "The Role of the Division Head in a Decentralized Nursing Service System," *Nursing Clinics of North America,* June 1973. Reprinted with permission.

Figure 7–3 Decentralized Nursing Service—Clinical Supervisors

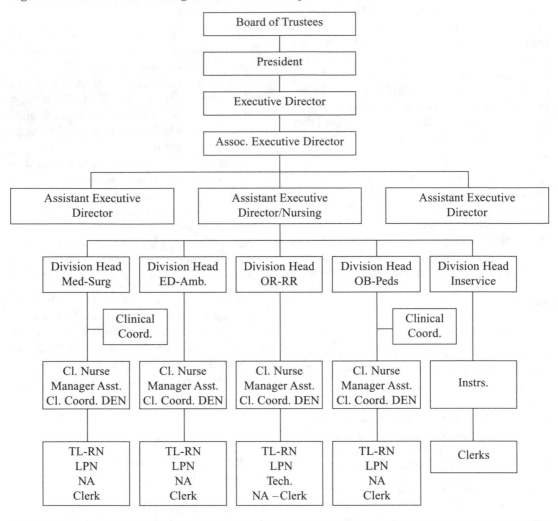

care complexity. Therefore, the management aspects will differ from unit to unit in material as well as human resource needs. The clinical nurse manager, as the first-level management person, has certain administrative duties: establishment of quotas for supplies and equipment for automatic delivery service, preparation of staff time schedules, evaluation of staff work performance, and initiation of staff disciplinary action. The clinical nurse manager is expected to make the day-by-day operational decisions that are specific to the individual unit. However, a most important element of these administrative duties is the sharing of information related to the management and operation of each and every unit

with the division head. Thus, the *lines of administrative responsibility* are clinical nurse manager to division head to the department head.

Clinical Responsibilities

The clinical advantage of a decentralized system is that the key figures in each division are clinically proficient. For example, the division head of medical-surgical nursing must be prepared educationally and with experience in the care of adult patients, while a maternal-child health background is essential for the division head of obstetrics and pediatrics. Another advantage of this system is the ability to use a clinical expert who has no administrative responsibilities, that is, the clinical coordinator. This person has the responsibility and the authority to make nursing decisions related to direct patient care. The clinical coordinator may function as a specialist with direct relationships to the patients and families, as a consultant to all staff members for improving nursing arts and skills, and as an evaluator of clinical nursing practice. Thus, the *clinical lines* of the organizational chart will follow from the clinical nurse manager on each patient care unit, to the clinical coordinator in an area of expertise, to the division head, and to the department head.

The Division Head

Since the division head has the responsibility and authority for both the management operations and the clinical practice within the specific division, methods must be established to receive unit input, refer information through proper channels, take appropriate action, and respond to staff. The division head is in the thick of a communication system that must connect all levels of nursing staff with top facility management and top management with all nursing staff. How does one individual meet these obligations? The first step is to establish a means of communicating within the individual division.

Intradivisional Communication

Of course, daily one-to-one contact between people is the most direct method of sharing information. However, this is impossible where patients and staff are numbered in the hundreds. Daily reports and weekly rounds will permit the average unit problems to be solved. Each morning and afternoon the division head meets with the clinical coordinators and the off-tour assistant clinical coordinators at the divisional intershift reports. During these times the off-tour patients and operational needs are discussed. Following the morning and prior to the afternoon report, a brief planning session between the clinical coordinators and the division head will allow for immediate clinical problems to be reviewed and extra supportive staff to be placed where the patient needs are greatest. General

management problems may also be processed through the various health care facility departments.

The division head schedules rounds with the clinical nurse managers of each unit weekly. Other members of the unit staff, nurses, and clinical coordinators are encouraged to join the rounds. At this time the unit operations are discussed and patients are reviewed.

Although reports and rounds are important for receiving information and establishing a close working relationship between individuals at the unit level, the *monthly operational council* is the most effective tool for intradivisional communication. The council consists of clinical coordinators, clinical nurse managers, representatives from the off-tour assistant clinical coordinators, and the registered nurse and licensed practical nurse staff. It is chaired by the division head. It is through this council that the division head is able to activate problem-solving techniques in a democratic atmosphere.

Interdivisional Communication

The second step in the decentralized nursing service communication system is a mechanism through which all division heads and the department head can effectively use the divisional input for planning patient care and operational management programs. Many nursing practice procedures and allied health care services are shared by all divisions. Therefore, a close interdivisional relationship must be developed. The executive council of nursing is the method most often used for communication. The participating members are the division heads and the clinical coordinators, and the council is chaired by the department head. This group is charged with the responsibility of identifying the strengths and weaknesses of the care delivered to patients. The information from the divisions' operational council meetings is pooled and more formalized fact-finding programs are generated.

In this decentralized system, the division head becomes the primary participant on the planning committees involving a specific clinical specialty area. Since the lines of communication within the divisions are so direct, the nursing input is realistic from a functional aspect. The division head is also in the advantageous position of promoting nursing to a peer relationship with the medical and administrative committee members rather than the subservient relationship that so frequently exists in a health care facility environment. This is sometimes a slow process, but eventually the clinical knowledge and managerial skills required of the division head in a decentralized nursing service system are recognized and accepted.

Budgetary Responsibilities

The department head rather than the division head is the representative to the executive finance committee. However, each division head is delegated the responsibility to prepare a projected yearly budget for his or her division. Fortunately, the inter- and intradivisional programs can provide necessary facts to justify certain budget requests. Since the nursing staff is the largest item in the facility's budget, the division head will use the information from the activity study to develop a staffing pattern.

The division head also meets with each clinical coordinator and clinical nurse manager to determine the major equipment needs. A written justification for additional hypothermia units, pacemakers, or other major items must accompany the request. The routine operational items are also adjusted. The division head makes an estimate of the operational costs by reviewing the expenditures for two previous years.

The final step in the budgetary procedure is to submit the total projected divisional costs with the justifications of the department head.

Using a Shared Governance Structure

Shared governance is a decentralized approach that allows nurses to retain influence about decisions that affect their practice, work environment, professional development, and personal fulfillment. An essential underlying belief is that, given the opportunity, environment, and framework, registered nurses will make appropriate and meaningful judgments in providing care and en-

acting their role as professionals. This organizational structure also requires practitioners to assume higher levels of accountability for patient care, clinical practice, and professional activities. By building on peer relations, governance can augment the professional practice model of a department of nursing by minimizing the isolation that a primary nursing system causes. Also, it enhances the staff's ability to take more responsibility and accountability for themselves and their peers. Its council structure fosters teamwork, thus allowing staff nurses a more active role in developing and implementing systems designed to achieve patient care outcomes and develop professional nursing practice.*

*Shared Governance Models***

There are a variety of shared governance models. The four most popular ones are the congressional, administrative, unit-based, and councilor models (see Figure 7–4).

The *congressional model* embodies all nursing staff and managers as being members of a nursing congress. A president and cabinet are elected, with at least half of the cabinet consisting of staff. Committees are formed to deal with nursing care issues related to quality assurance, education, and practice and human resources. The committees submit their work to the cabinet for action.

The *administrative model* creates practice and management structures. The work done by the councils is submitted to an executive council, composed of both staff and managers, for decisions. A forum may exist that looks at the work of the councils and makes recommendations regarding the integration of the work among the councils before the work is submitted to the executive council.

Source: Reprinted with permission from the January 1991 issue of *Nursing Management,* © Springhouse Corporation.

**Source:* Janette R. Yanko, Marge Hardt, and Jeanne Bradstock, "The Clinical Nurse Specialist Role in Shared Governance," *Critical Care Nursing Quarterly*, Vol. 18:3, Aspen Publishers, Inc., © November 1995.

Figure 7–4 Types of Shared Governance Models

Congressional

- All staff belong to congress.
- Structure is similar to federal government.
- Committees submit work to cabinet for action.

Administrative

- Practice and management structures exist.
- Forum integrates work of councils.
- Councils submit work to executive council for decisions.

Unit-Based

- Each unit establishes its own system.
- Multiple models may exist within one institution.
- There are no departmentwide coordinating activities.

Councilor

- Coordinating council coordinates activities on department level.
- Unit councils reflect department councils.
- Staff nurses are accountable for clinical decision making.

The *unit-based model* allows each unit to establish its own system of shared governance, thus encompassing many aspects of the different models.

The *councilor model* establishes councils that make practice-related decisions (see Figure 7–5). The councils are composed primarily of staff nurses with management and clinical nurse specialist (CNS) representation on each council. In addition, there is a management council composed of managers with a staff representative. The councils are accountable for practice, education, quality, and research. The management council is accountable for human, fiscal, and material resources.

Bylaws to Support the Governance Model*

One mechanism for building and supporting a professional governance model is the use of bylaws, which are simply rules that govern the internal affairs of an organization. Bylaws applied to any nursing structure should be congruent with the philosophy and goals of the corporate organization, but they should not remove the nursing professional's obligation to set standards

of practice and monitor compliance and quality within a defined practice arena.

The most important purpose of nursing bylaws in a shared governance structure is to legitimize the professional governance model of the nursing organization. Bylaws that are adopted by the professional organization and approved within the corporate structure include a governance model that will carry the necessary and legitimate authority to carry out its business. The existence of bylaws also means that the governance structure transcends individuals and does not dissolve as new leaders or executives enter the organization.

The bylaws should also describe the process of appointment to the professional nursing organization, including the process of applying for nursing staff privileges, the credentials necessary for membership, and the conditions and duration of the appointment. Further, the bylaws could delineate how the nursing staff will organize, integrate, manage, and evaluate the delivery of nursing care services. A description of how the nursing councils and committees operate and where the accountability for decision making rests could also be outlined.

Review of the nursing bylaws by the nursing coordinating council assists the governance structure in balancing the power and relationships among nursing councils and serves as an ongoing self-assessment and improvement process.

*Source: Kathryn J. McDonagh, "Nursing Bylaws: A Blueprint for a Professional Governance Model," *Aspen's Advisor for Nurse Executives*, Vol. 3:9, Aspen Publishers, Inc., © 1988.

Figure 7–5 Sample Decision Tree for Shared Governance

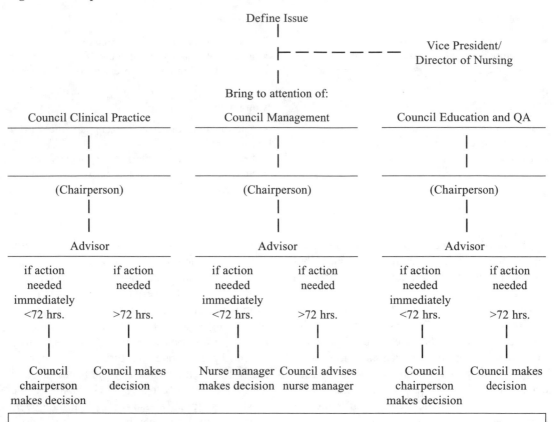

Key: Directing Issues to the Appropriate Council

The Council for Clinical Practice

— Clinical standards of nursing practice such as concerns about patient care
— Issues around role and responsibilities of the registered nurse
— Policies regarding nursing practice and resultant nursing care
— Peer review—evaluations
— Clinical ladder program
— Nursing standards

The Council for Education and Quality Assurance

— Nursing inservices/continuing education
— Preceptors
— Orientation
— Maintaining care plans, policies, procedures, care conferences
— Revision of nursing procedures

— Joint Commission review preparation
— Incident reports

The Council for Nursing Management

— Hiring/interviewing
— Staff conflicts
— Time requests/scheduling
— Policy making
— Nurse licensure

Nurse Manager

— Allocation of fiscal resources, including budgetary, operational, capital, and contingent financial resources essential to the practice of nursing
— Time cards
— Policy making <72 hours
— Back up for all of the above council activities

Source: Reprinted with permission from the January 1991 issue of *Nursing Management,* © Springhouse Corporation.

Nursing Bylaws—Key Components

- Philosophy of the professional nursing organization
- Definition of nursing
- Governance functions of the professional nursing organization
- Role of the professional nurse
- Professional nurse staff membership
- Credentials review process
- Description of the governance structure
- Discipline, appeals, and parallel levels processes
- Bylaw review and revision process

Further Decentralization: Empowerment Framework

Shared governance structures in nursing have begun a transformation paralleling that of the changing health care industry. Structures are evolving that reflect the changing values of organizational life, characterized by more fluid and open processes that increase and integrate the participation of all members of the patient care team.*

*Elements**

The staff empowerment model in health care has evolved in three distinct phases, moving from localized hierarchical staff empowerment models within nursing (nursing shared governance) to open integrated staff empowerment models in which cross-functional members of the health care team are franchised within a single empowerment framework (see Table 7–3). As organizations move through the phases of model devel-

---

Source: Jim O'Malley, "Organizational Empowerment: Moving Shared Governance beyond Nursing," *Aspen's Advisor for Nurse Executives*, Vol. 7.12, Aspen Publishers, Inc., © September 1992.

Table 7–3 Evolution of Staff Empowerment Models

Descriptors	Past	Present	Future
Model Definition	• Shared governance structures within nursing	• Separate shared governance structures within nursing and other clinical services (e.g., lab, pharmacy)	• Cross-discipline and functional teams within a single framework
Stage of Model Development	• Linear • Hierarchical	• Linear • Hierarchical	• Cross-functional teams • Integrated clusters
Degree of Empowerment	• Autonomous • Interdependence	• Autonomous • Interdependence • Coordination	• Autonomous • Interdependence • Coordination • Collaboration • Integration
Communication Modes	• Vertical • Horizontal • Need to know information	• Vertical • Horizontal • Focused on conflict	• Open • Direct • Automated networks
Decision-Making Processes	• Issues resolved via consensus	• Issues resolved via consultation and coordination	• Integrated team-based at point of service by collaboration

opment, the degree of empowerment, mode of communication, and decision-making mechanisms shift from hierarchical bureaucratic models to sociotechnical models characterized by a high degree of collaboration, integration, and cross-functional partnerships.

Redefining the Health Care Team. Decentralizing non-nursing structures and systems and developing multidisciplinary high-performing work teams are the key steps toward successful implementation of shared governance beyond nursing. The transformation from the hierarchical centralized structures in pharmacy, radiology, clinical laboratory, respiratory therapy, physical therapy, occupational therapy, speech therapy, and social services to a total staff-empowered organization will successfully move decision making for all clinical services to the point of care. The very definition of the patient care team will have to be expanded to include nonclinical services and departments such as dietary, medical records, and engineering, who also provide significant contributions to the patient care process.

Inherent in newly created empowerment structures is the potential for fragmentation and the need for coordination through centralization of defined functions within and across clinical as well as nonclinical services to ensure desired outcome attainment for the entire patient care organization. For these emerging empowerment systems to be truly successful, coordination must be individualized by function and discipline and assigned to the appropriate level of expertise within the patient care organization.

Reframing Perspectives and Values. Developing staff empowerment models beyond nursing to all of the clinical and support services will create a new patient care organization that will no longer have two-tiered management and staff systems. The current hierarchical, departmentally based systems will be abandoned and replaced with a newly empowered patient care organization that will radically defy traditional departmental boundaries. As the nursing leader, the nurse executive will need to reframe for the nursing organization a new perspective and value for each member of the newly defined patient care

team. Understanding that the services provided by the housekeeper and the admitting clerk and the plumber are corollary contributions to the services provided by the clinical pharmacist and the medical technologist and the clinical nurse will be the foundation for building a new patient care team. Making these quantum leaps in changing beliefs and values about each other's services will move health care organizations from merely a grouping of localized competing services to a coordinated and integrated high-performing patient care organization.

*Responsibilities**

Self-directed work teams that include multiskilled caregivers and support staff on patient

---

The activities of self-directed work teams include

- shared leadership and management activities
- management of production processes
- goal setting
- determination of work schedules
- review of team performance
- preparation and management of the unit budget
- coordination of interdepartmental work
- management of materials and supplier relationships
- acquisition of needed skills and knowledge
- hiring and participation in corrective actions
- quality assessment and improvement responsibilities

**Source:* Catherine E. Loveridge, "Organizational Design," in *Nursing Management in the New Paradigm*, Catherine E. Loveridge and Susan H. Cummings, eds., Aspen Publishers, Inc., © 1996.

care units often assume accountability for first-level management activities independent of the manager. In these structures, the manager, who often has responsibility for several units, consults with the staff regarding patient information, acts as a coach and facilitator for staff, and often learns of problem resolution and work group activities after strategies have been implemented.

Challenges for staff are inherent in self-directed work teams. In addition, managers who are responsible for patient care units with self-directed work teams also face the following challenges:

- managing multiskilled workers
- facilitating interdepartmental communication, problem solving, and organizational integration
- managing in old and new paradigms simultaneously
- transitioning their own role to a coach and facilitator
- orchestrating the three- to five-year transition to mature self-directed work teams
- providing team members with education and coaching related to organizational management functions and processes
- ensuring that individual and organizational outcomes are attained

A NEW ORGANIZATIONAL ENVIRONMENT FOR MANAGERS

As the health care delivery system continues to redefine itself, new kinds of relationships develop. Mergers, acquisitions, alliances, and partnerships are creating a new kind of organizational network that best positions the health care organization in a subscriber-based marketplace. (These connective relationships are discussed in greater detail in Chapter 37.)

On a theoretical level, nurse executives will have to operate on the partnership principle (see Table 7–4); on a practical level, they will have to handle the details of merging the nursing service.

Dealing with Mergers

As leaders on the management team of acute facilities, nurse executives will participate directly in merger-related activities. They will discover that in the more hard-edged mergers of today, the nursing department's performance is no longer judged by the local standards, or even compared with the limited number of facilities in a small health care corporation. Rather, nursing departments will be judged by the standards developed by fiercely competitive executives (including nurse executives) in acute care networks. Therefore, when health care facility mergers are imminent or in the early stages, nurse executives need a framework from which to chart their course. The extent of the merger adds to the complexity, a factor that is particularly important to nurse executives who are responsible for merging the patient care services. The outcome of the merger may be one health care facility with two campuses unless one facility is closed completely. The nurse executive's responsibility expands further when merging includes patient care services in several hospitals along with other facilities, such as urgent care centers or outpatient surgery facilities. In either instance, the process will be similar.*

Practical Steps**

Essentially, the role of the nurse manager is to cope with the employees' instinctive resistance or withdrawal and to channel workers' efforts into forming new work patterns—and new relationships that the workers will eventually see as profitable not only to the enterprise but also to themselves. Managerial power is best exerted in persuading staff members that change not only is

---

Source: Enrica Kinchen Singleton and Frankie C. Nail-Hall, "Charting the Course for Merger," *Journal of Nursing Administration*, Vol. 25:5, May 1995. J.B. Lippincott Company.

**Source:* Reprinted with permission from the December 1989 issue of *Nursing Management,* © Springhouse Corporation.

Table 7–4 The Partnership Principle

Perhaps there is no greater indicator of the emerging age than the notion of partnership. Partnership models mean forming unique relationships with different players. The problem for the manager with regard to these partnerships is that the rules within which competition once operated are no longer the rules of service in the prevailing marketplace. A different set of interactions, a higher level of dialogue, greater agreement on the protocols of service, and stronger relationships among the service providers are now required.

- The health care facility that was once the competitor down the street is more often becoming a part of the same service alliance, requiring integration of players not previously a part of the same system.
- The service structures are being reconfigured so that departmental structures are collapsing and other services and disciplines are now required to relate to each other in ways none ever considered possible or desirable.
- Managers are now responsible for broader areas of function as integration expands

their locus of control and challenges them to assume more of the activities of the organization that have an impact on the viability and success of the services that are provided.

- Many services are moving out of the hospital structure as reducing cost and accelerating health-related activities rather than sickness-related activities become the framework for service provision. Practitioners are not prepared for the change in focus in their relationship with each other and with those they serve.
- The skill base that was once required at the executive level now is needed at the point of service in organizational leadership, since decentralization and redesign around the service continuum require higher levels of decision making and leadership in the service arena.
- Reduction in the number of executive level roles in reengineering of the workplace is calling for more broad-based authority and independence in the service manager and results in higher levels of expectation and outcome than previously perceived for the role.

Source: Tim Porter-O'Grady, "Managing along the Continuum: A New Paradigm for the Clinical Manager," *Nursing Administration Quarterly*, Vol. 19:3, Aspen Publishers, Inc., © Spring 1995.

---

inevitable but also presents safer or broader options than they had before.

To determine just where they stand at the onset, nurse managers need to assess carefully the compatibility of the merging organizations. Traditional hierarchies create niches where deeply invested stakeholders heavily resist any changes that would alter their relationships and scopes of operational authority.

Further, every organization follows its own aging and learning cycles, which may bring "generational" conflicts to merging processes. If each organization is at a different stage of learning or maturity, attention must focus on evolving toward common ground. A clear picture of the present situation enables managers to reshape the organization in a sequence of activities that will dispel the influence of anxiety and uncertainty

while it builds a larger sense of competence, control, and commitment.

Priority I: Establish a common knowledge base. Nurse administrators need to introduce useful information on a realistic timetable with definite goals. Employees immediately need a clear, honest picture of why the merger is taking place, such as to increase market base, to diversify service offerings, or to strengthen purchasing power. Making the plans for reorganization quickly available is also a crucial step to turning everyone toward the desired direction. Therefore, nurse managers should arrange for exchange visits and meet to review one another's philosophy, standards of care, and goals, as well as policies and procedures in delivering care. Early, visible interest in pursuing common concerns signals to subordinates and superiors alike nurse managers' determination to prevent difficulties now rather than cure them later on. This is the time to learn the other health care facility's "personality" and to plan resolution of cultural mismatches.

As planning progresses, adopt a "plan, announce, act" pattern. Anticipate what staff areas are hardest hit and spend time accordingly. As soon as possible, inform and provide for those employees who will lose their present jobs. Mix employees as much as possible at all levels in the newly combined organization to eliminate "we/they" attitudes.

Priority II: Encourage a collaborative attitude. Effective collaboration develops from visible, persistent gestures of mutual respect and from open, direct communications. It is a good idea to concentrate early on blending the competencies of like staff members in the merging constituencies. How merged departments and unit managers handle job descriptions, staffing ratios, acuity systems, pay, and benefits profoundly influences the attitudes merged staff members will develop toward one another.

Priority III: Stabilize individual behavior. Comparing performance evaluations before and after mergers helps identify self-protective behaviors or those that indicate declining commitment. Concentrate on preventing or quickly resolving power struggles as well as on reassuring staff members who are considering leaving before giving the new regime a fair chance.

Priority IV: Develop new group identities and loyalties. Nurse managers of merging institutions should realize they have a relatively rare opportunity to strengthen nursing's position in the system as a whole—but only if they present a united front at corporate levels of decision and activity. Early joint activities among nursing departments and units can help establish positive networks, identify a common leadership group, and gather staff support for it. Sponsoring a community health fair or conducting a common research program helps draw groups together without threatening personal "turf."

In pursuing these priorities, nurse managers are, in effect, "unfreezing" old patterns and attitudes as painlessly as possible by introducing new information, challenges, and opportunities that put prevailing corporate cultures in a different light.

Chapter 8

Teamwork

TEAM-BASED ENVIRONMENT

Increasingly, health care organizations are being restructured around teams. This restructuring appears to be a comfortable "fit," since most of the work in health care organizations is already performed by groups of people responsible for different functions. As members of work teams, individuals end up with far greater knowledge and a better understanding of patient care needs than if they worked independently. When organized and developed effectively, multidisciplinary teams of caregivers will optimize the quality of care, and team members will be more satisfied with their work.

The range of team configurations can be quite extensive, but teams generally fall into the following categories, any one of which may be unit or department based or interdepartmental.

- *Patient care teams.* These can be multiskilled, using varied levels of skill within the same discipline (as in team nursing), or multidisciplinary, with team members crossing departmental lines to provide different functions (also called cross-functional teams).
- *Project-based teams.* These are formulated on a short-term or an ongoing basis for a specific purpose (quality improvement teams, process teams, planned change, equipment review task force).
- *Executive teams.* These cope with managerial issues and problems and may be empowered staff-level teams, as in shared governance, or administration-level teams.
- *Work group.* This is a general term often used with *team* to reinforce the concept that these people are grouped together to perform and control their work as a unit. Work groups are often designed to be self-directed or autonomous.

In general, the traditional command and control model of management is not effective with teams. If managers try to meet the challenges of leading and motivating work groups in traditional ways, the workers will continue to solve interconnected problems in a disconnected manner. Managers must set up conditions that release group potential, and the potential of each individual. This is essential when developing a team. Strong facilitation skills have never been in such demand, both from managers and from new team leaders. The new requirements are quickly making the traditional skills of managers obsolete and are challenging staff leaders new to participation in organizational decision making. Both managers and team leaders need the opportunity to develop, practice, and maintain new leadership competencies.*

The Manager's Role in the Emerging Team-Based Environment**

In the team-based approach to health care service delivery, managing the emerging relationship among various work groups creates a whole new set of challenges for the manager. In a team-based approach, the manager role is less directive and more facilitative. Expectation of leadership in this scenario calls for a broader commitment to development and growth of the staff in arenas like problem solving, effective communication, self-directed strategies, and quality-driven, problem-solving processes. There is considerably less focus for the manager on the content of work and increasing attention to the context of work and all that is necessary to support staff in their efforts.

Future managers will need to be well acquainted with database systems and the impact and management of great aggregates of information. The manager will be required to collect and generate much service and resource information for the clinical teams in order to provide them with the information they need to validate their work process and to evaluate their effort in terms of outcomes.

The manager's role in team effectiveness becomes a major focus of the position. Teams must be internally driven and self-directed if they are to maintain the relationships and integrity necessary to their work and affiliations. In the course of human relationships, however, there are breakdowns in communication, interaction, and effectiveness, all of which affect outcomes. The manager is constantly examining these characteristics and assessing the appropriate responses to them.

Pros and Cons of Teams*

A team is a highly interactive group of people who share a common goal and who work together to achieve that goal. As health care organizations become more complex, they depend more on the effectiveness of group efforts and cross-functional activities. Team building is therefore an activity that builds toward the future. It also provides considerable benefits.

- *Greater overall expertise.* The team development process helps refine a unit's diagnostic skills and increases the unit's ability to devise solutions. Teams are especially useful when they deal with methods, procedures, relationships, quality, productivity, problem solving, and decision making.
- *Synergy.* The total results are greater through team effort than what would be achieved by each member acting independently.
- *Higher morale.* The motivational needs of affiliation, achievement, and control are all satisfied.
- *Greater staff retention.* Employees are less prone to leave when they are members of teams.
- *Increased performance flexibility.* Performance flexibility can increase because there is less dependence on individuals.

On the down side, teams are not always needed. There are many responsibilities that can be handled as well or better by individuals. Persons who have unique professional or technical know-how or experience can handle specific situations faster without consulting others or getting a series of approvals.

Source: Adapted from Tim Porter-O'Grady and Cathleen Krueger Wilson, *The Leadership Revolution in Health Care: Altering Systems, Changing Behaviors*, Aspen Publishers, Inc., © 1995.

**Source:* Tim Porter-O'Grady, "Reengineering in a Reformed Health Care System," in *Reengineering Nursing and Health Care: The Handbook for Organizational Transformation*, Suzanne Smith Blancett and Dominick L. Flarey, eds., Aspen Publishers, Inc., © 1995.

Source: William Umiker, *Management Skills for the New Health Care Supervisor*, ed 2, Aspen Publishers, Inc., © 1994.

Work groups require start-up time, have a tendency to become bureaucratic, and may waste much time. When an enthusiastic focus group or task force turns into a standing committee, the topics often become repetitive and boring.

MANAGER'S ROLE IN TEAM DEVELOPMENT PROCESS

As a new team starts its work, the manager's first goals are

Reasons for Team Failure

- Breakdown in communications
- Failure to teach leadership skills to members of the team, resulting in the team being unable to respond to needs when a crisis occurs in the absence of the manager
- Lack of support, internal politics, hidden agendas, conformity pressures, favoritism, and excessive paperwork
- Too much closeness and team spirit, which shut the team off from the rest of the organization
- Competition among individuals for promotions, merit raises, bonuses, budgets, turf, resources recognition, and access to superiors
- Interdepartmental competition, which is self-defeating when there is deviation from organizational goals
- Unrealistic expectations
- Status quo barriers such as existing procedures, equipment, supplies, or environmental factors
- Disapproval or lack of action on suggestions or recommendations of team members
- Diminished enthusiasm due to lack of progress, failure to meet deadlines, setbacks, and bad results

---

- to help it define its roles, matching member expertise and interest with the process tasks
- to develop the team's operating policies
- to cross-train members in administrative and technical tasks

These activities merge into the *problem-solving* phase, where the focus shifts from tasks to process. The team will start to develop its unique mission and goals, which the manager will use to keep the team in focus and in action. Although problems and conflicts will occur throughout the life of a team, a manager's style of handling problems initially will be emulated and remembered by team members. If handled correctly, diversity and conflict can promote growth and encourage creativity. Whatever specific technique the manager uses, the overreaching problem-solving style should be to hear and appreciate differences, not try to reconcile them; to validate polarities, not try to reduce the distance between them; and to make it a practice not to avoid or confront extremes. The manager should put team energy into staking out the broadest common ground that all can stand on without compromise or force.

As trust builds and routine operations are understood, the team moves into its *peak learning phase*. It is motivated by achievement of short-term goals. Members teach other members, as well as being taught by others. The team has a unique sense of identity, learning from others' strengths and helping others improve weak areas. The team conducts most of the team's business. The manager serves primarily as consultant and advisor. Moving into the final stage of team development, members know how actions affect the whole and are fully capable of acting for the team. Informal leaders have emerged from the group. The appointed manager is now truly a resource, setting broad boundaries within which the team can function independently.*

Source: Suzanne Smith Blancett and Dominick L. Flarey, "Teams: The Fundamental Reengineering Work Unit," in *Reengineering Nursing and Health Care: The Handbook for Organizational Transformation*, Suzanne Smith Blancett and Dominick L. Flarey, eds., Aspen Publishers, Inc., © 1995.

Facilitation of Work Teams*

The Manager as Facilitator

The prevalent exhortation for leaders to build "team-based organizations" and to become effective "team builders" represents the current recognition that the outcomes of service are no longer directly produced by individuals working alone but result from the collective efforts of teams of sometimes diverse individuals.

Leaders who have developed expertise in interpersonal skills will be able to engage teams in solving the deep-rooted structure and process problems associated with the way care is delivered in a particular organization. (For assistance see Tables 8-1–8-4.)

In the health care workplace, leaders are increasingly challenged to lead temporary project teams as a flexible response to fluid changes in the environment. The critical nature of multidisciplinary problem solving, whole systems integration activities, and pluralistic work roles requires leaders who can make sure that teams remain productive in spite of the demands of their environment. As organizations move toward the use of self-directed work teams, leaders will be challenged to balance the coordinating efforts of multiple teams. These teams will not be able to be productive without concerted efforts by leaders acting in the role of facilitators.

PREPARING FOR TEAMS

The health care environment is used to teams as a way of dealing with emergencies, but not as a generalized mode of addressing day-to-day issues. The primary emphasis in health care organizations is on individualism. Therefore, management must sell the use of teams and provide their members with both basic and advanced training in how to make them effective. Facilitators must be available to help with the team process, even after training has been given. Often, teams are as much a way of getting people to talk with each other and to understand each other in highly compartmentalized organizations as they are agents of change. Management remains the primary agent of change, with teams available as their collaborators and colleagues.*

Team Leaders' Role**

Leaders must create an ambiance that features support and rewards for risk taking, creativity,

Source: Rebecca LaVallee and Curtis P. McLaughlin, "Teams at the Core," in *Continuous Quality Improvement in Health Care*, Curtis P. McLaughlin and Arnold D. Kaluzny, eds., Aspen Publishers, Inc., © 1994.

**Source:* William Umiker, *Management Skills for the New Health Care Supervisor*, ed 2, Aspen Publishers, Inc., © 1994.

Table 8–1 Facilitator Tool Kit

- *A set of warm-up activities.* Warm-up activities get team members involved in the task, clarify expectations about the work, and help members focus on the work.
- *A set of action methods.* To help teams make decisions, use methods such as brainstorming, nominal team techniques, mind-mapping, consensus building, win-win conflict resolution, and force field analysis.
- *Process observation tools.* Develop a standard set of tools to assist the organization in identifying common process issues blocking goal achievement.
- *Norm-setting guidelines.* The guidelines might be based on a set of effective behaviors that the team members agree to apply in their work. Have the team members review a sample list and then add their own. These might include statements about tardiness, confidentiality, respect, and so on.
- *Supervision processes.* Facilitators bring their own humanness to their work, which sometimes colors observations. Sessions led by a behavioral health specialist can help facilitators avoid turning their personal issues into team issues.

Source: Tim Porter-O'Grady and Cathleen Krueger Wilson, *The Leadership Revolution in Health Care: Altering Systems, Changing Behavior*, Aspen Publishers, Inc., © 1995.

Table 8–2 Sample Effective Leadership Questions for Team Workers

Helpful questions support individuals, teams, and the organization's common direction.

Purpose	Question
Support the concept of empowerment.	"Since you are closer to this process than we are, what are your findings and recommendations?"
Encourage individuals and groups to learn, share, and solve problems collaboratively.	"What information and people would be helpful to make improvements?"
Encourage decisions based on data.	"Can you explain the data to us?" "What do your data mean?"
Encourage ideas or theories for improvement while minimizing the risks of failure.	"That sounds like a good idea. Can you figure out a way to test it on a small scale?"
Demonstrate balance between people/ management and analytic/task issues.	"Do you have consensus of all the team members related to the flowchart of the current process?"
Convey and seek relationships relating to the organization's vision, values, missions, goals, and expected behaviors.	"How does this project relate to the organization's and department's mission and goals?"
Seek ways to help remove barriers perceived by the team or individuals.	"What barriers have you identified that we can help eliminate?"
Identify opportunities for improvement and focus on improvements.	"Can your team identify additional opportunities for improvement?"
Seek to understand.	"How did you reach this conclusion?"
Promote supportive behaviors.	"How can we or your manager help?"
Challenge ideas, not people.	"How can this idea be improved?"
Stimulate creative thinking and paradigm changes.	"What would you do if you had no constraints?" or "Can you think of other ways to improve this process?"
Support a culture of learning within an organization.	"What knowledge and skills would help improve performance?"
Support systems thinking.	"What impacts, if any, will your recommended changes have on other processes?"
Value people.	"What ideas do you have to provide greater opportunities for the people working in the process?"
Focus on customers.	"What input have you gathered from the patients, physicians, or other customers about this issue?"

Source: Adapted from Richard J. Coffey, Lauren Jones, Ann Kowalkowski, and James Browne, "Asking Effective Questions: An Important Leadership Role To Support Quality Improvement." *Journal on Quality Improvement.* Oakbrook Terrace, IL: Joint Commission on Accreditation of Healthcare Organizations, 1993, Vol. 19, no. 10. Reprinted with permission.

Table 8–3 Factors in Building High-Performing and Effective Teams

Success Factors	Pitfalls
• Empowerment	• Nonverbalized expectations
• Team cohesion	• Lack of information sharing
• Equality	• Lack of communication and direction
• Accountability	• Boredom
• Effective leadership	• No understanding of measurement tools
• Openness	• Inadequate incentive and recognition system
• Respect for each other	• Knowledge deficit or lack of understanding
• Recognition and acknowledgment	problem
• Positive communication patterns	• Not developing leadership skills
• Positive conflict resolution	• Avoidance of conflict
• Knowledge of the team building	
• Celebrating success	

Source: George Byron Smith and Elizabeth Hukill, "Quality Work Improvement Groups: From Paper to Reality," *Journal of Nursing Care Quality*, Vol. 8:4, Aspen Publishers, Inc., © July 1994.

Table 8–4 Team Development Flow Chart (Process Steps)

Do you perceive an opportunity to improve the —No→Consider other approaches to achieving desired levels of work group effectiveness of your work group through systematic team development activities?

|
Yes
↓

Do you feel you have the requisite knowledge —No→Read additional materials on team building and/or seek assistance from knowledgeable persons and skills to plan and implement a team development effort with your work group?

|
Yes
↓

Have you developed informational materials for —No→Develop from the literature a brief proposal on team building that describes the concept, its benefits, and your suggested approach to a program use by your work group that describe the purpose of team building, its advantages, and the development process itself?

|
Yes
↓

Based on informational materials and initial —No→Conduct additional discussions to clarify the concept and its advantages. Consider other approaches if discussions do not yield consensus discussion of team development, does your work group support implementing a team-building process?

|
Yes
↓

Is the necessary time for planning and imple- —No→Postpone implementation until staffing and workload conditions are favorable menting a team-building process available?

|
Yes
↓

continues

Table 8–4 continued

Has an agreed-upon systematic team development process been developed for the work
group?

—No→Work as a group using guidelines from the literature until an agreed-upon process can be
detailed.

|
Yes
↓

Has a nonthreatening process for resolving
conflict during the team development program
been agreed upon by the work group?

—No→Design and achieve consensus on a nonthreatening approach to managing conflict during the
team-building effort.

|
Yes
↓

Does the work group fully realize that team
development is a long-term process to
which members must remain committed to be
successful?

—No→Conduct additional discussions regarding long-
term benefits to enhance commitment to the
team-building process.

|
Yes
↓

Are work group members willing to undergo
self-evaluation through open discussions
on attitudes, feelings, conflicts, and related
matters?

—No→If an open, problem-solving climate cannot be
achieved in the initial planning sessions, seek
professional assistance or select another
approach.

|
Yes
↓

Are work group members and their leader willing to take the risks necessary to achieve tangible autonomy and shared power?

—No→If initial discussions do not produce a willingness to act autonomously, share power, and
take risks to achieve positive change, seek
professional assistance or select another
approach.

|
Yes
↓

Has the group developed effective work methods and patterns of interaction that are satisfying to the members?

—No→Evaluate work methods using management
engineering services if necessary. Hold periodic
group meetings that focus on work processes.

|
Yes
↓

Does the group periodically critique its performance and self-evaluate its role and accomplishments?

—No→Conduct management audits of the group's
work and discuss results in group sessions.
Focus on self-initiated improvements.

|
Yes
↓

Are members of the group pursuing personal
self-development in addition to the group's
efforts?

—No→Encourage and support continuing education
efforts.

|
Yes
↓

continues

Table 8–4 continued

Does the group ensure the infusion of new ideas and challenges in order to maintain its creative capacity?　—No→ Encourage and support intergroup interactions. Invite nongroup individuals to meet with the group to provide stimulation.

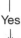

Yes
↓

Has the group established patterns of intergroup relations that are effective and satisfying?　—No→ Plan and carry out specific efforts to build effective linkages with other groups.

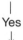

Yes
↓

Does evaluation of the team-building process reveal that it is meeting predetermined expectations?　—No→ Reexamine the process to identify and implement needed changes agreed to by the group.

Yes
↓
End

Source: Jerry L. Norville, "Team-Building Techniques for the Health Care Supervisor," in *The Health Care Supervisor: Effective Employee Relations*, Charles R. McConnell, ed., Aspen Publishers, Inc., © 1993.

openness, fairness, trust, mutual respect, and a commitment to safety and health. There must be opportunities for growth as well as security.

With the help of the team members, team leaders prepare mission statements, set goals, develop strategies and plans, design or improve work processes, provide resources, facilitate, coordinate, and troubleshoot.

Leaders must satisfy the affiliation needs of each team member. All employees want to be accepted by their colleagues. Leaders also encourage team members to train and coach each other.

The team as a unit and individuals on the team often participate in cross-functional activities. Team leaders must coordinate these activities with people in other departments and services.

Team leaders must know how to make their team effective and efficient, that is, how to make the team work smart. This cannot be accomplished without planning.

Good team leaders share certain characteristics (see Table 8–5).

Table 8–5 Characteristics of Good Team Leaders

- They provide a sense of direction and set high expectations and standards.
- They have both professional and team leadership skills.
- They are good role models. They cooperate with their counterparts in other departments, thus setting a good example.
- They provide feedback, both positive and negative.
- They criticize behavior, not people or personalities.
- They know their teammates individually.
- They are helpful and anticipate the needs and problems of their team members.
- They can answer most questions. When they cannot, they know where to get the answers.

Group Dynamics*

Understanding the dynamics of group norms, group processes, and group leadership may assist the team leader in developing and maintaining team performance.

Group Norms. It is important for the team leader to set team structure and identify the expected norms for groups. Group norms identify and define the team. The norms reduce ambiguity by providing guidance to the members. Some examples of group norms from effective teams include the following:

• Cooperation among team members is expected.
• Everyone has a role on the team and is provided with a clear expectation of his or her role.
• Decisions are made by majority rule or nominal group technique.
• Team members will be held accountable for assignments.
• Team members are expected to meet timelines and deadlines.
• Team meetings will begin on time and end on time.
• Competition between members and departments is not necessary.

The group norms evolve from the team's purpose and goals. The group norms can assist the team in attaining its quality improvement goals.

Communication Patterns. Team members' communication patterns and behaviors change as the team becomes more cohesive. During the initial stages of team building, communication patterns are generally directed toward the leader or facilitator. The sharing of ideas and problem identification is generally guarded and hesitant. However, the energy and motivation levels of the members are high. Members are highly motivated to solve the identified problem and to attain the

established goals. As the members become more comfortable and open with each other, a sense of group cohesiveness develops. The team reaches a sense of agreement on goals and expectations. Communication patterns become more evenly distributed as members interact with each other, instead of the team leader directing the communications. The group norms of the team become finalized and accepted. The team begins to deal with issues of conflict, team assignments, trust, and cohesiveness. To be effective, the members must remain focused on the established goals and objectives of the team. At this point, effective teams will begin to exhibit the following characteristics: effective problem solving, open sharing of opinions and perceptions, and attempts to include other members and provide positive support and reinforcement to each other.

Team Leadership. An effective team leader understands the concepts of leadership and the forces, scope, and limitations inherent within the leadership role. Influence, power, and authority are elements of leadership. These leadership elements have an impact on the team process. As the team becomes more cohesive, the elements of influence, power, and authority should become more evenly distributed among the other members. In effective teams, the leader plays a guide or facilitator role. The leader is also a team member and is able to present ideas, contribute solutions, and offer suggestions as can anyone else on the team.

Team leaders can develop basic skills to improve the likelihood of team effectiveness and success. The leader must develop the basic skills necessary to conduct meetings and facilitate team (group) processes. An important function of the team leader is to generate discussion about the team's mission, goals, and purpose. The leader must assist the team in remaining focused on the task in order to reach a consensus on important issues.

Finally, the climate and tone of the group is important to monitor. Individual members may have hidden agendas that may sabotage the group or decrease the effectiveness of the group. Nonverbal behaviors enhance or distract from the process. Team members need to be aware of their

*Source: George Byron Smith and Elizabeth Hukill, "Quality Work Improvement Groups: From Paper to Reality," *Journal of Nursing Care Quality*, Vol. 8:4, Aspen Publishers, Inc., © July 1994.

own nonverbal behaviors and how they impact the team's communication and performance.

The team leader must develop skills to conduct an effective group process. Learning how and when to use these skills is a function of experience, practice, feedback, and confidence in one's abilities to use the skills.

Evaluation of Group Behavior. In team building, it is important for the group to evaluate group behaviors. Having an understanding of group dynamics enhances the team's cohesion and effectiveness. An evaluation tool can be used to assist a team to monitor attributes that impact group effectiveness (see Table 8–6). The group evaluation worksheet can be used to assist members in understanding group dynamics. A member is chosen prior to the start of a team meeting to observe and record on the worksheet the attributes of the team's interactions. It is important that the observer member remain out of the current team meeting discussions so that he or she can remain objective.

The member who acts as observer is rotated each meeting to allow all members the opportunity to observe group interactions and behaviors and to develop a clearer understanding on how to use the evaluation tool. Allow five minutes at the close of the team meeting for discussion and evaluation of the observed attributes from the worksheet. The leader encourages the group to focus on the positive attributes and assist members to identify behaviors that would improve the identified negative attributes. Use the results from the evaluation tool for the team to identify strengths and weaknesses for future team performance and improvement.

Group Process Skills for Team Members*

Group process interaction is the way group members pool their abilities in a collaborative context to reach the best decision. The basic group process skills required include meeting skills, ability to generate ideas and reduce data to a usable form, and interpersonal skills of listening, participation, and conflict resolution. The next level of group processes relates to the evolution of mature group roles, problem solving, decision-making schemes, information sharing, communication, and conflict/negotiation strategies.

Group Roles. Accomplishing group tasks requires that certain group functions be performed and that group roles support them.

- *Individual roles* are played to satisfy personal needs unrelated to group tasks and unconcerned with group development or continuity.
- *Group task roles* can be assumed by any group member and are focused on problem-related tasks.
- *Group building and maintenance roles* are required of individuals concerned with the effectiveness and survival of the team.

Successful groups require different roles depending on the current stage of the task cycle or the level of maturity the group has reached (see Table 8–7). A high level of individual-centered role taking, as opposed to group-centered role taking, generally indicates a need for group self-assessment and further group process training.

Problem-Solving Skills. The problem-solving nature of many team tasks requires individual and group procedures that address the three phases summarized below:

Phase	Function
Orientation	Establishment of operating procedures Sharing of problem-related information Presentation of specialized/technical information
Evaluation	Analysis of problem Generation of alternatives Establishment of evaluation criteria Evaluation of alternatives Reconciliation of interests to achieve consensus
Control	Position group values/solutions within those acceptable to environmental powers Recommendation of alternatives Implementation of plan

Source: Adapted from Rebecca LaVallee and Curtis P. McLaughlin, "Teams at the Core," in *Continuous Quality Improvement in Health Care*, Curtis P. McLaughlin and Arnold D. Kaluzny, eds., Aspen Publishers, Inc., © 1994.

Table 8–6 Group Process Skills: Evaluation Worksheet

- Active listening
- Focusing discussions on the purpose
- Checking perceptions of the group
- Reflecting—the ability to convey the essence of what a team member has shared so that others can see it
- Clarifying—involves focusing on key underlying issues and sorting out confusing and conflicting feelings and thinking
- Summarizing—involves restating, reflecting, and summarizing major ideas and feelings by pulling important ideas together and establishing a basis for further discussion; used to summarize points of agreement and disagreement among team members
- Facilitating—by assisting the members to express their feelings and thoughts openly, and by actively working to create a climate of openness and acceptance in which members will trust one another and therefore engage in productive exchange of ideas, opinions, and perceptions
- Interpreting—entails offering possible explanations
- Questioning—is not overused, because members can become frustrated and annoyed with continued questions
- Confirming—restating a member's basic ideas by emphasizing the facts and encouraging further discussion
- Encouraging—in which the leader does not agree or disagree with a member's ideas but uses noncommittal words with positive tone of voice

Table 8–7 Types of Roles Played in Groups

Individual (Personal)	Task Related	Group Building
• Aggressor	• Initiator-contributor	• Encourager
• Blocker	• Information seeker	• Harmonizer
• Recognition seeker	• Opinion seeker	• Compromiser
• Self-confessor	• Information giver	• Gatekeeper and expediter
• Player	• Opinion giver	• Standard setter
• Dominator	• Elaborator	• Group observer and commentator
• Help seeker	• Coordinator	• Follower
• Special interest pleader	• Orienter	
	• Evaluator-critic	
	• Energizer	
	• Procedural technician	
	• Recorder	

Source: Rebecca LaVallee and Curtis P. McLaughlin, "Teams at the Core," in *Continuous Quality Improvement in Health Care*, Curtis P. McLaughlin and Arnold D. Kaluzny, eds., Aspen Publishers, Inc., © 1994.

Group dynamics and interpersonal relations can influence, interfere with, or inhibit problem solving. Some of the interferences are outlined in Table 8–8.

Information Sharing. Information sharing means the team takes advantage of an opportunity for improvement or solves a problem that requires access to and the ability to collect and pool information. The team must also know how to structure information to arrive at alternative solutions. In general, the greater the number and diversity of alternatives proposed and evaluated, the greater is the opportunity for selection of effective solutions.

Decision Making. Successful problem solving also requires the ability of the group to reach decisions. Efficient closure requires that the

Table 8–8 Factors That Interfere with Group Problem Solving

- Focus effect: in a rut, groupthink, tunnel vision
- Self-weighting effect: group members participating only to the level where they feel equally competent with other group members
- Judgment effect: judgments are being made but not expressed for fear that they will be perceived as criticisms
- Status inhibition effect: opinions are not being expressed because they are not in agreement with those of higher status group members
- Group pressure for conformity through implied sanctions
- Influence of strong personalities on group
- Overemphasis on group maintenance functions
- Pressure for speedy decisions

Source: Rebecca LaVallee and Curtis P. McLaughlin, "Teams at the Core," in *Continuous Quality Improvement in Health Care,* Curtis P. McLaughlin and Arnold D. Kaluzny, eds., Aspen Publishers, Inc., © 1994.

Table 8–9 Defining Consensus

- Reaching consensus involves a strategy different from one that would be used if the group were trying to achieve a unanimous or majority vote.
- Reaching consensus means developing an acceptable proposal that all team members can support and that none of the team members will oppose.
- Consensus is not a unanimous vote. A consensus may not represent everyone's first priorities.
  - A consensus is not a majority vote. It does not mean that only those in the majority will be happy with the result.
  - A consensus decision does not provide complete satisfaction for every team member. However, all members should agree with the decision.

Source: Adapted from Norbert Goldfield, Michael Pine, and Joan Pine, *Measuring and Managing Health Care Quality: Procedures, Techniques, and Protocols,* © Aspen Publishers, Inc.

---

group be able to make a final recommendation effectively. There is a direct relationship between group decision performance and the group's ability to (1) accurately understand the problems and (2) accurately assess the negative consequences of alternate choices.

Communication Techniques for Groups. Many of the interpersonal skills, including those on negotiation discussed in Chapter 28, are also applicable in group situations. What is most important in working in a group situation is reaching a consensus (see Table 8–9). It takes time to reach consensus. Other requirements include the following:

- active participation of all team members
- skills in communication: listening, conflict resolution, and discussion
- creative thinking
- open-mindedness and acceptance of differences

Model Process for Developing Self-Directed Work Teams*

The following is based on a National Seminars Group presentation entitled, "How To Build and Implement Self-Directed Work Teams."[1] It provides a functional model created to achieve a shared governance environment incorporating diverse role groups. The model encompasses the five-stage process.

The first stage is *structuring,* which demands assessment of group readiness. Is the commitment of the group apparent? Are resources available? In this stage, a plan is developed, and tasks

*Source: Beth Nocar-Bowen and Cynthia Ford, "Professional Practice and Role Diversity: A Team Concept for Patient Transportation Systems," *Critical Care Nursing Quarterly,* Vol. 18:3, Aspen Publishers, Inc., © November 1995.

[1]National Seminars Group. *How To Build and Implement Self-Directed Work Teams.* Shawnee Mission, Kan: Rockhurst College Continuing Education Center, Inc.; 1993.

are broken down among committees/teams. Each committee/team is to have representation from each discipline.

The second stage moves the group into a *settling phase*. In this stage, roles are clarified. Using available resources, staff members are educated and trained in the effective use of interpersonal, administrative, and technical skills.

The third stage, *problem solving (storming phase)*, is where the bulk of the work occurs. In this stage, a facilitator usually becomes necessary. The facilitator needs to be objective, unbiased, and therefore outside the team structure. A focus on objectives is necessary in this phase to keep team members directed.

The fourth stage is the *learning stage*. Achieving short-term results is important in this stage, because high morale comes from winning. Team members should understand the overall vision for the program. With this new confidence, each role group (e.g., nurse or paramedic group) is able and willing to train other roles. Teams of diverse roles also are able and willing to train other teams of diverse roles. Cross-training in skills and administrative tasks provides teams with a holistic picture, which enhances performance.

The fifth stage is the *performing phase*. In this stage, a change in the team members' self-perception becomes evident. Management moves from hands on to on hand.

A successful self-directed team environment can establish this process and outcome relationship in that the task orientation gives way to what is produced. Institution of the following eight components, fitting the acronym *MAXIMIZE*, can foster the creation of a successful self-directed team environment.

Process for Multidisciplinary Team Training and Competency*

Training teams to work under constantly revised visions of patient care delivery is a multi-

- *M*odel core values: Each member of the team is held accountable for practicing according to the values decided as a group.
- *A*ccept differences: Each role brings its own contribution and its own way of performing tasks. The inclination to mold one role into another must be avoided.
- "*X*" out negativism: Negative attitudes impede progress, deplete motivation, and cause others to lose sight of common goals.
- *I*nstill confidence: When individuals know that their peers have faith in their abilities, apprehension is minimized and performance is enhanced.
- *M*eet with a purpose: Each meeting must have a clear purpose, and a resolution or a plan for resolution must be developed by the end of the meeting.
- *I*nitiate conflict resolution: Different roles bring different views; conflicts inevitably arise. Each member needs to know or learn how to deal with conflict effectively since conflict resolution serves to clarify, strengthen, validate, revise, and improve initial concepts and plans.
- *Z*ero in on performance objectives: Through clear purpose, effective goals, a well-integrated operating structure, and sound leadership, the team can work competently and with quality.
- *E*njoy the ride!

faceted, complex process that must be interwoven throughout and beyond the transitional phase of any redesign project.

The purpose of training in a time of patient care delivery redesign is to facilitate change. Training is the process that aggregates health care workers from diverse backgrounds and facilitates the acquisition of knowledge, skills, and behavioral competencies fundamental to providing patient care and services at a foundation level of practice that is different from traditional methods of care delivery.

*Source: Patricia C. Parent, "Training and Competency within Patient Care Redesign," *Nursing Administration Quarterly*, Vol. 20:1, Aspen Publishers, Inc., © Fall 1995.

In a multidisciplinary effort, this training program is not the property of any individual or department. It is a collaborative effort of experts from all disciplines and positions within the institution who share a common goal to provide all partners in care with the information, knowledge, and skills needed to deliver competent care and services to patients in a transitional health care environment.

Training Goals

Initial training goals set up by one program are such that at the end of each training program, participants will be able to meet the following criteria:

- Identify their given role and behavioral expectations as described within the patient-focused care redesign framework.
- Demonstrate beginning interpersonal skills so as to practice in a collaborative partnership on their designated units with other partners in care.
- Demonstrate a foundation of knowledge and skills to function within the scope of their new partner role.

Team training is not focused on diluting or blurring professional roles. Training focuses on assessing and identifying tasks that can be shared among health care providers, in a reasonable and prudent manner, within regulatory guidelines. Training then focuses on planning and implementing competency-based programs that will allow multiskilled providers of health care and services to perform these tasks and functions in order to meet immediate patient needs and permit health care professionals to maximize their roles within their given scopes of practice. Finally, training focuses on evaluation of the training program and the development of employee evaluation tools to measure expected performance criteria.

Supporting the Cultural Change

Training must facilitate the transition of care delivery from the traditional fragmented, task-centered, discipline-specific, and department-focused mode to an integrated patient-centered process. The central focus of this process is patient outcomes, not tasks. These fundamental changes in the process of how care and services are delivered represent a major cultural change within the organization.

Cultural change is really the first and pivotal phase of the entire training process. People need to realize that not only is the organization going to change but the entire way they once performed in their given roles is going to undergo transformations.

It is essential that staff education and training begin once the decision to move into a team-based redesign has been affirmed. In this embryonic state, training content should focus on why the changes are going to occur, how they will affect individual jobs, what they will mean to each employee, and how they will affect functional groups. Employees need to know that they will be a vital part of the change process from its inception. Training sessions can take the format of open forums, staff retreats, staff focus groups, discussions at unit meetings, newsletters, information hotlines, and weekly bulletins.

Transitional support consists of informal sessions that focus on change process, the effects of change on individuals and functional groups, and coping mechanisms. This portion of training needs to begin during the informational phase, because it is the forum in which the information can be processed. These sessions can help individuals become aware that in spite of radical changes, each person possesses knowledge, skills, and performance qualities that are highly valuable resources in current and future marketplaces.

CROSS-FUNCTIONAL TEAMS IN HEALTH CARE ORGANIZATIONS

The promise of cross-functional teams in health care organizations is that the energies of team members will converge across departmental boundaries and individual interests in such a way that health care will be improved on a continuing basis.

A simple cost-functional team is a group of 6 to 14 persons from different work areas within an organization (representing different but related work processes or functions) whose purpose is planning, problem solving, or project activity undertaken for the quality improvement of goods and services.

More complex cross-functional teams, formed to deal with more complicated issues, include not only persons representing different functions within an organization but also individuals from different levels of the organizational hierarchy. Some cross-functional teams, for even more involved issues, may include vendors who provide an organization with supplies and the customers served by the organization.

There are several reasons for the use of cross-functional teams in health care organizations. The first of these reasons is the development of a comprehensive and indepth view of any situation through the pooling of knowledge and information. Second, once a situation is understood comprehensively in a detailed manner, and problems are identified, the cross-functional team is useful in devising an improvement of a situation or process. Third, the cross-functional team is quite effective in implementing changes and monitoring the effects of these changes.*

Succeeding with the Cross-Functional Team*

Health care managers and others in middle management are crucial to the success of cross-functional teams. Nurse managers bolster efforts to form cross-functional teams when they explicitly support the concept and the systems philosophy that undergirds cross-functional teams. There are, however, potential problems associated with cross-functional teams, such as the following:

- differential power among team members
- conflicts of interest arising from loyalty to others outside the team
- different assumptions about the issue under consideration due to previous experiences

- neglect of the norms under which cross-functional teams must operate if they are to be successful and disregard for valuable behaviors

These problems can be avoided.

First, those with organizational power must be selected for membership on a team not only because of their expertise and vision but also because of their maturity and experience working in groups.

Second, the group should monitor itself. After each session, members of the team should complete evaluation forms. One of the items in the form should refer to balanced participation of team members or the perceived dominance of one or two members of the team.

Third, the roles of leader of the team discussion and recorder of team minutes should rotate among team members. The recorder who stands before the group at the easel and transcribes the essentials of the team discussion can easily control the team by screening and interpreting what is said by team members.

Developing a Multidisciplinary Team Approach to Patient Care*

The steps required to move from individualistic to multidisciplinary activity start with improving the capacity of the organization to support a multidisciplinary approach. The following steps should be taken:

- Audit the organization for knowledge of and compliance with mission, goals, and objectives.
- Audit committee structures for information flow, problem resolution, outcomes, and documentation.
- Analyze the data collected for duplication, redundancy, and patient focus, and determine degree of nonsystems approach.

---

*Source: Leon McKenzie, "Cross-Functional Teams in Health Care Organizations," *The Health Care Supervisor*, Vol. 12:3, Aspen Publishers, Inc., © March 1994.

*Source: Sheila Lenkman and Ronald Gribbins, "Multidisciplinary Teams in the Acute Care Setting," *Holistic Nursing Practice*, Vol. 8:3, Aspen Publishers, Inc., © April 1994.

- Identify presence of parochial groups and chief characteristics as well as strengths and weaknesses.
- Identify predominant culture.

Action Plan

The following action plan highlights the general areas that must be addressed as the development of a multidisciplinary approach is undertaken.

Establish an environment for change. To accomplish this, the mission of the institution, rather than individualistic professional behavior, will need to play a central role in the development of values, beliefs, policies, and procedures. Some essential beliefs are "patient centered," "service oriented," and "continuous quality improvement." The mission should also provide support for several values that focus on managers and employees: the manager as a coach, leader, and facilitator; the availability of information to relevant parties, especially teams; the provision of needed training for a multidisciplinary approach; and support for innovative activity and risk taking.

Choose the organizational framework in which care will be given through teamwork. The goal will be to establish which structure most effectively fits what the institution and teams are attempting to accomplish. Some possible alternatives are total product line, modified product line, case management within traditional settings, and technician labor pools (cross-functional workers).

Determine barriers against successful teams. The more specific barriers that arise with the introduction of a multidisciplinary approach include territorial disputes, change seen as threatening group interests, perceived isolation from peers that occurs when one joins a team, fear and anger, negative personalization of the organization's reason for change, loss of status, and loss of power.

Establish opportunities and strategies for effective change. Change is frequently resisted because one or more of three elements is missing: (1) tension requiring search for new alternatives, (2) a clearly desired future state, and (3) specific action plans to achieve the future desired state. The action plans that are developed also need to pay attention to the commitment of the institution to individuals whose positions become obsolete in a multidisciplinary approach, the reward system that will support the new approach, and the benefits that are expected for the patient, employees, and the institution.

Embark on the educational and developmental phase of team building necessary for effective teamwork. The team is described as needing to learn how to trust and define boundaries first, and second, how to structure the group and foster a climate conducive to freedom of expression by members. In addition, the adaptation phase is completed when a team identity begins to form and members understand the contribution they each make. The third stage, the ability to negotiate through resolution of power and conflict issues, leads into the final and working stage. To hasten the process without losing effectiveness, the use of trained team facilitators is helpful.

Develop techniques to involve and support nonemployee physicians as they learn to work in a multidisciplinary context. Physicians will need to be respected, involved in the planning effort, and perceived as an asset. Physicians' estimate of management effectiveness and thus their willingness to engage in multidisciplinary team building is based on the following: what this is going to do for me, perception of impact on patient satisfaction, observation of the health care facility and its work environment, ease and convenience of association with the facility, and confidence in management capability.

Using a Collaborative Practice Committee*

Interdisciplinary collaborative practice committees can be set up in units or groups of units with like patient populations. Disciplines in-

---

Source: George D. Valianoff, Cynthia Neely, and Sharon Hall, "Developmental Levels of Interdisciplinary Collaborative Practice Committees," *Journal of Nursing Administration*, Vol. 7:8, July/August 1993. J.B. Lippincott Company.

volved in the care of the specific patient population or service line will vary depending on the specific needs; however, nursing, medicine, pharmacy, and social services should be involved in all committees. Disciplines that are not directly involved in the care of the specific patient population on a routine basis should be always accessible for consultation as needed. Further, as patient needs change and as the type of services delivered change, members can be added or removed as necessary.

The purpose of these committees is to facilitate discussions among multidisciplinary team members about strategies, methods, or processes that need to be changed, implemented, or revised to ensure delivery of quality services and care in a more efficient, beneficial, professional, and effective manner. In addition, the committees encourage an environment of customer service, continuous quality improvement, cost containment, and patient-focused care.

The chairperson of the committee will vary depending on the unit and the members. A physician, nurse manager, clinical nurse specialist, or staff nurse can chair the committee, or there can be cochairpersons. The nurse manager, however, is responsible for ensuring that the collaborative practice committee meets routinely and that agendas, minutes, and scheduling are handled appropriately. Minutes are distributed to all members and to administration, the patient care committee, the medical staff quality management committee, and the nursing practice and standards council.

MANAGEMENT TEAMS: EXTENSIONS OF THE MULTIDISCIPLINARY TEAM APPROACH

Collaborative Patient Care Management Team*

The development of a collaborative management team was, in part, an outgrowth of the suc-

cessful team model in patient care. The reasoning was that effectiveness as a department could be achieved by a coordinated approach to management that could maximize the relationships among individuals responsible for the smooth functioning of the unit. For example, in a radiation oncology process, four separate work groups, each with its own manager, come together to provide care: medicine, nursing, administration, and radiation therapy. Acknowledging that the work groups are interconnected and that shared responsibility promotes effectiveness, a model can be devised in which each manager's role is seen as equally important and valued, and in which the managers work together as a team. The team concept implies no hierarchy, and to this end titles can be adjusted to reflect equal status—physician manager (instead of division chief), nurse manager, therapist manager (instead of therapist supervisor), and administrative manager.

Avoiding Potential Pitfalls in a Collaborative Management Group*

In adopting a collaborative management model, thorny issues may arise. By anticipating the potential difficulties, the team can develop mechanisms to circumvent or resolve such concerns as the following.

Role Overlap. When everyone has a role in ensuring quality, the boundaries of responsibility can become blurred. Confusion can be avoided by clearly identifying who is handling a particular clinical or operational issue. That person brings the resources together, including other team members, and provides the leadership to see the issue through to conclusion.

Division of Labor. Although responsibilities are shared, the work may not be equally divided at all times. For example, many operational

*Source: Judith Kostka, Sandra Hall, Patricia Moran, and Jay Harris, "Collaborative Teams: Bridges for Clinical and Management Practice," Nursing Administration Quarterly, Vol. 18:4, Aspen Publishers, Inc., © Summer 1994.

*Source: Judith Kostka, Sandra Hall, Patricia Moran, and Jay Harris, "Collaborative Teams: Bridges for Clinical and Management Practice," Nursing Administration Quarterly, Vol. 18:4, Aspen Publishers, Inc., © Summer 1994.

changes are spearheaded by administrative managers. However, the manager carrying the bulk of the workload related to a particular endeavor can call in other managers as needed. This requires each manager to be attentive to the workload of the team and to offer assistance as necessary.

Availability. Since the team members come together as a functional whole, it can sometimes be difficult to keep momentum when a member is absent. Extra flexibility and planning is required in these circumstances. Frequent communication and advance planning regarding the division of responsibilities can make absences less of a problem.

Information Loops. An advantage to an interdisciplinary team is that each member obtains different information, which collectively benefits the department. Nevertheless, information loops are not equally efficient, and decision makers outside the team may not operate with the same collaborative, inclusive intent. It is necessary, therefore, for team members to provide information in two directions—to the team and from the team, keeping the vested interest of all members in mind.

Lack of Commitment/Lack of Fit. In certain circumstances, it can be difficult to engage all the necessary players in the collaborative process. Leverage can be used to encourage buy-in and to highlight possible gains. However, in some cases an individual may not be fully committed or may have a style of functioning that does not fit with the rest of the team. This can quickly become demoralizing and thought should be given to obtaining a better match. In practice, a collaborative model draws attention to both good and bad fits.

Executive Management Teams*

A major responsibility of the nurse executive is to function as a member of executive manage-

ment teams. This is becoming an increasingly critical responsibility as nurse administrators work more closely with all agency departments to provide cost-effective, quality nursing care.

For the most part, nurses are comfortable working with patient care teams and participating as effective team members. Nurse executives, however, usually have less experience and expertise in building and maintaining executive interdisciplinary teams.

Executive interdisciplinary teams differ from patient care teams in several ways. In executive teams, the focus of concern centers around the department or organization; for the patient care team, the focus is the overall welfare of the patient or client. Organizational bureaucracy, power, and politics directly affect the definition of and movement toward executive team goals; patient care teams can use social interactions and peer pressure to accomplish goals. Diplomacy, negotiation skills, and use of power based strategies or alliances are requisite skills of nurse executives in team building; facilitation skills that allow for sharing of knowledge and communication among peers are necessary for leadership of patient care teams. If the nurse administrator is to be effective in his or her role, these differences must be acknowledged and appropriate techniques employed to maximize team-building efforts.

Suggestions for Building Executive Interdisciplinary Teams

The welfare of the nursing profession may depend on the nurse administrator's ability to work with, build, and maintain effective interdisciplinary teams at the executive level. The following guidelines for building successful executive interdisciplinary teams provide suggestions for nurse administrators. The list includes principles that relate especially to executive interdisciplinary teams.

- Obtain political and organizational support for the proposal, plan, or anticipated goals from the chief executive officer or facility administrator.

Source: Mary J. Farley and Martha H. Stoner, "The Nurse Executive and Interdisciplinary Team Building," *Nursing Administration Quarterly*, Vol. 13:2, Aspen Publishers, Inc., © 1989.

- Keep conscious diplomacy in mind and contact potential team members to share a vision of positive outcomes that may occur as a result of team participation. It may be necessary to raise individual awareness of the problem or issue, keeping in mind that each potential team member will view participation from a "what's in it for me?" standpoint.
- Call a team meeting at a convenient time for all team members. An agenda should be sent to each member ahead of the meeting, and the meeting should be conducted in an expeditious manner.
- Clarify the purpose of the team, sharing all information available. Encourage participation as the group jointly sets clear, challenging, but realistic goals. Without clear, specific goals, the team has no measuring stick for accomplishments. Participation in goal setting contributes to commitment. Each member of the team ought to understand the goals and how he or she fits in the group efforts toward goal accomplishment.
- Seek commitment from each team member for accomplishment of team goals.
- Keep in mind that threats to individual power and/or protection of personal or departmental turf may influence behavior. Sensitivity to these needs along with good conflict management techniques will move the team forward.
- Create an atmosphere of cooperation and satisfying relationships. Praising team members and encouraging members to support each other enhance cooperation.
- Accept and appreciate the differences of the individual members and departments. Personal needs are part of the human condition.
- Communicate, communicate, communicate. Members of organizations are often apprehensive of executive team activities.

Chapter 9

Nursing Service Jobs

NURSING DEPARTMENT CHAIN OF COMMAND*

In an extensive survey, nurse administrators were asked to describe themselves and what they do. The nursing position definitions collated from their responses are presented below.

Director of Nursing. This title is given to the nurse who is administratively responsible for some or all nursing services in a health care institution. Director of Nursing may be the formal title given by the institution or a generic title for all heads of nursing services, regardless of their formal titles. Approximately 25 percent of the heads of nursing services have the title Director of Nursing. Other formal titles for the position include Vice President for Nursing and Executive Director of Nursing Services.

Nurse Executive.[1] This is the top-ranking member of the nursing administration team, responsible for nursing services and, in some health care

facilities, such support services as pharmacy and central supply. The usual titles for nurse executives are Director of Nursing and Vice President for Nursing. The nurse executive position is considered demanding because of the complex and dynamic nature of health care organizations, the high expectations of physicians and administrators, and the vulnerability of patients and nurses.

Most nurse executives rely on computer information systems and decision support systems to track operations and costs and to ensure that care delivered is of high quality and low liability. A nurse executive is responsible for the largest group of employees in a health care facility and is concerned with their supply and performance. Obtaining the most highly qualified nurses is a major responsibility, but educating and training nurses to ensure high standards of practice is equally important.

Also essential are good communication skills for dealing with staff, patients, guests, physicians, administrators, and union representatives. Delegating, negotiating, collaborating, and diplomacy skills are necessary because nurse executives are responsible for the single largest cost center of a health care facility. Knowledge of health care finances is a requisite for developing and maintaining budgets, managing cost distributions, and justifying expenditures for personnel, programs, and equipment. Identifying the

---

*Source: Excerpted from Richard Heyden and Beverly Henry, "Defining Nursing Administration Terms," *Aspen's Advisor for Nurse Executives*, Vols. 8:2–8:6, Aspen Publishers, Inc., © November 1992–March 1993.

[1]*Note:* More precise detail on the scope and accountabilities for nurse administrators as outlined by the Association of Nurse Executives is provided in Chapter 2.

nurses' contributions to an institution's productivity is important to justify the nursing resource requirement. The nurse executive usually has graduate-level education and experience as a practicing nurse (see Table 9–1).

Nurse Manager. This member of the nursing organization is directly responsible for the day-to-day operations of the one or more organizational units that, in hospitals, are usually called nursing units or patient care units. His or her major responsibility is implementing policy, handling problems, and disseminating information about patient problems and the allocation of human resources. Time is spent in obtaining and maintaining human, material, and information resources; acting as a resource for staff nurses; and integrating the work of the nursing unit into the institution's operational systems according to its overall strategic plan. Nurse managers handle conflict, plan for change, and develop the skills of those under their direction. A bachelor's degree is usually required, but a master's degree is preferred. Examples of titles for nurse managers include Head Nurse, Patient Care Coordinator, Unit Director, and Supervisor (see Table 9–2).

Nursing Supervisor. This nursing manager is responsible for coordinating patient care activities for a single work shift for 24 hours a day. A head nurse coordinates patient care on a single unit but the nursing supervisor usually coordinates the care on several units and, in small facilities, may coordinate care for all the units providing services, especially during evenings and nights. Nurse supervisors assign nursing personnel. Providing adequate personnel for all units, ensuring the delivery of safe care, and providing expert advice are among the key duties. Nursing supervisors are usually responsible on evening, night, or weekend shifts. Although they supervise staff, they usually do not schedule for the long term or hire employees.

Head Nurse. This is a practitioner in a first-level management position who has 24-hour responsibility, usually for one nursing care unit in an organization. The domain of responsibility includes nursing care, patient teaching, staff development, reporting, budgeting, evaluating, disciplining, and scheduling. The head nurse role varies by the type of governance; the traditions, philosophy, and goals of the institution; and the job description. Generally, however, a head nurse is responsible for the implementation, coordination, and evaluation of patient care. Head nurses are expected to implement and monitor administrative plans and policies, inform staff nurses about changes, and alert them to policies. They represent patient and staff needs to the next level of nursing administration and act as a resource to the nursing staff. The main administrative duties for a head nurse include productivity of operations, thorough resource staff management, staff development, and quality-of-care evaluation.

THE ROLE OF THE CONTEMPORARY HOSPITAL NURSE MANAGER*

The purpose of nursing management is to optimize the application of available nursing resources in the diagnosis and treatment of human responses to actual or potential health problems, such as self-care limitations, pain and discomfort, emotional problems related to illness and treatment, or strain related to life processes, including birth and death. When appropriately managed, nurses, in addition to providing nursing care, emerge as integrators of patient care services and facilitators of the efforts of members of the multidisciplinary team (see Table 9–3).

The nurse manager (also sometimes called the head nurse, clinical coordinator, or assistant director of nursing) helps coordinate the clinical nursing staff. The nurse manager's primary focus is operations. The nurse manager

- plans, prepares, and demonstrates accountability for the budget
- supervises the delivery of nursing care
- collaborates with ancillary, support, and interdisciplinary team members

*Source: Joan Gygax Spicer and Diane E. Nitta, "Nursing Organization and Management," *The AUPHA Manual of Health Services Management*, Robert J. Taylor and Susan B. Taylor, eds., Aspen Publishers, Inc., © 1994.

Table 9–1 Activities of the Nurse Executive

The nurse executive is responsible for organized nursing services and manages from the perspective of the organization as a whole. As the administrator of a significant component of health care organizations, the nurse executive exercises the authority inherent in positions to fulfill responsibilities to the profession, the health care consumer, and the organization.

1. Participates in the administration of the health care organization as a full member of the executive team.
2. Participates in the strategic and long-range planning of the health care organization.
3. Provides leadership in the determination of clinical and administrative nursing goals and directions.
4. Participates in the determination of functions and processes to achieve clinical and administrative goals.
5. Acquires and allocates human, material, and financial resources for specific functions and processes.
6. Evaluates and revises the systems and processes of organized nursing services to enhance achievement of identified desired client/family-centered outcomes.
7. Provides leadership in critical thinking, conflict management, and problem solving.
8. Provides leadership in human resource development and management.
9. Provides opportunities for consumer input into personal health care decisions and policy development.
10. Ensures the ongoing evaluation and innovation of services provided by organized nursing services and the organization as a whole.
11. Facilitates the conduct, dissemination, and utilization of research in the areas of nursing, health, and management systems.
12. Serves as a professional role model and mentor to motivate, develop, recruit, and retain future nurse administrators.
13. Serves as a change agent, assisting all staff in understanding the importance, necessity, impact, and process of change.

Source: American Nurses Association, *Scope and Standards for Nurse Administrators*, Publication No. NS 35, Copyright 1995 by the American Nurses Association. All rights reserved.

Table 9–2 Activities of the Nurse Manager

Nurse managers are responsible to a nurse executive and manage one or more defined areas of organized nursing services. In smaller settings, they may have responsibilities for management of the entire facility and its service.

1. Participates in nursing and organizational policy formulation and decision making.
2. Facilitates participation of staff in nursing and organizational policy formulation and decision making.
3. Accepts organizational accountability for services provided to recipients.
4. Evaluates the quality and appropriateness of care.
5. Provides guidance for and supervision of personnel accountable to the nurse manager.
6. Coordinates nursing services with the services of other health care disciplines.
7. Participates in the recruitment, selection, and retention of personnel.
8. Assumes responsibility for staffing and scheduling personnel. Assignments reflect appropriate utilization of personnel.
9. Assures appropriate orientation, education, credentialing, and continuing professional development for personnel.
10. Evaluates performance of personnel.
11. Participates in planning and monitoring the budget for their defined areas.
12. Participates and involves the nursing staff in evaluative research activities.
13. Fosters a climate conducive to educational experiences for nursing and other students.
14. Fosters peer review.

Source: American Nurses Association, *Scope and Standards for Nurse Administrators*, Publication No. NS 35, Copyright 1995 by the American Nurses Association. All rights reserved.

Table 9–3 Specific Competencies of a First-Line Manager

Structuring an Effective, Harmonious Workplace

☐ The first-line manager is the key player in determining and, in some instances, acquiring the staffing, equipment, and funding resources to deliver adequate, appropriate care, including
- setting fiscal priorities
- preparing, controlling, and monitoring a unit budget
- using budget data to make decisions
- identifying equipment resources needed
- ensuring equipment resources are present
- scheduling, monitoring, and protecting resources; determining staff mix; estimating patient workloads (quantifying care); and ensuring staffing reflects workload (workforce planning)
- recruiting, interviewing and selecting, and promoting staff

☐ Maintaining a suitable infrastructure entails allocating those resources appropriately to facilitate care provision, including
- setting unit goals
- organizing the unit
- identifying work to be done
- scheduling staff to reflect workload
- assigning staff appropriately to patients daily
- maximizing human resources
- monitoring activities on the unit
- coordinating work activities on the unit
- perceiving workload pressures on staff

☐ The first-line nursing manager's role in shaping the working environment also relates to enabling staff to establish and maintain social relations that ensure sufficient, well-coordinated patient care, which includes
- managing conflicts
- identifying and resolving staff problems
- using constructive confrontation skills
- handling grievances
- providing a forum for staff communication
- using motivational dynamics
- creating and maintaining a favorable working environment
- developing and maintaining staff morale
- building teams and coaching nurses in group dynamics skills

Assisting Nursing Staff

☐ The first-line manager envisions and sets expectations, assigns choices that foster professional growth, and achieves practice goals through modeling, counseling, and mentoring nurses in terms of their career stages, which includes
- developing standards of performance
- developing criteria for staff performance
- evaluating staff performance
- perceiving barriers to staff performance
- identifying and facilitating learning needs of staff
- assisting staff to maintain skills
- providing opportunities for staff development
- teaching staff
- identifying and developing staff potential
- counseling employees as to their performance
- acting as a teaching role model
- involving staff in research

Oversight of Clinical Practice Excellence

☐ The role of the first-line nursing manager is to get clinically excellent things done through others' endeavors. A nursing manager's personal commitment to clinical excellence is enacted in directing, coaching, and leading the staff at work, including
- identifying stress in staff and self
- performing under stress (stress management)
- initiating personal and professional growth and development
- developing and maintaining personal professional competence
- maintaining professional identity

General Competencies

☐ To undertake their many functions, managers in today's health care climate need certain general competencies, which include a knowledge of
- management information systems and computers
- changes in nursing care practices
- quality assurance activities, and total quality improvement techniques
- staffing models
- management and organizational behavior
- participative decision making
- delegation
- change theory
- communication skills, written and oral
- interviewing and counseling skills
- power and politics
- the research process

Source: Reprinted with permission from C. Duffield, "Role Competencies of First-Line Managers," *Nursing Management,* June 1992 issue, © 1992 Springhouse Corporation.

- recruits, selects, and trains personnel
- schedules resources
- evaluates staff members for promotion, transfer, disciplinary action, and separation of service
- serves as role model

ROLES FOR NURSES WITH ADVANCED TRAINING

Advanced Practice Nurses*

Of the 2.2 million registered nurses (RNs) in the United States, about 100,000 are considered advanced practice nurses (APNs). These nurses have received one to two years of advanced training beyond the four-year bachelor of science in nursing degree. Almost half of all APNs are engaged in primary care. The major categories of APNs include the following:

- *Clinical nurse specialists* (40,000). These nurses have earned a master's or doctoral degree in specialized clinical areas. They work in specialty practices such as cardiology, mental health, cancer, and neonatology and provide primary care for patients with chronic diseases such as diabetes and arthritis.
- *Nurse practitioners* (25,000). These nurses have two years of training and master's degrees from one of the 150 nurse practitioner programs. Most are working in primary care as members of multidisciplinary teams.
- *Certified nurse practitioners* (5,000). These nurses have 12 to 18 months of advanced training. This field is concentrated in obstetrics, gynecology, and midwifery.

Advanced practice nurses are considered an untapped resource for integrated health networks. With graduate-level training in clinical special-

ties, APNs have the competency and training to take on three important roles in managed care: (1) *team leader* of a multidisciplinary care team, (2) *case manager* and resource allocator for health maintenance organization (HMO) "covered lives," and (3) *physician substitute* to provide care in areas of physician shortage (e.g., primary care and geriatrics). In the last category, the acceptance of APNs is still controversial and clouded by economic competition. Physicians may resent the threat APNs present and, therefore, may oppose the use of APNs in independent roles by HMOs and integrated delivery networks.

Clinical Nurse Specialist*

The clinical nurse specialist (CNS) is an advanced practice delineation that indicates a higher intensity of knowledge in a specific specialty area and has unfolded mostly as an institutional practice. These primarily hospital-based specialists focus on some element of nursing care in an advanced practice format in a wide variety of specialty areas. Often, there are as many clinical nurse specialists in specialty practice delineations as there are divisions of practice. These individuals focus on a higher level of complexity and frequently play out the expert role in the delivery of these highly specialized clinical services. Therein lies the challenge of the role as well. Throughout the developments in the 20th century, the role of the CNS has responded to the changing needs and values of society.

In the literature, between 1965 and 1980 the CNS was described by nursing leaders as having the following four major role functions: practitioner, consultant, educator, and researcher. The bedside practitioner component of the role allowed the CNS to directly impact client outcome and improve nursing standards by acting as a role model for the staff nurse. The consultant role was

Source: Russell C. Coile, Jr., "Advanced Practice Nurses: A Critical Resource for Managed Care," *Russ Coile's Health Trends*, Vol. 7:7, Aspen Publishers, Inc., © May 1995.

Source: Adapted from C.E. Loveridge and S.H. Cummings, *Nursing Management in the New Paradigm*, pp. 469–470, Aspen Publishers, Inc., © 1996, and Takenburg and Rausch, "Redefining the Role of CNS," *Advanced Practice Nursing Quarterly*, Vol. 1, No. 1, pp. 37–48, Aspen Publishers, Inc., © 1995.

envisioned as providing expert clinical information to caregivers outside the immediate site of the specialist's practice. In the consultant role, the CNS could provide expert services either within the institution of practice or externally within the community as a representative of the institution. As an educator, the CNS was responsible for the education of both the client and family. Modalities for fulfilling this role include either individual teaching or group instruction, with the specialist in charge of material development and evaluation. The research aspect of the role has not traditionally been rewarded in the service setting.

Clinical nurse specialists have been looked at by hospitals as a luxury rather than as a requisite for high-level, high-quality, complex care. Even though care has become more intense and increasingly complex in institutions, the role of the CNS has not been greatly expanded. Often because specialization and advanced education in nursing practice are not of value to the institution, these roles have not been integrated into the nurse staffing process in unit-based clinical care. Furthermore, the use of CNSs has often been predominantly for roles other than in-depth practice activities. In many ways, the specialist has been taken away from advanced expert practice and placed into roles related to special programming, delegated functional management, quality improvement activities, and education and development as well as a host of special projects and support activities. The problem with this is that the nurse in advanced clinical specialty practice should have a primary focus on patient care. His or her frame of reference and functional value are in roles specific to patient care services. The use of these practitioners for other activities has made it challenging to define specifically their value within the context of patient care.

A 1986 survey by Robichaud and Hamric found that patient care (40%) rather than education (27%) consumed the majority of the role responsibilities of the CNS. However, the responsibilities of practice continue to be practitioner, educator, consultant, researcher, and change agent/executive, although the degree of involvement in each role varies with the individual and the institutional needs. Despite the setting, the focus of the CNS practice continues to be client-based.

By definition, the CNS has a major role in the delivery of innovative, cost-effective, quality care. Encompassed in this responsibility is the need to be current with innovations of the health care delivery systems as well.

The Case Manager*

Managed care and case management are not interchangeable concepts. Managed care is a system of cost containment programs; case management is a process. It is one component in the managed care strategy. The following definition of case management has been adopted by the Commission for Case Manager Certification (CCMC), the developers of the credentialing process for case managers: "Case management is a collaborative process which assesses, plans, implements, coordinates, monitors, and evaluates the options and services required to meet an individual's health needs, using communication and available resources to promote quality, cost-effective outcomes." CCMC goes on to clarify the role by stating that case management is not episodic or restricted to a single practice setting, but occurs across a continuum of care and addresses ongoing individual needs.

Throughout the course of care, the case manager works in four major areas of activity: medical, financial, behavioral/motivational, and vocational:

- Medical activities—Encompasses all those activities a case manager performs to ensure that the patient receives the most effective medical and nursing care, including:
  ——Contacting the patient in the hospital, in the rehabilitation unit, or at home

---

*Source: Catherine M. Mullahy, "Case Management and Managed Care," *The Managed Health Care Handbook*, Peter R. Kongstvedt, ed., Aspen Publishers, Inc., © 1996.

——Contacting the members of the medical treatment team (the physician, nursing staff, rehabilitation therapists, etc.) to discover the patient's course of progress and needs; utilizing the information in discharge planning and the initial needs assessment

——Arranging for all services required for discharge or relocation (equipment, home nursing care, therapy, transportation, transfer to another facility, home utilities, etc.); coordinating efforts with the primary nurse, discharge planner, or social services administrator to eliminate duplication of services and to conserve benefit dollars

——Visiting with the family

——Checking the home for safety factors and architectural barriers and arranging for any needed safety aids and modifications

——On follow-up, reevaluating equipment, ensuring that supplies are replenished, monitoring home nursing services, and arranging for equipment repair; evaluating activities of daily living, home programs, and modifications to treatment

——Identifying problems, providing health instruction, and referring the patient back to the physician or other health team member when appropriate

——Identifying plateaus, improvements, regressions, and depressions; counseling accordingly or recommending help

——Making personal visits or contacting the physician to clarify the diagnosis, prognosis, therapy, activities of daily living, expected permanent disability, and so on

——Assisting in obtaining payer authorizations for any modalities of treatment recommended

——Acting as a liaison between the physician and the insurance company when necessary

——Sharing pertinent information about the patient with the physician and working together with the physician to achieve the best outcome

● Financial activities

——Counseling the patient or family on budgeting and notifying creditors

——Identifying financial distress and referring the patient or family to appropriate community resources

——Helping the patient or family sort and prioritize unpaid bills

——Acting as a liaison among the insurance company, referral source, and patient to alleviate financial and other problems

● Behavioral/motivational activities

——Exploring the patient's feelings about himself or herself and his or her injury or illness and helping the patient with the associated trauma and frustration

——Monitoring the family's feelings regarding the patient's illness and observing the family's ability or inability to manage under new emotional stress

——Offering reassurance and information about the patient's condition

——If qualified, counseling in the areas of marital discord, role reversal, dependency, and sexual problems arising from the injury or illness

● Vocational activities

——Obtaining a history of education, employment, hobbies, and job skills and uncovering vocational interests and future goals

——If appropriate, overseeing psychovocational testing, work evaluations, schooling, on-the-job situations, transportation, and anything else needed to assist the patient in becoming or remaining gainfully employed

——Assisting the patient in using the recuperative period in a constructive fashion (studying, upgrading skills, preparing for job interviews, etc.)

——Visiting the patient's place of employment and talking with the personnel director or immediate supervisor about the employer's expectations and the patient's needs

——Completing a job analysis and discussing the possibility of the patient's return to work in the same job, perhaps after job modification or lightening of duties

——Sharing the above information with the physician at appropriate time

STAFF POSITIONS

Expanded Role Nurses*

Initially, an expanded role for nurses referred to the assumption of responsibilities previously associated with medical practice: obtaining health histories, performing physical examinations, ordering laboratory studies, making referrals, and the medical management of patients. Nurses from varying entry-level educational backgrounds were prepared for the expanded role through postbasic continuing education programs consisting of six to nine months of classroom work and clinical practice. Nurses practicing in the expanded role worked under medical supervision and medical authority.

Today, however, the scope of contemporary nursing practice has made aspects of the original model obsolete. These skills can now be considered part of the core of practice or common practice. For example, physical examination is taught in virtually every baccalaureate nursing program in the United States. Whatever the practice area, data collection using skills in physical examination and health history has become the cornerstone of nursing process and the first essential step in the professional standards of practice. Similarly, other activities, such as monitoring the course of an illness, interpreting laboratory or screening data, health teaching, counseling, initiating referrals, listening to and distinguishing normal from abnormal lung sounds, or administering prescribed IV medications, can all be considered established or common areas of practice and within the scope of practice.

Role of the Nurse as Collaborative Care Manager*

The care managers are clinical experts in the patient populations they represent. They are selected for their strong clinical skills as well as their leadership and "change agent" attitudes. The care manager position integrates the traditional roles of preadmission nurse, utilization review nurse, clinical expert, patient educator, and discharge planner into one role. Care managers are administratively exempt professionals who create their own schedules and work hours based on the needs of the patients, families, and physicians they serve. The daily interaction of the care manager with patients, physicians, and other health care disciplines must constantly be incorporated into the "big-picture view" of the patient populations they manage. They track and trend outcome data from individual encounters, aggregating it into valuable information that can be used to change care delivery and treatment plans for future patients. The care manager must keep up with the ever-changing delivery patterns, contractual obligations, and new technology in order to achieve the best demonstrated practice.

The role is most often misunderstood by the nursing staff. There is a perception that since the care managers are "seeing the patient," they will administer the treatment, ambulate the patient, and give the pain medication. This, of course, is not the case. The care managers do not replace the bedside clinician. They oversee and coordinate the continuum of care with emphasis on the processes and systems of care delivery and the relationship of the hospital to the bigger picture of the entire health continuum.

The skills and qualities that are necessary for care managers to be successful include:

- clinical expertise
- positive medical staff relationships
- economic savvy
- strong interpersonal skills
- ability to analyze data
- facilitation skills

---

*Source: Adapted from Hedy Freyone Mechanic, "Redefining the Expanded Role," Nursing Outlook, Vol. 36, No. 6, November-December 1988.

*Source: Clinical Maps for Acute Care: Managing Care through Collaborative Practice, Aspen Publishers, Inc., © 1996.

Generalist and Specialist Practice in the Expanded Role*

The central prerequisite is educational preparation. Nurses cannot practice in expanded roles if they hold narrow conceptualizations and understanding of the health issues confronting clients or if they perceive intervention primarily within a disease-oriented framework.

Generalist practice in the expanded role must begin at the baccalaureate level to meet the demands of the role. Similarly, advanced practice within a multisystem framework, with adjunct skills for practice in the extended role, requires in-depth theoretical knowledge, advanced clinical skills, and expertise that is attainable only through clinical specialization at the master's level.

Distinguishing between practice in the expanded role and advanced practice as a specialist also raises the issues of licensure and credentialing. If the expanded role requires educational preparation attainable only at the bac-

calaureate level, then licensing examinations and licensure must reflect this.

Redefining the expanded role with concomitant changes in licensure and credentialing has implications for reimbursement. As currently structured, certification and third-party reimbursement requirements limit direct access to insurance carriers to nurses certified as "nurse practitioners" who are practicing in "expanded roles." In contrast, regardless of educational preparation, knowledge level, degree of clinical expertise, or certification achievements, clinical nurse specialists and nurse generalists with certified advanced competencies are ineligible for direct reimbursement.

Differentiated Practice*

The American Nurses' Association began setting the national stage for differentiated practice with their 1965 position statement on entry into practice. It called for two distinct levels of registered nursing based on educational preparation and the resulting competencies acquired. Several years ago the National Commission on Nursing Implementation Project (NCNIP) thoughtfully examined the issue of differentiated practice and created a time frame in which to reach this goal.

In 1990 the American Academy of Nursing, in collaboration with the American Nurses' Association and the American Organization of Nurse Executives, convened a conference entitled Differentiating Nursing Practice: Into the Twenty-First Century. This gathering examined the concept of differentiated practice in the current health care crisis. Furthermore, various models of differentiation in the hospital setting and community were explored, and cost and quality outcomes were identified. Finally, the implications of differentiated practice for education and research were also addressed. Shared information provided ideas, new questions, and chal-

---

Defining the Expanded Role

A nurse practices in the expanded role in three ways.

- First, both in health promotion and protection and during episodes of illness, nurses view clients and their health concerns from an integrated multisystem perspective and intervene from this perspective in assuming primary care responsibility.

- Second, they maintain a collegial and collaborative relationship with other health team members.

- Third, acting with autonomy and authority, nurses assume full accountability for their actions.

Source: Adapted from Hedy Freyone Mechanic, "Redefining the Expanded Role," *Nursing Outlook*, Vol. 36, No. 6, November-December 1988.

Source: Rebecca J. Nelson and JoEllen Goertz Koerner, "Context," *Implementing Differentiated Nursing Practice*, J. Goertz Koerner and Karpicik, eds., Aspen Publishers, Inc., © 1994.

lenges for nursing to pursue as we plan how the profession will contribute to the public welfare during the next century.

Differentiated practice is referred to as a philosophy that focuses on the structuring of roles and functions of nurses according to education, experience, and competence. It establishes that the domain of professional nursing is broad, with multiple roles and responsibilities of various degrees and complexities. It assumes that nurses with different educational preparation, expertise, and background bring different competencies to the workplace. It seeks to ensure that the work of nursing is carried out by the most appropriate nurse in the most appropriate fashion. Comprehensive, cost-effective care is thus provided by the collective discipline of nursing through the integration of those services across the continuum of care into a synergistic whole.

Differentiated practice recognizes the contribution of all nursing personnel to patient care delivery as unique and valuable. It creates an integrative web of nursing practitioners across the health care continuum. When nurses contribute to patient care delivery by assuming differentiated roles, the aggregate contribution far surpasses that which could be delivered without such differentiation. This model provides the nursing profession with a vehicle to position nurses within the expanding care delivery system in a manner that is beneficial to the health and well-being of patients as well as the health and well-being of the profession and the industry.

Various rationales exist for differentiated practice. First, if properly carried out, it can serve to improve patient care and contribute to patient safety. Second, there is the benefit to be gained from a structure that enables the most effective and efficient utilization of scarce resources. Third, there is the opportunity to provide increased satisfaction for nurses themselves because they are better able to optimize their practice. Finally, differentiated practice provides the opportunity to compensate nurses fairly based on their expertise, contribution, and productivity. (See Table 9–4.)

Staff Nurse*

Job Duties. Renders professional nursing care to patients within an assigned unit, in support of medical care as directed by medical staff and pursuant to objectives and policies of the health care facility.

Performs nursing techniques for the comfort and well-being of the patient. Prepares equipment and assists physician during treatments and examinations of patients. Administers prescribed medications, orally and by injections; provides treatments using therapeutic equipment; observes patients' reactions to medications and treatments; observes progress of intravenous infusions and subcutaneous infiltrations; changes or assists physician in changing dressings and cleaning wounds or incisions; takes temperature, pulse, respiration rate, blood pressure, and heart beat to detect deviations from normal and gauge progress of patient, following physician's orders and approved nursing care plan. Observes, records, and reports to nurse manager or physician patients' condition and reaction to drugs, treatments, and significant incidents.

Maintains patients' medical records on nursing observations and actions taken, such as medications and treatments given, reactions, tests, intake and emission of liquids and solids, temperature, pulse, and respiration rate. Records nursing needs of patients on nursing care plan to ensure continuity of care.

Observes emotional stability of patients, expresses interest in their progress, and prepares them for continuing care after discharge. Explains procedures and treatments ordered to gain patients' cooperation and allay apprehension.

Rotates on day, evening, and night tours of duty and may be asked to rotate among various clinical and nursing services of the institution. Each service will have specialized duties, and the staff nurse may be known by the section to which assigned, such as Staff Nurse, Obstetrics

---

*Source: *Job Descriptions and Organizational Analysis for Hospitals and Related Health Services*, U.S. Training and Employment Service, Department of Labor, 1971.

Table 9–4 Model for Differentiating Nursing Practice Roles

	Clinician/Case Manager	*Team Leader*	*Staff Nurse*
Educational preparation	Postbaccalaureate	Baccalaureate	Associate degree
Structure of practice	Direct long-term relationship with clients for determination and coordination of nursing care across multiple settings	Continuous responsibility for clinical leadership of nursing staff in specific, structured care context, such as institutional settings or service agencies	Time and place-limited responsibility for delegated care of assigned clients
Role responsibilities	Primary relationship with client for the purpose of identifying health care needs and facilitating client's decision making regarding action to be taken	Transformation and interpretation of prescribed medical and nursing care according to individualized, client-centered needs	Implementation of delegated medical and nursing care for specific clients according to plans developed by nursing clinician and team leader
	Communication and collaboration with nurses In various settings where client is being cared for regarding relationship of immediate care to long-term perspective	Matching of client's needs with staff abilities Integration of nursing care within interdisciplinary context	Communication of observations regarding client's condition and effectiveness of care
	Collaboration with other health professionals to facilitate client's access to needed resources		

Source: Reprinted from "Toward an Integrative Model of Professional Practice," by M.A. Newman, 1990, *Journal of Professional Nursing, 6,* p. 171. Copyright 1990 by W.B. Saunders Company. Reprinted by permission.

or Staff Nurse, Pediatrics. May serve as a team leader for a group of staff rendering nursing care to a number of patients.

Assists in planning, supervising, and instructing licensed practical nurses, nursing aides, orderlies, and students. Demonstrates nursing techniques and procedures, and assists nonprofessional nursing care personnel in rendering nursing care in unit.

May assist with operations and deliveries by perparing rooms; sterilizing instruments, equipment, and supplies, and handing them, in order of use, to surgeon or other medical specialist.

Education, Training, and Experience. Graduation from an accredited school of nursing and current licensure by state board of nursing.

Orientation training in specific unit only; no experience required beyond that obtained in school of nursing.

NURSE ASSISTIVE/EXTENDER PERSONNEL

Institutional Goals

Many health care facilities have moved toward the creation of roles designed to complement and support the role of the professional nurse and patient care teams. These supportive and complementary roles have been given several labels, including *nursing technicians, nurse extenders, nonlicensed support staff, partners in practice,* and several other institutionally oriented titles. Institutions use assistive personnel to achieve the following goals.*

Provide a model that promotes and fosters the professional nurse having the time and authority for the management of patient care processes. In this model, the assistive health care worker possesses the necessary skills to carry out selected technical, less complex, and more routine activities involved in the patient care process and selected tasks of maintaining the patient care environment. The achievement of this goal fosters the professional nurse focus on the patient care management process and the more complex aspects of the patient care process.

Capitalize on the unique skills of the professional nurse. These skills are related to the higher level cognitive activities of analysis, synthesis, critical thinking, and moral reasoning, which are necessary to carry out the processes of assessment, diagnosis, intervention in the more complex and unpredictable aspects of care, and evaluation of care processes and outcomes. By using assistive/supportive staff in a critical care area, more time and focus can be given by the professional nurse to the cognitive/knowledge aspects of the patient care process.

Decrease the total cost of staff delivering care and maintaining the patient care environment. The cost of support staff is less than that of professional members, thereby enabling the total cost of staff to decrease. The decrease in cost must be measured and financially evaluated in relation to defined outcomes, including length of stay, complications, readmissions, and other forms of rework. A true decrease in the cost of staff salaries and benefits expense must be measured by outcomes achieved.

Differentiate the roles of the professional nurse in critical practice areas of responsibility, authority, and accountability as based on knowledge, skills, competency, and legal definitions of roles and the type and level of care required.

These goals can become the criteria for consideration in the development of the role responsibilities, skills required, and qualifications for the assistive/support staff position.

Definitions of Nurse Extenders*

Various types of nurse extenders have been reported in new models of nursing practice. (One major study found over 65 titles applied to the range of personnel who would qualify as assistive personnel.)

Using Unlicensed Assistive Personnel

Unlicensed assistive personnel (UAPs) are, and will continue to be, used in most health care settings. It has been suggested that if UAPs participate in direct care, a framework for training and supervising them must be in place and the terms related to the use of UAPs must be understood (see Tables 9–5 and 9–6).

Source: Sally Knox, Jan Gharrity, and Brydie Baker, "The Successful Utilization of Nonlicensed Assistive Staff in a Critical Care Area," *Critical Care Nursing Quarterly,* Vol. 18:3, Aspen Publishers, Inc., © November 1995.

Source: Cecile A. Lengacher and Patricia R. Mabe, "Nurse Extenders," *Journal of Nursing Administration,* Vol. 23:3, March 1993, J.B. Lippincott Company.

Table 9–5 Using Patient Care Assistants

Key Components of Patient Care Assistant
Training Program

- Being a team member
- Safety needs of the patient
- Infection control
- Positioning and transfers
- The elderly patient
- The stroke patient
- The hypertensive patient
- The diabetic patient
- Meeting nutritional needs
- Skin care
- Bowel and bladder care

Tasks that R.N.s Would Give Up

Nonnursing functions
- Transportation
  - –Trips to pharmacy
  - –Trips to central supply

- –Moving furniture
- –Moving patients
- –Delivering water pitchers, dietary trays
- Unit operations
  - –Cleaning utility room
  - –Stocking supply carts
  - –"Stuffing" charts
  - –Answering telephone
  - –Nursing functions

Selected aspects of patient care
- –Routine vital signs
- –Ambulating patients
- –Bed baths
- –Morning care
- –Bedtime care
- –Assisting patient to bathroom
- –Turning patients
- –Feeding patients
- –Oral hygiene
- –Answering call lights

Source: Sandra C. Hesterly and Margaret Robinson, "Alternative Caregivers: Cost-effective Utilization of RNs," *Nursing Administration Quarterly*, Vol. 14:3, Aspen Publishers, Inc., © 1990.

Table 9–6 Limitations of Unlicensed Assistive Personnel

A large number of employees in the nursing service are grouped under the title of auxiliary nursing personnel; these include nurses' aides, orderlies, and technicians. Auxiliary nursing personnel generally go through at least a hospital orientation training program before assuming their nursing duties with patients. Some states require a formal training program for nurses' aides. They do not need to be graduates of a formal education program, nor are they licensed or certified. These personnel generally are assigned duties by the graduate nurse, staff nurse, or head nurse. Specific limits to interventions that may not be delegated to unlicensed personnel are outlined in each state and vary according to their law. The more common restrictions include:

- medication administration

- any procedure that requires piercing of the skin (as in drawing blood or giving injections)
- surgical asepsis
- tube feeding
- suctioning

Many states strictly prohibit the delegation of the administration of medication, but several states are recognizing that this is appropriate in some settings. Group homes for the developmentally or mentally disabled, community settings for the physically handicapped, group homes for the elderly, and long-term care facilities are all examples of areas where assistive personnel may be allowed to administer medication. These circumstances include the involvement of the RN in the training and supervising of the assistive personnel.

Source: Adapted from I.D. Snook, *Hospitals: What They Are and How They Work,* Aspen Publishers, Inc., © 1992 and R.I. Hansten and M.J. Washburn, *Clinical Delegation Skills: A Handbook for Nurses,* Aspen Publishers, Inc., © 1994.

- *Traditional extender model:* assistive personnel to the registered nurse, including the nursing assistant, unit assistant, ward clerk, orderly, housekeeping staff, and dietary aide
- *Nontraditional extender model:* assistive positions to the registered nurse that require extra training; includes the electrocardiogram technician, monitor technician, phlebotomy technician, and corps members
- *Traditional extender in partnership model:* assistive personnel to the registered nurse, including the traditional extender as a partner in patient care with a registered nurse (nursing assistants and licensed practical nurses)
- *Nontraditional extender in partnership model:* assistive personnel to the registered nurse, including the use of a nontraditional extender as partner in patient care with a registered nurse (primarily patient care and critical care technicians)

Framework for Using UAPs *

The following framework for supervision has been suggested by the American Association of Critical Care Nurses (AACCN):

- definition of nursing support personnel as unlicensed individuals who are not professional nurses but who are accountable to and work under the direct supervision of a professional nurse to implement specifically delegated patient care activities
- clearly delineated and monitored patient care standards
- administrative systems that establish accountability for ensuring that the use of support personnel complies with established standards of care

- written job descriptions that clearly delineate duties, responsibilities, qualifications, skills and supervision of support personnel
- competency-based performance expectations and mechanisms for ongoing performance appraisals
- appropriate orientation and training of support personnel in line with performance expectations and role responsibility
- clearly defined mechanisms to ensure all nursing support personnel are directly supervised by and responsible to professional nurses
- careful monitoring and evaluation of the impact of nursing support personnel on adherence to care standards and patient outcomes

Differentiation of Activities—Workload Redistribution *

Appropriate use of assistive personnel will result in workload distribution. Workload distribution evaluates the roles of the nursing team members, helps allocate the workload more effectively, promotes teamwork, defines what care is delegated, and specifies the registered nurse's responsibilities for care assigned to nursing assistants and other assistive personnel.

The nurse manager must determine which activities require the professional expertise of a registered nurse and which tasks may be performed by ancillary personnel and then redistribute the work accordingly. When planning to redistribute the workload, consideration should be given to the following questions:

- What is the risk management and liability for each level of caregiver?
- Who is the least expensive worker to perform a specific task?

Source: Reprinted with permission of *AACN News,* American Association of Critical-Care Nurses, "Clinical Practice," The American Association of Critical-Care Nurses, January 1996.

Source: Adapted from Cynthia Allen Abbott, "Strategies for Integrating Unlicensed Personnel into the Perioperative Setting," in *The Manual of Operating Room Management: An Administrative and Patient Care Resource,* Cynthia Spry, ed., Aspen Publishers, Inc., © September 1992.

- How much supervision must the nurse provide the assistive personnel?
- Will an expanded role for the assistive personnel (e.g., health care technician) influence recruitment of department nurses?
- Will an expanded role for the assistive personnel have an impact on collective bargaining?

To identify activities that can be performed by assistive staff/technicians, management and staff must identify all the activities of nursing practice and then separate them into non-nursing and nursing activities. Non-nursing activities do not involve direct patient care and do not require nursing skills. Non-nursing activities include tasks such as cleaning, running errands, clerical duties, and maintaining stock, and other maintenance activities. Nursing activities are those that directly involve the patient, such as patient transfer and preoperative skin preparation. Nursing activities require specialized knowledge, judgment, and skill.

AMBULATORY MANAGEMENT POSITIONS: OUTPATIENT CLINICS*

Many hospitals have expanded their nursing division by developing outpatient clinics. Depending on the extent of the clinic network, the major responsibilities are to the chairperson of the department of nursing.

Director of Outpatient Clinics

- Assigns nursing technician personnel and provides adequate staffing of all outpatient clinics.
- Supervises all nursing technicians assigned to the outpatient clinics where there are no charge nurses.
- Inspects clinics daily and identifies the necessity for rotation of personnel in general therapy clinic and emergency department,

for training, and for adjusting schedules to provide for competent patient care at all times.
- Keeps nurse managers informed of special abilities of technicians or other pertinent items of special interest.

Charge Nurse—Clinics

General Therapy Clinic

- Assesses and identifies patients' health problems and needs.
- Assists with or initiates emergency lifesaving procedures.
- Provides health teaching for patients and families.
- Assists with research related to the improvement of the delivery of health care services.

Surgical Clinic

- Plans, organizes, directs, coordinates, and evaluates all nursing functions in the surgical specialty clinics.
- Screens patients and refers them to appropriate physicians, clinical specialists, or hospital departments.
- Identifies patients' nursing care needs and problems and practices nursing to meet established goals.
- Maintains accurate records of nursing assessments, plans, and care.
- Is self-directing in practice; makes professional judgments, counsels and teaches patients, families, and coworkers.

Obstetrical-Gynecological Clinic

- Directs and coordinates all nursing activities in the obstetrical-gynecological clinic.
- Provides health services, which include health education, maintenance, prevention, and early case finding.
- Plays an important role in interpretation of treatment, making diagnostic reports, giving emergency care, taking patients' histories, and initiating charts.

Source: Russell C. Swansburg, *Management of Patient Care Services,* C.V. Mosby Co., © 1976. Reprinted with permission of the author.

EDUCATIONAL POSITIONS*

Director of Staff Development (Inservice/Education Coordinator)

Job Duties. Plans, develops, and directs program of education for all nursing service personnel, and coordinates staff development with nursing service program.

Develops, schedules, and directs orientation program for professional and auxiliary nursing service personnel. Develops instructional materials to assist new staff in becoming oriented to the health care facility's operational techniques. If not scheduled by human resources department, schedules facility tours and addresses by administrative staff to acquaint new staff with overall operation and interrelationship of facility services. Determines effectiveness of orientation materials and procedures through practice sessions. Sets up demonstrations of nursing service equipment to acquaint staff with new equipment and make them more familiar with established equipment.

Plans, coordinates, and conducts regular and special inservice training sessions for nursing staff to acquaint them with new procedures and policies and new trends and developments in patient care techniques and to provide opportunity for individual members to develop to their full potential.

Keeps current on latest developments by attending professional seminars and institutes and reading professional journals. Assists nurse managers and head nurses in planning and implementing staff development programs in their units. Keeps bulletin boards current by listing information on seminars and institutes and promotes appropriate staff attendance at these professional meetings. Plans training sessions for supervisory staff members.

May participate with committees in writing and maintaining policy and procedure manuals and nursing service forms. Reviews suggestions

submitted by nursing service staff for changes or clarification in policies and procedures.

Writes annual reports on activities and prepares plans for future activities. Prepares budget requests.

Education, Training, and Experience. Graduation from an accredited school of nursing and current licensure by state board of nursing; graduation from a recognized college or university with specialization in education; bachelor's degree required. Experience as head nurse, nurse manager, or nurse educator.

It would be a positive advantage for the director of staff development to have had professional experiences that would encompass clinical, teaching, and supervisory practice within a large, active nursing service organization. It is important that the director be "service minded" and familiar with the needs and problems of service staff. The director should have a broad and thorough knowledge of nursing skills that would enable him or her to appraise the quality of nursing care being given as well as to assess the abilities enabling an individual nursing practitioner to meet the expectations of a specific job.

Nurse Educator

Job Duties. Plans, coordinates, and carries out educational programs (theoretical and practical aspects of nursing) to train ancillary nursing personnel.

Prepares and issues trainee manuals (which describe duties and responsibilities of nursing assistants) to be used as training guides. Familiarizes new employees with physical layout of the facility and facility policies and procedures, organizational structure, etiquette, and employee benefits. Plans educational program and schedules classes in basic patient care procedures, such as bedmaking, blood pressure and temperature taking, and feeding of patients. Teaches nursing aides and orderlies nursing procedures by demonstration in classrooms and clinical units and by lectures in classrooms, using aids such as motion pictures, charts, and slides. Observes trainees in practical application of procedures. Secures cooperation of nurse managers and head

---

*Source: Job Descriptions and Organizational Analysis for Hospitals and Related Health Services, U.S. Training and Employment Service, Department of Labor, 1971.

nurses to assist in teaching their specialty; coordinates training with all nursing service units to maintain consistency in practice and establish relationships, to give scope to the educational program, and to point out variations of duties required by different units and on different shifts.

Prepares, administers, and scores examinations to determine trainees' suitability for the job. Makes recommendations to nursing service regarding placement of trainees according to test scores and practical application performance. Evaluates trainees' progress following training period and submits report to nursing service for further processing. Conducts meetings with trainees and with nurse managers to discuss problems and ideas for improving nursing service training program.

Education, Training, and Experience. Graduation from an accredited school of nursing and current licensure by state board of nursing; advanced training in teaching methods and supervision.

One year's experience as head nurse or nurse manager.

Nursing Instructor: Inservice

Job Duties. Plans, directs, and coordinates inservice orientation and educational program for professional nursing personnel.

Assists director of staff development in planning and carrying out program of staff development. Confers with director of staff development to schedule training programs for professional nurses already on the staff, according to departmental work requirements. Lectures to nurses and demonstrates improved methods of nursing service. Lectures and demonstrates procedures, using motion pictures, charts, and slides.

Orients new staff members and provides inservice refresher training for professional nurses returning to nursing service.

Instructs volunteer workers in routine procedures such as aseptic practice and blood pressure and temperature taking.

Education, Training, and Experience. Graduation from an accredited school of nursing and current licensure by state board of nursing; advanced training in teaching methods and supervision.

One year's experience as head nurse or nurse manager.

NON-NURSING JOBS ON THE UNIT*

Some nursing administrators have sought relief from responsibilities that fall outside of direct patient care by inserting a non-nursing person into the nursing service organizational structure—the unit supervisor. The unit supervisor is intended to provide administrative direction in the patient unit while the nursing staff retain full control over patient care.

Unit Supervisor

Job Duties. Supervises and coordinates administrative management functions for one or more patient care units.

Supervises clerical staff and ensures accomplishment of administrative functions on a 24-hour basis by scheduling working hours and arranging for coverage of nursing care unit by non-nursing personnel. Performs human resources management tasks by orienting and training new staff. Evaluates performance of assigned workers by checking for quality and quantity.

Inventories and stores patients' personal effects either within the unit or in the health care facility vault.

Establishes and maintains an adequate inventory of drugs and supplies for the unit.

Coordinates with other departments such as housekeeping and maintenance to maintain a unit that is hygienically safe and functional. Checks for cleanliness of the unit and reports discrepancies to the appropriate supervisor. Performs daily maintenance inspection, and through proper

---

Source: Job Descriptions and Organizational Analysis for Hospitals and Related Health Services, U.S. Training and Employment Service, Department of Labor, 1971.

channels initiates minor facility improvement projects.

Maintains close contact with medical and surgical reservations in regard to admissions, transfers, discharges, and other services. Serves as liaison between the specific patient care unit and other departments. Reviews special tests at the end of shift.

Ensures that the medical record is completed in accordance with the standards of the Joint Commission on Accreditation of Healthcare Organizations. Ensures facility compliance with Medicare requirements insofar as certification and related administrative matters are concerned. Checks charts of patients scheduled for surgery or other special procedures to verify completeness of orders of consent, preparation orders, and lab results and for necessary signatures.

Greets, directs, and gives nonprofessional factual information to patients, visitors, and staff from other departments.

Participates in projects, surveys, and other information gathering activities approved by facility management.

Education, Training, and Experience. One year of college or equivalent.

A minimum of one year's supervisory experience.

On-the-job training in coordinating non-nursing services for the assigned nursing units.

Unit Clerk (Floor Clerk, Nursing Station Assistant)

Job Duties. Performs general clerical duties by preparing, compiling, and maintaining records in a nursing unit.

Records name of patient, address, and name of attending physician on medical record forms. Copies information, such as patients' temperature, pulse rate, and blood pressure, from nurses' records. Writes requisitions for laboratory tests and procedures such as basal metabolism, X-rays, electrocardiograms, blood examinations, and urinalysis. Under supervision, plots temperature, pulse rate, and other data on appropriate graph charts. Copies and computes other data, as directed, and enters on patients' charts. May record diet instructions. Keeps file of medical records on patients in unit. Routes charts when patients are transferred or dismissed, following specified procedures. May compile census of patients.

Keeps record of absences and hours worked by unit staff. Types various records, schedules, and reports and delivers them to appropriate office. May maintain records of special monetary charges to patients and forward them to the business office. May verify stock supplies on unit and prepare requisitions to maintain established inventories. Dispatches messages to other departments or to persons in other departments and makes appointments for patient services in other departments as requested by nursing staff. Makes posthospitalization appointments with patients' physicians. Delivers mail, newspapers, and flowers to patients.

Education, Training, and Experience. High school graduation or equivalent, including courses in English, typing, spelling, and arithmetic, or high school graduation supplemented by commercial school course in subjects indicated.

No previous experience is required.

Chapter 10

Nursing Service Standards and Policies

NURSING SERVICE STANDARDS

Nursing service standards created by the various professional organizations and governmental agencies concerned with quality health care can be of immense value to the director of nursing by serving as a framework for departmental evaluations. The difficulty is in deciding which set of standards to use—though in some instances there is no choice. State and city regulations or the "voluntary" criteria linked to an accreditation process, as with the Joint Commission on Accreditation of Healthcare Organizations, are often backed by sanctions, legal or otherwise. The standards most often referred to by nursing administrators are those of the American Nurses' Association.

There is, however, an ever-increasing number of nursing specialty organizations that have been busy formulating practice standards in their area of expertise. A partial list of organizations that may be consulted for standards includes the American Association of Critical Care Nurses, American Association of Nurse Anesthetists, American Nephrology Nurses' Association, American Radiological Nurses Association, Association for Practitioners in Infection Control, Association of Operating Room Nurses, Inc., Association of Rehabilitation Nurses, Intravenous Nurses Society, Nursing Association of the American College of Obstetrics and Gynecology, National Association of Neonatal Nurses, National Association of Orthopedic Nurses, National Nurses Society on Addictions, Oncology Nursing Society, and Society of Gastroenterology Nurses and Associates, Inc.

The function of established standards is to supply professionally desirable norms against which the department's performance can be viewed. Once areas for improvement have been identified, the criteria continue to serve in setting directions for corrective action. The process is not complete until the decisions for improvement are transformed into a plan of action and implemented. And even later, at the time of reassessment, the original data collected can be used as a baseline for measuring progress against the standards.

American Nurses' Association Standards

The American Nurses' Association (ANA) developed a series of generic standards that may provide a basis from which nursing can further generate or modify standards to meeting its particular needs. The ANA provides two major kinds of standards.

1. *Nursing service standards* focus on those elements, conditions, or results believed essen-

tial to the effective and efficient management of any nursing service or department. Established series of standards for nursing range from the education of nurses to the administration of nursing services. Specific standards include standards for continuing education in nursing; guidelines for staff development; nursing staff requirements for inpatient health care services; and roles, responsibilities, and qualifications for nurse administrators.

2. *Nursing practice standards* focus on those elements, conditions, or results believed to be indicative of quality nursing care. The ANA's Congress for Nursing Practice has developed and published standards of practice in 10 areas: nursing practice, community health nursing practice, geriatric nursing practice, maternal-child health nursing practice, psychiatric-mental health nursing practice, medical-surgical nursing practice, emergency department nursing practice, cardiovascular nursing practice, orthopedic nursing practice, and operating room nursing practice.

Overview: Joint Commission Accreditation Standards

The Joint Commission on Accreditation of Healthcare Organizations (Joint Commission) can trace its roots to a 1918 American College of Surgeons program that established standards, evaluated care provided in hospitals, and granted accreditation for those hospitals meeting the standards. Those standards set the first formal requirement for review and evaluation of the quality of patient care. In 1951, the American College of Surgeons joined with the American College of Physicians, the American Hospital Association, the American Medical Association, and the Canadian Medical Association to form the Joint Commission on Accreditation of Hospitals. The early emphasis was on processes and structures for delivering care rather than on outcomes.

Today, in its most recent reorganization of accreditation requirements, the Joint Commission has reformulated its standards. The *Accredita-*

tion Manual is no longer organized into chapters based on distinct departments or disciplines such as surgical services, radiology, and laboratory. Now, the manual is divided into three sections related to functions critical for patient care (see box).

Though there are requirements set for the nursing service as an essential "structure with functions" (see Table 10–1), the criteria pertinent to the nursing process are found in a number of chapters, not just one.

The objective of these changes is to stimulate and reinforce a cross-functional (multidisciplinary) approach to performance and performance improvement across the entire health care organization. The emphasis is on overriding professional boundaries and constructing a collaborative approach to delivering patient care services.

Joint Commission Accreditation Manual Standards

Patient-Focused Functions

Patient Rights and Organizational Ethics
Assessment of Patients
Care of Patients
Education
Continuum of Care

Organizational Functions

Improving Organizational Performance
Leadership
Management of Information
Management of Human Resources
Management of the Environment of Care
Surveillance, Prevention, and Control of
  Infection

Structures with Functions

Governance
Management
Medical Staff
Nursing

Table 10–1 Requirements for Nursing as a Structure

NR.1 Nursing services are directed by a nurse executive who is a registered nurse qualified by advanced education and management experience.

NR.1.1 If the organization's structure is decentralized, an identified nurse leader at the executive level provides authority and accountability for, and coordination of, the nurse executive functions.

NR.2 The nurse executive has the authority and responsibility for establishing standards of nursing practice.

NR.2.1 *The nurse executive and other nursing leaders participate with leaders from the governing body, management, medical staff, and clinical areas in planning, promoting, and conducting organizationwide performance-improvement activities.*

NR.3 *Nursing policies and procedures, nursing standards of patient care, and standards of nursing practice are*

NR.3.1 developed by the nurse executive, registered nurses, and other designated nursing staff members;

NR.3.2 defined in writing; and

NR.3.3 approved by the nurse executive or a designee(s).

Source: © *1995 Accreditation Manual for Healthcare Organizations.* Oakbrook Terrace, IL: Joint Commission on Accreditation of Healthcare Organizations, 1994. Reprinted with permission.

To allow more latitude in how these relationships and improvements are structured, the Joint Commission no longer mandates specific processes and methods to be used in implementing the standards. It is the responsibility of the health care facility's leaders to be knowledgeable about the intent, content and requirements of the standards in all the chapters that may pertain to their scope of responsibility.

*Preparing for the Survey**

Hallmarks of the Joint Commission's new survey process are an increased emphasis on education, useful and timely feedback, and better service to surveyed organizations. Each organization has a Joint Commission liaison person assigned to it to facilitate preparing for the survey. Six months prior to the survey, a survey planning packet will be sent to the organization containing guidelines for the survey process, a survey planning questionnaire, documents for review, and a generic agenda.

The on-site survey process has been designed to assess whether correct processes not only are performed, but are performed well or whether, if necessary, they are being improved. The focus of the survey is performance, both organizationwide and multidisciplinary in scope. The methodologies employed during the survey include (1) interviews with patients, families, and staff; (2) observation through tours of the entire facility; and (3) review of documents. The document review session orients the surveyors to the health care facility's practices, provides an early indication of compliance with the standards, and prepares the surveyors for the interactive portion of the survey. The facility determines which documents will be reviewed and the method of organizing the documents.

In preparing for the survey, the organization should conduct a self-assessment using the scoring guidelines and should conduct a mock survey. In addition, it is imperative to have practice sessions for staff interviews, leadership interviews, open and closed medical records reviews, and presentation of performance improvement projects. There are many publications available from both the Joint Commission and private organizations that can provide a framework and documents for conducting the self-assessment and mock surveys.

Source: Jacqueline B. White, "Preparing for the Joint Commission on Accreditation of Healthcare Organizations Survey," in *The Manual of Operating Room Management: An Administrative and Patient Care Resource*, Cynthia Spry, ed., Aspen Publishers, Inc., © October 1995.

NURSING SERVICE POLICIES

Policies are the guides to thinking and action by which managers seek to delineate the areas within which decisions will be made and subsequent actions taken. Policies spell out the required, prohibited, or suggested courses of action. The limitations on actions are stated, defined, or at least clearly implied.

Source: Joan Gratto Liebler, Ruth Ellen Levine, and Jeffrey Rothman, *Management Principles for Health Professionals*, ed 2, Aspen Publishers, Inc., © 1992.

Policy Formulation*

There are three general areas in nursing that require policy formulation: (1) areas in which confusion about the locus of responsibility might result in neglect or malperformance of an act necessary to a patient's welfare; (2) areas pertaining to the protection of patients' and families' rights, such as right to privacy, property rights; and (3) areas involving matters of human resource management and welfare.

It is not necessary that policies always provide detailed directions for action on every issue. Perhaps, for some issues, *specification of where the responsibility resides is the most pertinent consideration.*

Occasionally one hears that a policy is "just a guideline, not a rule calling for rigid enforcement." The implication seems to be that one can choose to follow a different course, that the policy is simply a suggestion. This might at least in part be reasonable at certain levels of functioning, but at others such an approach could generate chaos, particularly when the very reason for the existence of such policies may be to avoid the possibility of individual choice of action. The extent to which a policy will not be followed to the letter or might even be ignored

*Source: M.M. Cantor, "Policies . . . Guidelines for Action," *Journal of Nursing Administration*, May-June 1972. Reprinted with permission.

entirely will likely depend on the difficulty of its implementation and the degree to which individuals are led to believe that departmental policies do not constitute mandatory matters.

If a policy is developed with attention to its feasibility within the actual setting, there should be little occasion for individuals to deviate from or ignore it. If the persons who have the information needed to make decisions in individual situations are given appropriate degrees of latitude, and those who are not equipped to deviate are given clear directions to follow explicitly, little difficulty should be experienced in maintaining strict implementation of policy.

Setting the expectation that a policy must be followed and holding to that expectation are essential for effective use of policies. If a policy is deemed necessary to achieve a particular purpose, then one ought to assume that it should be followed. If it appears not to matter whether or not individuals follow it, then one might well question the need for it.

There could be several reasons why a policy is not or cannot be implemented. If a policy fails to take into account the constraints within a situation then one can expect that it will not be implementable. A policy that requires isolation of individuals with wound infections would not be implemented on an area in which there exist no such accommodations. A policy that requires that only a registered nurse shall perform certain functions, when in fact registered nurses are not always available, is doomed from the beginning. The decision to change the policy to allow for discrepancies in the situation as opposed to modifying the situation so that the policy can be implemented is a serious one. One must be careful not to assume that, because a policy is not currently being implemented, the policy should necessarily be changed. If the situation is such that the policy as it stands is not implemented and that serious consequences might occur as a result, it would appear that the situation must be changed to ensure that the policy is followed.

The criteria by which one can judge the appropriateness of departmental policies have to do with the degree to which they facilitate the achievement of the goals of the department. Poli-

---

Wording and Flexibility of Policies

Policies permit and require interpretation. Language indicators, such as "whenever possible" or "as circumstances permit," are expressions typically used to give policies the flexibility needed. Policies should be somewhat futuristic in that they are meant to remain in force, with little change, for long periods of time. In any age of rapid social change, it is helpful to think in broad terms, anticipating change. It also helps to set aside the normal biases that stem from describing the way things are now. Contradictions within policies and between policies and their related procedures should be avoided. The careful development of procedure, in addition to a comparison with related policy statements, is an essential step.

Source: Joan Gratto Liebler, Ruth Ellen Levine, and Jeffrey Rothman, *Management Principles for Health Professionals*, ed 2, Aspen Publishers, Inc., © 1992.

---

cies that do this will probably contain the characteristics listed in Table 10–2.

Nursing Service: Mission, Philosophy, and Objectives*

Purpose or Mission

Each institution exists for a specific purpose or mission and to fulfill a specific social function. For health care institutions this means health care services to maintain health, cure illness, and allay pain and suffering.

Defining mission or purpose allows nursing to be managed for performance. It describes what it will be and what it should be. It describes the constituencies to be satisfied. It is the profes-

---

*Source: Russell C. Swansburg, *Management of Patient Care Services*, The C.V. Mosby Co., 1976. Reprinted with permission of the author.

Table 10–2 Criteria for Evaluating Appropriateness of Policies

- The purposes of the policies can be stated in terms of the effects to be achieved as a result of their formulation and implementation.
- The expected consequences of the policies can be shown to be instrumental in achieving the objectives of the department.
- The content of the policies is directly related to their stated purposes and reflects the due consideration given to relevant factors in their formulation.
- The amount of direction included is based on the level characterizing the position in which the implementation must occur.

---

sional nurse manager's commitment to a specific definition of purpose or mission.

Philosophy

Philosophy describes vision, what the nursing service manager sees the nursing service as and what he or she believes it to be. The written statement of philosophy explains the beliefs that determine how the mission or purpose is achieved; it gives direction to achieving purpose. Philosophy is abstract, and, with the mission or purpose statement, it sets the character and tone of service.

[The content areas in Table 10–3 are found in most comprehensive nursing philosophies. If the division has no strong values concerning a given content area, the area may be omitted in the philosophy statement.]

Objectives

Objectives are concrete and specific statements of the goals that the nurse manager of the department of nursing plans to accomplish. They are action commitments through which the mission or purpose will be achieved and the philosophy or beliefs sustained. They are used to establish priorities. They should be stated in terms of results to be achieved and should focus on the production of health care services to clients.

Table 10–3 Nursing Philosophy: Typical Content Areas

Nursing Values

____ A specific nursing theory, incorporated or given by reference to another document

____ Nursing practice values, which may or may not include commitments to various practice models and assignment systems

____ Nursing education values, with respect either to staff education, to education of students, or both

____ Nursing research values, with respect to active research programs, to the application of research findings of others, or both

____ Relationship of nursing practice to nursing administration or institutional administration

____ Nursing management values (may include commitments to particular modes of management, e.g., participative management)

Patient Relationships

____ Relationship of nursing or the nursing division to the client (or patient)

____ Perceived rights of clients and significant others in relation to patient care and health-related choices

____ Values related to human rights and other beliefs about patients/people

____ Relationship of nursing to patient outcomes, their achievement, and measurement

Professional Relationships

____ Relationship of nursing to the rest of the organization, which may include reference to its modes of operation

____ Relationship of nursing staff with other health professionals or to other nurse professionals to the goals of other departments (e.g., to research goals of medicine or placement goals of social service)

____ Relationship of the nursing division (or its members) to professional nursing—organizational or conceptual

____ Relationships of nursing to other institutions of health care (coordinative and cooperative relationships)

____ Relationship of nursing to the extended client world (e.g., the community or the society)

____ Relationship to other value systems (e.g., religious beliefs or societal preferences)

Other Values

____ Values related to employee rights or concepts of professional and occupational behavior

____ Values related to promotions, retentions, and transfers within the organization

____ Values related to ethical conflicts and related nurse decision making

Source: Barbara Stevens Barnum and Karlene M. Kerfoot, *The Nurse as Executive*, ed 4, Aspen Publishers, Inc., © 1995.

Objectives are similar to the philosophy of the department of nursing because both support the mission or purpose: Philosophy states beliefs and values, and objectives state specific and measurable goals to be accomplished. Both must be functional and useful—alive.

Areas for Objectives. Objectives are the fundamental strategy of nursing, since they are the end product of all nursing activities. They must be capable of being converted into specific targets and specific assignments so that nurses will know what they have to do to accomplish them.

Objectives become the basis and motivation for the nursing work necessary to accomplish them and for measuring nursing achievement.

Management must balance objectives. Some will be short range, with their accomplishment in easy view or reach. Others will be long range, and some may even be in the "hope to be accomplished" target date timetable. The budget is the mechanical expression of setting and balancing objectives.

In nursing, all objectives should be performance objectives. They should provide for existing nursing services for existing patient groups. They should provide for abandonment of unneeded and outmoded nursing services and health care products. They should provide for new nursing services and health care products for existing patients. They should provide for new groups of patients, for the distributive organization, and for standards of nursing service and performance.

Objectives are the basis for work and assignments. They determine the organizational structure, the key activities, and the allocation of people to tasks. Objectives make the work of nursing such that it is clear and unambiguous, the results are measurable, there are deadlines to be met, and there is a specific assignment of accountability. They give direction and make commitments that mobilize the resources and energies of nursing for the making of the future.

NURSING SERVICE POLICY MANUAL

Setting up a policy manual for the nursing service, and keeping it current, involves a lot of work, but the result is well worth the time and effort involved. Writing and organizing it require concentrated thought, and the result is usually clearer, more realistic policies. Since departmental policies must reflect the policies of the health care facility, the carefully thought out manual defines the scope of departmental responsibility within the facility. The manual becomes a tool for orienting staff, a reference when unexpected problems arise, a foundation on which to develop administrative procedures, and a firm basis for discussion when differences occur. Conflicts and issues are easier to settle in terms of policy than in terms of personalities; the basis of the conflict becomes the point of discussion and not who is to blame for it.

Setting Up a Policy Manual

Some manuals contain a combination of policies and administrative procedures. Others are limited to policies only. When the two are mixed, it is often difficult to be sure what is policy and what is procedure, and the manual may become bulky with lengthy instructions and sample forms. But whatever will work best for the individual department should be included.

Here are a few suggestions from the American Hospital Association (AHA) to keep in mind when writing policies and organizing them into a manual.

- Use concise, simple language; keep it easy to understand and next to impossible to misunderstand.
- Remember that policies are guides for making decisions about what to do, so keep them realistic and be sure they truly reflect the objectives of the department.
- Organize the manual as simply as possible so that it will be easy to use. Give thought to indexing, to dating entries, and to the need for keeping it up-to-date. Provide for incorporating policy changes into the manual.
- Plan for periodic review of policies, and set up a timetable for such review.
- In reviewing, evaluate effectiveness and workability; review experiences of staff in carrying out the policies; and verify that policies are being followed.
- Be objective about changes; do not let policies become sacred.
- When changes are made, provide for informing all personnel.[1]

Checklist for a General Nursing Service Policy Manual*

The suggested checklist in Table 10–4 is intended as a guide in developing nursing service policies. Though it can scarcely be all-inclusive, it is an indication of the type of material that should be included in a policy manual.

A similar manual should be prepared for each clinical unit and should include those items pertinent to that area.

---

[1]"Practical Approaches to Nursing Service," *AHA*, Vol. 1, No. 1, Summer 1962.

*Source: Sister Jean Marie Braun, S.C.S.C., "A Checklist for Nursing Service Policy Manual," The Catholic Health Association. Reprinted with permission.

Table 10–4 Checklist for a General Nursing Service Policy Manual

PART I. INTERNAL NURSING SERVICE

I. Accidents
A. Care
1. Who
a. Patients
b. Personnel
c. Visitors
2. Where
3. Whose responsibility
B. Reporting
1. Forms
a. Number of copies
b. Who fills out
c. Who receives
2. Oral
a. Who
b. What office
c. Telephone number
C. Precautions to prevent

II. Admissions
A. Receiving patients
1. Information obtained
2. Instructions given
B. Notifying
1. Intern
2. Doctor
3. Other departments

III. Autopsies
A. Obtaining permission
1. By whom
2. From whom—
relationship
3. Witness
B. Arrangement
1. By whom
2. Use of morgue

IV. Breakage
A. Classification
B. Responsibility
C. Reporting

V. Bulletin boards
A. Location
B. Posting of information
1. What
2. Who
C. Removing information

VI. Communicable diseases
A. Types accepted
B. Where placed

C. Cared for by whom
D. Reporting
E. Immunization of
personnel
F. Isolation techniques
1. Concurrent
disinfection
2. Terminal disinfection
3. Gowning and
masking
4. Disposal
a. Food
b. Linen
c. Waste
G. Visiting

VII. Complaints
A. How handled
1. Type
a. Patient
b. Personnel
c. Visitors
2. Kind
a. Routine
b. Emergency
B. Action taken
1. By whom
2. When

VIII. Consents
A. Obtaining
1. By whom
2. From whom
a. Husband and wife
b. Parents
c. Emancipated
minors
3. For what
a. Legal
responsibility
b. State regulations
4. Witness
B. Filing

IX. Consultations
A. List of required
B. List of appropriate

X. Deaths
A. Notifying
1. Who
a. Doctor
b. Family

2. By whom
B. Care and identification
of body
C. Care of personal
belongings
D. Death certificate
1. Making out
2. Signing

XI. Discharge
A. Time
B. Notifications
C. Checking of clothes and
valuables
D. Accompaniment of
patient

XII. Doctors
A. Relationship with
B. What to do if they
cannot be contacted

XIII. Doctor's orders
A. Automatic stop orders
B. Cancellations—surgery
cancels all previous
orders
C. Telephone
D. Oral

XIV. Documents, legal
A. Types
B. Notary public
1. When necessary
2. Where obtained
C. Who may witness

XV. Emergency
A. Definition
B. Use of available beds
C. No available beds

XVI. Elevator service
A. Where
B. Who

**XVII. Equipment and
supplies**
A. List
1. Expendable
2. Nonexpendable
B. Care
C. Lending
D. Repairing
E. Requesting

continues

Table 10–4 continued

**XVIII. Fire regulations;
    evacuation; disaster**
A. Drills
  1. Frequency
  2. Plan
    a. Who in charge
    b. Departmental
      instructions
B. Prevention
  1. Hazards
  2. Extinguishers
    a. Location
    b. Use

XIX. Funeral directors
A. Notification
  1. By whom
  2. How selected
B. Release of body

XX. Flowers
A. Delivery
  1. To facility
    a. When
    b. Where
  2. To patient

XXI. Interns and residents
A. Relationship with
B. Notification of
  1. When
  2. Where

XXII. Information
A. Nature of facility
  information
B. Publication
  1. When
  2. What
  3. By whom
  4. To whom
    a. Press
      1) Name
      2) Telephone
        number
    b. Police
      1) Station
      2) Telephone
        number

  c. Relatives

XXIII. Linen
A. Distribution
B. Requesting
C. Damaged

XXIV. Lost and found
A. Where kept
B. How long
C. Whose
  1. Patients
  2. Personnel
  3. Visitors
D. Whose responsibility

XXV. Meetings
A. Frequency
B. Purpose
C. Types
D. Members
E. Minutes

XXVI. Mentally ill
A. Admission
B. Notification
C. Restraints
D. Supervision
E. Transfer

XXVII. Messenger service
A. Who served
B. By whom
C. Where
D. When

XXVIII. Night security guard
A. Services
B. How contacted

XXIX. Nursing care
A. Borderline functions
  1. Administration and
    preparation
    a. Intravenous fluids
    b. Blood transfusions
    c. Removing sutures
    d. Applying traction
    e. Acute cardiac care
    f. Other
B. Charting

  1. Forms used
  2. Red and blue ink
  3. Things to note
C. Daily assignments
  1. By whom
  2. Where
  3. When
D. Dentures
  1. Identification
  2. Responsibility
E. Emergency drug supply
  1. Contents
  2. Responsibility
  3. Location
F. Ice water
  1. Where obtained
  2. Who allowed
G. Kardex
  1. Use
  2. Sample form
H. Lights out regulations
I. Medications
  1. Card system
    a. Color
    b. Responsibility
    c. Checking
  2. Errors
    a. Correction
    b. Reporting
J. Oxygen
  1. When given without
    an order
  2. Storage of equip-
    ment
  3. Care of equipment
K. Property of patient
  1. Responsibility
  2. Placement

XXX. Patients
A. Relationship to
B. Booklet of privileges
  1. Activity
  2. Postal service
  3. Questionnaires
  4. Radios and televi-
    sions

continues

Table 10–4 continued

a. Renting
b. Time limit
c. Use in wards
5. Smoking
6. Telephones
7. Tipping
8. Visiting

XXXI. Photography
A. Requesting
B. Consent
C. Ownership

XXXII. Private duty nurses
A. Cancellation
B. Engaging
C. Obligations to facility
1. Reporting
2. Following regula-
tions
D. Supervision
E. Evaluation
F. Remuneration

**XXXIII. Reasonable and
due care**
A. Definition
B. Explanation
C. Legal implications

**XXXIV. Release from
responsibility**
A. Abortions
B. Discharges without
order
C. Use of electric pads
D. Valuables

XXXV. Reports
A. Forms
1. Number
2. Where kept
3. Where sent
4. Types
B. Responsibility

XXXVI. Reporting
A. On and off duty
1. Information given
2. Who present

B. Leaving unit
1. When
2. To whom

XXXVII. Restraints
A. When applied
B. Whose order

XXXVIII. Safety
A. Dangerous materials
1. Drugs
2. Poisons
3. Radioactive sub-
stances
B. Proper labeling
C. Control
1. Equipment and
appliances
2. Temperatures
3. Infections
D. Side rails
1. Age range
2. Conditions
3. Type of patient
4. Where obtained
5. By whom
E. Explosions
F. Smoking
1. When
2. Where
3. Who
G. Disposal
1. Broken objects
2. Closed cans
H. Electric cords

**XXXIX. Soliciting and
vending**
A. Tips and gifts
1. When accepted
2. By whom
B. Vending
1. When
2. Who

XL. Suicide
A. Reporting
1. To whom
2. By whom

B. Forms necessary

XLI. Suspicious persons
A. Who to notify
B. Telephone number

XLII. Telephone
A. Use
1. Personal
2. Patients
3. Visitors
B. Handling of incoming
and outgoing calls

**XLIII. Taxi or ambulance
service**
A. Service
B. How obtained

XLIV. Transfer of patients
A. Within the facility
1. Clearing house
2. Reasons
3. Special care units
B. From facility
1. Who contacted
2. Responsibility

XLV. Unusual occurrences
A. Report
1. To whom
a. Day
b. Evening
c. Night
2. Number of copies
a. Where sent
b. By whom
B. Emergency action

XLVI. Visitors
A. Hours
B. Number
C. Children
D. Special requests

XLVII. Wills
A. Drawing up
B. Witnessing
1. Who
2. When

continues

Table 10–4 continued

PART II. INTERDEPARTMENTAL POLICY

Interdepartmental policies are in keeping with overall facility policies, thus ensuring unity and harmonious relationships among departments. The nursing unit will endeavor to make good use of the professional and technical services that render help to the patient. This requires a clear understanding of how these services can be carried out smoothly to the betterment of all concerned. Coordination of all their activities in obtaining the same final goal may be reached by the use of written policies.

I. Admitting office
A. Admissions
  1. Type of patients
  2. Time
    a. Elective surgery
    b. Medical care
  3. Reservations
    a. When made
    b. How long
  4. Identification of patient
    a. How
    b. When
  5. Signing of consents
  6. Accompanying patient to unit
B. Transfers
  1. Requests
  2. Departments to be notified
C. Discharges
  1. Notification
  2. Request for transportation

II. Barber and beautician service
A. Arrangements
  1. How contacted
  2. Time
    a. Bed patients
    b. Ambulatory patients
B. Remuneration
  1. Paying patients
  2. Service patients

III. Blood bank
A. Obtaining
  1. Written requisition
    a. What information
    b. Number of copies
  2. Issuance
    a. By whom

    1) Day
    2) Evening
    3) Night
    b. Rechecking information
B. Reactions
  1. Who notified
  2. Records filed
C. Replacement
  1. Time
  2. Who
  3. Where

IV. Cafeteria
A. Hours
B. Late meals
C. Who may use
D. Removal of food

V. Cashier's office
A. Notification of discharge
B. Checkout time
C. Information given
D. Valuables
  1. Safekeeping
  2. Receipt

VI. Dietary
A. Requisitions
  1. New diets
    a. Therapeutic
    b. House
  2. Extra nourishments
  3. Discharge diets
  4. Change in diet
  5. Late meals
B. Tray service
C. Dish room

VII. Electrocardiograms
A. Requisition
  1. Routine
  2. Emergency
B. Bed or ambulatory patients

VIII. Health service
A. Hours
B. Types of service
  1. Routine
  2. Emergency
C. Who may use

IX. Housekeeping
A. Assignments
B. Inspections
C. Responsibility
D. Cleaning of patents' rooms
  1. How notified
    a. Daily
    b. After discharge
  2. Precautions to be taken

X. Laboratory
A. Requisition
  1. Routine orders
  2. Emergency orders
    a. Who to call
    b. Where
B. Charting
  1. Hours
  2. By whom
C. Manual for nurse's responsibilities

XI. Laundry
A. Issuance
  1. Routine
  2. Emergency
B. Disposal of soiled linen
C. Special items
  1. Uniforms
  2. Patients' clothes
D. Safeguards

XII. Maintenance
A. Requisitions
  1. Routine
  2. Emergency

continues

Table 10–4 continued

B. Inspection of units
C. Movable articles, care of

XIII. Medical library
A. Hours
B. Who may use
C. Overdues

XIV. Medical record library
A. Medical record
   1. How compiled
   2. Whose property
   3. Return of completed record
   4. Previous admissions
   5. Nurse's responsibility
B. Late reports
C. Release of information

XV. Occupational therapy
A. Hours of service
B. Requisitions
C. Kinds of activities
   1. Ambulatory patients
   2. Bed patients

XVI. Patient's library
A. Hours
B. Time limits
C. Service
   1. Ambulatory
   2. Bed patients
D. Overdue books
E. Damage or loss of books

XVII. Personnel department
A. Requisition for personnel

   1. Replacement
   2. New employee
B. Interviewing
   1. Preemployment
   2. Postemployment
C. Recordkeeping
D. Assistance given personnel
   1. Counseling
   2. Grievances
   3. Health and welfare program
   4. Training
E. Job analysis and specifications
F. Personnel policies
G. General orientation

XVIII. Pharmacy
A. Hours of service
   1. Day
   2. Evening
   3. Night
B. Ordering of drugs
   1. Unit supply
   2. Prescription orders
C. Narcotic and barbiturate regulations
D. Label changing
E. Inspection of stock drugs and solutions on units
   1. How often
   2. By whom
F. Safety precautions

XIX. Physical therapy
A. Hours of service
B. Requisitions

C. Types of treatments

XX. Purchasing department
A. Hours of service
B. Requisitions
   1. Routine
   2. Emergency
   3. Types
   4. Number of copies
C. Back orders

XXI. Social service
A. Hours of service
B. Referrals
   1. By whom
   2. Who
C. (Contact) agencies contacted

XXII. X-ray
A. Requisition
   1. Information necessary
   2. Time
      a. Routine
      b. Emergency
         1) Who contacted
         2) Where
B. Preparation of patient
   1. Details in procedure manual
      a. Prepared by X-ray
      b. Kept on nursing units
C. Notification of unit
   1. Before and after X-ray
      a. Who
      b. When
   2. Cancellation of X-ray

Source: Sister Jean Marie Braun, S.C.S.C., "A Checklist for Nursing Service Policy Manual," The Catholic Health Association. Reprinted with permission.

Table 10–5 The Nursing Service Procedure Book: A Model for Contents

continues

Table 10–5 continued

continues

Table 10–5 continued

continues

Table 10–5 continued

Section	Subject Index	Section	Subject Index
4	Surgery, Minor		Wheelchair
4	Swan Ganz (Pulmonary Artery Cath)	1	Tub Bath, Routine
1	Teeth and Mouth, Care of	2	Tub Bath, Therapeutic Skin
1	Temperature Reducing Sponge Bath	7	Turning Patient after Spinal Fusion
1	Temperature Taking	1	Unit, Cleaning of Patient's
1	Temperature Taking (Ivac Electronic Thermometer)	1	Urinal, Giving and Removing
2	Therapeutic Tub Bath (Dermatology)	8	Urine Specimen Collection (Catheterized)
7	Thomas Splint, Use with Buck's Extension	9	Urine Specimen Collection (Pediatrics)
2	Thoracocentesis	1	Urine Specimen Collection, Single Voided
2	Topical Medication, Application of		
5	Tracheostomy, Care of Patient with	1	Urine Specimen Collection, 24 Hour
1	Transportation of Patient on Stretcher	10	Vaginal Douche
		10	Vaginal Douche, Solutions for
1	Transportation of Patient in	1	Valuables, Care of Patient's

Source: Reprinted with permission of Cook County Hospital, Chicago, IL.

Communication of New Policies*

Distribution

New or revised material should be distributed as soon as possible after it is approved and ready for distribution.

Manuals or individual policies/procedures may be mailed to persons/places listed on a need-to-know distribution sheet. Interoffice mail, hand delivery, or pay envelope issue are methods for dispensing the materials.

A memorandum should be attached to any manual material that is distributed. It should contain the date of distribution, an explanation of the subject, and directions for posting, indexing, adding, deleting, and filing. Even if the material is hand delivered and the instructions are carried out by the person who delivers the material, the memorandum should be posted on the department bulletin board as a reminder that new material is to be implemented.

Implementation of New Policies and Procedures

A new manual or revised individual policies and procedures bring about changes, sometimes suddenly. If staff are not prepared for these changes, discord, confusion, and resentment may result.

Suggestions for implementation include both the understanding that a mandate exists and that a positive approach to change is important. The following are some implementation suggestions.

Distribute new or revised policies and procedures to the entire staff at the same time. Ask staff members to read and demonstrate that they understand and can perform them. Their signing that they have read and do understand the information places the responsibility on them.

Hold a conference or meeting in small departments to discuss and demonstrate new policies and procedures. This can be done as a part of regular meetings that are held weekly or monthly.

Have a procedure demonstration day. All participants are given a copy of the procedures so they can follow along as demonstrations are

*Source: Reba Douglass Grubb, *Hospital Manual: A Guide to Development and Maintenance*, Aspen Publishers, Inc., © 1981.

made. Return demonstrations from the group also are used to reinforce learning.

Each participant is given an unsigned posttest, including a few questions from each procedure. At the close of the session, these are analyzed and the questions that were answered incorrectly are emphasized in the next sessions. If too many questions were missed on one procedure, this indicates that further instruction is needed or that the procedure needs to be rewritten.

Staff who were unable to attend the regular sessions should be scheduled to attend another or work the "buddy system" with one who is experienced in the procedure. Released time for this education program is provided for each employee.

Place the complete manual on each unit. Discuss one or two revised or new policies and/or procedures at each conference or department meeting until the manual has been reviewed by all employees. This would be difficult for a large department or if the manual is large.

Ask staff of one nursing unit to demonstrate a procedure to another unit. That unit then demonstrates the procedure to another unit; this continues until all units have participated in a learning session.

Videotape a procedure and hand out written copies of the process. Let the staff follow the videotaped action. The tape may be shown as often as necessary.

Chapter 11

Nurses and the Law

PRIMER ON THE LAW*

Nurses have a legal and an ethical duty to practice nursing according to a professional nursing standard of care. Nurses are required to use the same degree of knowledge and skill as reasonably prudent nurses would use under the same or similar circumstances and, if they fail to do so, they can be sued for malpractice by the injured plaintiff.

The Distinction between Negligence and Malpractice

Negligence is the failure to exercise the degree of care that a reasonably prudent person would exercise under the same or similar circumstances. *Malpractice* (professional negligence) refers to negligent acts committed by a person in his or her professional capacity. It is defined as any professional misconduct, unreasonable lack of skill or fidelity in professional or fiduciary duties, evil practice, or illegal or immoral conduct. There are fundamental differences be-

tween a lawsuit based on a charge of negligence and a lawsuit claiming malpractice. In a malpractice suit:

- The act of negligence must have been committed in the course of carrying out a professional responsibility.
- The statute of limitations is generally shorter than for negligence.
- The standard of care will be tested in reference to the behavior of other nurses.
- The testimony of an expert witness is usually required to prove the standard of care.

When professionals are sued for malpractice they are accorded these added protections; however, they are not available to nurses in jurisdictions where the courts do not recognize that the nurse's actions are those of a professional. The legal concept of professionalism has traditionally considered a profession to require (1) a rigorous and systematic educational program for practitioners, (2) a code of ethics, (3) a strong research program, and (4) a certain authority and prestige associated with the field. The nursing profession has the altruism and the code of ethics and is improving in the area of research; however, in prestige and authority it is still lagging behind other professions.

---

*Source: Carmelle Pellerin Cournoyer, *The Nurse Manager & the Law*, Aspen Publishers, Inc., © 1989.

Elements Required To Establish Nurse Liability

To establish a claim of negligence or malpractice, a plaintiff is required to introduce proof of the four elements of negligence: (1) duty; (2) breach of the duty, which is the failure to meet the required standard of care; (3) causation; and (4) injury.

Duty

The courts have stated that in negligence cases, the duty is always the same, to conform to the legal standard of care or reasonable conduct in the light of apparent risk. The plaintiff must first prove that the person charged with negligence is under a legal duty to exercise due care. There is no legal duty to come to the aid of another unless a legal relationship exists.

A nurse's duty toward a patient is established by providing evidence that the nurse was employed by the health care organization in which the plaintiff was a patient. The nurse's duty arises in the context of the nurse-patient relationship, in which the nurse has a legal and an ethical duty to the patient. Once a duty is acknowledged, the plaintiff must establish the scope of the duty that the nurse was obligated to provide. The plaintiff must prove that the nurse failed to act as a reasonably prudent nurse would have acted under the same or similar circumstances. To do this, the plaintiff must introduce evidence of the standard of care that was required; in other words, the plaintiff must demonstrate how the nurse should have acted under the circumstances.

Standard of Care

Although jurisdictions continue to treat nursing malpractice as ordinary negligence, the trend is to hold nurses to a professional standard of care. The plaintiff can prove the standard of care, and the nurse's failure to meet that standard, by the introduction of documentary evidence and the testimony of expert witnesses.

The type of documents that are usually used to prove the standard of care include the following:

- American Nurses' Association (ANA) standards of nursing practice, the standards that are published by the specialty professional nursing organizations, and the Joint Commission on Accreditation of Healthcare Organizations' standards

- statutes and administrative codes such as the nursing practice act and regulations, the federal hospital regulations, and the applicable health care facility licensing standards and regulations

- facility bylaws and facility policy and procedure manuals relevant to the standard of nursing practice within the institution

Expert Witness Testimony. The standard of care in a nursing malpractice action must be established by expert witness testimony. The general rule is that witnesses can testify only as to the facts; their opinions and conclusions are not admissible. On the other hand, expert witnesses are presented for the purpose of eliciting their expert opinion as to the matter being litigated. Unlike regular witnesses, expert witnesses seldom have direct, personal knowledge of the actual facts and circumstances of the case. They have generally reviewed the record and formed an opinion as to the nurse's conduct. Both the plaintiff and the defendant may present expert witness testimony. The trial court first determines that the expert witness is competent to testify as an expert on the subject. The court must be satisfied that the testimony to be presented is the kind that requires special knowledge, skill, and experience. The purpose of the expert witness's testimony is to help the jury understand the professional or technical issues that are being litigated. The expert witness is subject to cross-examination by the attorney for the opposing side. The jury decides how much weight and credence to give to the expert witness's testimony.

Traditionally, the standard of care required of health care professionals was that degree of care ordinarily exercised by health care professionals of similar knowledge and skills in the same or similar community. The application of a community standard of care, commonly referred to as the locality rule, is rapidly being replaced with the recognition of a national standard of care so that expert witnesses can be hired from anywhere in the country. The practice of nursing, however, may involve situations in which there are several different, equally safe and efficient ways of performing a procedure. There is no liability if the nurse has followed the approach used by a respected minority of the profession.

Causation

Proximate cause or legal cause requires that the plaintiff prove that a reasonably close connection exists between the defendant's conduct and the plantiff's injury. Many lawsuits are lost by plaintiffs who are unable to prove the causal relationship. Proximate cause requires a two-pronged inquiry.

1. Is the defendant's conduct the cause "in fact" of the plaintiff's injury? Two tests are used to answer this question. First, could the injury have occurred "but for" the defendant's conduct? An example would be a nurse's negligent administration of an overdose of medication that results in the patient suffering an adverse reaction. Second, was the defendant's conduct a material and substantial factor in bringing about the injury? This issue is critical when there is more than one defendant.

2. How far will the law extend the responsibility for the defendant's conduct to the consequences that have occurred? Foreseeability of the risk of injury is the criterion used to determine the limits of the defendant's liability. If the defendant's failure to foresee the consequences of the action is proven to be a direct cause of the patient's injury, legal causation is established.

Injury

In negligence actions, plaintiffs are required to prove that they suffered physical, emotional, or financial injury. The plaintiff is compensated for the injury by an award of money damages that the defendant is ordered to pay. Types of damages include nominal, actual or compensatory, and punitive damages.

Nominal damages are a minimal sum that is sometimes awarded to vindicate a technical right; however, nominal damages cannot be obtained in a negligence action where no actual loss oc-

curred. *Actual* or compensatory damages are the losses sustained by the plaintiff and include medical costs, loss of earnings, impairment of future earnings, and past and future pain and suffering. *Punitive* damages, which are also called exemplary damages, are designed to punish the defendants and deter others from following their example.

LIABILITY ISSUES

Scope of Practice Responsibilities*

Although the nursing director's duties vary from state to state, directors are generally responsible for the supervision, provision, and quality of nursing care; coordination and integration of nursing services with other patient care services; development of job descriptions for nurses and nurses' aides; development of nursing service procedures; selection of nursing staff members; and development of orientation and training programs (see Tables 11–1 and 11–2).

Nursing Administration

Although a nursing manager is liable for his or her own negligent acts, the employer is liable for the negligent acts of all employees, including managers (e.g., directors of nursing, assistant directors of nursing, and head nurses). Managers are not liable under the doctrine of *respondeat superior* for the negligent acts of those being supervised. They have the right to direct the nurses who are being supervised. In a health care facility, the nursing administration's powers are derived directly from the facility's right of control.

A manager who knowingly fails to supervise an employee's performance or assigns a task to an individual he or she knows, or should know, is not competent to perform can be held personally liable if injury occurs. The employer will be liable under the doctrine of *respondeat superior* as the employer of both the manager and the in-

---

Source: George D. Pozgar, *Legal Aspects of Health Care Administration*, ed 6, Aspen Publishers, Inc., © 1996.

Table 11-1 Actions To Help Meet Nursing Administrative Legal Obligations

The two major legal responsibilities that civil law imposes on nurses and nurse managers are to (1) maintain the standard of nursing care and (2) respect the rights of patients and staff. The following behaviors demonstrate some of the responsibilities that nurse managers must assume in order to fulfill their legal obligations to the patient and to the employer.

- Hire, supervise, and evaluate the nursing staff.
- Evaluate interaction with the non-nursing staff.
- Develop mechanisms for resolving professional conflicts.
- Participate in the credentialing and evaluation process.
- Provide for nursing staff competency through education.

- Evaluate the nursing staff and the level of nursing care being provided to patients.
- Discipline nurses found to be incompetent, reporting to the state board when necessary.
- Respect nurse's right to fair and equitable treatment under the employment agreement.
- Respect the nurses' legal and constitutional rights.
- Promote an environment of mutual respect and cooperation between health care professionals.
- Implement and maintain the current standard of nursing practice.
- Participate in the risk management process.
- Respect patient's right to consent or to refuse to consent to treatment.

Source: Carmelle Pellerin Cournoyer, *The Nurse Manager & the Law*, Aspen Publishers, Inc., © 1989.

Table 11-2 Helpful Advice for Health Professionals

- Do not criticize the professional skill of another publicly. Use appropriate, available reporting mechanisms when the skill of another is to be challenged.
- Maintain complete and adequate patient care records.
- Provide each patient with good care comparable with national standards.
- Seek the aid of consultants when indicated.
- Check that informed consent is obtained for diagnostic and therapeutic procedures.
- Do not be afraid to ask questions.
- Practice in the fields in which you have been trained.
- Participate in continuing education programs.
- Maintain all confidential communication without violation.
- Report equipment failures promptly. All patient equipment should be checked frequently for safety.
- Do not be rigid or impersonal. Develop a relationship with the patient in which, for example, the patient begins to say, "That's

my nurse." Likewise, the nurse should say, "That's my patient."
- Be confident and professional in the presence of patients. A professional who is not self-confident and constantly complains about coworkers, physicians, and the institution will only serve to make patients more insecure and suit prone.
- Investigate patient incidents promptly.
- Maintain incident reports separately from patients' records. Incident reports prepared by a health professional, placed in a patient's record, and given to the administration are not protected by attorney-client privilege. If incident reports are prepared only for the attorney to provide legal services, they could be regarded as privileged communications.
- Be a good listener and allow each patient sufficient time to express fears and anxieties.
- Above all, be compassionate and understanding to each patient and to one another as individuals.

Source: George D. Pozgar, *Legal Aspects of Health Care Administration*, ed 6, Aspen Publishers, Inc., © 1996.

dividual who performed the task in a negligent manner. The manager is not relieved of personal liability even though the employer is liable under *respondeat superior*.

In determining whether a nurse with supervisory responsibilities has been negligent, the nurse is measured against the standard of care of a competent and prudent nurse in the performance of supervisory duties.

Physicians' Care and Nurses' Liability*

Nurses have the responsibility to observe the conditions of patients under their care and report any significant findings that may adversely affect a patient's well-being to the attending physician. If a physician should fail to respond to a call for assistance and such failure is likely to jeopardize a patient's health, the matter must be brought to the attention of the nurse manager, chief of the appropriate service, or administration. Failure to exercise this duty can lead to liability for the nurse, as well as the health care facility, under the doctrine of *respondeat superior.*

A health care facility's policies and procedures should prescribe the guidelines for staff members to follow when confronted with a physician or other health professional whose action or inaction jeopardizes the well-being of a patient.

Failure to take correct telephone orders can be just as serious as failure to follow, understand, and/or interpret correctly a physician's orders. Telephone orders are necessary because of the nature of a physician's practice. Nurses must be alert in transcribing orders because there are periodic contradictions between what physicians claim they ordered and what nurses allege they ordered. Orders should be repeated, once transcribed, for verification purposes. Verification of an order by another nurse on a second telephone is helpful, especially if an order is questionable. Any questionable orders must always be verified with the physician initiating the or-

der. Physicians must countersign all orders—this should be a firm rule of the health care facility. Nurses who disagree with a physician's order should not carry out an obviously erroneous order. In addition, they should confirm the order with the prescribing physician and report to the nurse manager any difficulty in resolving a difference of opinion with the physician.

Dealing with Inappropriate Physician Orders*

Depending on your state's laws or practice acts, you may have a legal obligation to report any incidents that may lead to the harm of a patient. In any event, you have an ethical obligation to report incompetence, malpractice, and misconduct to the appropriate licensing agency. It is, however, improper to go directly to a patient with adverse information about the individual's attending physician or other provider.

When faced with these situations, nurses should first decide if the patient is in immediate danger. If the answer is yes, one is obligated to bring the matter first to the attention of the provider and try to resolve the matter. If the provider is unwilling to alter his or her behavior, the problem should be taken up with the individual's supervisor, peer review committees, or state licensing agency. Even if the immediate situation has been corrected and the error is of such significant magnitude as to be incompetence or if the provider repeatedly engages in such behavior, then one is obligated to bring it to the attention of the appropriate authorities to ensure that the provider's activities are reviewed and do not jeopardize patients in the future.

Evidence of Care: Documentation**

Nurse charting is an important reflection of the nursing care provided to the patient. The

---

*Source: George D. Pozgar, *Legal Aspects of Health Care Administration*, ed 6, Aspen Publishers, Inc., © 1996.

*Source: D.L. Flarey and S.S. Blancett, *Handbook of Nursing Case Management: Health Care Delivery in a World of Managed Care,* Aspen Publishers, Inc., © 1996.
**Source: George D. Pozgar, *Legal Aspects of Health Care Administration,* ed 6, Aspen Publishers, Inc., © 1996.

document contains clinical data, both objective and subjective, that are used for ongoing patient care. In the end, it serves as legally viable evidence of that care.

Documentation may be legally risky if it is not executed properly. Not only may the patient record be legally insufficient to be relied on in a court case, but it could be legally damaging through improper entries or omissions. To avoid these problems, a documentation entry must meet the conditions explained and summarized in the following box.

The use of computerized patient records may eliminate most of the problems connected with poor entries such as illegibility and corrections, but others may arise connected to patient confidentiality. Nursing managers and administrators should organize inservice programs that discuss the security needed for computerized charts of patient care; the responsibility for maintaining confidentiality, accuracy, and completeness of data; and the procedures for accessing and signing off on computerized documentation.

Employee Rights and Employment Law*

Few managers need to be reminded that legal actions related to employment are increasing. This increase seems to stem from two general causes, or, perhaps more appropriately, two forces in modern American society. These forces, each adding to the strength of the other, are

- the population's rising consciousness of individual rights
- legislation regulating terms and conditions of employment to legally ensure equal treatment for all persons

More employees now tend to speak up when they believe they have been wronged, and they know resources are available to provide them with advocacy and assistance. Since many employment practices that were once legal are now against

---

Source: Charles R. McConnell and Marion Blankopf, "Managing a Discrimination Case," *The Health Care Supervisor,* Vol. 8:1, Aspen Publishers, Inc., © September 1989.

A documentation entry must:

- be in accordance with professional standards
- be appropriate to the patient's needs
- include a description of situations that are out of the ordinary
- provide specific details of patient assessment and intervention
- be timely and chronologically organized
- be complete; contain application of standard measures as well as extraordinary interventions
- be consistent with other documents
- include standing orders
- not include risk-related information
- show no bias or dissension among caregivers

On manual patient records there are a number of errors to avoid when making entries or corrections.

- Do not insert lines between entries.
- Do not use "white-out" or show different handwriting.
- Do not write illegibly.
- Do not allow time gaps (i.e., omitted entries).
- Do not use inappropriate or unidentifiable signatures.

---

the law, it stands to reason that many perceived acts of discrimination will become formal charges of discrimination.

Unlawful discrimination is discrimination on the basis of age, race, sex, disability, national origin, pregnancy, religion, sexual orientation, or retaliation.

Any manager at any level in the organization can be drawn into a discrimination case. Once named and involved, he or she will have no choice but to participate. A complaint charging an organization with discrimination will ordinarily name one or more agents—in this case, managers—of the organization who participated in the alleged discriminatory acts. Thus, any manager can become involved in a discrimination case at any time. For this reason, it is useful to keep in mind some typical problems and decisions that may arise at various stages of a discrimination case.

Prevention: The Precomplaint Stage

Since you usually do not know a complaint is going to arrive until it does indeed arrive, you might think of the precomplaint stage as the consideration of everything you should have been doing all along, including those critical elements you may not have thought of at all until after a complaint actually arrived, such as the following:

- Keep the lines of employee communication open, taking deliberate steps to be sure that your availability and attitude truly support the open-door policy that your organization probably espouses.
- In dealing with problems of employee performance, document your efforts at working with those employees who are falling short of meeting the normal requirements of the job.
- Examine every significant personnel action—warning, suspension, demotion, termination, or change of shift or job assignment—for its legal implications before it is implemented.
- If you maintain anecdotal note files on your employees, do so with great care. Anecdotal note files are extremely helpful and often necessary, but they can be extremely troublesome in a discrimination case. Since anecdotal files cannot hurt you if they do not exist, periodically purge your anecdotal files of outdated or irrelevant material. However, never destroy or discard a document once legal action has been instituted.
- Thoroughly observe the documentation requirements of your job. Use the forms that are supposed to be used in the way they are supposed to be used. A discrimination case

involves paper, often in massive amounts, and added problems and extra expense arise because of documents that are incomplete, undated, unsigned, illegible, or missing.

You can, of course, do everything absolutely correctly and still receive a discrimination complaint. Still, it is far better to cover all bases at all times and thereby either minimize your chances of receiving a complaint or have all the proper moves documented to support your defense against charges that might arise.

INFORMED CONSENT

Basically, as developed through the courts, there are three elements of informed consent: (1) information or knowledge, (2) competence, and (3) voluntariness. All three must be present to have valid informed consent from a patient.

Information or Knowledge*

In order for the patient to make a valid decision as to the treatment decision, the patient must be given adequate information to consider. Health care providers are responsible for communicating with patients and informing them of the diagnosis, prognosis, available alternatives to the treatment recommended, the risks and benefits of the treatment options, and the risks of not accepting treatment.

There are actually two different standards applied by courts in determining whether sufficient information was provided to the patient. Most states have adopted one of these two approaches through either statute or case law. The older, traditional standard is known as the "reasonable physician standard" or "professional standards approach." In states that have adopted this standard, a health care provider is only required to give a patient that information that another similar health care provider would have disclosed under the same or similar circumstances.

---

*Source: Martha D. Nathanson, *Home Health Care Law Manual*, Aspen Publishers, Inc., © 1996.

- explanation of the patient's diagnosis, condition, or illness
- description of the nature and purpose of the proposed treatment
- description of any expected risks or consequences of the treatment
- estimation of the probability that the proposed treatment will be successful
- disclosure of any appropriate alternatives
- explanation of the consequences or probable outcome if the treatment is not accepted

---

The Intent of Informed Consent

- The fact that consent is given does not automatically establish that the consent was informed.
- Express or implied consent must be given after the patient has receive sufficient information to make an informed choice.
- It is important to remember that consent is a process, not a document. The document merely codifies and reflects the culmination of the process.
- Written consent alone, without true disclosure and an opportunity for dialogue between the provider and the patient, is generally inadequate.
- Consent forms were developed primarily as a means of establishing that informed consent did in fact occur. However, such forms have been recognized as an important component of the process, as many states mandate that consent forms be used as a part of the decision-making process.

Source: J. Phillip O'Brien, Michael R. Callahan, and Jamie A. Savaiano, "A Practical Approach to the Doctrine of Informed Consent," in *Health Care Ethics*, Gary R. Anderson and Valerie A. Glesnes-Anderson, eds., Aspen Publishers, Inc., © 1987.

Competence

The law presumes that an adult over 18 years of age (in most states) is legally competent and capable of giving valid consent for medical treatment. However, the patient must be of sound mind and free from any legal or mental impediments that would prevent making a binding decision concerning his or her health care. Therefore, if the patient has a court-appointed guardian or is a minor, the patient may not be legally competent to give consent for treatment. Each state's laws should be checked for exceptions provided for treatment of minors.

The consent of any other person with an impairment to his or her legal faculties will not be considered sufficient to be considered legally valid. This restriction includes a person under the influence of drugs or alcohol that might affect mental status. Stress, shock, or dementia may also inhibit one's capability to make a competent, legally valid decision.

Voluntariness

In order for the patient's consent to be voluntary, the patient must freely elect to undergo the proposed treatment without any sort of physical or psychological coercion. If the health care provider intimidates, threatens, or coerces the patient in any way, there could be a lack of valid consent. Medication given to the patient without the patient's knowledge represents another example. Consent induced by fraud, misrepre-

The second, and more liberal, standard is known as the "reasonable patient standard." Under this newer standard, a court will seek to determine whether or not a patient should have been informed about a particular risk or alternative based on what the average reasonable patient would have wanted to know. The significance or materiality of the disclosure is examined from the patient's point of view. Unless the patient is given information on alternatives that are available (often information that is usually only known to the health care provider), he or she may not actually be given a choice.

The type of information that must be provided to the patient includes the following:

sentation, or furnishing false information will likewise be invalid and illegal.

Disclosure*

Generally a physician or other health care provider must disclose the following categories of information to a patient: (1) diagnosis, (2) nature and purpose of the proposed treatment, (3) risks and consequences of the proposed treatment, (4) probability that the proposed treatment will be successful, (5) feasible treatment alternatives, and (6) alternatives and prognosis if the proposed treatment is not given. Although this is the generally accepted list of items, the list may be expanded to include all information that the physician knows or reasonably should know would be material to the patient's decision-making process.

Medical Experimentation and Research

Patients consenting to treatment ordinarily consent to procedures and treatments that are used customarily. If innovative or experimental procedures are to be used, the physician must disclose the pertinent information to the patient and obtain appropriate consent. Federal, state, and local laws on human experimentation and the protection of human subjects contain guidelines that health care facilities must be aware of and comply with as applicable. These laws contain specific safeguards for research subjects and guidelines for obtaining informed consent.

Nursing Roles in Informed Consent**

The nurse often becomes involved in consent issues almost immediately after the first physician-patient interaction that is focused on obtaining informed consent. If the physician has given the patient the needed information prior to admission, the nurse may first become involved when the intern does an intake interview to gather clinical data. Such interviews often lead to the patient and nurse discussing what treatment the patient will receive.

Nurses identify five roles they can assume as forms of active involvement.

Watchdog. This role serves to monitor informed consent situations. Nurses often accompany the patient to witness the consent. They also confer about and report what they saw as violations of the consent process. In this role, they attempt to establish and maintain clear limits regarding their ethical obligations to patients, physicians, and the institution.

Advocate. Nurses assume this role to mediate on behalf of patients. As a part of this role, it is important to bring crucial new or additional information to the physician or researcher from the patient or family. For example, the patient's rationale for certain choices and decisions can function to recast the meaning of events and expose the underlying values at play. As advocates, nurses also support the decision-making process per se and the decision made by the patients.

Resource Person. As resource persons, nurses collect, dispense, and report information about all alternatives available, guide patients regarding their informational needs, and clarify the features of consent that the patients misunderstood or overlooked.

Coordinator. Nurses can explore implications for and observe direct and indirect effects on the patient and family. They can integrate treatment and care with the workings of the system so as to try to ensure necessary time for working through any issues that might arise about informed consent.

Facilitator. Nurses can clarify and validate differences in perspective between parties involved in informed consent. They can discuss with patients and families such topics as long- and short-term consequences of choice, suffering, and pain, as well as psychological and physical benefits. As facilitators, they try to build in

---

Source: William F. Roach, Jr., Susan N. Chernoff, and Carole Lange Esley, *Medical Records and the Law*, ed 2, Aspen Publishers, Inc., © 1994.

**Source:* Anne J. Davis, "The Clinical Nurse's Role in Informed Consent," *Journal of Professional Nursing*, Vol. 4, No. 2, March–April 1988.

opportunities for reevaluation at a later stage. And finally, they assume the responsibility of getting the team together to discuss aspects of specific situations, including those of informed consent, that raise issues that need to be discussed.

Other Consent Issues

Judging Competency*

In the President's Commission for the Study of Ethical Problems in Medicine and Biomedical and Behavioral Research report, the Commission refers to competency as decision-making capacity. The Commission spelled out the components of decisional capacity: the possession of a set of values and goals, the ability to communicate and understand information, and the ability to reason and deliberate.

Competency assessment usually focuses on the patient's mental capacities, specifically the mental capacities to make a particular medical decision. Does this patient understand what is being disclosed? Can this patient come to a decision about treatment based on that information? How much understanding and rational decision-making capacity is sufficient for this patient to be considered competent? Or how deficient must this patient's decision-making capacity be before he or she is declared incompetent? A properly performed competency assessment should eliminate two types of error: (1) preventing competent persons from deciding their own treatment and (2) failing to protect incompetent persons from the harmful effects of a bad decision.

Refusing Medical Treatment

The Patient Self-Determination Act provided legislative support to the expression of a patient's consent to or refusal of medical treatment (general and specific) even when the patient is no longer able to verbalize them. These directions can be spelled out in several different types of documents.

- *Advance medical directives:* Written instructions expressing an individual's health care wishes in the event of incapacitation.
- *Durable power of attorney:* Legal instrument enabling an individual to act on another's behalf. In health care, it is often a part of the advance medical directive and permits and directs another to make medical decisions on behalf of the patient.
- *Health care proxy:* Document that delegates the authority to make one's own health care decisions to another when one has become incapacitated or is unable to make his or her own decisions.
- *Living will:* Document in which an individual expresses in advance his or her wishes regarding the application of life-sustaining treatments in the event he or she is unable to do so at some future time (due to illness or incapacitation).

The legislation is very particular about how facilities must establish policies for accepting, managing, and respecting these documents.

Consent to Treating Minors*

The task of determining the appropriate party from whom to obtain consent to treatment of pediatric patients can be confusing because of the impact of single parents, joint custody agreements, teenage parents, emancipated minors, mature minors, unmarried parents, and custodians/relatives without formal guardianship status. Although state consent laws vary, some common issues can be addressed.

Source: James F. Drane, "The Many Faces of Competency," *Hastings Center Report,* Vol. 15, No. 2, April 1985.

Source: Barbara Grand Sheridan, "Risk Management in the Pediatric Setting," *The Risk Manager's Desk Reference,* Barbara J. Youngberg, ed., Aspen Publishers, Inc., © 1994.

Recognition that a consent issue exists is primary to averting a claim based on failure to authorize treatment. Parents can sue physicians for any unauthorized nonemergency medical treatment of a child. The risk manager should determine whether minors in the state are considered legally capable of giving consent and whether limitations and/or restrictive circumstances in which a minor can be legally capable in some specific situations but not in others exist. Knowledge of relevant requirements will facilitate the establishment of specific protocols to address the multiple situations that can be encountered.

The risk manager can be proactive by providing the admitting staff with accurate consent policies for pediatrics, repetitive in-service activities, and access to risk management staff when questions arise. Written guidelines are preferable. When special family circumstances such as custody battles exist, hospitals should have mechanisms to ensure that the physician and nurse have administrative support to ensure they will be able to provide medical services that are *in the best interest of the child*. Parental animosity or family fighting should never be allowed to compromise the care of a child. If a family situation becomes threatening to a health care provider, administration should seek to involve social services or legal counsel and ascertain the appropriateness of placing the child under custody of a state guardian who can ensure that parental hostilities will not negatively impact care of the child.

PROFESSIONAL LIABILITY INSURANCE

Determining the Need for Coverage*

An increasing number of lawsuits are being filed against nurses. For many nurses, the un-settled question is whether to purchase professional liability insurance.

Reasons given for seeking coverage beyond that provided by a health care facility employer include the following:

- In the event of litigation, the facility, not the nurse, makes any decisions about settlement or defense, so the nurse's best interests may not be represented.
- If the court determines that the nurse acted outside the scope of employment, he or she is unprotected.
- If the nurse does, in fact, practice outside the facility's job description (professional committees, outside speaking, educational work), the facility coverage does not apply.
- Facilities have the right to seek reimbursement from the nurse for claims paid as a result of negligence.
- Personal assets may in some cases be attached to satisfy a judgment, or wages may be garnished.
- Health care facility insurance is frequently a claims-made policy. This type of policy will cover the nurse only while he or she is employed by the facility, not years later when the claim is in court.
- The cost of insurance is relatively small in relation to the peace of mind the insurance provides.

Because nurses are in a high-risk field, they should maintain job descriptions that accurately reflect scope of responsibilities. Each nurse should determine the dollar limits of any facility liability coverage and whether the coverage is of a claims-made or occurrence type. Knowledge of the institution's recent history in litigation involving nurses will provide a background for supplementary insurance decisions (see Table 11–3).

Source: Sister Rosann Geiser and Karen Fraley, "Perinatal Outreach: Liability Issues," *Journal of Perinatal and Neonatal Nursing*, Vol. 2:3, Aspen Publishers, Inc., © 1989.

Table 11–3 Deciding on Professional Liability Insurance

Reasons To Obtain Insurance	Reasons Not To Obtain Insurance
• Nurse is responsible for every action undertaken or omitted. • Facility could seek countersuit if nurse is negligent. • No coverage is provided for actions outside of job description. • With claims-made policy, no coverage is provided after leaving facility. • Nurse lacks control if RN representation includes facility and physicians and has no part in decision to settle or defend. • Nurse is self-employed, serves on professional committees, or does volunteer work. • Cost is relatively minimal for protection provided.	• Nurse is practicing within scope of duties; facility covers. • Fear of countersuit is unrealistic. Dollars gained in countersuit by facility may cause negative effect on RN recruitment and retention. • Potential for damage recovery increases risk of lawsuit. • Potential conflict exists over percentages of compensation to be paid by nurse and facility as separate policyholders. • Potential conflict exists between nurse and facility attorneys.

Source: Sister Rosann Geiser and Karen Fraley, "Perinatal Outreach: Liability Issues," *Journal of Perinatal and Neonatal Nursing*, Vol. 2:3, Aspen Publishers, Inc., © 1989.

Conditions of a Professional Liability Insurance Policy*

Each insurance policy contains a number of important conditions. Failure to comply with these conditions may cause forfeiture of the policy and nonpayment of claims against it. Generally, insurance policies contain the following conditions.

Notice of Occurrence. When the insured becomes aware that an injury has occurred as a result of acts covered under the contract, the insured must promptly notify the insurance company. The form of notice may be either oral or written, as specified in the policy.

Notice of Claim. Whenever the insured receives notice that a claim or suit is being instituted, notice must be sent by the insured to the

---

Source: George D. Pozgar, *Legal Aspects of Health Care Administration*, ed 6, Aspen Publishers, Inc., © 1996.

insurance company. The policy will specify what papers are to be forwarded to the company. Note that failure to provide timely notification in accordance with the terms of a policy may void the insurer's obligation under the policy. It may not matter that the insurer has in no way been prejudiced by the last notification. The mere fact that the insured has failed to carry out its obligations under the policy may be sufficient to permit the insurer to avoid its obligations. Where the insurer has refused to honor a claim because of late notice and the insured wishes to challenge such refusal, a *declaratory judgment* action can be brought asking a court to determine the reasonableness of the insurer's position.

Assistance of the Insured. The insured must cooperate with the insurance company and render any assistance necessary to reach a settlement.

Other Insurance. If the insured has pertinent insurance policies with other insurance companies, the insured must notify the insurance company in order that each company may pay the appropriate amount of the claim.

Assignment. The protections contracted by the insured may not be transferred unless permission is granted by the insurance company. Because the insurance company was aware of the risks the insured would encounter before the policy was issued, the company will endeavor to avoid protecting persons other than the policyholder.

Subrogation. Subrogation is the right of a person who pays another's debt to be substituted for all rights in relation to the debt. When an insurance company makes a payment for the insured under the terms of the policy, the company becomes the beneficiary of all the rights of recovery the insured has against any other persons who may also have been negligent.

Changes. The insured cannot make changes in the policy without the written consent of the insurance company. Thus an agent of the insurance company ordinarily cannot modify or remove any condition of the liability contract. Only the insurance company, by written authorization, may permit a condition to be altered or removed.

Cancellation. A cancellation clause spells out the conditions and procedures necessary for the insured or the insurer to cancel the liability policy. Written notice is usually required. The insured person's failure to comply with any of the conditions can result in nonpayment of a claim by the insurance company. An insurance policy is a legal contract, and failure to meet the terms and conditions of the insurance policy may result in breach of contract and voidance of coverage.

Chapter 12

Ethics

ETHICAL STEWARDSHIP OF NURSING ADMINISTRATORS

The nursing administrator's primary ethical responsibility is to ensure safe patient care. Running a close second is the responsibility to make the risks of nursing practice tolerable and the acceptance of duty safe— both personally (proper pay and benefits) and professionally (proper support and recognition)—for the nurses who design and deliver care to vulnerable patients.

In any health care organization, however, resources are inevitably limited because of the unlimited uncertainties that heavily burden both economical and ethical administration by creating risks and dilemmas.

Like all their administrative predecessors and models, nursing administrators derive their political and social advantages and privileges from their power to allocate the limited resources assigned to their discretion.

Role of the Nurse Executive in Setting Ethical Priorities*

Given the complexity of ethical issues in today's health care institution, what should the

nurse executive do? He or she must look simultaneously at ethical implications of nursing practice and of institutional policies and strategies. He or she also needs to keep current on legal precedents that may have an effect on ethical decision making in the institution.

The *Code for Nurses* produced by the American Nurses Association (1985) serves as a general guideline, presenting broad ethical principles generally accepted in this country, as well as offering brief explanations for each principle. Unfortunately, the principles are too broad to suggest specific actions to be taken. Take, for example, the item, "The nurse assumes responsibility and accountability for individual nursing judgments and actions." Few would argue with the principle, but it serves little purpose in solving an issue of accountability.

For the subordinate staff, the nurse executive can set up structures that prevent the staff nurse from being caught in the middle between his or her own convictions and the orders of others with more power in the institution. There should be a channel by which nurses can refuse to participate in treatments or in patient management strategies when to do so presents them with valid moral crises. The structure should be devised so that a nurse can refuse participation for personal ethical reasons without being faced with threat or coercion. Certainly, the nurse should not face

*Source: The Nurse As Executive, Aspen Publishers, Inc., © 1995.

psychological (or other) penalties for enacting his or her own personal code.

The nurse executive also may elect to provide inservice education to make nurses more able to make effective discriminations in cases of ethical decision making. One case study was instructive on this point. A nurse was extremely upset when a liver available for transplant went to another patient rather than to hers. The nurse clearly had assumed an advocacy position for her patient but failed to understand that the mere fact that he was *her* patient was not sufficient rationale for the hard choice that had to be made.

As new laws are enacted to cover new problems, the nurse executive must keep informed. Both changes in the law and in case decisions setting new precedents are important. When major changes occur, the nurse executive will need to review divisional and institutional policy for conformance with the new dictate.

Ethical Considerations in Patient Care*

The Massachusetts Nursing Association has formulated guidelines for nursing staff and managerial actions to promote ethical behavior in the provision of nursing services.

Responsibilities

All nurses are expected to recognize their responsibilities toward their patients. Nurses have a responsibility to recognize when the care and safety of a patient is in jeopardy. This recognition is grounded in the application of sound concepts of patient care, taking into account differing but valid practice techniques. Nurses have a duty, as moral agents, to intervene to prevent harm to patients. Nurses should seek the least harmful and least disruptive methods of ensuring patient protection. Nurses who are employed in institutions or groups have a responsibility to make every effort to use and exhaust the internal reporting mechanisms before notifying

public agencies or the general public; such notification is generally referred to as "whistleblowing." Nurses should seek to minimize harm to colleagues and the institution as well as patients. In crisis or emergencies, a nurse's first and overriding responsibility is to patients.

Nursing Administrator/Manager Actions

- Promote a climate in which employees are encouraged to report those situations that may adversely affect the delivery of quality care.
- Identify those persons or those practices that may cause actual or potential harm to the patient.
- Establish mechanisms for reporting and handling instances of incompetent, unethical, or illegal practice.
- Maintain confidentiality in appropriate circumstances.
- Respond to those situations that involve unacceptable practices by determining through investigation that a problem exists, including verification and documentation of facts.
- Respond further to unacceptable practices by taking actions to halt the harmful practice, such as the following:
  - reporting facts in accordance with established institutional processes
  - ensuring that practitioners receive appropriate notification and referral if a pattern of unsafe practice occurs
  - ensuring appropriate notification and counseling to the injured party if there has been actual or potential injury to the patient
  - adhering to institutional disciplinary policies and procedures when just and appropriate

Staff Nurse Actions

- Identify and confront those individuals on the health care team whose clinical practice clearly presents a danger to the health or safety of the client under their direct or indirect care.

- Report to the appropriate authority the individual whose unethical or unsafe practice has been confronted without an acceptable solution.
- Recognize the necessity of further reporting if the problem is not resolved at the initial reporting level.
- Participate in the development of specific procedures for identifying and reporting incompetent, illegal, or unethical practice.

Determining Whether an Act Is Right or Wrong*

A nursing manager needs to recognize when he or she is faced with a situation that involves a moral issue. A balance has to be maintained between classifying all decisions as moral judgments and totally neglecting the ethical implications of any action.

How can a manager be certain of the rightness or wrongness of an action or decision? Three schools of thought provide guidance for determining whether an act is right or wrong.

The first holds that *people should do what is right.* This view assumes knowledge of basic human rights and right conduct (i.e., right to self-determination and well-being, right to know, right to privacy). A right decision is one made in accordance with the person's rules, codes, and rights. This presents a conflict when (1) there is little agreement concerning these rules of conduct, (2) there is a conflict between personal values and the decision's perceived benefit or the survival of a department or institution, or (3) there is a contradiction between two rules, for example, the dilemma posed in respecting someone's confidential communication when that person intends to harm someone else.

The second view holds that *a moral course of action is that which provides the greatest benefit to those people affected by the action.* In simple terms, this view states that rightness or wrongness is relative to outcome (whereas the first school emphasizes that one should do what is right regardless of the circumstances). This view assumes knowledge of a decision's benefit and also requires the difficult task of weighing and balancing the consequences for one person against those for others.

A third (less prominent) view suggests that *what is right is what is in the best interest of the person choosing the course of action.* This view advances an individualistic stance and suggests that the "end justifies the means."

To maintain a higher degree of objectivity in decision making, a nurse manager might need to examine his or her values and exercise caution in applying these values.

In addition to recognizing issues that involve values, the nursing manager must make decisions that involve ethical concerns. These decisions can be made and ethical issues can be resolved to some extent through collaboration with institutional resources, such as ethics committees, and the use of a decision-making process that carefully identifies an ethical component in analyzing and arriving at a decision.

Types of Ethical Conflicts*

Ethical dilemmas occur when a solution to a conflict encroaches on the interests and welfare of another. For example, society's inclination toward prolonging life may conflict with the patient's autonomy to make decisions about his or her care. Among critically ill patients, such dilemmas most frequently center around four ethical conflicts: autonomy versus paternalism, duty (deontological approach) versus outcome (teleological approach), justice versus utilitarianism, and veracity versus fidelity.

Autonomy versus Paternalism

Autonomy refers to the right of the patient to self-determination and freedom of choice. Au-

Source: Gary R. Anderson and Valerie A. Glesnes-Anderson, "Ethical Thinking and Decision Making for Health Care Supervisors," *Health Care Supervisor*, Vol. 5:4, Aspen Publishers, Inc., © 1987.

Source: Ginger Schafer Wlody, "Technology, Ethics, and Critical Care," in *Advanced Technology in Critical Care Nursing*, John M. Clochesy, ed., Aspen Publishers, Inc., © 1989.

tonomy asserts that humans have incalculable worth, deserve respect, and have the right to self-determination. If a competent patient makes a clear statement about his or her wishes, then those wishes should be respected. Freedom of choice requires that full information be given to the patient; thus, informed consent is defined as the right of competent adults to accept or refuse medical treatment on the basis of full information.

Paternalism, on the other hand, claims that beneficence (doing good for others, being helpful) should take precedence over autonomy. Beneficence also involves balancing the benefit of some therapy with the burden of it. For example, in the paternalistic approach a health care worker makes a decision for the patient, saying "It's in his best interest." This type of conflict (autonomy versus paternalism) occurs frequently in the area of technology related to treatment decisions. If a patient needs a technological therapy that the physicians view as lifesaving but the patient views as unnatural and unbearable, he or she may make an informed decision that the benefit does not outweigh the psychological and physical costs. The patient may then refuse the therapy.

Justice versus Utilitarianism

Justice demands that people have an opportunity to obtain the health care they need on an equitable basis. Utilitarianism states that the morally right thing to do is that act that produces the greatest good (for the greatest number of people, or society).

The current situation, in which there are expensive or limited resources, has forced health care leaders to review outcomes of care. Critically ill patients use vast amounts of resources, including staff, time, space, highly sophisticated equipment, and pharmacological products. Provision of intensive care to critically ill patients ultimately has effects on other patients (the moderately ill) from whom resources may have been diverted. Therefore, clear benefit should be gained by the critically ill patient to justify the vast expenditures of resources.

Conflicts in this area arise because some physicians and nurses want to provide every avail-

able therapy for their patients, even though the cost (psychological and financial) may outweigh the benefits or eventual outcome.

Veracity versus Fidelity

The concept of veracity refers to truth telling, honesty, or integrity. The nurse, as a professional, has an obligation to tell the truth. Fidelity is related to trust, or to the promises we make. Professional nurses promise to care for a patient to the best of their ability. The American Nurses' Association Code of Ethics puts forth the ethical standards for professional nurses and sets the standards for a trust relationship between the nurse and the patient.

As the nurse carries out this trust relationship and strives to deliver safe, quality care to the patient, conflicts may arise with other responsibilities the nurse has (e.g., to perform a painful or potentially dangerous procedure). Veracity conflicts with fidelity in these situations. Telling the patient truthful information that could cause the patient distress may conflict with protection of that patient.

Professional Integrity versus Remaining True to One's Own Ethical and Moral Beliefs

Conflicts between professional integrity and remaining true to one's own ethical and moral beliefs occur in various situations. Such conflicts might result in objecting to delivering certain types of treatment or to caring for certain types of patients.

The best-known examples include nurses' participation in abortion when this procedure conflicts with their own religious and/or philosophical beliefs and nurses' caring for patients with acquired immune deficiency syndrome (AIDS). Nurses, however, have traditionally removed themselves from the specific job situation to spare themselves the daily conflict. This becomes necessary because management cannot function in a situation in which individual nurses are saying such things as, "I don't think homosexuality is right; therefore, I cannot take care of this patient with AIDs."

Factors Affecting Ethical Issues and Ethical Decision Making*

The factors that influence ethical decision making are delineated below.

Patient Needs. Are the patient's physiological needs being met even though the patient has a terminal disease? Does the intensive care unit (ICU) "dump" (i.e., transfer) the patient out of the unit as soon as he or she is listed as a "no code" or "do not resuscitate"? The family may view the situation this way: One minute the physician in the ICU is doing everything he or she can to preserve the patient's life, and the next minute fewer and fewer resources are used. Families sometimes value care in relation to the cost and intensity of resources used rather than what the patient needs.

Disease Processes. Which disease processes are affecting the patient? Is a given disease process reversible? Is it terminal? Is it superimposed on a chronic, irreversible process? For example, does the patient have multiple sclerosis and pneumonia?

Patient Rights. Is the nurse familiar with the American Hospital Association's *Patient Bill of Rights*? Does the hospital have a policy? The patient should be consulted and, if possible, participate in decisions that affect his or her care. If the patient is not competent, does the next of kin or guardian have the opportunity to participate in the decision-making process? The patient has the right to privacy and to competent care and the right to informed consent regarding special procedures.

Patient Feelings and Wishes. It is the patient's right not only to have informed consent but to have his or her wishes followed. If the patient wishes to have a living will or to be considered "do not resuscitate" and is hopelessly ill, these wishes should be honored and carried out according to health care facility policy.

Family Wishes. A major focus in recent years has been the promotion of greater patient and family participation in decision making. Frequently, although the patient is alert and competent, the family, or a specific member, will disagree with the patient, usually "putting the patient's feelings down" or disregarding them. This occurs especially if the patient is anoxic, is losing consciousness, or has a disability. Family members, because they may have been the patient's caregivers, lose sight of the patient's right to self-determination. Health care workers frequently assume this type of attitude.

Treatment Team. The treatment team is usually composed of the nurse, physician, respiratory therapist, social worker, and nutritionist. More and more often in large medical centers an ethicist, or a person who acts as an ethicist, is involved in addressing ethical dilemmas with the treatment team and family.

A nurse might consult an ethicist when there are conflicting ideas about what to do in a situation because of different values or principles (a nurse may not be sure whether to support the patient's freedom of choice or the patient's health needs).

Society. Societal changes in attitudes toward access to care, death, people with disabilities, and the concept of informed consent are all important factors that influence ethical decision making.

Resource Allocation. Shortages of staff, equipment, and other resources affect the decision-making process.

Legal Issues and Facility Policies. The nurse must be aware not only of facility policies related to all these issues but also the legal requirements of the state in which he or she is working. For example, nurses should be familiar with facility policies on resuscitation, withdrawal of life support, care of the brain-dead organ donor, and levels of care for the terminally ill patient.

Source: Ginger Schafer Wlody, "Technology, Ethics, and Critical Care," in *Advanced Technology in Critical Care Nursing*, John M. Clochesy, ed., Aspen Publishers, Inc., © 1989.

ETHICS COMMITTEE

The Institutional Ethics Committee*

An institutional ethics committee varies considerably among institutions. Some committees have diverse functions, such as discussing general ethical topics, reviewing and formulating facility policy, educating staff, and providing ethics case consultation. Some committees limit their activities to one or more of these functions. The quality of the ethics committee's performance in any activity, though, directly relates to the expertise of its membership.

For an ethics committee to perform effectively, especially when offering ethics case consultation, the members must be educated in ethical theory and practice. Participating nurse members also must be educated about their roles and functions within the committee.

The Essentials of Clinical Ethics Needed by Committee Members

A prospective ethics committee member should clearly understand the crucial elements of clinical ethics. The member should understand how to (1) accurately identify ethical conflicts, (2) relate ethical practices to current case law and state and federal statutes, (3) discuss ethical issues appropriately using the vocabulary of ethics, (4) logically and objectively approach ethical analysis, and (5) openly discuss, debate, and resolve ethical issues brought before the ethics committee.

Identifying Ethical Conflicts

An ethics committee member should be able to identify, analyze, and resolve ethical problems. A committee member should clearly distinguish between ethical and "problem patient" dilemmas. For example, cases might be referred for an ethics consultation that involve communication

*Source: Ray Moseley and Mary Harward, "Educating Ethics Committee Members: Programs and Networking," in *Health Care Ethics: Critical Issues for Today's Health Professional*, John F. Monagle and David C. Thomasma, eds., Aspen Publishers, Inc., © 1994.

problems or personality conflicts between physicians. An ethics committee may choose to participate in analysis and resolution of these cases but should understand that they involve disputes between physicians and not ethical problems.

Relating Law and Ethics

The relationship between the law and ethics also should be clear to all committee members. Of course, the ethics committee members should be familiar with pertinent case and state law, since many laws and legal cases regarding medical care are rooted in ethical analysis. Despite this connection, it is naive to believe that the law will unambiguously resolve ethical dilemmas for ethics committees.

Using the Language of Ethics

Members of ethics committees should be conversant in the language of clinical ethics. Most health care areas use specialized language to clarify life and death issues; thus, diseases, symptoms, medicines, and procedures are discussed in highly technical language to ensure precise, focused communication. Members of ethics committees should understand the precise meaning and ethical ramifications of terms such as *terminal, futile, extraordinary, informed consent, autonomy,* and *competence*.

Analyzing Ethical Dilemmas

Ethical analysis is more complex than a "matter of opinion." First, ethical theory and case analysis can be used to evaluate the validity of an argument in supporting a position. Specifically, one should analyze the logic, consistency, and accuracy of any argument. If the case is discussed using the method of analogy, the appropriateness of the analogy should be reviewed. Second, many ethical problems, especially those found in medicine, are extremely complex. Ethical analysis will raise questions about the medical indications of any recommended therapy; patient preferences; quality-of-life issues; and contextual factors such as the personal opinions of patients, family members, and health care providers; institutional policies; economic factors; and societal influences. Frequently, the answers to these questions are not clearly known, and often decisions must be made without all of the facts. This problem should not discourage but rather stimulate a committee to search for facts and to carefully and expertly analyze the identified ethical issues.

Discussing Ethical Issues Openly

Ethics committee members also must be receptive to open discussion and disagreement. A fundamental practice of clinical ethics is acceptance and encouragement of open debate regarding an ethical problem, as long as that debate is based on logical, consistent, and accurate reasoning.

Along with acknowledging the occurrence of disagreements, members of ethics committees should strive to be open-minded and objective.

Methods of Educating the Ethics Committee

Most health care facility staff and ethics committee members will have no formal background or education in ethical theories, case analysis, and practices. One of the primary functions of the committee is to ensure appropriate education for the members and the staff, including physicians, nurses, other clinical staff, and administrators. Several venues for adult education are available to accomplish these goals.

The ethics committee can maintain a pertinent library on ethical issues that is readily available to committee members and facility staff. The readings should be current and chosen carefully for content and readability. Journal articles also are useful but should be carefully selected.

The American College of Physicians publishes an ethics manual that provides an excellent reading list. Many articles related to ethics are now published in the clinical journals such as the *New England Journal of Medicine,* the *Journal of the American Medical Association, Annals of Internal Medicine,* the *Journal of General Internal Medicine,* and the *Journal of Family Practice.*

Select committee members may want to focus on a particular area of expertise, review that area, then educate the other members about the topic. Such topics could include facility policy; current state legislation and case law regarding ethical issues, especially refusal and withdrawal of treatments; the Patient Self-Determination Act

and its implications; the process of ethics case consultation; management of the dying patient; and informed consent.

Many ethics committees find a monthly or bimonthly conference on ethical topics within the health care facility to be a useful forum for educating staff. Medical ethics or medical humanities departments are available to provide conferences and/or workshops at local facilities and can be of assistance in getting an ethics committee started.

In many cases, ethics committees are joining together to form regional or statewide networks. The organization of this network may aid others in establishment of similar networks.

Functions of the Ethics Committee*

There is increased pressure to create formal mechanisms for conflict resolution and policy development in health care facilities. Ethics committees can be helpful in dealing with ethical issues. They can also be used to mend the seams of the delivery system to better ensure continuity of care as well as continuity of patients' wishes. However, questions as to their value, role, and scope need to be answered fully. Also, existing committees can become stagnant and purposeless and need revitalization.

Establishing an ethics committee—an institutional forum for addressing a wide range of ethical issues—is not always an easy task. Like many innovative mechanisms for addressing controversy, an ethics committee may be feared as potentially too influential, and its role may be reduced from problem solving to identification of and education about ethical issues.

An ethics committee must be provided with certain "tools of the trade." Members need to be familiar with key ethical and legal principles and how to define issues, test provisional decisions, and offer advice. They need up-to-date materials and other resources. Developing a small library of books or articles is a sensible way of increasing members' knowledge and skills.

---

*Source: Dennis A. Robbins, *Ethical and Legal Issues in Home Health and Long-Term Care,* Aspen Publishers, Inc., © 1996.

Although models can be used for developing policies, going through the process of development themselves is important for committee members so that they understand why the specific language was employed. Understanding this will help them perform their advisory role and reduce the chance of conflict. For example, if the committee chooses not to use the words "heroic measures" and replaces them with something more appropriate, the reason behind the choice is important, particularly when a caregiver approaches the committee for advice and uses "heroic measures" to define the issue. The committee hopefully will be able to explain that heroism implies sacrificing oneself or putting oneself in danger for a noble cause and that therefore "heroic measures" is inappropriate for referring to procedures that do not more than prolong the dying process. Being supplied with that insight might be extremely helpful to the staff member who has come to the committee for advice.

Typical ethics committee members include the following:

- the director of nursing
- the medical director
- the head of the agency or facility
- the director of social work
- the director of pastoral care
- representatives from managed care and/or management company organizations (if appropriate)
- representatives from other community post-acute care providers (e.g., long-term care facilities and home health agencies)
- representatives from referring institutions (e.g., hospitals and clinics)
- dietitians and other appropriate health professionals

To play their proper role, ethics committee members must

- gain some sense of what ethics is all about
- understand the role, scope, and charge of the committee

- identify the strengths and weaknesses of the committee
- master problem identification, problem solving, and conflict resolution techniques
- know how to test and refine provisional decisions or recommendations
- recognize that there will not necessarily be clearly defined right and wrong answers but that the problem-solving process itself can be helpful and illuminating
- learn how to clarify or flesh out important components of a problem and explore an array of solutions to identify the most appropriate one
- recognize that getting together to talk about a problem and merely feeling better as a

---

Objectives for a Nursing Bioethics Committee

- To provide a structural format for professional nurses to increase their knowledge of applied ethics
- To assist nurses in assuming ethical responsibilities and making judgments as professionals affecting change
- To influence the development of policies on health care standards within the profession and institution
- To serve as a resource to individual clinicians and managers whose responsibility for high-quality nursing care spans patients, families, and the community
- To develop support within the system for nurses' active participation in ethical decision making
- To serve as the group from which nursing representation will be selected to serve on the facility's multidisciplinary ethics committee

Source: Barbra J. Edwards and Amy M. Haddad, "Establishing a Nursing Bioethics Committee," *Journal of Nursing Administration*, Vol. 18, No. 3, March 1988.

result is not a sufficient response to the problem

- understand the ethical and legal issues that often arise in case discussion and policy development

SPECIAL ETHICS ISSUES

Contemporary View of Ethical Problems

Many ethical issues confront the nurse in the performance of his or her professional role as a health care provider. These issues vary over time. Some, like those associated with the indiscriminate prolongation of life by using life-sustaining technology, became such festering issues that they were addressed by society at large. The resulting legislation was introduced in the form of the Patient Self-Determination Act. It then became an obligation of the health care facility to honor the advance directives formulated by an enlightened patient population. But ethical dilemmas never go away. Some of the current ethical issues covered in a guide for health care providers are outlined in the following box.

The most overriding concern among nurses, however, is on the horizon: the potential ramifications from the cost constraints enacted under a managed care system. It is possible that awareness of the potential problem and the establishment of guidelines will prevent speculation from becoming a reality.

Allocation of Scarce Health Care Resources*

Health care delivery probably has reached a point at which some form of rationing or restriction must be invoked even though society lacks moral agreement about how, or to whom, to deny

*Source: Mychelle M. Mowry and Ralph A. Korpman, *Managing Health Care Costs, Quality, and Technology: Product Line Strategies for Nursing*, Aspen Publishers, Inc., © 1986.

Current Ethical Issues

- Reproductive issues
- Autonomy of patient decision making
- Advance directives
- AIDS care
- HIV-positive status
- Futile therapy situations
- Genetic screening counseling
- Human genome research
- Fetal diagnosis therapy
- Embryo implantation
- Prenatal screening and drug use
- Conducting research in emergency or acute care situations
- Quality of life and the patient
- Physician-assisted suicide
- Health care access
- Nutritional fluid support
- Persistent vegetative status (PVS)
- Drug policy conflicts
- Surrogacy and health care decisions
- Technology—extent of use
- Transplantation of organs

---

medical services. Medical triage is being used in a covert fashion. Patients are "allowed" to die, physicians are deciding who shall receive high-tech medical treatments, and cost and delay inevitably kill many who cannot get access to quality health care. The ethical issues can no longer be avoided. Perhaps the most urgent ethical problem is that most health care providers sidestep such questions.

Many ethical issues involve clinical organizational support decisions where there are competing claims for scarce resources. Nurse executives should create forums for dialogue with each other and with appropriate representatives from other disciplines to begin to address these issues. In relation to their role in "distributive justice," nursing administrators can ask three basic questions.

- Do they have a moral responsibility to identify and resolve ethical issues related to the distribution of scarce nursing resources?
- If so, what kind of knowledge base do they need to enhance their moral reasoning about how to allocate these scarce nursing resources?
- How, then, can they apply this knowledge base to distributive justice problems arising out of their nursing and administrative practice?

These are meant to be used as a springboard from which many other questions and issues will be raised.

Nursing professionals essentially have a moral obligation to guard the allocation of resources so that the care and safety of patients is not compromised. There is a large body of ethical knowledge and principles on which nurses can base and apply moral reasoning about these issues.

Structuring Ethical Relations with Patients

Assisting Patient Self-Determination*

Although the nurse is obligated to act in the best interests of the patient, it is the patient and not the nurse who decides what those "best interests" are. The role of the nurse, however, goes beyond that of merely protecting patients against institutional encroachments on their freedom of choice. It involves actively assisting patients in the exercise of self-determination—helping them to clarify values and beliefs, to develop their understanding of self and of the situation, and to make decisions based on their own goals and wishes.

Three models of practice that may have some relevance for how nurses structure their relationships with patients have been described. The first

is the *engineering model*, which consists of giving the patient only the facts, usually emphasizing "scientific facts," and allowing the patient to decide. The provider in this model believes that it is improper to get involved in values concerning patient situations and often is unaware of how his or her own values influence the nature of transaction.

The *priestly model* of practice is paternalistic in orientation. The provider expects the patient to follow directions given and operates on the basis of "I know best." A variant of this model is the maternal form, which often assumes an ultraprotective stance toward the patient while at the same time setting absolute standards for the patient's performance.

The *contractual model* of practice provides for shared decision making by the provider and the patient and assumes that both parties have obligations and obtain benefits from their shared endeavors. The contractual model appears to be most suitable for the nurse-patient relationship given nursing's primary goals. Establishing contractual arrangements by mutual consent and the ongoing process of evaluating progress and making decisions about new courses of action depends on both parties being willing to exchange information and to validate their observations, so that the next step can be taken toward the agreed-upon goals. The process of helping the patient to make decisions that incorporate the patient's own values and concepts of self and health demands far more of nurses, both intellectually and interpersonally, than simply making decisions on behalf of the patient.

The education of nurses who are responsive to the moral as well as the technical components of professional work requires an interpersonal environment that does more than distribute knowledge and promote conformity to established professional norms. It should promote the exercise of self-determination and personal growth of students in a holistic sense through a milieu that encourages independence of observation, originality of thought, dissent from established opinion, tolerance for differences in viewpoint, and respect for the rights and contributions of others.

---

*Source: Reproduced from J.Q. Benoliel, "Ethics in Nursing Practice and Education," *Nursing Outlook,* 1983, Vol. July/August, with permission from Mosby-Year Book, Inc.

The Language of Clinical Ethics*

The following terms, formulated for an ethical approach to patient self-determination, represent respect for the privacy and autonomy of all patients as well as the responsibility of the physician and institution.

- *Life-sustaining treatment:* any medical procedure or intervention (including, but not limited to, dialysis, medication, artificial hydration/nutrition/ventilation, and resuscitation) that supplants or supports a vital function to delay the occurrence of death
- *Competent:* possessing the ability, based on reasonable medical judgment, to participate in treatment discussions and to understand and appreciate the nature and consequences of a treatment decision
- *Incompetent:* lacking the ability, based on reasonable medical judgment, to participate in treatment discussions and to understand and appreciate the nature and consequences of a treatment decision
- *Effect:* a measurable change on some portion of a patient's anatomy, physiology, or chemistry
- *Benefit:* to cause an improvement in the patient's prognosis, comfort, or well-being
- *Futile treatment:* treatment that provides only a measurable *effect* on some part of the patient (e.g., blood pressure, kidney function) without providing a *benefit* such as improved prognosis, relief of pain, and well-being; treatment that through clinical studies or experience has failed to work in a majority of cases; treatment that merely preserves permanent unconsciousness, prolongs dying, or fails to end total dependence on intensive medical care
- *Terminal condition:* an incurable or irreversible condition (including permanent vegetative state, dementias, and amyotrophic lateral sclerosis) caused by injury, disease, or illness, which, without the application of life-sustaining procedures would, within reasonable medical judgment, produce death, and where the application of such procedures serves only to postpone the moment of death of the patient; a condition in which the prospects for recovery of quality of life (as defined by the patient/family) are so minimal that the patient's care requires preoccupation with intensive medical treatment to the exclusion of other life goals

Competent Patients*

A competent adult patient's wishes concerning his or her person may not be disregarded. The court in *Erickson v. Dilgard* was confronted with a request by the hospital to authorize a blood transfusion over the patient's objection. The court recognized that the patient's refusal might cause his death, but it would not authorize the blood transfusion, holding that a competent individual has the right to make this decision even though it may seem unreasonable to medical experts.

The court in *In re Melideo* held that every human being of adult years has a right to determine what shall be done with his or her own body and cannot be subjected to medical treatment without his or her consent. When there is no compelling state interest that justifies overriding an adult patient's decision, that decision should be respected.

In the Illinois case of *In re Estate of Brooks*, the court held that competent adult patients without minor children cannot be compelled to accept blood transfusions that they steadfastly have refused because of religious beliefs. In this case, the patient had made her beliefs known to her physician and the hospital before consenting to any medical treatment. She was aware at all times of the meaning of her decision and had signed a statement releasing the hospital and her attend-

---

*Source: Adapted from "Guidelines for Refusing, Withholding, or Withdrawing Life-Sustaining or Futile Treatment," Courtesy of St. David's Health Care System, Austin, Texas.

*Source: George D. Pozgar, *Legal Aspects of Health Care Administration*, ed 6, Aspen Publishers, Inc., © 1996.

ing physician from liability for any consequences of her refusal to accept a blood transfusion.

Only a compelling state interest will justify interference with an individual's free exercise of religious beliefs. Application of this principle in *Application of President & Directors of Georgetown College, Inc.*, involved a pregnant patient at the Georgetown Hospital. The hospital was granted a court order authorizing blood transfusions because the patient's physicians said they were necessary to save her life. The patient and her husband had refused authorization because of their religious beliefs. To learn whether the woman was in a mental condition to make a decision, the judge asked her what the effect would be, in terms of her religious beliefs, if the blood transfusions were authorized. Her response was that the transfusions would no longer be her responsibility. In its decision, the court stressed that it was convinced she wanted to live. Furthermore, according to the woman's statement, if the court undertook to authorize the transfusions without her consent, she would not be acting contrary to her religious beliefs. The effect of the court order preserved for Mrs. Jones the life she wanted without sacrificing her religious beliefs.

The Court of Appeals of the District of Columbia noted in *In re Osborne* that the state's concern for the welfare of the children could override a patient's decision to refuse treatment for religious reasons. However, the court found in this case that the patient had made sufficient financial provisions for the future well-being of his two young children, so they would not become wards of the state if he should die. Under the circumstances, the court held that there was no compelling state interest to justify overriding the patient's intelligent and knowing refusal to consent to a transfusion because of his religious beliefs.

The New Jersey Supreme Court took the position in *John F. Kennedy Memorial Hospital v. Heston* that the state's power to authorize a blood transfusion does not rest on the fact of the patient's condition or competence; it rests on the fact of the state's compelling interest in protecting the lives of its citizens, which in this case was sufficient to justify overriding the patient's determination to refuse vital aid.

The New York Supreme Court, Suffolk County, in *Fosmire v. Nicoleau*, issued an order authorizing blood transfusions for a patient who had refused them. The plaintiff applied for an order vacating the supreme court's order. The New York Supreme Court, Appellate Division, held that the patient's constitutional rights of due process were violated by the supreme court's issuing an order authorizing blood transfusions in the absence of notice or opportunity for the patient or her representatives to be heard. The rights of a competent patient to refuse medical treatment, even if premised on fervently held religious beliefs, is not unqualified and may be overridden by compelling state interests. However, a state's interest in preserving a patient's life is not inviolate and in and of itself may not, under certain circumstances, be sufficient to overcome the patient's express desire to exercise her religious belief and forgo blood transfusion. The appellate division held in part that the state's interest would be satisfied if the other parent survived.

The court of appeals went further by stating that "[t]he citizens of the state have long had the right to make their own medical care choices without regard to their medical condition or status as parents." The court of appeals held that a competent adult has both a common-law and statutory right under Section 2504 and 2805-d of the Public Health Law to refuse life-saving treatment. Citing the state's authority to compel vaccination to protect the public from the spread of disease, to order treatment for persons who are incapable of making medical decisions, and to prohibit medical procedures that pose a substantial risk to the patient alone, the court of appeals did not that the right to choose was not absolute.

In the final analysis, if there is no compelling state interest to justify overriding a patient's intelligent and knowing refusal to consent to a medical procedure because of his or her religious beliefs, states are reluctant to override such a decision.

Part III

Administration

Chapter 13

Financial Managing and Budgeting

INTRODUCTION TO BUDGETING

Overview: Elements and Participants*

Budgeting is regarded by many as the primary tool that health care facility managers can use to control costs in their organizations. The objectives of budgetary programs, as designated by the American Hospital Association, are:

- to provide a written expression, in quantitative terms, of the policies and plans of the health care facility
- to provide a basis for the evaluation of financial performance in according with the plans
- to provide a useful tool for the control of costs
- to create cost awareness throughout the organization

The budgetary process encompasses a number of interrelated but separate budgets. This chapter discusses the budgetary process and the relationships among specific types of budgets.

*Source: William O. Cleverley, *Essentials of Health Care Finance,* ed 3, Aspen Publishers, Inc., © 1992.

Roles in the Health Care Facility Budgeting Process

The governing board's involvement in the budgetary process is usually indirect. The board provides the goals, objectives, and approved programs that are used as the basis for budgetary development. In many cases, it formally approves the finalized budget, especially the cash budget and budgeted financial statements; these are critical in assessing financial condition, which is a primary responsibility of the board.

The chief executive officer (CEO) or administrator of the health care facility has overall responsibility for budgetary development. The budget is the administrator's tool in the overall program of management by exception, which enables the CEO to focus only on those areas where problems exist.

The primary function of the *comptroller* or *budget director* is facilitation. The comptroller is responsible for providing relevant data on costs and outputs and for providing budgetary forms that may be used in budget development. He or she is not responsible for either making or enforcing the budget.

The head of a responsibility center is usually the designated administrator of the department. Responsibility centers are the focal points of control. Managers of departments should be actively involved in developing budgets for their assigned areas of responsibility and are responsible for meeting the budgets developed for their areas.

A special budgetary committee is often used to aid in budget development and approval. It is usually composed of several department managers, headed by the comptroller or administrator. A committee structure such as this can help legitimize budgetary decisions that might appear arbitrary and capricious if made unilaterally by management.

Financial Responsibilities and Nurse Managers

Changes in third-party reimbursement, the economics of the nursing and medical professions, organizational diversification, and rising competition make it imperative that managers be well versed in and allocate sufficient time to financial management. Unless nurse managers develop a functional competency in financial management, they may be unable to contribute to financial issues involving their nursing program or organization.

If nurse managers expect to adopt a financial perspective commensurate with their managerial and clinical skills, it follows that they must first learn basic financial concepts and techniques. Such knowledge is a prerequisite to nurse leadership. A solid grounding in financial basics allows nurse managers to acquire power and to participate jointly (with other non-nursing managers) in key decision processes.*

*Constraints on Nursing Budgets and Resources**

Decisions about budgets and financial plans, for example, are constrained by many factors outside nursing services.

First, the philosophy of the CEO and the governing board relative to expenditure increases,

capital outlays, equipment acquisition, or cost control affects financial decisions for the nursing program.

Second and third, nursing's profile as a revenue generator (or revenue consumer) influences the extent to which funds are allocated for program growth. Nursing is often viewed as a consumer of resources rather than a revenue generator. Nurse managers need to demonstrate how nursing expenditures enhance other service units (e.g., laboratory, radiology, and surgical services) that are revenue earners. In this manner, nursing establishes rights to its fair allocation of resources.

A *fourth* factor constraining financial plans is the extent to which the proposed plans are cost-effective. This cost-effectiveness is related to nursing's reputation as a credible financial manager. The credibility of proposed budgets is linked to the credibility of nurse managers as financial planners. It is also supported by past efforts at attaining budgets.

Fifth, decisions about nursing expenditures and annual budgets by key decision makers are affected by the perceived thresholds of safe clinical practice.

Other factors affecting financial plans—quality of care and state-of-the-art practice—are related to safe clinical practice. Nursing programs are expected to produce high-quality care and to maintain safe clinical practices. Hence financial planning hinges on documentation (of quality or low risk) to justify resource expenditures.

Further, resources used in the budgeting process influence financial planning by nurse managers. Reports, information, data files, historical schedules, and similar resources ultimately determine the accuracy of proposals. Consequently, they represent another factor constraining financial plans. This information is usually provided by financial personnel who may not understand the considerations and trade-offs surrounding clinical practice. Nurse managers work with financial officers in guiding their understanding of how nursing functions as an individual financial entity. The final step suggests that expected outcomes from nursing activities influence decisions about allocations to nursing services.

---

*Source: Judith F. Garner, Howard L. Smith, and Neill F. Piland, *Strategic Nursing Management: Power and Responsibility in a New Era,* Aspen Publishers, Inc., © 1990.

In sum, nurse managers should attempt to control various factors in presenting a solid financial plan to health care decision makers. Financial management is predicated on basics. Without basic knowledge of financial skill areas, it will be difficult if not impossible for nurse managers to contribute an enlightened perspective on nursing services to the rest of the organization.

Delegating Details of Financial Management*

The expansion of the planning, designing, and communicating role places the executive and manager in the role of consistently determining priorities between the overall survival needs and the day-to-day operational details. For most nurses experienced in management, however, the past taught a sometimes painful lesson: The nursing department that did not become very proficient and knowledgeable in budgeting and attentive to day-to-day fiscal management paid a high price in terms of respect, authority, and overall autonomy. Therefore, the delegation of the financial operation of a nursing department must be very carefully planned and managed.

Preliminary Executive Decisions. Initially the executive, in determining what can be delegated, must define the current system, or lack thereof. The following questions should be asked:

- Who is currently doing what?
- Is it effective?
- Are the most qualified doing the components that match their skills?
- Is the work being done by various members of management producing good data for decision making?
- Are decisions being made based on data or are the data being ignored?
- Do the multiple reports currently being received provide useful, accurate data or meaningless numbers?

The size and complexity of the health care facility will also enter into any review of the current situation. Should an operations component be established that consists of a highly qualified non-nurse who will centralize many functions, or will the activities be spread across several existing positions?

The desired goal for the executive determined to delegate financial operational processes is to receive timely, brief, accurate reports that show actual performance relative to all budgets, with variances and the rationale for them. In addition, the executive needs to know when trends are developing that will affect current budgeted units of service as well as future budgets. The executive cannot delegate the vital role of initiating the budget.

Whether the presentation takes place in the form of a management retreat or a series of one-on-one meetings, there are key issues that the executive must address.

- Do nursing data accurately reflect the finance office's projections?
- Will the projected revenues enable the department to continue the same delivery of care methods?
- Are the existing skill mixes affordable?
- Do the projected revenues indicate departmental restructuring?

What Can and Cannot Be Delegated. Once these and other similar questions are answered, the actual personnel budget preparation can be delegated. The formula for full-time equivalent (FTE) and benefit calculation, education, and governance requirements is approved by the executive.

The responsibility for designing the departmental plan of care and reviewing the unit plans of care cannot be delegated. The critical issue of the design of the standards of care that result in quality outcomes cannot be delegated in the large sense. If the standards are inappropriate or poorly monitored, the final responsibility rests with the nurse executive.

The capital and supply budgets can be delegated once the following planning and operational questions have been answered:

Source: Sheila Lenkman, "Delegating Responsibility for Financial Operations," *Aspen's Advisor for Nurse Executives*, Vol 5, No. 3, Aspen Publishers, Inc., © December 1990.

- What new services are proposed that will require expenditures in these areas?
- Are there changes in revenue projections that will require a major review of supply usage?
- What supplies can be standardized to reduce cost?
- What major purchases are needed to increase operational and clinical efficiency?

Once budget preparation has been delegated and the budgets approved, either secretaries or a designated person can pull together data to provide the executive with the information that is needed. The executive role is to design the format in which the information will be presented, set the parameters that indicate a need for immediate management concern and action, and communicate to all managerial staff how this management tool is to be used.

The executive, depending on the competencies of the delegated staff member, may also have to research all sources of data that are useful to the operational monitoring. The research should include a discussion with the involved departments about where they obtain the information.

- Is it based on monthly or payroll time frames?
- Is it actual midnight or adjusted census?
- If adjusted, what is the formula?
- What types of patients are included?
- Are any left out because of software design limitations?
- Are staff who are working innovative and creative shift schedules being shown as working overtime because the system is unable to reflect what is actually occurring?

Requests for explanation of variances provided to managers should be simple and, as much as possible, use a "fill in the blanks" type format to reduce the managerial time involved. Information provided to managers for explanation is helpful if it shows clearly the relationship between dollars, hours of care, and census.

For example, if dollars are higher than budget but nursing care hours per patient are as budgeted, the following may have occurred:

- use of agency workers at higher salaries
- use of float/overtime at higher salaries
- use of richer skill mix

If the dollars are less than budgeted but the nursing care hours per patient are the same, then a cheaper skill mix than budgeted has been used. If actual acuity recorded is higher than budgeted but the dollars and care hours delivered are as budgeted, then it will be necessary to check on outcomes, falls, incidents, errors, morale, retention of staff, and complaints. If over a long period of time there are no untoward incidents, it indicates the budget was higher than necessary.

In a nutshell, the nurse executive must ensure the design of a system, appropriately delegate responsibilities, and consistently monitor financial performance. The larger issue of the planning and critical analysis of all budget inputs, prompt management actions, communication, and discussion with managers cannot be delegated.

THE BUDGET PROCESS

For our purposes, a budget will be defined as the systematic documentation of one or more carefully developed plans for all individually supervised activities, programs, or sections. These individually supervised cost centers, frequently referred to as responsibility centers, are coordinated into a departmental budget. Departmental budgets are further consolidated into a health care institution's master budget.

Many CFOs, recognizing the budget's importance as a management tool, have identified and assigned one individual to be the organization's budget director. The budget director, who usually reports to the CFO, is responsible for the entire budgetary control program and may also serve as the chairperson of the budget committee.

Budget Committee and Its Role*

The budget committee generally consists of a representative cross section of the major functional areas or divisions within the institution, with the designated budget director usually serving as the chairperson. Budget committees frequently include, among others, those who hold the following positions:

- *Director of Nursing.* This position is responsible for the major function of most health care institutions and also accounts for one of the largest, if not the largest, proportion of the institution's expenses and revenues.
- *Director of Human Resources.* This position is responsible for administering the institution's salary and wage program, including its hiring and firing policies. Since in most health care institutions salaries and wages constitute well over 50 percent of the organization's total operating expenses, the director of human resources is a valuable member of the budget committee.
- *Director of Materials Management.* This position represents the other half of the operating expense equation, the non-salary-and-wage expenses. The director of materials management provides knowledge of inflation trends; new market products; purchase and trade discounts; fixed asset requirements; and the requirements for receiving, storing, processing, pricing, and distributing the institution's operating supplies.
- *Director of Engineering and Plant Operations.* This position is responsible for the institution's building(s) and equipment, including repair and maintenance. The director of engineering and plant operations can provide a wealth of information about such things, as well as experience in new construction, remodeling, utilities efficiency, and other areas of concern.

- *Chief of Medical Staff.* This position represents the other half of the patient care equation, the medical staff. It is imperative that the physicians be represented in the budgetary planning and control process. They are not only the institution's major consumers, but they can be its best marketeers and salespersons. The medical staff, who are on or near the "cutting edge" of medical technology and therapy, can assist in identifying new procedures, treatments, and other related services that can benefit the institution and the community it serves.
- *Chief Executive Officer, Chief Operating Officer, and/or the Chief Financial Officer.* All three frequently serve as ex officio members of the budget committee. Their attendance at meetings and active interest in the budget committees's activities add credibility to the budget process and help to keep top management aware of the budget process, its direction, and the anticipated results.

Management Approaches to Budgeting*

The two basic approaches commonly used in generating a budget are the unilateral approach and the multilateral approach. The unilateral approach places the whole responsibility on one or two persons who are (usually) members of administration, are financially oriented, and have a general knowledge of departmental activities and needs. Since there is virtually no involvement by other members of the organization's personnel, a budget that meets management's goals and objectives can be generated within a short time period.

The multilateral or participative approach can be a very cumbersome and slow process, because it requires that all individuals who are responsible for any revenue/cost center be involved in generating the budget as it applies to their areas. Although slow, this approach has its advantages.

Source: Allen G. Herkimer, *Understanding Health Care Budgeting*, Aspen Publishers, Inc., © 1988.

Source: Allen G. Herkimer, *Understanding Health Care Budgeting*, Aspen Publishers, Inc., © 1988.

The department managers are being "sold" on the budget during their involvement in the mechanics of the budgeting process, and since they helped to generate the budget, they will make every effort to promote it and to operate within its established standards.

There are times when the unilateral approach may be necessary or especially desirable. If, for example, a budget program is urgently needed for a new service or acquisition, one person may be assigned the task of unilaterally generating a budget quickly. Another example is if an organization's management has never before had a budgetary control program. In such a situation, the faster a budget is developed and implemented, the better. Experience has shown, however, that the success of the program is more often assured if middle management participates from the beginning and that the multilateral approach is generally preferable.

Cost Centers*

The nurse executive needs to identify cost centers. A cost center is the smallest functional unit for which cost control and accountability can be assigned under the existing accounting system. Ideally, each separate functional unit in the nursing division should have its separate account for expenses. For example, a nursing service budget should make it possible to charge each separate patient floor for the actual supplies used on that single unit. Logically, a head nurse cannot be held responsible for costs on his or her unit unless they are identified and separated from costs accrued by other nursing units.

The personnel budget is the largest single expense for the nursing unit, if not for the organization as a whole. Therefore, considerable care should be given to learning exactly how the nursing department formulates its staffing pattern and how specific variables affect the work unit. Staffing will be affected by several variables, including the nursing care delivery model in place, the rate of turnover, the acuity of the patient population, length of stay, fluctuations in census, numbers of experienced nurses versus new graduates, continuing education requirements, and staff mix. Nurse managers need to use their judgment when making staffing decisions as they relate to the budget. Enough flexibility should be built into the budget to accommodate the day-to-day reality, as opposed to the ideal staffing plan.

Budget Planning

Factors in Budget Planning*

Nursing service needs are determined by many factors, which the staff should be aware of as budget planning proceeds.

1. The type of patient (medical, surgical, maternity, pediatric, communicable disease, chronically ill), the length of stay, and the acuteness of the illness.
2. The size of the facility and its bed occupancy. It takes more staff in a *large* facility than it does in a small one to care for the same number of patients.
3. The physical layout of the facility, the size and plan of the ward—open ward, small units, private ward.
4. Personnel policies established to cover

- salaries paid to various types of nursing personnel, including pay for overtime
- the length of the workweek and work period as well as flexibility of hours
- the extent of vacation, statutory holidays, and sick leave
- provision for service education programs, including instructional staff as well as relief staff
- provision for development of staff through university preparation, refresher courses, and so forth

*Source: Adapted from Barbara S. Barnum and Karlene M. Kerfoot, *The Nurse as Executive*, ed 4, Aspen Publishers, Inc., © 1995 and Barbara S. Barnum and Catherine O. Mallard, *Essentials of Nursing Management*, Aspen Publishers, Inc., © 1989.

*Source: *Nursing Service Budget*, National League for Nursing, Pub. No. 22, 1957. Reprinted with permission.

5. The grouping of patients. For example, specialized units, such as neurological services and intensive care units, will have differing needs.

6. Standards of nursing care. The kind and amount of care to be given as it affects the number of hours of bedside care, for example, assisting the patient with a fracture to adjust to the degree of independence of which he or she is capable; health teaching, including methods of adjusting to normal living in the community.

7. The method of performing nursing procedures, simple or complex; the method of record-keeping and charting, for example, whether or not all routine procedures such as baths and back rubs must be charted, all medications must be recorded in the nurses' notes, a worksheet and checking system are in use.

8. The proportion of nursing care provided by professional nurses as compared to that provided by auxiliary personnel.

9. The availability of graduate and allied personnel and the utilization of both groups according to competencies and preparation.

10. The amount and quality of supervision available and provided; the efficiency of job descriptions and job classifications.

11. Method of patient assignment, for example, team nursing.

12. The amount and kinds of labor-saving equipment and devices: intercommunication systems; carrier and pneumatic tube systems; electronic monitor for determining vital signs, and so forth.

13. The amount of centralized service provided: sterile supply, central oxygen service, postoperative recovery room, messenger and porter service, linen service, including distribution of linen.

14. Whether or not non-nursing functions such as clerical, dietary, housekeeping, messenger, and porter services are the responsibility of the nursing department.

15. The nursing service requirements of ancillary departments: clinics, admitting office, health service, emergency department, and so forth. These activities may be included in the responsibilities of the nursing department but should not be charged to nursing.

16. Reports required by administration, whether simple or complex.

17. Method of appointment of medical staff, size of staff, activities of medical staff, kind and frequency of treatments and orders.

18. Affiliation with a medical school. Inexperienced medical students need more equipment and supplies.

19. The presence of a school of nursing.

*Steps in Budget Planning**

Preparation of the budget package can be divided into eight activities.

1. *Productivity goal determination.* The director of nursing services and the head nurse determine the unit's productivity goal for the coming fiscal year.
2. *Forecast workload.* The number of patient days expected on each nursing unit for the coming fiscal year is forecasted.
3. *Budgeted patient care hours.* The number of hours expected to be used in patient care for the patient days is forecasted.
4. *Budgeted patient care hours and staffing schedules.* The budgeted patient care hours are reflected in recommended staffing schedules by shift and by day of the week.
5. *Planned nonproductive hours.* Hours for vacation, holiday, education leave, sick leave, and the like are budgeted for the coming year.
6. *Productive and nonproductive time.* To aid in the planning process, a graph is used to show head nurses and assistant head nurses how the level of forecasted patient days and therefore the staffing requirements are expected to move up and down during the year. Productive time is the time spent on the job in patient care, administration of the unit, conferences, educational activities, and orientation.

Source: J.N. Althaus et al., *Nursing Decentralization: The El Camino Experience,* Aspen Publishers, Inc., © 1981, based on "Planning and Budgets: Magic or Math" by John Fleming in *Maintaining Cost Effectiveness,* Elsie Schmied, ed., Aspen Publishers, Inc., © 1978.

Steps 7 and 8, "supplies and services" and "capital budget," are concerned with nonlabor expenses.

These eight steps result in a total budget package that goes to the director of nursing services for review. Upon his or her preliminary acceptance of this budget, it is sent to the accounting department, where the forecasted patient days are turned into expected revenue. The budgeted productive and nonproductive time is extended into dollars, as are the costs for supplies and services and other operating expenses that will be allocated to a given nursing unit for the coming year. A pro forma operating statement is then returned to the director of nursing who then reviews it with the head nurse. When the director and head nurse accept the budget, it is returned to the accounting department and forwarded with the rest of the health care facility budgets to administration and the board of directors.

Preparation and Presentation*

The director must be aware of any special instructions available from administration about preparation of data and the annual procedure for budgeting and must inform the committee and unit personnel responsible for budget preparation. He or she must also obtain a copy of the facility calendar budget, which will provide sufficient information for internal budget planning and a timetable of proposed activities. The nursing budget committee initiates a calendar based on the facility calendar, which will also serve as a schedule to outline activities leading to the preparation and completion of the nursing budget. (See Figure 13–1.)

Past operations records need to be analyzed, and the overall master staffing plan must be reviewed. Each nurse manager should work with his or her head nurses to determine the staff requirements for each unit. They should consider such factors as (1) assurance of standards according to the philosophy and objectives of the health care facility and the department of nursing, (2) past experiences of the unit, (3) anticipated needs for the unit, and (4) percentage of unit occupancy.

The estimation of staff for each unit should also include, for example, provision for vacation, sick leave, holidays, average amount of illness per staff member, and on-call pay. The number of hours of nursing care and nursing service hours per patient should be estimated from the total.

As these figures are identified for each unit within the nursing department, there emerges a visible method of interpreting nursing care needs to the nursing budget committee and later to administration.

Consideration should next be given to any new activities that will occur within a unit or have some bearing on the overall department, such as new services for patient care, changes in inservice educational programs, or changes in other departments that affect the nursing services required.

A review of the number of nursing hours per patient per day should be done to determine whether the amount of care provided was comparable to what is considered minimal for safe nursing care. The record of hours may be maintained by the nursing office or data processing office and must be available to nursing administration. Each nurse manager and head nurse should receive a monthly report of nursing hours and should have a cumulative record from the previous fiscal year to review. These figures must be scrutinized, moreover, to find out whether the quality of nursing care met the predetermined standards of care and whether it could be maintained by using other levels of personnel, with fewer professional personnel, through a pre-arrangement of duties and responsibilities—for example, by adding unit clerks to the evening tour of duty.

The next step in the preparation of the budget is to ascertain the amount and kind of supplies needed for the operation of each nursing unit, or those which are for total departmental use. A review of the last fiscal year's expenses provides data for planning. For budgetary purposes, the year's expected expenses can be divided by 12

---

*Source: Marie DiVincenti, *Administering Nursing Service*, Little, Brown and Company, 1978. Copyright © 1978 by Little, Brown and Company. Reprinted with permission.

Figure 13–1 Annual Budget Plan for Department of Nursing

SCHEDULE / ACTIVITIES	JUL	AUG	SEP	OCT	NOV	DEC	JAN	FEB	MAR	APR	MAY	JUN	WHO WILL DO/HELP
1. Establish Obectives for the Fiscal Year (July to June)	■												Dir. of Nursing, Assoc. Director
2. Identify Key Issues	■												Dir. of Nursing, Assoc. Director, Pt. Care Coords.
3. Analyze Performance and Resources		■											Dir. of Nursing, Comptroller, Pt. Care Coords.
4. State Basic Assumptions				■									Pt. Care Coords., Dir. of Nursing
5. Set Unit Objectives					■								Pt. Care Coords., Unit Staff
6. Develop Program Strategies and Action Plans							■						Pt. Care Coords., Unit Staff
7. Forecast Income							■						Comptroller
8. Develop Operational Plans								■					Pt. Care Coords., Unit Staff
9. Prepare Budget Recommendations									■				Pt. Care Coords., Dir. of Nursing, Assoc. Director
10. Submit Budget; Review, Revise, and Secure Approval										■			Dir. of Nursing, Assoc. Director, Pt. Care Coords.

Source: Adapted from J. Ganong and W. Ganong, "APB for Nursing Administration," *Journal of Nursing Administration*, May-June 1973. Reprinted with permission.

or, where possible, calculated month by month. Generally, a 5 to 10 percent increase in cost of supplies is figured because of rising prices. Each unit should identify its needs in writing. Each nursing unit also submits a list of its own capital expenditure needs, and they are compiled into the total departmental requests.

As each nurse manager or head nurse completes the preparation of the proposed budget, he or she meets with the nursing budget com-

mittee to make a formal presentation of the unit's financial request. The purpose of the session is to review the operating and capital expenditures and allow for an explanation and justification of unit requests. Topics to be discussed include (1) staffing requirements, with a justification if additional staff are needed; (2) general impact of supplies needed for use; (3) capital equipment to be replaced or requested, with documented justification, and other items requiring financial assistance; and (4) in some situations, specific recommendations for equipment and supplies prepared by the nursing unit staff with the chief of staff.

The unit budgets are approved as recommended, or revisions may be requested by the committee. Once the unit budgets are reviewed, classified, and summarized, the next step is to examine the departmental nursing budget appropriation and the actual expenditures for the current year, using information furnished by the accounting department in conjunction with the statistical data, such as average daily census per unit per service for the past year and anticipated census for the fiscal budget year; percentage of bed occupancy by months; average length of patient stay for the past year; total patient days and outpatient visits; nursing service hours per patient per day; number of employees divided into their various classifications; and expenses for supplies.

A comprehensive budget presentation reflects administrative skills in budgeting and finance (see Table 13–1). This demonstration of the ability of the nursing service to produce a fiscally responsible budget is ultimately conducive to budget acceptance.

The Review and Approval Process*

Competition, bargaining, and compromise in the allocation of scarce resources (personnel, money, and space) occur in the review and approval phase of the budget process. It is important for the manager to have the necessary facts to support budget requests; control records to demonstrate fluctuations in the workload, staffing needs, equipment usage, and goal attainment are essential sources of such information.

The internal approval process begins with a review of the department's budget by the department head's immediate budget officer. Compli-

---

*Source: Joan G. Liebler, Ruth Ellen Levine, and Jeffrey Rothman, *Management Principles for Health Professionals,* ed 2, Aspen Publishers, Inc., © 1992.

Table 13–1 Components of a Contemporary Nursing Department Budget Presentation

An effective, convincing nursing department budget presentation for administration and finance should include the following items:

- An *introduction* that includes the *strategic plan focus* areas of the budget such as
  –the improvement of the quality, effectiveness, and acceptability of service
  –the maintenance of sufficient, qualified staff to support this service
  –the implementation of effective management and systems to support this service
- A *supporting cost benefit analysis* of the budget noting the eventual cost savings or revenue enhancements to be realized through improved patient caring including decreased patient waiting times, decreased length of stay (LOS), elimination of agency nurses, reduction of excessive overtime, improved continuity of care, and so forth
- *Methodologies* used, such as cost per patient day analysis and zero base budgeting
- *Breakdown* of the personnel and operating budgets prepared by individual clinical directors
- *Service budget* presentations
- A *budget summary* of the nursing department, indicating
  –percentage increase or decrease by service
  –the relationship to current and projected service trends and programs as noted in census data
  –projected revenue effects of new programs

Source: Anne L. Felteau, "Tools and Techniques To Effect Budget Neutrality," *Nursing Administration Quarterly,* Vol. 17, No. 4, Aspen Publishers, Inc., Summer 1993.

---

ance with guidelines is checked; justifications for requests for exceptions are reviewed. The organization's designated financial officer (usually the comptroller) may assist the chief executive officer in coordinating the department budgets into the master budget for the organization, but the chief executive officer is the final arbiter of resource allocation in many instances.

In the present political climate, there is increasing insistence on cost containment, and a cost containment committee may be involved in the budget review process. Current voluntary efforts contribute to the routinization of this aspect of budget review. Cost-containment committees vary in structure and mandate, but their tasks typically include advising, investigating, and even participating in the implementation of cost-containment measures. Such a committee should have the questioning attitude as its primary philosophical stance; data are scrutinized and compared in an effort to identify areas where cost can be contained.

The final approval for the total budget is given by the governing board. In practice, a subcommittee on budget works with the chief executive officer, and final, formal approval is then given by the full governing board, as mandated in the organizational bylaws and/or charter of incorporation.

The budgets of organizations that receive some or all of their funds from state or federal sources may be subject to an external approval process, for example, by the state legislature or the federal Bureau of the Budget. There is a certain predictable drama in the budget process, which becomes more evident in the external review process. There is a tacit rule that budgets are padded, because budget requests are likely to be cut. The manager attempts to achieve a modicum of flexibility in budget maneuvering through overaim. There is also a necessary aspect of accountability, however. The public more or less demands that federal or state officials take proper care of the public purse. Even as clients (the public) seek greater services, they want cost containment, especially through tax relief. Public officials, then, must in fact dramatize their concern for cost containment, partly by a highly specific review of budget requests and a refusal to approve budgets as submitted.

On the other hand, should an agency request a budget allocation that is the same as, or less than, that of a previous year, it might be seriously questioned whether the agency is doing its job. At best, the manager must recognize the subtle and overt political maneuvers that touch the budget process.

BUDGET APPROACHES

1. Zero-Base Budgeting*

Zero-base budgeting or zero-base review, as some like to call it, is a way of looking at existing programs. Zero-base budgeting assumes that no existing program is entitled to automatic approval. Many individuals have identified automatic approval with existing budgetary systems that are based on prior-year expenditure levels.

Zero-base budgeting looks at the entire budget and determines the efficacy of the entire expenditure.

Zero-base budgeting is a process of periodically re-evaluating all programs and their associated levels of expenditures. Management decides the frequency of this re-evaluation and may vary it from every year to every five years.

Although most decision makers agree with the concept of zero-base budgeting, in practice it poses two significant questions:

- What arithmetic should be used in zero-base budgeting?
- Who should be involved in the actual decision-making process?

In each case, the answers are important to the success or failure of the zero-base budget program.

Arithmetic of the Zero-Base Budgeting Process

Nearly everyone would agree that cost benefit analysis should be the arithmetic of zero-base budgeting. There are two important issues involved in the application of cost benefit analysis to zero-base budgeting programs: (1) Are the services that are presently provided being delivered in an efficient manner? (2) Are these services being delivered in an effective manner in terms of the organization's goals and objectives? A procedure for quantitatively answering these two questions involves seven sequential steps:

Source: William O. Cleverley, *Essentials of Health Care Finance,* ed 3, Aspen Publishers, Inc., © 1992.

1. Define the outputs or services provided by the program/departmental area.
2. Determine the costs of these services or outputs.
3. Identify options for reducing the cost through changes in outputs or services.
4. Identify options for producing the services and outputs more efficiently.
5. Determine the cost savings associated with options identified in steps 3 and 4.
6. Assess the risks, both qualitative and quantitative, associated with the identified options of steps 3 and 4.
7. Select and implement those options with an acceptable cost/risk relationship.

2. Fixed or Static Budget*

Currently, the fixed or static budget is the most common budgetary approach. This budget is based on a fixed annual level of volume activity (i.e., number of patient days, tests performed) to arrive at an annual budget total. Usually, these totals are then divided into 12 equal parts for each month of the year. The primary weakness in this approach is that it does not allow for seasonal or monthly variations. To illustrate, assume a nursing station has 36 beds and the nurse manager and head nurse anticipate a 75 percent patient occupancy and a staffing requirement of 4.2 nursing hours per patient day. The nursing salary budget would be developed as follows:

- total capacity: 36
- projected percent of occupancy: 75 percent
- projected average daily census: 27
- project calendar days: 365
- projected annual patient days: 9,855
- average nursing hours per patient days: 4.2
- annual nursing hours requirement: 41,391
- average hourly rate: $7.50
- annual nursing costs: $310,433

*Source: Allen G. Herkimer, Jr., *Understanding Hospital Financial Management*, ed 2., Aspen Publishers, Inc., © 1986.

- average monthly patient day census: 822
- average monthly nursing hours requirement: 3,449
- average monthly nursing costs: $25,869

However, this approach is frequently used to prepare a department's initial budget. This is especially true when there is relatively little historical data on which to project seasonal volume variations. Obviously, this is the simplest budget to prepare, but most managers feel it is too difficult to compare, evaluate, and relate to the department's actual performance, since the fixed budget does not allow for volume variations in the initial plan.

3. Flexible Budget

The flexible budgeting approach establishes relevant ranges of volume activity. A relevant range of activity represents the range of volume or production units from a low point to a higher point. Expanding on the above illustration, assume the nurse manager and the head nurse establish the variations for patient census or occupancy level options indicated in Table 13–2.

Revenue and expense budgets are then prepared to reflect the average revenue and expenses (i.e., staffing requirements) for each of the three volume options. The monthly flexible nursing salary budget would be computed as shown in Table 13–3.

In reality, three individual budgets are prepared to reflect the hourly and salary requirements for the various volume levels or relevant

Table 13–2 Patient Volume and Range of Activity

Volume Options	Total Patient Pay Capacity	Volume Percent	Range of Activity Patient Days
1	36	60–75%	22–27
2	36	76–89%	28–32
3	36	90% & over	33–36

Table 13–3 Computation of Flexible Nursing Salary Budget

$$
\begin{array}{c}
\text{Budgeted quantity} \\
\text{of nursing} \\
\text{time per patient day}
\end{array}
\times
\begin{array}{c}
\text{Budgeted} \\
\text{nursing hourly} \\
\text{rate}
\end{array}
$$

$$
\times
\begin{array}{c}
\text{Actual number} \\
\text{of patient days}
\end{array}
=
\begin{array}{c}
\text{Flexible budget for} \\
\text{nursing salaries}
\end{array}
\quad (3)
$$

Source: Steven A. Finkler, "Flexible Variance Analysis Extended to Patient Acuity and DRGs," *Health Care Financial Management*, Vol. 10, No. 4, pp. 21–34, Aspen Publishers, Inc., © 1985.

---

ranges of activity. These ranges of activity will facilitate the fitting of budget-level requirements to actual performance of the nursing unit.

The two primary disadvantages of this budgeting approach are that it requires more preparation and maintenance time and that it establishes a range of activity rather than pinpointing the actual volume of activity.

4. Variable Budget

The variable budget approach allows the department manager and nurse managers to pinpoint the budget plan to the actual performance volume. In practice, the variable budget approach establishes a formula to enable the generation of a control budget that is directly related to volume activity. It is computed by using predetermined standards or budgeted rates and multiplying these rates by the actual volume. This eliminates variances that might occur due to volume differences.

To develop a variable budget, each cost item must be classified into one of the following categories:

- *fixed costs*—those that remain essentially constant in the short run, irrespective of changes in output volume
- *variable costs*—those that vary directly (in proportion) with changes in output volume

- *semi- or step-variable costs*—those that are neither fixed nor variable

This variable budget approach is frequently referred to as dynamic cost control. It is effective in departments where it is difficult to budget workload volume, such as nursing, but it requires a considerable amount of preparation, maintenance time, and cost.

5. Rolling or Moving Budget

The rolling or moving budget concept is basically an expansion on any of the above-mentioned budgeting approaches. Under this method, the most recent month or quarter is deleted and a new project is added for a corresponding month or quarter, so that the budget continually projects a fixed period of time, usually a minimum of a year.

The rolling or moving budget approach is especially effective in a department or facility that is exceptionally dynamic as far as costs and volume changes are concerned. Also, this concept ties very nicely into the belief that the budget is a management tool and must be continually monitored and updated.

6. Program Budget

The program budget approach can be very effective when a department manager is interested in projecting estimated revenue and expense of a specific new program.

The program budget is usually developed separately from the conventional budgetary process and simply serves to supplement the overall department budget. Frequently, the time period for a program budget is over the anticipated life of a program or piece of equipment. The program budget concept is a very effective management tool to determine the cost or benefit of a specific project or program, but the concept should never be considered as the replacement for a budgetary control system.

Variance Analysis Concept

Monthly analysis of significant budget variances has a twofold purpose. First, it acts as a control by requiring managers to identify any potential problem areas. Potential problem areas, once identified, are further analyzed. Second, the reports represent a historical account of whatever creates a significant unfavorable variance. The manager and the administration become very knowledgeable about the major spending patterns within the institution.*

*Action To Be Taken****

Interpretation of the reported results involves not only the identification and justification of specific variances but also the interpretation of the impact that these contributing causes will have on the various levels of cost behavior.

Each of the variances will have some impact on the overall cost behavior. Management's key role is to identify the type of variance, the probable duration of the contributing cause, and the corrective action that must be taken. The information in Table 13–4 provides a course of action to be taken based upon specific variances.

TYPES OF BUDGETS

In generating a budget, most institutions project costs of activities in three categories: manpower costs, operational costs, and capital expenses.

1. Operating Budget Overview***

The operating budget estimates and determines how much money it will cost to keep a specific nursing unit open next year. The budget estimates future requirements and expenses for personnel, supplies, and other items necessary to the functioning of the unit, which is identified as a cost center. It may also include estimated revenues from patients and other sources.

Formulation of the operating budget should begin months before the beginning of the new fiscal year to provide sufficient time for planning and forecasting. Before beginning to plan an expense budget, the year-to-date report of expenditures during the current fiscal year must be reviewed. This report often provides only six or eight months of information; therefore, it must be annualized to project expenditures for the entire year. Then judgments must be made about future directions for the unit. Will any major changes be made in programs or services that might have an impact on the expense budget?

2. Labor Budget: Demonstration

To illustrate how the labor budget system works, a description of a typical budget process at a typical hospital follows. This account will explore the creation of a labor budget by Shirley, the head nurse of 2-East, a 34-bed surgical unit.

To start, Shirley and her staff have agreed to a 95 percent productivity goal. They have reviewed the census forecast and have found a typical yearly pattern has been predicted. There is no forecast for any changes in the patient mix or the major/minor surgery mix.

To determine the total number of full-time equivalents that are needed based on the productivity goal and anticipated census, Shirley uses a budget worksheet. She takes into account the hours of patient care needed, the vacation and holidays that the staff will accumulate during the coming year, the average amount of sick time used, and other significant factors that will require additional coverage. (An illustration of the procedure is presented in Figure 13–2.)

Upon completion of the budget worksheet, the number of FTEs has been determined: 13 FTEs for the day shift; 9.8 FTEs for the evening; and 5.6 FTEs for the night. A department total of 28.4 FTEs will be required for patient care. Shirley now compares that number with the cur-

---

*Source: Donald F. Beck, *Basic Hospital Financial Management*, ed 2, Aspen Publishers, Inc., © 1989.

**Source: Robert B. Taylor, Jr., "Budget Reporting and Control," *Topics in Health Care Financing*, Vol. 5:4, Aspen Publishers, Inc., © 1979.

***Source: Arlene N. Hayne and Zeila W. Bailey, *Administration of Critical Care*, Aspen Publishers, Inc., © 1982.

Table 13–4 Coping with Different Types of Variances

1. Price Variance (Labor)

Management Action

- Determine reasons causing increase in wages and determine if wage increase is permanent or temporary.
- Determine if substitute for labor is acceptable *and* available.
- Determine if wage and salary framework is structured and competitive with other facilities.
- Determine impact (if any) on profitability.

Unit Action

- Assist staff in identifying alternatives to current staff disciplines.
- Align available staffing to actual staff needs more closely.

2. Price Variance (Supplies)

Management Action

- Determine reasons causing price increase and if price increase is permanent or temporary.
- Determine availability of substitute supplies.
- Determine feasibility of reducing price through bidding process or other purchasing techniques.

Unit Action

- Reexamine supply use by specific volume indicator and reevaluate cost behavior trends.

3. Efficiency Variance (Productivity)

Management Action

- Determine reasons causing increase/decrease in labor component and assess impact of patient mix, service mix, and the like.
- Determine if labor variance is permanent and, if so, reassess impact of change as cost behavior.
- Examine fringe benefit program and other contributing reasons if variance is due to substantial incurrence of nonproductive labor.

Unit Action

- Change in required labor component will necessitate reexamination of cost behavior.
- Determine impact, if any, on profitability.

4. Capacity Variance

Management Action

- Determine reasons for increase/decrease in level of use and identify degree of permanence.
- If permanent increase/decrease, assess need for reallocation of resources and reexamine cost behavior.

Unit Action

- Identify specific course of action that can be used to correct (if adverse capacity variance) or sustain (if favorable variance) change in capacity.

---

rent number of employees and determines the number of people she needs to hire for each shift, if any. Two questions have been answered: *(1) How many staff members should be hired to care for these patients? (2) How many staff members should be scheduled on day shift, evening shift, and night shift?*

Now Shirley must ascertain how many staff members should be assigned to each shift each day of the week. The management engineer will review with Shirley last year's historical census pattern. The census by day of the week has been kept and graphed by the management engineer and will help to determine the most frequent census level for each day of the week for the coming year. The recommended weekly staffing schedule worksheet (Table 13–5) is used to translate the expected census level each day into

Figure 13–2 Labor Budget Worksheet

NURSING UNIT: _____*2 EAST*_____   BUDGET PERIOD: _____

ANNUAL PATIENT DAYS: *9795*

AVERAGE DAILY PATIENT DAYS: *26.9* @ *5.09* H.P.D. *4.84* @ *95% Goal*

AVERAGE DAILY PRODUCTIVE HOURS *1369* ÷ 8 = *17.12* STAFF x 1.4 = *23.%* FTE's

AVERAGE DAILY PRODUCTIVE HOURS BY SHIFT

	HOURS		STAFF		FTEs
DAY	*44* : *60.24*	÷ 8	*7.83*	x 1.4 ·	*10.54*
EVE	*36* : *49.29*	÷ 8	*6.16*	x 1.4	*8.63*
NITE	*20* : *29.38*	÷ 8	*3.42*	x 1.4	*4.79*

NON-PRODUCTIVE TIME COVERAGE

SHIFT	HOLIDAYS		E.L.	VACATION	FTES
	HR/ PROD FTE FTE HRS	HR/ PROD FTE FTE HRS	HR/ PROD FTE FTE HRS	HR/ WK WK HRS	HR/ HRS FTE FTE
DAY	56 x *10.54* = *590.2*	16 x *10.54* = *168.6*	24 x *7.4* = *177.6*	*32.8* x 40 = *1312*	*2243.4*/2000 = *1.12*
EVE	56 x *8.62* = *482.7*	16 x *8.62* = *137.9*	24 x *6.2* = *148.8*	*18.2* x 40 = *728*	*1497.4*/2000 = *.75*
NITE	56 x *4.79* = *268.2*	16 x *4.79* = *76.6*	24 x *3.2* = *768*	*16.4* x 40 = *656*	*1077.6*/2000 = *.54*

FTES

	DAY	EVENING	NITE
1. PRODUCTIVE	*10.54*	*8.62*	*4.79*
2. VACATION/ HOLIDAY/EL	*1.12*	*.75*	*.54*
3. AVE. SICK TIME	*.473*	*.237*	*.147*
4. ADMINISTRATIVE	*.87*	*.2*	*.1*
5.			
6. TOTAL FTES HIRED (1 thru 5)	*13.0*	*9.8*	*5.6*
7. EDUCATION	*.11*	*.05*	*.05*
8. ORIENTATION	*.145*	*.2*	*.1*
9.			
TOTAL BUDGETED FTES (1 thru 4-7 and 8)	*13.26*	*10.06*	*5.73*

DEPARTMENT TOTAL BUDGETED FTES	*29.05*

Table 13–5 Recommended Weekly Staffing Schedule Worksheet

UNIT __2-EAST__   CENSUS DATA PERIOD _____

	AVE. CENSUS	H.P.P.D. x CENSUS	HOURS/ DAY	STAFF (÷ by 3)	DAY x 44%	PM x 36%	NITE x 20%
SUNDAY	23.88	5.09	121.55	15.19	6.68	5.47	3.04
MONDAY	27.79	5.09	141.45	17.68	7.78	6.36	3.54
TUESDAY	29.89	5.09	152.14	19.62	8.37	6.85	3.80
WEDNESDAY	30.03	5.09	152.85	19.11	8.41	6.88	3.82
THURSDAY	29.42	5.09	149.75	18.72	8.24	6.74	3.74
FRIDAY	26.16	5.09	133.15	16.64	7.32	5.99	3.33
SATURDAY	22.06	5.09	112.29	14.04	6.18	5.05	2.81
TOTAL FTE'S: (SUM ÷ 5 SHIFTS/FTE)					10.6	3.7	4.8

Source: Courtesy of Health Share for the Texas Hospital Association, Austin, Texas.

Table 13–6 Recommended Weekly Staffing by Shift and Day

UNIT __2-EAST__   BUDGET YEAR _____

Recommended Time Schedule

	SUN	MON	TUE	WED	THU	FRI	SAT		Full-Time / Part-Time Mix	FT	PT
AVE. CENSUS	24	28	30	30	29	26	22				
DAYS	6	7	7/8	8	8	8	6/7	DAYS	RN	5	4
									LVN		2
									NA	2	
									CUS	1	
PMS	5	6	7	7	6/7	6	5	PMS	RN	4	5
									LVN		
									NA		2
									CUS		1
NITES	2/3	3/4	4	4	4	3/4	2/3	NITES	RN	2	2
									LVN	1	
									NA	1	
									CUS		

the required staff for each shift each day. This information is then transferred to a recommended weekly time schedule (Table 13–6), which represents a midpoint or core staffing guide per shift per day for the coming year.

Another question has also been answered: *How much will the staffing needs vary by day of the week?*

There is one remaining question: *How much and when can vacation time be scheduled?* In order to answer this question, Shirley and her staff review the forecasted workload (converted to productive patient care hours). The workload is distributed across the year by accounting period and reflects the amount of staff necessary for patient care. The difference between the FTEs required for patient care (28.4) and the total FTEs (29.05) reflects when and how much vacation time may be scheduled; thus the forecasted census is translated into the required number of nursing care hours by pay period.

The result is the expected number of patient care hours required by shift each pay period across the year to take care of the expected patient census. Shirley adds this information on a

staff planning graph, which shows how the workload varies by pay period across the year. The graph also shows, from the budget worksheet, the number of FTEs that are available for patient care as well as for providing coverage for administrative, education, orientation, vacation, holiday, and average sick time. The difference between the staff available and the expected patient care requirements is the time available to give the staff their vacations and holidays as well as coverage for these other functions. Thus the last question has been answered:— *How much vacation time can be scheduled and when?*

Finally, when the vacation and holiday time is scheduled on a personnel budget-by-position form, the labor portion of 2-East's budget is completed.

3. Capital Expenditure Budget

The capital expenditure budget outlines the need for major equipment or physical changes in the plant requiring large sums of money. If an item exceeds some arbitrary amount—for example, $100—it is classified as a capital expenditure. The ceiling is established by administration.

These expenses are figured on a capital expenditure worksheet (Table 13–7). After conferring with the assistant head nurses and the director of nursing, the head nurse will plan for the purchase of new equipment and/or the replacement of existing equipment. The capital expenditure worksheet includes a description of the item, the importance and urgency of its acquisition, and other requested information. Head nurses are required to indicate in which quarter the equipment should be purchased and to specify annual equipment needs for the following two years. The capital expenditure worksheets are used by the purchasing agent and health care facility administration in developing a capital expenditure budget for the next three years.

4. Supplies and Services Budget

The use of medical and nonmedical supplies is based on the forecasted patient days for the coming year. The average cost of medical and nonmedical supplies is determined from the preceding year's expense plus the expected inflationary increases.

Purchased services are based on historical information and reflect any service contracts particular to that unit. The input for this budget is primarily from accounting data that the head nurse reviews. He or she may make changes based on anticipated changes in the type and amount of supplies required for the coming year. The major tool in figuring the supplies and services budget is the nonlabor expense worksheet.

AUTOMATED FINANCIAL REPORTS: A BUDGETARY DECISION SUPPORT MODEL

A computer record of financial data allows the manager to generate a multitude of reports. These can be used as instant references on an as-needed basis to monitor performance. However, the value of such instantly available reports reflects the relevance of the format in which data are collected. If constructed properly, the system will offer substantial support to financial decision making in the nursing department.

For example, the automated financial system implemented at one hospital has provided the foundation for evaluating the needs of nursing units while balancing allocation and deployment of resources. It uses a financial tracking and monitoring program designed to analyze, monitor, and provide the means for nurse leaders to understand and meet their scope of financial responsibilities.

The financial tracking and monitoring system contains a performance evaluation measure that compares standards, goals, or budget targets with actual performance. It enables quick identification of deviating performance. Further, it provides a trend analysis mechanism for analyzing and comparing past results and projections of future activity with the current situation. The budgetary decision support model is applicable and adaptable to any health care organization.*

Groundwork for Budget Performance Review*

1. Indicators

Several key indicators need to be analyzed and monitored to ensure successful budgetary performance. The set of indicators does not need to

*Source: Adapted from Kathi Kendall Sengin and Alejandra M. Dreisbach, "Managing with Precision: A Budgetary Decision Support Model," Journal of Nursing Administration, Vol 25, No. 2, February 1995. J.B. Lippincott Company.

Table 13-7 Capital Expenditure Worksheet

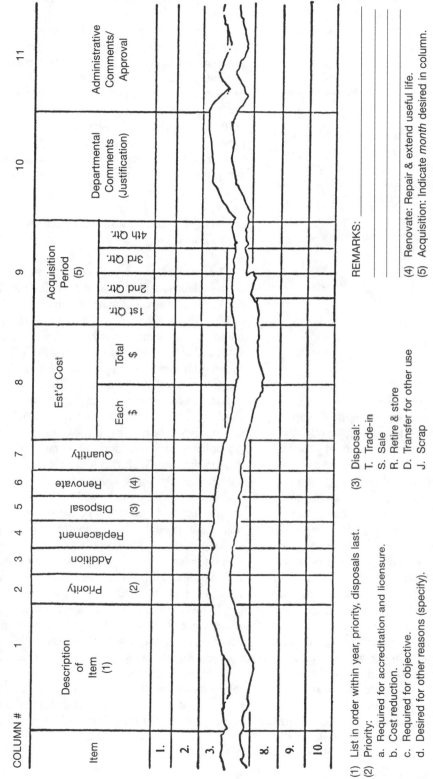

COLUMN #	1	2	3	4	5	6	7	8		9				10	11
	Description of Item (1)	Priority (2)	Addition	Replacement	Disposal (3)	Renovate (4)	Quantity	Est'd Cost		Acquisition Period (5)				Departmental Comments (Justification)	Administrative Comments/ Approval
								Each $	Total $	1st Qtr.	2nd Qtr.	3rd Qtr.	4th Qtr.		
1.															
2.															
3.															
8.															
9.															
10.															

(1) List in order within year, priority, disposals last.
(2) Priority:
  a. Required for accreditation and licensure.
  b. Cost reduction.
  c. Required for objective.
  d. Desired for other reasons (specify).
(3) Disposal:
  T. Trade-in
  S. Sale
  R. Retire & store
  D. Transfer for other use
  J. Scrap
(4) Renovate: Repair & extend useful life.
(5) Acquisition: Indicate *month* desired in column.

REMARKS:
_____
_____

be extremely onerous. Indicators required to keep track of the nursing department's budgetary performance of the division need to focus on two fundamental questions:

- What are we trying to measure?
- Does this analysis report need to be done at all?

Key budgetary indicators (see box) help the department plan and track the course of yearly activities. In addition, they provide early warning signs or "red flags" of areas that may require additional evaluation or intervention.

Key Budgetary Indicators

- Patient volume
- Occupancy rate
- Patient acuity
- Direct hours/patient day
- Paid hours/patient day
- Salary cost/patient day
- Nonsalary cost/patient day

The success of an operating budget planning process depends on understanding the fundamental assumptions to be used in preparing the budget, such as projected patient volume and types of programs to be offered for the coming year. Nursing managers participating in the budget development need to incorporate current operational and financial knowledge for areas within their control. Planning may be based on an incremental budget process in which prior-year expenditures are taken as the base and changes for the forthcoming year, such as a percentage increase for salaries or supply inflationary projection, are added to the base. As a result of intense scrutiny of expenditures by health organizations, the nurse manager may be asked to undertake the process of a zero base budget, in which there is no automatic approval of programs, but a review of the efficacy of all expenditures. Both budgetary processes require a clear and comprehensive picture of the existing conditions and expenses of the patient care delivery.

Figure 13–3 is structured as a framework displaying the relationship among all types of operational and economic elements that need to be evaluated and incorporated into the budgetary process. The nurse manager incorporates into the budgetary process the effect of changes in volume, case mix, staff, and skill mix of the employees. Increase in supply prices and sophistication of technology also may impact productivity, resource consumption, and expenses.

2. Budget Planning and Development Reports

The planning and development of the budget are based on a number of inputs, beginning with the key indicators. Once the key indicators are defined, a *unit staffing cost projection report* is completed. This report is prepared as a spreadsheet and identifies the unit staffing for both the Monday through Friday period and the weekend. There is a section in the spreadsheet that addresses the cost of the replacement factor for the staff replaced when using benefit time. Another section shows the incremental salary cost of paying holiday premiums during a number of holidays in the year. With this powerful but simple spreadsheet, the nurse manager may change or update the report quickly with any new information that may affect the performance of the unit, such as staff mix, number of employees, and hourly rates. This report gives a concise, accurate picture of the cost of staffing the unit. It also provides the nurse manager with the ability to experiment with different scenarios and obtain instantaneous data of how these changes affect the bottom line. This type of simulation becomes extremely useful when projecting the cost and impact of assumptions for developing the budget, such as patient days, percentage of salary increases, changes in staffing mix, number of holidays, or any other changes that need to be evaluated for the salary budget projection on the specific patient care unit.

Figure 13–3 Relationship of Operational and Economic Elements of the Patient Care Unit

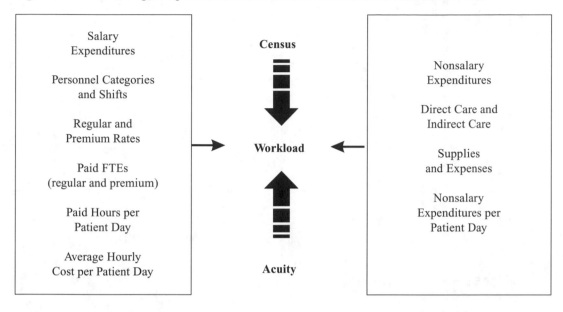

A second report lists the *staffing guidelines* that were developed for the specific needs of each patient care unit. The staffing guidelines are developed directly from the staffing cost projection report. The type and quantity of staff required to meet projected patient care needs per shift are displayed graphically. The requirements are based on the actual average patient acuity on the specific patient care unit.

Changes in patient acuity are reflected in the direct and total paid hours per patient care. The staffing guidelines are used throughout the fiscal year to provide guidance to the nurse manager, staffing coordinators, and other nursing leaders when allocating and assigning staff to patient care units. The staffing guidelines assume that there is no change in patient acuity from that predicted. When changes in patient acuity occur (as documented by the daily acuity sampling) the appropriate adjustment is made. This report also is used during the year to compare actual and predicted staffing levels to identify variances for each of the individual units.

The third report completed during the budget planning process is the *unit specific position con-*

trol. It documents the budgeted full-time equivalents available to the nurse manager throughout the fiscal year. It contrasts budgeted positions to those actually filled and allows the nurse manager to quickly determine the type and percentage of filled/vacant positions. When this information is aggregated for the nursing division, it provides a current overview of the staff of the nursing division. The position control is updated as modifications occur.

Finally, the fourth component (Table 13–8) is the *actual unit-based budget*. The unit budget incorporates staff mix, actual salaries, projected increase, nonproductive coverage, holiday pay, shift differentials, and other institution-specific benefits and financial incentives. Completed budgets are submitted to the finance division for final resource allocation and approval.

3. Budget Implementation and Monitoring Reports

Evaluation and monitoring of division performance in comparison with the budget uses analyses and reports produced by the financial

Table 13-8 Sample: Unit Salary Budget Breakdown

Professional Staff	Hours	FTEs	Base Hourly Wage	Adjusted Hourly Wage	Shift Difference	Base w/ Difference Jul/Dec	Base w/ Difference Jan/Jun	Incentive Program	Total Salary W/Difference	Shift Difference
HN-Cohen, C.	80.00	1.0	$22.00	$23.10	$1.00	$22,880.00	$24,024.00	$0.00	$46,904.00	$0.00
RN-Bagley, P.	60.00	0.8	$18.50	$19.43	$1.00	$14,710.80	$15,432.30	$0.36	$30,143.46	$0.00
RN-Varghese, S.	80.00	1.0	$18.75	$19.69	$1.10	$21,861.84	$22,934.34	$0.36	$44,796.54	$4,072.41
RN-Tutt, M.	80.00	1.0	$19.50	$20.48	$1.15	$23,322.00	$24,468.10	$0.00	$47,810.10	$6236.10
RN-Carter, B.	32.00	0.4	$16.50	$17.33	$1.00	$7,013.76	$7,356.96	$0.36	$14,371.06	$0.00
RN-Beuno, M.	32.00	0.4	$16.50	$17.33	$1.10	$7,550.40	$7,927.92	$0.00	$15,478.32	$1,407.12
RN-Vacancy, E.	32.00	0.4	$16.50	$17.33	$1.15	$8,065.82	$8,480.50	$0.36	$16,526.69	$2,155.66
Total Professional	396.00	4.95	$18.32	$19.24		$105,404.62	$110,624.12		$216,030.19	$13,871.29
Nonprofessional Staff						Jul/Sep	Oct/Jun			
US-Smith, A.	80.0	1.0	$7.75	$8.14	$1.00	$4,030.00	$12,694.50	$0.00	$16,724.50	$0.00
US-Palmer, N.	32.00	0.4	$8.15	$8.56	$1.00	$1,695.20	$5,339.88	$0.00	$7,035.08	$0.00
Total Nonprofessional	112.00	1.40	$7.95	$8.35		$5,725.20	$18,034.38	$0.00	$23,759.58	$0.00

Nonproductive Time

Professional	Hours		Base Hourly Wage		Shift Difference
Sick	4		$158.40		$3,960.00
Vacation	20		$792.00		$19,800.00
Holiday	12		$475.20		$11,880.00
Education	1		$79.00		$1,980.00
Subtotal			$1,504.80		$37,620.00
Nonprofessional					
Sick	4		$44.80		$627.20
Vacation	15		$168.00		$2,352.00
Holiday	12		134.40		$1,881.60
Education			11.20		$156.80
Subtotal			358.40		$5,017.60
Total			1,863.20		$42,637.60

Incentives		Adjusted Hourly Wage		Incentive Program	Totals
Holiday Premium	Professional	$2,826.57	Nonprofessional	$800.00	$3,628.57
Night Bonus	Professional	$2,121.43	Nonprofessional	$0.00	$2,121.43
Sick-Time Buyback	Professional	$2,475.00	Nonprofessional	$392.00	$2,867.00

Rationale:

Impact or Results:

Total Division Salary Costs

	PRO	NON-PRO	TOTAL
Salary	$216,030.19	23,759.58	$239,789.77
Holiday	2,826.57	800.00	$3,628.57
Nonproductive Time	37,620.00	5,017.60	$42,637.60
Orientation	1,980.00	235.20	$2,215.20
SICK-TIME INCENTIVES	4,596.43	392.00	$4,988.43
OVERTIME PREMIUM	12,112.94	1,918.49	$14,031.44
TOTAL	275,166.13	32,122.87	$307,291.00
BENEFIT:	$76,822.75	Total with Benefits:	$384,113.75

Source: Demonstration developed by Robert Wood Johnson University Hospital Nursing Division. Kathi Kendall Sengin and Alejandra M. Dreisbach, "Managing with Precision: A Budgetary Decision Support Model," Journal of Nursing Administration, Vol. 25, No. 2, February 1995.

tracking and monitoring system of the nursing division. An overtime report is prepared from the data compiled by the labor distribution report. The report may be compared with a standard, past pay periods, or other clinical areas.

A monthly report can be produced on a unit's patient acuity, census, and workload (defined as acuity × census). For each activity, the actual monthly result is compared with a budget or standard measure. This comparison is valuable by itself, and additional information from the previous months provides an added feature for understanding and reviewing the trended activity of the unit.

A graphic presentation is made of the number of FTEs paid per pay period of the year at the regular rate, and the other line depicts the total of paid FTEs for the pay period. This graphic report is superior to reports that show long columns of unit names and FTE numbers by pay period.

Another performance monitoring report is the holiday premium report. It compares the actual occupancy and acuity, number and mix of staff that worked during the holiday, with the standards or average experience of the unit during several previous holidays. This report provides a comprehensive picture of the activity of the patient care unit during the holidays.

4. Budgetary Performance and Decision-Making Reports

The financial management system arranges data that can be the basis for meaningful managerial decisions. The decision system identifies areas requiring investigation and, potentially, for one unit from one period to another. For example, a nurse manager could identify the equipment most frequently rented and then explore options such as capital purchase, equipment substitution, and agreements for equipment/lease purchase.

Another area shows a seasonality pattern of patient days identified for the past years for a patient unit. This recurring event forewarns the nurse manager to "save" budgetary dollars during the rest of the year to fund higher staffing levels and higher nonsalary requirements dur-

ing the months of higher volume. Identification of seasonality trends has provided the capability for the nurse manager to plan for additional demand placed on the staffing resources, such as strengthening the per diem pool.

The information obtained from the analyses and reports has proved to be a strong foundation for the decisions made by nursing leadership during the course of daily operations. The goals of the system are to assist nursing leadership in successfully performing their managerial roles by providing a tool that:

- minimizes risk and uncertainty of daily operations
- provides for better decision-making capabilities
- assigns priorities
- reviews and measures performance based on budgets and past patterns
- evaluates the progress of new programs
- assesses the effectiveness of solutions being implemented to deal with current problems

COSTS

Controllable and Real Costs*

Besides knowing the nature of each cost, the nurse executive may want to differentiate *controllable costs* from *real costs* before making managerial decisions. The *real cost* of a project will include all the labor, materials, and administrative overhead required for the project's enactment. In contrast, the *controllable* costs are those that would not exist if the project were eliminated.

Suppose, for example, that the nurse executive and the staff development director create a case management nursing education project. Suppose that the secretary for the staff development department devotes one-fifth working time to the project; also assume that one regular instructor is assigned for 50 percent time to the

---

Source: Barbara S. Barnum and Karlene M. Kerfoot, *The Nurse as Executive,* ed 4, Aspen Publishers, Inc., © 1995.

project. The project will include 10 hours of lecture by an outside expert and the distribution of materials on case management to program attendees. It is anticipated that the program will be offered to 40 nurses on work hours, for a total of 30 hours by each nurse for the total course.

In this example, real costs would include distributed materials, salaries (proportional) of the secretary and the staff development instructor, time of the staff development director, and the total time of the outside expert. Real costs also would include salaries of the employees for the hours that they are attending the program, administrative overhead (proportion of overhead charged to the staff development department), and depreciation of any audiovisual equipment used in the classroom. Charges also might be calculated for use of a classroom.

Many of these costs would be eliminated if the executive only considers controllable costs. For example, if the in-house instructor were a full-time employee, the salary would have been paid even if the employee were not involved in this project; the same is true for the secretary and the staff development director. Only the fees of the outside expert would be listed as controllable costs. Cost of materials are also controllable costs, but salaries of employees attending the course would only be counted if they actually were replaced on their units for the time of class learning. Similarly, if the classroom belonged to the staff development department and did not need to be rented from another source, then its cost would not be considered.

It is important that the nurse executive have a good idea of both real and controllable costs for major projects in the division. Real costs in some cases and controllable costs in other cases will be dominant in the decision making. At other times, the nurse executive will wish to compare these costs. Some nurse executives repeatedly lose money on projects because they forget some real costs involved. For example, if a nurse executive contracts to run a new clinic on funds sufficient only for controllable costs, then he or she will have to find support for administrative overhead elsewhere. Such expenses, if not considered when a budget is set, may make a funded project a major expense to the organization in terms of real costs.

For some projects, it is important to have a *unit cost* as well as a *total* project cost. A unit cost tells what it will cost to turn out a single "unit" of production. What comprises the unit of production will vary from circumstance to circumstance. For example, the absolute cost of running a labor and delivery function may not tell the executive as much as would a figure that describes average cost per delivery. Similarly, cost per clinic visit and cost per employee hired may have more significance than the report of a total cost. A *unit cost* is one that is reported in terms of one unit of production, whether that unit be a patient, a surgical experience, a student, a visit, or any other item determined to be appropriate to the subject under consideration.

It is particularly important to calculate unit costs if fees are to be associated with costs. In this way, it is possible to determine what to charge the clinic patient per visit, what to charge the nurse for attending a continuing education course, or what to charge the patient for use of the surgical suite. In the resource-driven model with the reality of decreasing resources, the cost-per-unit-of-service methodology is an excellent productivity measure for benchmarking. As the volume goes up, the challenge is to hold cost as stable as possible. Similarly, when the volume drops, the challenge is to maintain the cost per unit of service and not to let the ratio of costs to unit of service escalate. Therefore, this measure is significant for assessing productivity.

The nurse executive will discover that some unit costs vary depending on the volume. It becomes expensive to staff an emergency department with two nurses if few patients wander in; costs of their salaries are covered if there is a high or normal volume of emergency department traffic. Costs per unit of production usually go down as volume increases, although the relation may not be exact. (Step or proportional costs may be involved.)

Often, there is a critical volume at which costs invested in the project are recovered, and it is important that such volumes be determined. For example, the fee for a staff development offering to outsiders may be determined based on a certain volume of attendees. If that volume is not achieved, the program may lose money. Certainly, the staff development director will need to learn how to calculate break-even costs, as will any other nurse manager who is involved in fee setting when volume affects profit or loss.

Cost Benefit/Cost-Effectiveness Analyses

Distinctions*

Cost benefit and cost-effectiveness analyses are primarily analytical techniques used by the manager in making decisions. By their use it is possible to select what is considered to be an optimal approach from a group of feasible alternatives.

In cost benefit analysis, generally one seeks to value all inputs (i.e., costs) and all outcomes (i.e., benefits) in dollars. Cost benefit analysis can assist in setting priorities across programs with substantially different outcomes and in the process yield an estimate of the net dollar value associated with each course of action. Cost-effectiveness analysis, on the other hand, can help in choosing among alternative means of achieving a given, presumably desired, outcome possessing a single measure of effectiveness. The price paid to accomplish the more powerful cost benefit analysis, however, is high, for in valuing all benefits the question of subjectivity arises, such as valuing human life or quality of life in dollars. Despite the conscientious efforts of analysts to attack these issues, many decision makers may not find such valuations palatable.

Finally, a still simpler form of economic analysis is the comparative cost analysis. In this case, the benefits from two projects are presumed or known to be indistinguishable; the choice may be made on costs alone.

Cost-Effectiveness Analysis*

In cost-effectiveness analysis, the following concepts are most important:

- There are alternative ways to accomplish an objective and the manager must select the optimal alternative, which may not be the least costly one.
- There must be at least two alternative ways to accomplish a task in order to undertake cost-effectiveness analysis.
- Cost-effectiveness analysis is not cost reduction; it is optimization of an approach to a specific goal or set of goals.

From a managerial standpoint, cost-effectiveness analysis is directed by two basic economic considerations: (1) a minimum expectation that in either social or economic terms, for the program being undertaken, there will be a dollar of return for each dollar of investment, and (2) an optimal expectation that one dollar plus some additional increment of economic or social return will accrue for each dollar of investment.

A cost-effectiveness analysis is ultimately reduced to a series of models. These models, which are frequently but not always complex, set out alternatives and indicate the anticipated return of each alternative relative to a given level of investment.

A disciplined look is taken in order to fully analyze information, alternatives, and problems and, where possible, take advantage of various new technological developments that are available.

The initial step is to delineate clear and specific objectives by asking why it is necessary to do a given task and what is expected in return for the undertaking. Managers should not merely decide to reduce condition X by 20 percent or

*Source: Analysis of New Health Techniques. Health Planning Information Series, DHHS, Pub. No. (HRA) 80-14014, 1980.

*Source: Royal A. Crystal and Agnes W. Brewsterm, "Cost Benefit and Cost Effectiveness Analyses in the Health Field: An Introduction." Reprinted, with permission of the Blue Cross Association, from *Inquiry*, Vol. 3, December 1967, pp. 3–13. Copyright © 1966 by the Blue Cross Association. All rights reserved.

**Guidelines for Use of Cost
Benefit/Cost-Effectiveness Analyses**

Following are 10 principles of analysis that could be used to guide the conduct, evaluation, or use of cost benefit/cost-effectiveness studies:

1. *Define the problem.* The problem should be clearly and explicitly defined and the relationship to health outcome or status should be stated.
2. *State objectives.* The objectives of the new approach being assessed should be explicitly stated, and the analysis should address the degree to which the objectives are (expected to be) met.
3. *Identify alternatives.* Alternative means to accomplish the objectives should be identified and subjected to analysis. When slightly different outcomes are involved, the effect this difference will have on the analysis should be examined.
4. *Analyze benefits/effects.* All foreseeable benefits/effects (positive and negative outcomes) should be identified and, when possible, measured. When possible, and if agreement on the terms can be reached, it may be helpful to value all benefits in common terms in order to make comparisons easier.

5. *Analyze costs.* All expected costs should be identified and, when possible, measured and valued in dollars.
6. *Differentiate perspective of analysis.* When private or program benefits and costs differ from social benefits and costs (and if a private or program perspective is appropriate for the analysis), the differences should be identified.
7. *Perform discounting.* All future costs and benefits should be discounted to their present value.
8. *Analyze uncertainties.* Sensitivity analysis should be conducted. Key variables should be analyzed to determine the importance of their uncertainty to the results of the analysis. A range of possible values for each variable should be examined for effects on results.
9. *Address ethical issues.* Ethical issues should be identified, discussed, and placed in appropriate perspective relative to the rest of the analysis and the objectives of the technology.
10. *Discuss results.* The results of the analysis should be discussed in terms of validity, sensitivity to changes in assumptions, and implications for policy or decision making.

Source: Cost Effectiveness Analysis of Medical Technology, Office of Technology Assessment, Pub. No. (OTA)H-125, August 1980.

add 50 new beds. Rather, they should ask why the department should be doing this and what the real short- and long-range objectives are. After the objectives have been determined, the cost-effectiveness approach evaluates the alternatives, asking, "To attain this objective, how many alternatives and what types of alternatives are available? Do we have only one way to do the job? Are there two or more alternatives open to us?" It is necessary next to specify what resources are required for each alternative—resources in terms of people, money, equipment, and facilities.

The analyst then prepares cost-effectiveness models for each alternative and also determines the criteria to be used for the selection of the preferred alternative or alternatives.

As the cost-effectiveness models are built, several pertinent measurements will be used in making a decision and will form parts of the model. These include

- measures of effectiveness—the criteria that indicate how well the alternative satisfies the objectives
- measures of operational use—the criteria for consideration of alternatives in light of the other responsibilities that must be undertaken
- measures of personnel and equipment needed—the determination for each alternative of the number and kinds of people and equipment required
- cost factors
- measures of cost—the determination of cost for each alternative way of doing the job and the manner in which cost will be measured

Cost Benefit Analysis*

There are clear advantages to performing a cost benefit analysis. It provides a systematic and consistent approach to the evaluation of alternative actions. It avoids subjective judgment by requiring explicit (numerical) statements regarding the values of all recognized effects attributed to the various interventions. It takes a total view of the allocation decision, as opposed to that of a dollar cost alone. Finally, it yields an explicit appraisement of the net value of undertaking the preferred alternative.

Steps in Analysis. Cost benefit analysis uses the following sequential steps:

1. articulation of a clear, unambiguous statement of the decision faced and objectives sought by the health planner
2. identification of alternative actions or programs that satisfy stated objectives
3. identification separately of the costs and benefits associated with the proposed undertaking and each alternative action
4. quantitative evaluation of all costs incurred and benefits returned for each action

5. comparison of alternatives against explicit decision criteria to yield the preferred program

The Cost Benefit Study*

As part of the evaluation of new ventures or new systems, a well-executed cost benefit study supports administrative efforts to gain a competitive edge. The study provides the basis for sound decision making: It identifies both the actual costs of the present system and the estimated costs of the proposed system or venture. By comparing the two sets of costs, administrators can determine the extent of tangible and intangible benefits, as well as the range of risks and opportunities, associated with an impending decision.

The cost benefit study provides both the raw data that help drive the decision-making process and the basic plan for ensuring a favorable return on investment from that decision. The principle reasons administrators choose the cost benefit study are to:

- Identify the costs of the present system.
- Document the constraints in the present system (these become the opportunities with the new system).
- Document the favorable features in the present system (these become the risks with the new system).
- Identify the costs of the proposed system.
- Identify the benefits of the proposed system.
- Identify the mandatory requirements for the proposed system.
- Develop an action plan for benefits realization.
- Validate the benefits and the action plan.

Types of Benefits. Identified benefits fall into two broad categories: tangible and intangible.

---

*Source: *Analysis of New Health Technologies*, Health Planning Information Series, DHHS, Pub. No. (HRA) 80-14014, 1980.

*Source: Mike Sullivan, "The Cost/Benefit Study: A Competitive Edge," *U.S. Healthcare* (formerly called *HealthCare Computing and Communications*), May 1987, © 1987 Health Data Analysis, Inc.

Tangible benefits, in turn, can be further subdivided into economic and noneconomic. A tangible *economic* benefit is one that can be quantified in terms of dollars and has a direct relationship to the proposed system or venture. A tangible *noneconomic* benefit is one that is directly related to the proposed system or venture but is not readily converted to dollars, such as an improvement in the quality of patient care.

Intangible benefits, on the other hand, are not easily converted to dollars and, at best, have an indirect relationship to the proposed system or venture (see Table 13–9).

FTE Reduction versus Cost Avoidance. Of the five basic types of tangible economic benefits, the identification of FTE reduction versus FTE cost avoidance is, perhaps, the most controversial.

The labor costs associated with the major nursing tasks in the present or manual system must be compared to the estimated costs to perform these same tasks in the proposed system. The difference between the two sets of costs is the identified savings or benefits—the FTE reduction or cost avoidance.

In Table 13–10 the actual time it takes a nurse to perform major tasks in the present system is compared to the estimated time it would take the nurse to perform the same tasks in the proposed system. Timings and volumes are based on an eight-hour shift, a staffing ratio of one to five, an average daily census of 30 patients, and an average acuity of three (on a scale of one to five).

Reading from left to right, the first column shows time in increments of 40 minutes. Reading from bottom to top, note that the first five elements constitute the major, time-consuming tasks, while element six represents a group of minor tasks. To significantly impact nursing, the proposed system must impart tasks in the first five areas.

In comparing the proposed system column with the present system column, tasks two, three, and five are the ones impacted for a combined labor savings of 90 minutes per nurse. As previously noted, with a staffing ratio of one to five and an average daily census of 30 patients, the individual savings is multiplied by six nurses for a total saving of 540 minutes per shift (days).

Of the identified 540 minutes on the day shift, 480 minutes are FTE reduction while 60 minutes are FTE cost avoidance.

To realize the benefits from the FTE reduction and the cost avoidance, administration must have an action plan in place ready to be implemented.

Table 13–9 Tangible Economic Benefits

Personnel	Material	Equipment	Purchased Services	Revenue Enhancements
• FTE reduction • FTE cost avoidance	• Forms and supplies • Inventory reductions	• Typewriters and copiers • Terminals and printers • Computers	• Agency personnel • Maintenance services	• Bad-debt reduction • Capture of late/lost charges • Reduction of days in accounts receivable

Table 13–10 Daily Nursing Activities, by Elapsed Time

MINUTES	PRESENT SYSTEM		PROPOSED SYSTEM	
480		100%		100%
440	6. Other Tasks (118 min)		7. Savings/Benefit (90 min)	
400				81%
		75%		
360	5. Report (33 min)		6. Other Tasks (118 min)	
		69%		
320	4. Assessments (70 min)			57%
280			5. Report (12 min)	
		54%		54%
240	3. Charting (75 min)		4. Assessments (70 min)	
200				
		38%		40%
160	2. Medications (84 min)		3. Charting (50 min)	
				29%
120			2. Medications (40 min)	
		21%		21%
80	1. Treatments (100 min)		1. Treatments (100 min)	
40				
0				

ESTABLISHING THE COST OF NURSING SERVICES

The Importance of Accurate Cost Measurement*

Careful identification of nursing costs is essential for several reasons. First, nursing salary costs represent a large percentage of overall health care facility operating costs. Nursing salaries in a typical community hospital, for example, usually represent about 20 percent of the hospital's total inpatient operating cost. Further, for particular types of patients, the cost of nursing care can easily represent more than 30 percent of the total cost of care.

Second, knowledge of nursing salary costs is essential for the preparation of accurate budgets and financial forecasts. How many nursing hours will be required in the next fiscal year, and what will be the associated costs? These two questions can be answered systematically if good nursing cost data by patient type are available. If the health care facility plans to start a new service, such as a free-standing urgent care center, nursing cost accounting data can be extremely useful in developing a projection of needed nursing hours and salary dollars.

Third, the identification of nursing costs by patient type is essential for case mix management. Are nursing costs increasing because more cardiovascular surgery and fewer ear, nose, and throat patients are being treated? If the obstetrics product line is expanded by 10 percent, how

*Source: Paul L. Shafer, Betsy J. Frauenthal, and Catherine Tower, "Measuring Nursing Costs with Patient Acuity Data," *Topics in Health Care Financing*, Vol. 13:4, Aspen Publishers, Inc., © 1987.

much will nursing salary costs increase? If nursing salary cost information is developed at the diagnosis-related group (DRG) or International Classification of Diseases, 9th edition, Clinical Modification (ICD-9-CM) level, then the answers to these questions will be readily available.

Approaches*

The first step in cost allocation is to determine the unit of analysis for classifying patients within relevant cost categories. The most commonly used units of analysis have been day of service, diagnosis (medical or nursing), timed functions, or nursing workload units as measured by patient classification system (PCS). The most frequently used cost categories have been cost per patient or length of stay (LOS), cost per patient care unit, and cost per DRG.

The significant variation in the amount of daily nursing care needed by different types of patients has important implications regarding the accuracy of alternative methods for costing nursing.

There appear to be four major approaches for allocating nursing service costs: (1) per diem or costs per day, (2) costs per diagnosis, (3) costs per relative intensity measure (RIM), and (4) costs per nursing workload unit based on PCS.

Per Diem Method of Cost Accounting

Per diem or cost per day is the oldest method of allocating resources. It has been used for rate setting and internal managerial control. This cost is calculated by dividing the total nursing costs by the number of patient days for a selected time period. Nursing costs consist of the salaries and fringe benefits for clinical and administrative nursing personnel. This method has been criticized as being inadequate, because it does not accurately represent types of patients and because patient days vary widely in terms of resource consumption.

Source: Loucine M.D. Huckabay, "Allocation of Resources and Identification of Issues in Determining the Cost of Nursing Services," *Nursing Administration Quarterly,* Vol. 13, No. 1, Aspen Publishers, Inc., © 1988.

Cost per Diagnosis

Diagnosis-based methods of accounting for nursing costs attempt to reduce the variability in nursing care requirements by using information above the case mix. The DRG system and several other case-mix methods have used medical diagnoses to group patients. Some have also used the nursing diagnosis to group patients and calculate cost per diagnosis. Still others have used the American Nurses' Association's nursing care standards for classifying patients according to nursing care requirements. In one study, nursing diagnosis was a better predictor of nursing care requirements than DRGs based on medical diagnosis. Nursing diagnosis explained two times as much variance as medical diagnosis (DRG) in predicting nursing time.

A system for the development of 23 nursing care categories (NCCs), one for each of the 23 major diagnostic categories from which DRGs are derived, is advocated by Leah Curtin, past editor of *Nursing Management.* To stress the nursing aspect of the care and treatment process for DRGs, Curtin also proposes that a detailed nursing care plan, called a nursing care strategy (NCS), be developed for each of the 467 DRGs. Within each NCS, patient care requirement levels may be assessed using a PCS.

Others have advocated that costs for delivering nursing practice be calculated not on the basis of actual practice, as measured by PCSs for staffing, but on the basis of time required to achieve an institution's standard of care.

Cost per Relative Intensity Measure

Another method of cost allocation using case-mix information is the RIM. A RIM is an arithmetic abstract that serves as a proxy for charges in detailing nursing resource use. A RIM is actually one minute of nursing resource use. The method through which RIMs are costed and ultimately allocated to DRG case-mix categories involves a three-step process. First, the cost of a RIM is calculated. A RIM is obtained by dividing the total nursing costs for the health care facility by the total minutes of care estimated or nursing resources used to provide care to all patients. Second, the number of minutes used by the total facility population is determined, including the usual corrections for downtime, such as sick leave, vacation, fatigue, less than maximum efficiency of new employees, and so on. Third, the cost of care for each patient is calculated by multiplying the RIM by the minutes of care required by the patient as estimated by the appropriate equation. Unlike the PCS, which looks at staffing needs per shift, the RIM method measures the time spent by nursing personnel in performing nursing and non-nursing tasks during the patient's entire stay.

Cost per Nursing Workload Unit Based on Patient Classification System (Patient Acuity)

Nursing workload–based methods are primarily used to forecast staffing needs. Acuity-level staffing allows nursing managers to staff nursing units shift by shift based on the individual needs of the patients. This method of staffing replaces the more conventional method of determining nurse staffing requirements of the unit based on the daily census.

An increasing number of health care facilities use patient data for allocating nursing costs to DRGs by using the following procedure to calculate the nursing cost:

1. The PCS is used as usual.
2. Patient classification statistics are converted in required hours of care for the course of the patient's stay.
3. Patient care hours are then translated to dollar cost.
4. Patients are classified into DRGs.
5. Nursing care costs for patients in selected DRGs are compiled and analyzed in many different ways.

Another method of obtaining workload data recommends assigning nursing functions for patients in each DRG into three categories: daily essential functions common to all patients, physician-dependent functions, and nursing-independent functions. Cost analysis can then be cal-

culated for each of these functions, for patient care units, and for each DRG. This type of workload analysis will provide a useful pricing approach but entails additional data collection.

The following material demonstrates costing of nursing services based on a patient classification system.

Comparison of DRG and Acuity Approaches*

Variability of Nursing Costs by Diagnosis

Only in recent years has the technology been in place to evaluate nursing's contention that patients in different illness categories require different amounts of daily nursing care. It is often true that patients within the same illness category also require different levels of daily nursing care. The development and widespread use of DRGs have provided health care facilities with the nomenclature needed to consistently designate these illness categories.

As shown in Table 13–11, there is a significant difference in the actual amount of daily nursing care for patients in selected DRGs. Table 13–12 presents the calculation of average daily nursing cost used for the patient acuity approach.

At one hospital, estimates of the cost of daily nursing care based on the patient day approach were compared to estimates of daily nursing costs for six selected DRGs. The results of the analysis are presented in Table 13–13.

The analysis indicates that the patient day approach is fairly accurate if the patients within a DRG have an average acuity level. If, on the other hand, patients in a particular DRG have extremely high or extremely low acuity levels, then the estimates of daily nursing salary costs based on the patient day approach can be significantly inaccurate.

Source: Paul L. Shafer, Betsy J. Frauenthal, and Catherine Tower, "Measuring Nursing Costs with Patient Acuity Data," *Topics in Health Care Financing*, Vol. 13, No. 4, Aspen Publishers, Inc., © 1987.

Table 13–11 Comparison of Average Nursing Care Requirements for Patients in Six Selected DRGs

Selected DRG		Average Length of Stay	Estimated Nursing Staff Hours per Day	Overview of Required Nursing Care
No.	Description			
138	Cardiac arrhythmia >69 and/or comorbidity and complication (CC)	20.1	2.5	Initially this type of patient is in an intensive care unit where high concentration of time is required. Once the arrhythmia is controlled the patient is moved to a medical/surgical unit, where the nursing activity is primarily observational and patient education and discharge instructions are carried out.
36	Retinal procedures	3.3	8.5	These patients require nursing assistance with certain physical activities because of their impaired eyesight. Nursing time is also used for frequent monitoring of vital signs as well as prevention of potential complications and education of the patient prior to discharge.
296	Nutritional and miscellaneous metabolic >69 and/or CC	6.6	11.7	The nursing activities related to the treatments received in this DRG include education, assessment of the gastric system, monitoring of elimination, monitoring of laboratory work, care of the intravenous catheter, and close observation of daily weights and fluid balance.
197	Total cholecystectomy >69 and/or CC	13.2	12.2	Initially the patient is uncomfortable and requires pain medication and positioning. Nursing activities include frequent initial vital signs, dressing checks, gastric assessment, fluid monitoring, and prevention of postoperative complications.
87	Pulmonary edema and respiratory failure	7.3	27.0	The patients in this DRG are in an acute life-threatening situation requiring immediate and intense medical and nursing intervention.
210	Hip and femur procedures >69	14.9	20.3	The patients in this DRG require significant nursing care due to their age, lack of initial mobility, and inability to perform activities of daily living. These factors make the patient totally dependent on nursing personnel.

Nursing staff hours include nurse manager, clinical coordinator, head nurse, registered nurse, licensed practical nurse, nursing aide, and unit clerk time.

Table 13–12 Evaluation and Patient Days as a Basis for Costing Nursing Services

| | | | Direct Nursing Salary Costs | | | | |
	Selected DRG		Estimate Using Patient Days as Costing Basis ($)	Estimate of Actual Cost ($)	Difference ($)	Full Cost per Day ($)	Difference as a Percent of Full Cost per Day (%)
No.	*Description*	*Medical (M) or Surgical (S)*					
138	Cardiac arrhythmia >69 and/or (CC)	M	74.91	23.03	51.88	166.78	31.1
36	Retinal procedures >69 and/or CC	S	172.80	75.46	97.34	472.62	20.6
296	Nutritional and miscellaneous metabolic >69 and/or CC	M	74.91	104.26	(29.35)	378.30	(7.8)
197	Total cholecystectomy >69 and/or CC	S	83.34	113.07	(29.73)	486.66	(6.1)
87	Pulmonary edema and respiratory failure	M	136.03	285.48	(149.45)	924.05	(16.2)
210	Hip and femur procedures >69 and/or CC	S	102.31	197.14	(94.83)	673.24	(14.1)

Source: Paul L. Shafer, Betsy Frauenthal, and Catherine Tower, "Measuring Nursing Costs with Patient Acuity Data," *Topics in Health Care Financing*, Vol. 13, No. 13, Aspen Publishers, Inc., © 1987.

Table 13–13 Calculation of Average Daily Nursing Cost with Patient Acuity Approach

Calculation of cost per patient acuity point:

Cost per patient acuity point	=	Annual nursing salary cost for nursing unit	÷	Patient acuity points for all patients seen on unit during year

Calculation of average daily patient acuity points for patients in DRG:

Average daily patient acuity points for patients in DRG	=	Patient acuity points for all patients in DRG	÷	Patient days for all patients in DRG

Calculation of average daily nursing cost for patients in DRG:

Average daily nursing cost for patients in DRG	=	Cost per patient acuity point	×	Average daily patient acuity points for patients in DRG

Source: Paul L. Shafer, Betsy Frauenthal, and Catherine Tower, "Measuring Nursing Costs with Patient Acuity Data," *Topics in Health Care Financing*, Vol. 13, No. 13, Aspen Publishers, Inc., © 1987.

Patient Acuity Systems*

Patient acuity, or classification, systems are management tools designed to measure or forecast the nursing time required to care for individual patients.

Acuity-level staffing results in a more accurate matching of nursing resources to patient needs. By clearly defining the resource requirements of each patient on a nursing unit, an acuity system can assist the nursing department in most efficiently allocating the staff to the various nursing units.

Barriers to Implementation

If the patient acuity approach for identifying nursing costs is significantly more accurate than the patient day approach, why then is it not used more frequently? Some reasons why the method is not used are as follows:

- The patient acuity system lacks credibility in the eyes of fiscal service personnel. Frequently, fiscal service personnel either have minimal knowledge of the nursing department's patient acuity system or have doubts about the quality of information derived from the system.
- Patient acuity data are not being collected regularly or are not summarized in a manner useful for cost accounting. Frequently, the nursing department will collect patient acuity data on an ad hoc basis. For cost accounting purposes, however, comprehensive patient acuity data must be collected for each patient. Similarly, difficulties arise if patient acuity data are not summarized correctly. For staffing purposes, the nursing department will aggregate patient acuity data by nursing unit. For cost accounting, however, patient acuity information must be summarized by individual patient.

*Source: Paul L. Shafer, Betsy J. Frauenthal, and Catherine Tower, "Measuring Nursing Costs with Patient Acuity Data," Topics in Health Care Financing, Vol. 13, No. 4, Aspen Publishers, Inc., © 1987.

- Acuity information is voluminous and frequently never leaves the nursing department. It is also difficult to enter data into the cost accounting system. A system must be in place to integrate the clinical information with the health care facility's financial system to ensure that nursing information for every patient is regularly entered into the cost accounting system.

Recommendations for Smooth Implementation

The following actions will facilitate the implementation of patient acuity-based costing in the nursing department:

- Fiscal services and nursing must work closely together to develop needed patient acuity data.
- New billing statistics must be developed and used for patient acuity information.
- Patient acuity information must be collected each day for each patient.

First, for cost accounting, the fiscal service department will want to ensure that patient acuity information obtained from the nursing department is well documented, timely, and accurate. Fiscal services must clearly articulate these goals to the nursing department and provide the nurses with the resources they will need to achieve these goals. For example, to enhance the documentation, timeliness, and accuracy of the patient acuity system, the nursing department may need to implement some or all of the following:

- Hire a patient acuity coordinator.
- Develop new patient acuity forms.
- Implement an inservice education program related to the patient acuity system.
- Implement a rigorous data audit process for the acuity system.

The second factor needed for smooth implementation of patient acuity–based costing for nursing is the capture of patient acuity data in the health care facility's patient billing system. In most hospitals, for example, the charge for nursing services is included as part of the routine room and board charge automatically generated based on the midnight census. Consequently, hospital billing systems have not needed to capture patient acuity data. It is recommended that fiscal service personnel develop new billing statistics that will facilitate the daily entry of patient acuity data into the billing system.

It is advantageous to establish a separate billing statistic for acuity data for each nursing unit or service. In addition, it is necessary to have separate charge codes for each nursing unit or service; this accounts for the different nursing care factors that are either directly or indirectly associated with each unit or service.

Third, it is also recommended that acuity information for all patients be collected and entered into the billing system each day. Nursing, data processing, and fiscal service personnel will want to work together to develop an appropriate operational process for entering acuity information into the billing system on a daily basis. Once this is achieved, management will be able to compute the average patient acuity measure per patient per day, per patient per length of stay, by nursing service, and by DRG or major diagnostic category.

Variable Billing for Nursing by Patient Classification*

With the added complexity introduced into health care by the prospective payment system and diagnosis-related groups, some health care providers have reevaluated the idea that the daily room rate should include nursing care costs. Nursing managers assert that "hotel services"— the costs of housekeeping and dietary services (room and board)—are fixed costs that should be the same for all patients. Nursing care, on the other hand, is a variable cost: Some patients require much more care than others. Thus some

---

Source: Mehmet Kocakulah, Norma Hagenow, and Francine Cope, "The True Costs of Nursing Care," *Health Progress,* December 1990.

administrators have separated nursing costs from fixed room and board and instituted variable billing for nursing care.

Existing System

Option A in Table 13–14 is a simplified version of a patient's actual bill, used as an example throughout this discussion. The first item on this bill is a semiprivate room at $178 per day for six days. This daily rate is based on overhead costs (room and board) and nursing care, but in setting the rate, providers also consider competitive rates and what insurance companies define as "reasonable and customary" rates.

In a proposed new system, the cost of nursing care is separated from the overhead, using the

---

Table 13–14 Comparison of Billing Options

OPTION A: STANDARD PATIENT BILL

Service	Cost	Percent of Total Bill
Medical/surgical/ gynecological semiprivate bed ($178 per day)	$1,068.00	34%
Pharmaceuticals	564.85	18
Supplies	493.72	15.7
Diagnostic tests	197.90	6.3
Operating and recovery room services	813.50	25.9
Total charges	$3,137.97	

OPTION B: VARIABLE BILLING WITH NURSING COST BREAKDOWN

	Unit Cost	Unit	Total
Semiprivate bed	$106.80 ×	6 =	$640.80
Nursing care			
Class I days	57.71 ×	2 =	115.42
Class II days	73.38 ×	3 =	220.14
Class III days	88.34 ×	1 =	88.34
Class IV days	338.69 ×	0 =	
Nursing care total			$423.90

Hospital Corporation of America's (HCA's) patient classification system. Placement in a nursing classification—Class I, II, III, or IV—is based on assessment of the indicators for nursing intervention and the patient's need for assisted daily living. As patients improve and progress to the next class, they require less nursing care. Thus, one day at a Class IV level will cost much more than one day at a Class III level.

In addition to allocating labor, these four classifications help managers monitor nursing productivity. A major efficiency indicator in nursing throughout the United States is *hours per patient day* (HPPD). A recent HCA regional hospital audit indicated the following average number of hours per class per patient day for *direct nursing care* on a general surgery unit:

> Class I—2.54 hours
> Class II—3.42 hours
> Class III—3.89 hours
> Class IV—14.90 hours

Direct care reflects activities at the patient's bedside; the audit included two other components—indirect care and constant time—which encompass nursing activities performed away from the bedside.

Indirect care includes all paperwork, documentation, medication preparation, patient transportation, and so forth. *Constant time*, or unit management time, includes on-site education, committee work, administrative duties, and personal time. The total constant time is assigned equally to each patient independent of classification.

For each nursing area, researchers have determined standard hours for direct, indirect, and constant care. The result is *productive hours per patient day*. The figure varies according to nursing area. For example, in the general surgery unit the internal audit revealed the following figures for a Class II patient:

direct care (DC)	+	indirect care (IC)	+	constant time (CT)	=	total productive HPPD
3.42	+	1.48	+	0.3	=	5.2

From this foundation, already in place and fully computerized, one can derive the cost of nursing care simply.

Determining a Variable Cost

By building on the existing system, providers can determine a variable labor cost for each patient class. They can obtain the additional unit-specific data easily from routine payroll or operations reports. They can add nonproductive time (benefit hours, based on historical data for the unit) to the previous example to determine *total nursing hours* paid for one Class II surgical patient.

total HPPD (DC + IC + CT)	+	benefit hours (12% of productive time)	=	total paid hours
5.2	+	0.624	=	5.824

Total hours paid multiplied by the average hourly rate on the surgical unit gives the *variable nursing care cost* for a Class II patient for one day.

total paid hours	×	average hourly rate	=	variable cost
5.824	×	$10.50	=	$61.15

Using this method, managers can determine labor cost for each department. The *range* on the surgical unit according to patient classification is as follows:

> Class I—$48.09
> Class II—$61.15
> Class III—$73.62
> Class IV—$282.24 (1:1 patient to nurse ratio)

To complete the transition to variable billing, one adds an arbitrary *profit margin* (in this case 20 percent) to the labor cost.

	labor cost	+	20% profit	=	total daily rate
Class I	$48.09	+	$9.62	=	$57.71
Class II	$61.15	+	$12.23	=	$73.38
Class III	$73.62	+	$14.72	=	$88.34
Class IV	$282.24	+	$56.45	=	$338.69

Adding this proposed variable billing for nursing care hours to the patient bill in Option A (Table 13–14), one can determine the totals shown in Option B (room and board rate was reduced by 40 percent because it no longer contained the nursing care costs). Total charges for nursing care added to the other charges shown in Option A now total $3,134.67—almost exactly the same as the actual bill. The only difference is that in the actual bill, hotel and nursing costs were 34 percent, whereas the proposed bill shows the costs of the bed were $640.80 (or 20 percent) and nursing was $423.90 (or only 13.5 percent).

As Option A shows, with 20 percent profit, nursing is still only 13.5 percent of the total bill (consistent with research indicating nursing care ranges from 11 percent to 21 percent of total charges billed). This percentage is characteristic of all medical-surgical nursing care costs. In addition to showing that nursing care is cost-effective, billing by classification provides clearly documented evidence, supported by nursing notes, of the costs a health care facility incurs in providing care.

Nursing Benefits

Viewing nursing as a profit center, one can evaluate a nursing manager's performance on the basis of business goals. When nursing staffs are recognized as income producers who have increased influence in decision making, they will cease to be the major target in cost-containment programs and will no longer be perceived as an economic drain.

Also, nursing revenues could directly fund programs for nursing in need of subsidy: continuing education for nurses, career opportunities to reward professional development, incentive programs to encourage efficiency in patient care, and nursing research, which has already saved organizations much money.

Cost accounting increases the accountability, professionalism, and control of nurse managers. Identified costs are more manageable, and the department's and the facility's efficiency in-

creases. Administrators can evaluate departmental performance based on analysis of costs and budget variances. Because nursing costs are derived from valid classification systems, third-party payers may be further persuaded to correlate prospective reimbursement with nursing costs.

FISCAL CONTROL

Manager Education for Monitoring and Controlling Resources*

Data for budgeted positions are usually conveyed by department managers who, in turn, depend on the nurse managers for information. Education of the department manager in fiscal operations and enforcement of responsibility and accountability for performance will maximize the nurse administrator's fiscal control (see Table 13–15).

The most fundamental aspects of salary budget development, monitoring, and control must be clearly and accurately relayed. The department's standard, in hours or dollars per patient day, must be understood, including the relationship to volume or units of service. This standard, typically based on average acuity for the department, should be broken down into an allocation for each shift. Based on departmental acuity and volume, a clear guideline is given for staffing, even in the absence of the department manager. Using this guideline, decisions can be easily calculated and traced to the individual decision maker. A cumulative shift report encompassing the 14-day pay period documents fiscal compliance with the departmental standard and in most cases is readily accepted and understood by staff.

The issues of budgeted skill mix, overtime, per diem pay, and registry usage should be thoroughly discussed so that there is an understood

Source: Thomas R. Soule, "Attaining Financial Control in Nursing: Three Basic Factors," *Aspen's Advisor for Nurse Executives*, Vol. 6, No. 8, Aspen Publishers, Inc., © 1991.

Table 13–15 Outline of Manager Education Regarding the Control of Resources

Salary Education

- Human Resource Monitoring/Control
- Written Human Resource Utilization Standards
- Monthly Salary Expense Analysis
- FTE Analysis/Projection

Nonsalary Education

- Nonsalary Subaccounts
- Monthly Analysis—Variance Reporting
- Review of Charging Practices
- Nonsalary Standards Development
- Noncapital Purchase Planning

Responsibility

- Clarify Responsibilities
- Document Expectations
- Incorporate into CBPE

Accountability

- Clarify Accountability
- Provide Consistent Feedback
- Provide Positive Support
- Enforce Accountability

Source: Thomas R. Soule, "Attaining Financial Control in Nursing: Three Basic Factors," *Aspen's Advisor for Nurse Executives,* Vol. 6, No. 8, Aspen Publishers, Inc., © 1991.

priority for making decisions. Standards for staff utilization, overtime, registry, and so forth, should be clearly defined in writing in order to provide guidance and consistency. Manager feedback based on review of staff utilization and compliance with the department staffing standards is essential. In some cases—depending on how acuity is validated and how frequently acuity and volume are measured, by shift or 24-hour period—solid and objective rationales for variances can be obtained. Control will be expedited with the implementation of written control standards.

As managers' expertise in controlling and monitoring staffing hours develops, efforts can be redirected to the broader picture of salary expenses. Specifically, the relationship of the monthly costs in salary accounts to hours used can be evaluated and analyzed. Full participation in projecting yearly units of service and departmental FTEs and positions should be a common expectation for department managers.

Nonsalary Expenses

The second key area for manager education should focus on departmental nonsalary operating expenses. As with salary expenses, managers should participate in their budgeted yearly allocations in all subaccounts. Managers must be educated in each specific subaccount—what is costed to it and who will be charging against those accounts. All managers should gain expertise in correctly reading the monthly departmental expense reports and identifying unfavorable variances.

Monthly variance reports, based on investigation and identified rationales for unfavorable variances, should be routine and documented. Some of the most meaningful learning will take place when departmental charges from the multitude of internal and external sources are confirmed.

True savings and cost reductions will surface when charging practices are scrutinized by investigating managers. Noncapital supplies and equipment maintenance controls deserve attention. Frequently allocations by support or ancillary services (e.g., pharmacy or central service) are incorrect, inconsistent, or simply cannot be supported by a sound fiscal rationale. Incorrect practices in ordering and charging out to the cost centers can be put back on track so that nursing operations can be fairly and objectively evaluated. Managers cannot buy-in on their responsibilities unless charging practices truly reflect reality.

Standards for the subaccounts reflecting volume-affected consumable supplies should be considered. By simply involving the managers in evaluating prior monthly costs (dividing actual expense by units of service) for the period, numerical standards can be developed. From these standards for nonsalary expenses, future targets can be adapted according to control or reduction plans. If nurses review in order to use better, more cost-effective product brands or to develop a less wasteful system, a lasting financial impact will occur.

Other categories that can be reviewed are noncapital minor medical and nonmedical equipment. A fundamental planning of purchases can be achieved by encouraging a listing of planned purchases consistent with departmental goals. This is not to say that only planned events will occur. But with a sound process, the consistent and equal allocation of monies for emergencies can be accomplished based on the equipment intensivity of the service.

Responsibility

The education of department managers in salary and nonsalary monitoring and control practices will be effective only if accountability and responsibility are clarified up front. If department managers do not accept responsibility for what is expected of them in controlling their departments' expenses, no amount of financial education will help. Further, even if the monitoring and control responsibilities are readily assumed, they will be of little value unless each manager is held accountable for fiscal decisions he or she makes.

One of the most acceptable methods for clarifying the monitoring and control responsibilities is identification of expectations, in writing, with the management group. It is an opportunity to spell out, discuss, and negotiate exactly what responsibilities must be performed by the manager—until consensus is reached. Timing of reports, acceptable rationales for variances, and implementation of solutions are just a few standards that should be covered. With minor rewording, these standards become a criterion-based performance evaluation.

Accountability

Accountability follows the acceptance of the responsibility. In some cases, it enforces responsibility. The message must be clear that managers *will* be held accountable for decisions that they and their staffs make. Staffing decisions, supply purchases, and implementation of cost-effective programs and projects require consistent feedback, which enforces the accountability expected. A positive, supportive, mentoring approach is necessary during the learning phase. Over time, feedback becomes more direct, and accountability for meeting budgetary standards is heightened. Manager buy-in may be encouraged with a pay-for-performance system, monetarily recognizing those managers who have become masters at the art of fiscal control.

Chapter 14

Management of Patient Care

BASIC NURSING CARE DELIVERY SYSTEMS

Overview

Within the context of nursing practice, the framework for providing nursing services is an important consideration. The system used to deliver nursing care gives the objective observer some idea of the context of care delivery and the philosophy of the organization. Whether it be functional, team, primary, or some modification of one of these, each system reflects a particular philosophy and the way that professional practice of nursing unfolds. The organization must commit itself to a delivery system that will articulate in practice the philosophy, beliefs, and standards that are applied to nursing care and that are acceptable to the institution. While it is argued that some nursing care delivery systems reflect a higher level of professional nursing practice than others, the decision about which system is most effective and most representative of the resources, skills, and abilities of a particular institution's nursing professionals must be made realistically. Appropriate structural and practice strategies can be undertaken within any nursing care system that preserves and promotes high standards of practice. With an understanding of all constraints and pursuing all possibilities avail-

able to the nursing organization, the highest level of practice effectiveness must be demanded by the practitioners themselves. It is in that context that any choice of an appropriate nursing care system should be addressed (see Figure 14–1).*

Delivery Systems Defined**

A nursing delivery system is a set of concepts defining four basic organizational elements. The definitions of these elements are based on principles that are in turn based on fundamental values. These fundamental values will ultimately determine the quality of the product. If the workers are not valued as independent decision makers by the definers of the principles of work organization, independent decision making will not be characteristic of their practice. If the definers do not believe the average staff nurse has the ability to manage a patient's care (to be distinguished from clinical ability), the system will not give decision-making authority to staff nurses.

---

*Source: Timothy Porter-O'Grady and Sharon Finnegan, *Shared Governance for Nursing: A Creative Approach to Professional Accountability*, Aspen Publishers, Inc., © 1984.
**Source: Marie Manthey, "Definitions and Basic Elements of a Patient Care Delivery System with an Emphasis on Primary Nursing," in *Patient Care Delivery Models*, Gloria Gilbert Mayer, Mary Jane Madden, and Eunice Lawrenz, eds., Aspen Publishers, Inc., © 1990.

248

Figure 14–1 Nursing Practice

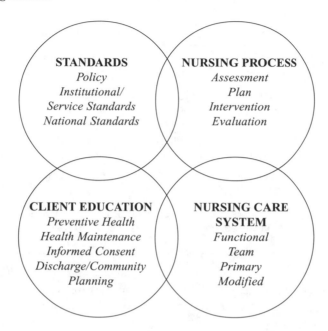

The four fundamental elements are

- clinical decision making
- work allocation
- communication
- management

These four elements are the cornerstones on which a delivery system is built. The more clearly they are articulated, the better they will be. (See Table 14–1.)

Roles are developed to function within the framework of the delivery system, and that framework impacts the functions in such a way as to support or prohibit various behaviors. For example, imagine a well-qualified, competent nurse functioning one day as a primary nurse, the next as a team leader, and the third day as the medication nurse. The knowledge contained in his or her brain and the skill reflected in his or her hands-on practice and verbal interactions will differ dramatically depending on the *role* created to fulfill the functions assigned in the context of the expectations inherent in the delivery system.

There is another major way the delivery system impacts work performed and the worker's experience of it. When work is allocated according to tasks rather than patients, a body of knowledge about the patients is simply not accumulated by the staff. This absence of knowledge has a negative impact on the clinical decisions that need to be made. In addition, the absence of patient information severely impacts the quality of data communicated. Data communication is one of the major sources of evidence available after the fact to judge the quality of performance. Delivery system design is the framework within which roles are developed and clinical knowledge is required and formulated.

The Mechanics of Delivering Nursing Care*

The continuous search for improvement in the delivery of nursing care has provided adminis-

---

Source: Marie Manthey, "Definitions and Basic Elements of a Patient Care Delivery System with an Emphasis on Primary Nursing," in *Patient Care Delivery Models*, Gloria Gilbert Mayer, Mary Jane Madden, and Eunice Lawrenz, eds., Aspen Publishers, Inc., © 1990.

Table 14–1 Comparison of Delivery Systems: Essential Elements

	Case Method	Primary Nursing	Team Nursing	Functional Nursing
Decision Making	24-hour responsibility	24-hour responsibility	8- to 12-hour shift responsibility	8- to 12-hour shift responsibility
Scope of Responsibility	Small groups of patients assigned by various designations	Small groups of patients from same geographic area	Large groups of patients from same geographic area	Large groups of patients from same geographic area
Focus of Patient Management	Managing critical pathways	Providing total patient care	Coordinating and planning care	Supervising delegated tasks

Source: Joan Gygax Spicer and Diane E. Nitta, "Nursing Organization and Management," in *Manual of Health Services Management*, Robert J. Taylor, ed., Aspen Publishers, Inc., © 1994.

trators with four basic model systems: case, functional, team, and primary care. The construction and mechanics of each system reflect a shifting emphasis in the service provided by health care personnel and in the roles of the patient.

The oldest method of delivering nursing care is the *case system*, where one nurse is involved in nursing observation and care of a single patient. Considered a one-to-one relationship, this method is used today primarily for assignments in intensive care units and for educational demonstrations with student nurses.

The most frequently adopted method is the *functional system*, which focuses on the number of tasks that must be provided to the overall patient population and assigns qualified personnel to the appropriate task. This division of labor is based on the assembly line production concept found in industry. In the nursing unit the breakdown of activities is translated into patient care assignments that are specific for each staff member: to provide hygienic care, to distribute medication, to administer treatment or therapy, to instruct the patient, to keep records, and so on. The central authority resides in the charge nurse, who processes all major communications. Though this system has been favored as an economic measure, comparisons of cost-effectiveness indicate other combinations of nursing care delivery systems are equal to and sometimes superior to the functional method. More impor-

tant, nurses frequently chafe under this partial involvement, limited to only one aspect of the patient's total health care. Patients are often confused by the endless flow of different caregivers.

The *team system* modifies the depersonalized, skilled-worker approach in a format that focuses on individualized patient health care. Adopted in the 1950s, this system employs a cluster of health care personnel whose varied skills are directed by a team leader to provide total services for a specific patient case. The formation of a team is a cooperative and collaborative venture that involves a professional nurse capable of leadership and health personnel who are technically proficient in their respective roles and capable of participation in a group effort. The care of the patient is conceived of as a group task, with observations, interpretations, and evaluations mutually investigated and shared. The team leader's responsibility is to coordinate, supervise, and engage the full participation of coworkers in the construction and implementation of nursing care plans for the well-being of the patient.

A more recently developed care delivery method is the *primary care system*, which recalls some of the features of the case system but assumes added dimensions in the nurse's increased responsibility in areas such as coordination and range of patient coverage. The primary nurse has full, 24-hour-a-day, continuous accountability for planning, evaluating, and directing the nursing care of a patient case. The primary nurse establishes a direct relationship with the patient, collecting and assessing data, forming plans, making decisions, and representing the patient's total needs in the coordination of activities with other health personnel and disciplines. When the primary nurse is off duty, his or her relief nurse continues to act in accordance with the care plan he or she has developed. More than one patient case is usually assigned, though the number varies with the nature and treatment of nursing services required and the number of support personnel and systems available in the health care facility. The assignment of patient cases is usually the responsibility of the nurse leader, who attempts to match professional expertise or special interests with cases. Occasionally the primary nurse is allowed to pick and choose his or her own patients.

In practice, these basic models of nursing care delivery systems have been adapted and altered in new combinations to suit different department needs. Since the team and the primary care systems are the more current and more variable modes of delivering nursing care, further details and information will be provided below. (*Note:* For a comparison of nursing care delivery systems, see Figure 14–2 and Table 14–2.) The text then provides more details on several of the distinctive features in each system as well as modified versions.

Team Nursing*

Objectives

The objectives usually stated for team nursing are to provide

- adequate staff for good care
- good experiences for staff members
- good personnel policies to maintain morale

Assignments

Charge nurses make assignments of team leaders. They assign both team members and workloads to individual teams. Team leaders further break down the workload assignments within the teams. A team member should be able to do the following: (1) when reporting for duty, obtain a written assignment; (2) receive an oral or taped report on the team's patients; (3) take orders from nursing care plans and physician's order sheets; (4) orally review assignment with team leader and organize his or her assignment on a written assignment sheet. The following items should be considered in making team nursing assignments:

- quantitative workload: total direct and indirect patient care activities
- qualitative workload: specialized needs of patients
- available staff, including experience level of staff
- personal factors or qualifications and abilities of staff
- division of work, including limiting the physical work of registered nurses
- geography of unit
- continuity of care
- type of assignment: team, case, primary nursing, or functional method
- availability of clerical and housekeeping personnel

Primary Nursing Concepts and Structure

Philosophy *

Primary nursing provides comprehensive and continuous patient care from admission to dis-

Source: Russell C. Swansburg, *Management of Patient Care Services*, The C.V. Mosby Co., © 1976. Reprinted with permission.

Source: Linda Burnes-Bolton et al., "A Cost Containment Model of Primary Nurses at Cedars-Sinai Medical Center," in *Patient Care Delivery Models*, Gloria Gilbert Mayer, Mary Jane Madden, and Eunice Lawrenz, eds., Aspen Publishers, Inc., © 1990.

Figure 14–2 A Pictorial Presentation of Nursing Care Structures

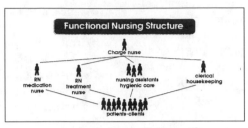

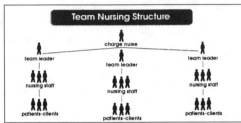

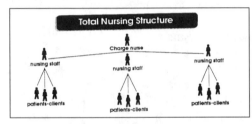

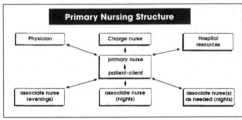

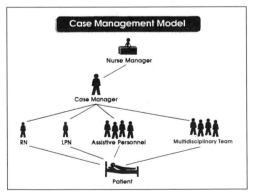

Note: Total nursing structure is also called "total patient care" and signifies a staff of only registered nurses to supply all patient needs. (This is popular in intensive care units, emergency departments, and neonatal care.) It differs from primary nursing care in that the primary nurse has 24-hour responsibility even though associate nurses do care for the patient on various shifts.

Source: Ruth I. Hanston and Marilynn J. Washburn, *Clinical Delegation Skills*, Aspen Publishers, Inc., © 1994.

Table 14–2 Working Features of Various Methods of Delivering Nursing Care

Factor	Method of Nursing Care		
	Functional	Team	Primary
Assignments	Head nurse or nursing coordinator assigns to staff members tasks that fall within their job descriptions.	Team leader assigns to team members tasks that fall within their job descriptions.	Head nurse or nursing coordinator assigns individual patients to professional nurses, matching the patients' needs to the nurses' skills.
Assessment, planning, and evaluation	Related to a specific need of each patient; done by any member of the nursing staff; no continuity.	Related to specific needs of each patient; done by the team leader; a limited continuity depending on how long a person remains team leader.	Related to specific needs of each patient; done by the primary nurse; maximum continuity, since primary nurse remains throughout patient's stay on unit.
Implementation	Different members of the nursing staff do tasks for a given patient.	Each team member does tasks for all patients, according to job description; the team leader often does medications and charting for the team.	Each primary nurse delivers total care to all assigned patients. ("For the first time I feel that somebody knows who I am.")
Documentation	Staff members make notations on only those actions or aspects of care done by them. *or* A staff member is assigned to "chart" for a given number of patients; usually no nursing care plan is in evidence.	Team leader usually documents care for patients cared for by most, or all, team members; sometimes a team member makes certain entries on patient charts; the team leader documents the nursing care plan.	Each primary or associate nurse documents care given to each assigned patient during shift; the primary nurse documents the nursing care plan.
Reporting at end of shift	A charge nurse gives report on patients to another charge nurse; most of the information shared is based on reports of other workers.	The team leader gives report on the group of patients to the oncoming team; most of the information shared is based on reports of other workers.	The primary nurse gives report on each assigned patient to oncoming nurse who will care for the patient; the nurse who reports has interacted directly with all the patients about whom reports are given.

continues

Table 14–2 continued

Factor	Method of Nursing Care		
	Functional	Team	Primary
Responsibility for planning care	No one person is responsible for planning unless this is assigned as a functional task to a specific registered nurse for a given period.	The team leader is responsible for planning the nursing care for the assigned group of patients.	The primary nurse is responsible for planning the nursing care of all primary patients, from the time they are admitted to a nursing unit until they are discharged from that unit.
Responsibility for providing care	Nursing care is delivered in a fragmented manner, with many staff members interacting with the patient as the various tasks are done.	As in functional nursing, delivery of nursing care is a "mixed bag."	The primary nurse directly delivers all nursing care to the primary patients when on duty.
Decentralization of authority, for continuous decision making and follow up of nursing care	Totally decentralized—decisions are made on basis of separate tasks done by individual staff members for each patient on the unit.	The team leader makes final decisions about nursing care for the patients in the group on basis of feedback (some of which is lost) from team members.	Each primary nurse makes final decisions about nursing care for the assigned patients.
Accountability			
For professional actions	Professional nurses are each answerable for their own professional actions.	Professional nurses are each answerable for their own professional actions.	Professional nurses are each answerable for their own professional actions.
For coordination and outcomes of nursing care	No one nursing staff member is answerable for the coordination and outcomes of nursing care; the head nurse often answers to everyone for the entire staff.	The team leader, who plans care but often does not give it, is answerable for the care of each patent in the assigned group and for the coordination and outcomes of nursing care.	The primary nurse who plans and delivers the care to each assigned patient is answerable for the coordination and outcomes of nursing care.

continues

Table 14–2 continued

| Factor | Method of Nursing Care | | |
	Functional	Team	Primary
For follow up on patient problems	Physicians, administrators, and other interdepartmental personnel can rarely pinpoint responsibility for follow up on problems.	The team leader is responsible for follow up on patient problems, which are often generated by other staff.	The primary nurse is responsible for follow up on problems of assigned patients.
"Passing the buck"	Passing the buck prevalent.	Moderate amount of "buck passing" due to change in staff assignments from day to day.	Minimal, if any, passing the buck because of constancy of staff assignments to same patients.
Comprehensiveness of care, in terms of: *Patients' needs*	Not possible; focus of care is on tasks, not on the patient as a unique individual with a broad spectrum of needs and resources.	Theoretically, and sometimes actually, possible, since team members are expected to communicate ideas related to patient needs and nursing action to meet those needs; a united approach is the goal; however, plans are often designed with minimal patient/ family input, and focus is on nursing action rather than on patient goals.	Inherent in the system, because continuity in same nurse/same patient relationships is maximized; focus of nursing care is on patient goals rather than on nursing action.
Documentation	Nursing care regimens are rarely documented, so individual approaches are inconsistent.	Documented nursing care plans are encouraged but can rarely be demanded, because nursing caseload is too large.	Documented nursing care plans are mandated and are facilitated by smaller caseload of each nurse and by constancy of assignment.
Communication: *Between nurses and patients or clients*	Patient, family, and significant others find it difficult to	Patient, family, and significant others may be confused	Patient, family, and significant others can clearly identify

continues

Table 14–2 continued

| Factor | Method of Nursing Care | | |
	Functional	Team	Primary
	identify a nursing staff member with whom to relate on a continuing basis.	as to identity of the nursing staff member to whom questions and problems may be directed.	the nurse and can share ideas, feelings, and problems freely with this person.
Between nurses and staff of other departments	Physicians, administrators, and interdepartmental staff address questions and problems to nurses or to head nurse on unit, but often satisfactory answers are delayed or are not available.	Same as in functional nursing, except team leader rather than head nurse may be consulted.	All communications are directed to the primary nurse for each patient. Satisfactory answers are more likely to be forthcoming. Persons may find difficulty in locating specific nurses.
Between nurses and supervisors	Instructions often have to be repeated because of changes in staff assignments and lack of consistent documentation of nursing care plans.	Same as in functional nursing.	Dramatic decrease in repetition of instructions for particular patients due to constancy of assignments and mandatory care plans.

Source: Donna R. Sheridan, Jean E. Bronstein, and Duane D. Walker, *The New Nurse Manager*, Aspen Publishers, Inc., © 1984.

charge by using the same registered nurse (primary nurse) to coordinate, evaluate, and provide direct patient care (the registered nurse uses the nursing process in planning this care). The patient's and family's involvement in care encourages a trusting nurse-patient relationship, thereby promoting continuity and effective discharge planning.

Peer accountability, review, and support are integral parts of the primary nursing system and they result in a continuous evaluation of patient care. In primary nursing, the responsibility (and authority) to make decisions about patient care devolves to the individual nurse. This responsibility allows the nurse to act as a change agent and patient advocate.

*Structure**

The *primary nursing coordinator* is a registered professional nurse who assumes 24-hour-a-day, seven-day-a-week responsibility and accountability for activities of an assigned nursing unit, with the main focus on patient and nursing staff needs. The *primary nurse* is a registered professional nurse responsible and accountable for (1) the nursing process for a specified num-

---

**Source:* Linda Burnes-Bolton et al., "A Cost Containment Model of Primary Nurses at Cedars-Sinai Medical Center," in *Patient Care Delivery Models*, Gloria Gilbert Mayer, Mary Jane Madden, and Eunice Lawrenz, eds., Aspen Publishers, Inc., © 1990.

Major Areas of Primary Nurse Responsibility

There are three major areas of responsibility. First, the primary nurse is responsible for making available the necessary clinical information others need for the intelligent care of the patient in the nurse's absence. This means the nurse not only must be knowledgeable but also must be able to recognize what information is essential for the others to have.

Second, the primary nurse is responsible for deciding how nursing care shall be administered and for making available to other nurses the instructions for care. Instructions left by the primary nurse are to be followed by others caring for the nurse's patients in his or her absence unless an alteration is dictated by a change in a patient's condition. When that happens, the nurse's instructions may be modified to deal with the new situation. Otherwise, they are to be followed by the staff members who care for the patient on the other shifts.

The third major area of responsibility is discharge planning. The primary nurse is responsible for ensuring that the patient and family (if the family will be caring for the patient at home) have been prepared to provide safe and effective care. If the patient is being transferred to an agency that employs nurses, the primary nurse is responsible for communicating any information needed for a smooth transition.

Source: Marie Manthey, "Definitions and Basic Elements of a Patient Care Delivery System with an Emphasis on Primary Nursing," in *Patient Care Delivery Models*, Gloria Gilbert Mayer, Mary Jane Madden, and Eunice Lawrenz, eds., Aspen Publishers, Inc., © 1990.

cian. The *associate nurse* is a registered professional nurse who, in the absence of the primary nurse, assumes responsibility and accountability for maintaining individualized quality nursing care for a designated number of patients for an eight-hour period. Keystones of primary nursing are

- continuity of patient care
- centrality of the patient
- responsibility to the patient
- patient advocacy
- centrality of the patient's lifestyle and family
- emphasis on health (in the sense of wellness)
- patient education
- accountability to peers, the patient, and the physician
- goal directedness
- job fulfillment and retainment
- nurse practitioner autonomy
- patient inclusion in planning care

Certain advantages of primary nursing are clear. Nurses who are aware of their patients' diagnoses and the ramifications become more involved with their patients. Continuity of care is fostered by uninterrupted care planning   shift to shift, nurse to nurse, and health care facility to home.

Patients realize that someone knows them as individuals from certain cultural and social backgrounds. Primary patients have opportunities to express their needs and concerns, and they will usually feel confident that their nurses will integrate these needs into their care.

Head nurse positions in primary nursing become ones of quality control, management of people, and staff development. Decentralizing decision making to the bedside requires a unit leader who has assessed the staff's capabilities, provided for their learning, and allowed and trusted them to function as independently as possible.

Staff nurses will have intense involvement with a consistent group of primary patients instead of a superficial knowledge of (and consequent superficial involvement with) a whole team. In converting to primary nursing from the team

ber of patients, including but not limited to assessing patient needs and planning, implementing, and evaluating all aspects of patient care; (2) the delivery of care 24 hours a day from admission to discharge; and (3) participation in a communication triad between patient and physi-

system, two more caregivers are gained—the team leaders. This brings a potential for growth of clinical skills, collaboration with other health team members, and satisfaction from direct patient care.

*Patient Assignment Method**

Three patterns have been described: geographic, individual, and promotional. Principles to consider in any method are

- equal caseload depending on staff ability and hours
- optimal match between patient need and staff competence made at admission or within 24 hours and maintained through patient's stay unless:
  - a patient-nurse personality conflict exists that cannot be resolved
  - the nurse is going onto a block of nights or on vacation
  - the patient condition changes beyond the capability of the primary nurse
  - the patient requests a change
  - the patient transfers to a room that is inconvenient for the primary nurse
- a variety of patient conditions for staff growth, identified and visible to patient, family, nurses, physician, and other staff
- the geographic location of rooms

There are advantages and disadvantages to each of the three systems, as shown in Table 14–3. There is no perfect system. Considering all the unique variables, one or a combination of methods can be chosen, keeping the main principles in mind.

Duration of Assignment. Some nurses misunderstand the primary nursing assignment to be absolute, never changing. If difficulties occur between the nurse and patient, there is reluctance to discuss a possible change, because the nurse might feel exposure of the situation would reflect inadequacy.

---

*Source: Karen Ciske, "Misconceptions about Staffing and Patient Assignment in Primary Nursing," *Nursing Administration Quarterly*, Vol. 1, No. 2, Aspen Publishers, Inc., © 1977.

Table 14–3 Methods of Patient Assignment

Geographic Method

Advantages	Disadvantages
1. Stable, patients easy to keep track of	1. No guarantee of fair caseload
2. Easier to have consistent secondary coverage	2. Loses patient who transfers to another district
3. Well organized	3. Unclear who is accountable when off duty for long stretch
4. Easier for health team to learn who has what patient	

Individual Method

Advantages	Disadvantages
1. Caseload fair	1. Much time spent in making original and daily assignment
2. Variety of cases	
3. Can be maintained when readmitted	2. Wasted steps if patients for any nurse are spread through unit
4. Control by head nurse	

Promotional Method

Advantages	Disadvantages
1. Screening process, only for best professionals	1. Large caseload
2. Viewed as more status	2. Much delegation of direct patient care
3. Stimulates staff to show competence	3. Cost of positions
4. Increased role clarity	4. Holds back advancement if more nurses are ready to be promoted than positions available
5. Reward of increased pay	

A solution to this is the head nurse's surveillance of all assignments. The head nurse is ultimately responsible for quality of care. Supervision and education can be provided through patient rounds, chart and care plan audits, conferences, and so on. When nurses want to change patients, problem solving can help staff see their situations more objectively, learn from them, and possibly stay with the patients rather than requesting reassignment.

When patients are readmitted, the choice to remain primary nurse with a patient should be left to the nurse. Many times, the patient's condition will have deteriorated, as with patients who have cancer. It could be stressful for the primary nurse to resume care for such a patient, depending on caseload, emotional reaction to the declining condition, hours, or skills required. When given the option, most choose to remain primary and receive satisfaction in continuing the relationship, even if the patient is dying. However, most nurses appreciate having an "out" in case they need it.

OTHER OPTIONS FOR DELIVERING NURSING CARE

New structures of organization and new systems of applied practice have been evolving that, while they may not demand that the executive deny the value of traditional approaches, will require leaders to understand how those approaches are undertaken, the framework within which they were applied, the systems out of which they operate, and the outcomes they achieve. Without building those processes into the deliberations regarding the most appropriate and effective ways of delivering health care services, the nurse executive and other leaders are disadvantaged by their own traditional approaches and belief systems about health care, the role of the nurse, and other professions' roles in making decisions regarding direction, values, and service structures for the future.*

Managed Care and Nursing Case Management**

Nursing case management, with its foundation of *managed care,* is a clinical system for the

strategic management of cost and quality outcomes (see Table 14–4). Managed care and case management provide patients and their families with a collaborative plan based on standards of care, yet individualized by groups of clinicians who have expertise in their "case types." Continuity of care is accomplished by managed care. Continuity of providers across an entire health care facility is achieved through group practices that provide case management.

The basic components of managed care, as manifested in the New England Medical Center, a major trendsetter for this system, are

- *standard critical paths*, which are used as adjuncts to care plans
- *critical paths*, which are used as bases for change-of-shift reports
- *analysis of positive and negative variances* from the critical path
- *timely case consultation* for the caregiver "inheriting" a complex patient care situation
- *health care team meetings* initiated, conducted, and followed up by nursing
- *variances aggregated, analyzed and addressed* by the unit's nurse manager

Structure for Case Management

Nursing case management relies on the unit-based systems of managed care but goes one step further to identify the specific nurses and physicians who will be accountable for the financial and clinical outcomes of designated patients. There are several components.

The first component, *accountability* for outcomes, is achieved at the staff nurse level through a combination of primary nursing, managed care, and formal group practice.

Paramount to the nursing case management model is the *use of caregiver as case manager* (except for training or volume-overload situations). This component differentiates the model of New England Medical Center hospitals from others in which the case manager may be a nurse but is not involved in the direct care of the patients being managed. *Nursing case management results in ultimate decentralization inasmuch as*

Source: Tim Porter-O'Grady, *Reorganization of Nursing Practice: Creating the Corporate Venture,* Aspen Publishers, Inc., © 1990.

**Source:* Karen Zander, "Managed Care and Nursing Case Management," in *Patient Care Delivery Models,* Gloria Gilbert Mayer, Mary Jane Madden, and Eunice Lawrenz, eds., Aspen Publishers, Inc., © 1990.

Table 14–4 Ground Rules for Case Management

- Every designated patient will be admitted to a formally prepared group practice composed of an attending physician and staff nurses from each of the units and clinics likely to receive the patient.
- Each nurse in the group practice will give direct care as the patient's primary or associate nurse while the patient is on his or her geographic unit.
- Every group practice will assign one of its nursing members to be the case manager who works with the attending physician in evaluating an individualized case management plan (CMP) and critical path for each patient.
- A critical path for the whole episodes of care will be used to manage the care of every designated patient, both at change-of-shift report and during group practice meetings.
- The nurses in the group practice will meet on a weekly basis at a consistent time and place and maintain a patient roster.
- Each nurse member of the group practice will communicate immediate patient care issues with the attending physician while

the patient is on his or her own unit. The assigned case manager will work through the group and the attending physician for nonemergent issues.

- Negative variances from critical paths and/or CMPs require discussion with the attending physician and possibly a case management consultation.
- The group practice will meet to discuss care patterns, policies, specific patients and variances, research questions, and updated knowledge at their own predetermined intervals (e.g., monthly, bimonthly). Minutes will be taken for reference by members who cannot attend.
- Nurse members of the group practice will negotiate a flexible schedule that accommodates the needs of their case-managed patients and collaborative practices *as well as* the needs of their units.
- Responsibility of the case manager begins at notification of patient's entry into the system and ends with a formal transfer of accountability to the patient, family, another health care provider, or another institution.

Source: Copyright © Karen Zander, Department of Nursing, New England Medical Center Hospitals, 1988.

---

it delegates accountability for clinical and financial outcomes to specific staff nurses. To accomplish this, the staff nurse, as case manager, is placed in a case-based matrix at the patient care level (see Figure 14–3). That is, there are *formal registered nurse/physician group practices.* The staff nurse works with certain physicians individually or as a member of a multiunit group of primary nurses. The case manager is both a member of a unit-based staff and a member of the group practice.

The fourth component encompasses new methods for *actively involving patients and their families* in every phase of care. This includes pre- and posthospitalization phone calls, giving patients copies of their critical paths, using patient portfolios, including patients (when indicated) in team meetings, negotiating meaningful outcomes and discharge plans, and involving them in audits of their responses to interventions.

Figure 14–3 Patient Care–Level Matrix for Case Management

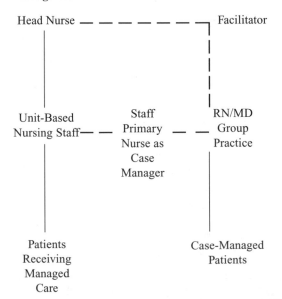

Table 14–5 Responsibilities in Case Management Modality of Care

Professional

Registered nurse—Case manager responsibilities
- Patient shift assessments
- Admission database
- Patient teaching
- Discharge planning
- Discharge summary
- Nursing care plans
- Care planning conferences
- Walking rounds with team caregivers for beginning and end-of-shift reports
- Making rounds with physicians for collaboration of care and making physician phone consults
- Insertion of feeding tubes
- Administration of IV medications—nows and stats
- Charting—summary
- Working with concurrent review
- Communication with team members about changes in plan of care
- Patient acuity
- Follow-up phone call to patient after discharge
- Patient rounds at least twice during shift for goal sharing and problem solving
- Patient presentation at interdisciplinary care conferences
- Reviewing lab work
- Shift patient-team assignments
- Communicating with physicians to coordinate care and solve problems
- Checking patient orders for accuracy

Technical

Licensed practical nurse (LPN)—Medication/treatment nurse responsibilities
- Administration of PO, SQ, and IM medications, both routine and prn
- Tube feedings
- Foley catheter insertions
- Routine IV maintenance and hanging fluids
- Heparin flushes on INTs
- Charting as appropriate
- Telemetry battery changes

Helper

Nurse extender (PCA, GN, GPN, LPN) responsibilities
- General hygienic care
- Beds and baths
- Vital signs
- Intake and output
- Ambulation of patients
- Feeding patients
- Minor treatments as defined by training nurse
- Charting (when appropriate)

Note: PO, by mouth; SQ, subcutaneous; IM, intramuscular; INT, in the vein; PCA, patient care assistant; GN, graduate nurse; GPN, graduate practical nurse.

Source: Nancy Barton, Ruth Kunkle, Annette Tucker, and Deborah Robinson Bailey, "Redesigning Care Delivery: Another Definition of Managed Care," *Nursing Administration Quarterly*, Vol. 17, No. 4, Aspen Publishers, Inc., © Summer 1993.

Variant on the Existing Structures

Differentiated Practice

Differentiated practice, as developed by the National Commission on Nursing Implementation Project, is a care delivery system that combines the model of primary nursing for all clients with a case management model for the chronically ill or for those with no support system in the home. Its goal is to place nursing in a strategic position to influence health care facility operations and medical practice. Some of the potential benefits of differentiated nursing practice include effective deployment of nursing staff into emerging new roles, shared governance that facilitates staff nurse involvement in the clinical decision-making process, and increased clinical management skills, resulting in integration and continuity of care and substantial cost savings.*

Aspects of Differentiated Practice**

The *differentiated practice model* is a system designed to provide distinct levels of nursing practice based on defined competencies that are incorporated into job descriptions. General guidelines for the concept are as follows:

- Current registered nurse (RN) practice will be the minimum level at which differentiation of RN competencies will be established.
- Competencies will be consistent with the minimum expectations for the associate degree (ADN) and baccalaureate degree (BSN) levels in the education sector.
- Nurse satisfaction will improve, and thus so will retention, because the authority, responsibility, and accountability for the planning and provision of high-quality, cost-effective nursing care is placed at the staff nurse level.

- Differentiated competencies will be time- and setting-free and will be applicable to nursing practice in any setting.
- Differentiated levels of practice will, in the future, be supported by separate licensure laws and regulatory requirements.

The differentiated competencies for the registered nurse (ADN and BSN) can be developed based on the principles of differentiated educational preparation. The competencies of the currently practicing licensed practical nurse can be defined and presented in the same format as the ADN and BSN competencies.

The differentiated practice model displayed in Figure 14–4 shows the three major and three minor role components of nursing practice. The three major components—provision of direct care, communication, and management of care—make up the model, and their intersections form the three subcomponents. Direct client care intersects with communication to form patient teaching. Communication intersects with management of care to form coordination with other disciplines. Management of care intersects with direct care to form delegation of care. As shown by the placement of the ADN and BSN circles, the complexity of decision making in the nursing process is the basis for the differentiated levels of practice.

Once the scope of competencies is delineated, the levels of practice, as differentiated by complexity of client, timelines, and structure of the setting in reference to the nursing actions described in the competencies, can then be quantified and documented in the form of competency-based job descriptions specific to each institution or agency.

Nurse Extender Concept*

The nurse extender concept, as a complement to primary care nursing, has become popular since 1985. The nurse extender and technicians model became popular because health care fa-

*Source: Virginia Del Togno-Armanasco, Susan Harter, and Nannette L. Goddard, "Cost and Quality: Are They Compatible?" in The Encyclopedia of Nursing Care Quality Volume I: Issues and Strategies for Nursing Care Quality, Patricia Schroeder, ed., Aspen Publishers, Inc., © 1991.

**Source: Judy Blauwet and Patty Bolger, "Differentiated Practice in an Acute Care Setting," in Patient Care Delivery Models, Gloria Gilbert Mayer, Mary Jane Madden, and Eunice Lawrenz, eds., Aspen Publishers, Inc., © 1990.

*Source: Sally Knox, Jan Gharrity, and Brydie Baker, "The Successful Utilization of Nonlicensed Assistive Staff in a Critical Care Area," Critical Care Nursing Quarterly, Vol. 18:3, Aspen Publishers, Inc., © November 1995.

Figure 14–4 Model for Differentiated Practice Roles

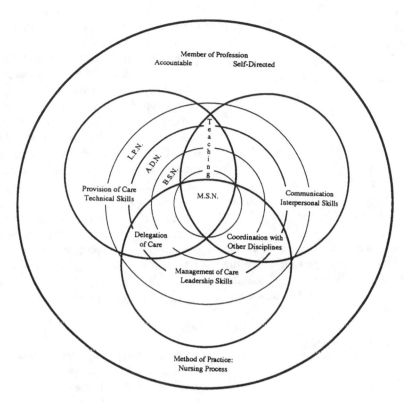

Source: Associate Degree Nursing; Facilitating Competency Development. Copyright by Midwest Alliance in Nursing and W.K. Kellogg Foundation. Reprinted with permission.

cilities experienced difficulty in finding a sufficient supply of registered nurses for primary nursing staff. In the 1990s, assistive/supportive nurse extenders continue to be used because of the need for cost-effectiveness and the need to focus the activities of the professional nurse on the more complex, unpredictable, and critical elements of care that are most related to positive outcomes, compliance with desired processes, and patient satisfaction.

The cost perspective of the assistive/support role is salient to the operational criteria for success in critical care areas. The *nurse extender, partners in practice,* or *assistive/support role* offers opportunities to modify the traditional 100 percent RN staffing based on careful scrutiny of patient needs.

A project designed to create a new assistive/ supportive role in a nursing unit must give spe-

cific consideration to several factors that are primary to successful implementation. These factors can serve as a checklist of questions to ask in the early conceptualization and actual development of the new role. Several of these factors and related questions have relevance for any area in which such a program might be implemented. The salient factors for consideration in designing the assistive/supportive role are

- acuity of patient care needs
- safety factors in care processes and the patient care environment
- actual savings with the change
- additional responsibilities for registered nurses with nonlicensed staff
- specific task and intervention responsibilities for which the registered nurse has relief

- actual cost of care per unit/trends in costs over the past few years
- integration of the assistive/supportive staff into a professional practice model
- alteration in the practice model to accommodate the assistive/supportive staff
- alteration in the role of the practicing nurse to accommodate the assistive/supportive staff
- relationship of the change to the management/governance structure
- philosophy and values of patient care and management within the organization, the nursing organization, and the unit

These and other factors as determined by the specific organization and the unit for which the newly defined roles are being created may be used as a basis for discussion and formulation.

NURSING CARE PROCESS

Components*

Following is a brief outline of the components of the nursing process: assessment, planning, implementation, and evaluation. (See Figure 14–5.)

Assessment

The assessment component begins with the nursing history and health assessment and ends with a nursing diagnosis. The purpose of assessment is to identify and obtain data about the client that will enable the nurse and/or client or family to designate problems relating to the client's wellness and illness. If problems exist, then the first step toward solving them is to identify them. The nurse becomes involved with basic human needs that affect the total person rather than one aspect of that person, one problem, or a limited segment of need fulfillment. The nurse

validates, organizes, categorizes, compares, analyzes, and synthesizes the data obtained about the client and makes one or more judgments based on these data. Either no problem exists that demands the intervention of the nurse or another member of the health team, or the precise identification is made of all problems (nursing diagnoses) that need to be resolved so that the client can experience optimum wellness. Problems are stated in terms of client problems and result when basic human needs are either not met or are met inadequately. Making a nursing diagnosis requires a high level of intellectual skill. It is a most strategic aspect of the nursing process and concludes the assessment component. Without a nursing diagnosis there is no reason to continue on into other components of the process. (See Table 14–6.) There will be no basis for planning or intervention nor any basis for evaluative judgments about the client's problems.

Planning

The planning component begins with the nursing diagnosis. It is during this component that plans are made with the client to deal with his or her problems as diagnosed. The four purposes of this component are (1) to assign priority to

---

Figure 14–5 The Nursing Process

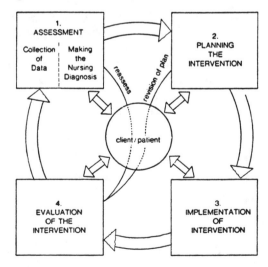

Source: Phyllis E. Jones, "A Terminology for Nursing Diagnoses," *Advances in Nursing Science*, Vol. 2, No. 1, Aspen Publishers, Inc., © 1979.

Source: Reprinted with permission from H. Yura, "Climate to Foster Utilization of the Nursing Process," *Providing a Climate for Utilization of Nursing Personnel*, © 1975, National League for Nursing.

Table 14–6 Aspects of the Nursing Care Process

Nursing Diagnosis	Nurse-Initiated Treatments and Interventions
• Assists in organizing, defining, and developing nursing knowledge • Aids in identifying and describing the domain and scope of nursing practice • Focuses nursing care on the patient's responses to problems • Prescribes diagnosis-specific nursing interventions that should increase the effectiveness of nursing care • Facilitates the evaluation of nursing practice • Provides a framework for testing the validity of nursing interventions • Provides a framework for developing a system to direct third-party reimbursements for nursing services	• Observing, assessing, and monitoring patient condition • Providing comfort measures in pain and in positioning • Monitoring and assisting in problems related to physiologic functions of hydration, nutrition, respiration, and elimination • Assisting, giving direction, or supervising activities of daily living • Teaching and counseling • Instructing and performing actions to prevent infection, injury, or complications of the disease process • Providing emotional support • Providing a therapeutic milieu • Referring to appropriate resources and, when appropriate, instructing the patient in how to access and use resources

Source: Charold L. Baer, "Nursing Diagnosis: A Futuristic Process for Nursing Practice," *Topics in Clinical Nursing*, Vol. 5, No. 4, Aspen Publishers, Inc., © 1984.

the problems diagnosed; (2) to differentiate problems that could be handled by the client and/or members of the family and those that need to be referred to other members of the health team or handled in conjunction with health team members; (3) to designate specific actions and the immediate, intermediate, and long-term goals of these actions, as well as expected behavioral outcomes for the client; and (4) to write the problems, actions, and expected outcomes on the nursing care plan or the problem-oriented client record. The planning phase terminates with the development of the nursing care plan, which is the blueprint for action, providing direction for implementing the plan and providing the framework for evaluation. This phase draws heavily on the intellectual and interpersonal skills of the nurse.

Implementation

Once the nursing care plan has been developed, the implementation component begins. Depending on the nature of the problem and the condition, ability and resources of the client, as well as the nature of the action planned, the client or family, the nurse and client, the nurse alone, or nursing team members who are to act or function under the nurse's supervision may be designated to implement the nursing plan. Implementation may be accomplished by the nurse, assisted by nursing team members or in cooperation with health team members. Any one or a combination of or all of these situations may prevail; in any one situation, some planned actions may be accomplished by the client, some by the nurse, and others by nursing team members. The implementation component of the nursing process draws heavily on the intellectual, interpersonal, and technical skills of the nurse. Decision making, observation, and communication are significant skills to enhance the success of action. While the focus is action, action is intellectual, interpersonal, and technical in nature.

During the implementation phase, the viability of the nursing care plan is tested. The phase concludes when the nurse's actions are completed and the results of these actions and the client's reaction to them are recorded. The quality of the recording about the client and what the nurse chooses to document give direct evidence of the status of goal achievement and individual client reactions. The recording designates the status of and the direction for continued problem solving. The appropriateness and direction of the nurse's actions are determined by the client's behavioral change in the direction of expected behavioral outcome.

Evaluation

Evaluation, the fourth component of the nursing process, follows the implementation of designated actions. Evaluation is always expressed in terms of achieving expected behavioral manifestations within the client. Since specific nurse actions are planned to solve client problems, any judgment about how these problems are being resolved should originate with the client. Evaluation is the natural intellectual activity completing the process components because it indicates the degree to which the nursing diagnosis and nursing actions have been correct. The entire focus of the nursing process is goal directed. The process is systematically geared to solve diagnosed client problems: Specific nurse actions are prescribed that will most successfully induce a specific behavioral effect that will denote that the client's problems have been resolved. Evaluation helps the nurse and the client to determine which problems have been resolved and which need to be reprocessed (including reassessment, replanning, and implementation), and evaluation helps them to diagnose any new problems. The need for nursing research is inherent in the nursing process to test strategies and their effectiveness in bringing about the expected behavioral changes in the client, accounting for the influencing variables related to the client's individuality.

NURSING DIAGNOSIS*

A nursing assessment should focus on the chief complaint of a patient, any actual or po-

tential life-threatening problems, the primary medical diagnosis, or the immediate care needs mentioned on the typed plan of care provided in a particular setting. The *nursing assessment* contains physical, psychosocial, environmental, functional, learning needs, and health care management information regarding a patient during an episode of illness or injury.

Collection of ongoing assessment data can focus on particular problem areas based on the actual and potential health care problems a patient is exhibiting at the time of assessment.

- An *actual health problem* is a current problem that exists at the time of assessment.
- A *potential health problem* is a possible complication of an existing health problem that is not yet an actual problem.

Data are collected from a patient's previous health record, current health history, physical examination, and test results, and from interviews with the patient, family, and caregivers.

An initial assessment is documented when a patient is admitted for care at a health care organization. Since assessment is ongoing, information will be added to a patient record as more data are collected. A nurse will gather and document more information as the nurse-patient relationship develops, as contact with the patient increases over a period of time, and as new needs and problems arise. Depending on an organization's documentation procedure, a nurse will record information on a reassessment form, ongoing assessment flowsheet, or in nursing progress notes.

In determining what to assess, a nurse should note

- patient health care needs, problems, and complaints
- potential complications related to physical condition or psychological state
- learning needs
- pertinent factors to consider for discharge planning

Assessment data can be multidimensional due to the holistic nature and needs of a patient and

*Source: Adapted from Ellen Thomas Eggland, *Nursing Documentation Resource Guide*, Aspen Publishers, Inc., © 1993.

Purpose of Assessments

An assessment is used as a core of information to determine

- the patient's actual and potential health care problems
- patient resources to manage care after discharge
- eligibility for care, particularly in third-party reimbursement programs
- factors related to legal protection or liability
- patient acuity

---

family. Data can be gathered in relation to the following general areas:

- physical status
- psychosocial status
- family relationships and caregiving
- cultural influence
- environmental aspects
- functional capabilities
- patient priority of needs
- patient/family expectations of health care services

Family relationships and caregiving capability/willingness and resources are also assessed because determining learning needs and making discharge plans begin at admission to a health care organization.

Assessment Models

Nursing assessment formats can be a framework of general multidimensional areas focused on health care problems, body systems, and functional abilities oriented to a particular health care setting, type of patient, or high risk for injury.

Assessment forms include similar content, although they come in a wide variety of formats. Content can be clustered differentially, however,

depending on a model used to categorize data to be collected.

Traditionally, health care organizations determine their format according to specific needs of patients they service or to documentation they wish to capture. While the most frequently used model is still the medical model, some organizations are revising their assessment forms according to Gordon's Functional Health Patterns model or North American Nursing Diagnosis Association (NANDA) taxonomy. These classification systems for nursing diagnoses, when applied to an assessment, create a logical, consistent framework for data to flow easily from assessment to care plan. (See Table 14–7.)

Almost every health care organization has a slightly different format for documenting an assessment. In any format, however, there are usually two components: a nursing history and a physical examination. Some organizations have separate history and physical forms; others combine a history and brief physical into a single assessment form. Some health care organizations give a different name to their assessment form. An assessment form is sometimes called an (nursing) admission form, a database, or an initial (nursing) assessment.

DOCUMENTATION OF CARE AND OUTCOMES: THE CARE PLAN

Nursing diagnoses and resultant interventions are integral to the practice of nursing. Based on the exercise of the nurse's professional judgment, a nurse clinically assesses a patient, derives a nursing diagnosis, and determines the appropriate intervention. Documentation in the patient's record should reflect delivery of this nursing process. In a subsequent action for medical malpractice, the court and the jury will review the patient's records and, as stated, could also review the health care facility's established standards.*

Source: Edna M. Koch, "Legal Implications of Standards," in *The Encyclopedia of Nursing Care Quality Volume II: Approaches to Nursing Standards*, Patricia Schroeder, ed., Aspen Publishers, Inc., © 1991.

Table 14–7 Chart of Assessment Models

Body System Model	Gordon's Functional Health Patterns	NANDA Taxonomy
EENT (Ears, eyes, nose, throat)	Health perception-health management	Exchanging
Respiratory	Nutritional-metabolic	Communicating
Circulatory	Elimination	Relating
Gastrointestinal	Activity-exercise	Valuing
Neurological	Sleep-rest	Choosing
Urological	Cognitive perceptual	Moving
Musculoskeletal	Self-perception Self-concept	Perceiving
Reproductive	Role-relationship	Knowing
Integumentary	Sexuality-reproductive Coping-stress tolerance Value-belief	Feeling

Source: Ellen Thomas Eggland, *Nursing Documentation Resource Guide*, Aspen Publishers, Inc., © 1993.

Purposes of Patient Care Documentation

- Communicates vital information about a patient's health status to other health care providers
- Acts as a basis for planning and continuity of care
- Serves as the primary source of information for monitoring and evaluating the quality of patient care rendered
- Provides information for utilization review and reimbursement decisions
- Identifies training needs
- Serves as a resource for research and education
- Serves as a business and legal document
- Provides substantive evidence on whether care rendered met the legal standard of care
- Memorializes informed consent to treatment and patient wishes regarding life-sustaining measures in the event of a patient's incapacitation ("advance directives")

Source: Ronald W. Scott, *Legal Aspects of Documenting Patient Care*, Aspen Publishers, Inc., © 1994.

Standardized Care Plans*

Standardized care plans that are individualized for a patient and used uniformly and completely by the nursing personnel are an enhancement to the quality of patient care and to the defensibility of a case in the event of medical malpractice litigation. In the busy atmosphere of a health care facility, standardized care plans provide pre–thought-out and developed approaches that assist the nurse in providing quality patient care. The plans serve as a forced checklist for assessing, evaluating, and intervening to alleviate a patient's problem, to maintain a certain health level, or to promote a desired patient outcome. A structured, systematic implementation of the nursing care process evolves as the nurse complies with the institution's individualized patient care plans.

*Source: Edna M. Koch, "Legal Implications of Standards," in *The Encyclopedia of Nursing Care Quality Volume II: Approaches to Nursing Standards*, Patricia Schroeder, ed., Aspen Publishers, Inc., © 1991.

New Directions: Documenting Care without a Care Plan

The traditional nursing care plan for the patient was intended to help organize and facilitate the documentation of that care. But since the Joint Commission on Accreditation of Healthcare Organizations no longer mandates a separate care plan as such for accreditation, health care organizations are seeking effective ways to include planned care in documentation without a separate care plan. Some innovative uses of documentation tools and formats have resulted, thus facilitating the documentation of the patient's actual status, interventions, and responses to that care.

Guidelines. Guidelines address a nursing diagnosis or a nursing management problem. Specifics of planned care are documented on the guidelines.

A nursing order flowsheet (which can be called a guideline flowsheet) is used to list guidelines for a particular patient. For example, a patient with a pressure ulcer could have the following guidelines documented on the nursing order flowsheet: Follow pressure ulcer guideline, follow infection control guideline, follow pain management guideline. A guideline flowsheet with columns for dates can also be used by nurses to document the fact that guidelines were followed on specific dates and shifts.

Protocols. Protocols for interdisciplinary care can be used in the same manner as guidelines. An interdisciplinary order flowsheet, called a protocol flowsheet, can be used to list protocols to be followed for a particular patient.

PIE progress notes. Problem, intervention, and evaluation (PIE) notes incorporate planned care into daily nursing notes. After an assessment is documented, a problem list of four to five problems is documented. Nursing progress notes are documented in a PIE format. Each nursing diagnosis intervention is documented in nursing notes in categories of problem, intervention, and evaluation. A 1, 2, 3, 4, or 5 before the P, I, or E indicates what problem is the topic of the entry. For example, Problem 1 listed on a problem list is

"Impaired thermoregulation," and IPE indicates an evaluation or patient outcome of interventions for the problem of impaired thermoregulation. Planned care is implied in the intervention portion of the PIE progress note. Planned care can be supported by policy and procedure manuals on standards of care for patients with specific diagnoses. Standards of care are general principles or statements on nursing care.

Problem-Oriented Record with SOAP-IER Progress Notes. A problem list is documented after admission assessment, and daily nursing notes include topics of clinical data categorized as (S)ubjective data and (O)bjective data; nursing intervention categorized in (A)ssessment and (P)lan, (I)ntervention, (E)valuation, and (R)evision. Planned care is implied in the plan portion of the SOAP-IER note. Planned care can be supported by policy and procedure manuals on standards of care for patients with specific diagnoses.

Case Management Critical Paths. Critical paths are protocols with timelines indicated to present a definite plan for care on specific days or visits of care. For example, on postoperative day (POD) 3, nurse will instruct patient in self-administration of IV analgesia (a planned intervention), and on POD 5 patient will state pain is at or below level 5 on a 0 to 10 scale (a patient outcome). Planned care is evidenced on the case management guideline that presents standards of care for a procedure or diagnosis; daily activities with expected time frames are concisely documented on a critical path. (See the next section for a more detailed discussion.)

Charting by Exception. This documentation system focuses on documentation of abnormal conditions. Guidelines or standards of care can represent planned care, and SOAP-IER notes reflect ongoing care planning.

Focus Charting. Focus charting can include a separate initial care plan, or a focus list; ongoing planned care is shown in the nursing notes categorized (D)ata, (A)ction, (R)esponse. Planned action is implied in the action phase of the nursing progress note. Patient outcomes are shown in the response.

Nursing Intervention List. Based on the Nursing Interventions Classification (NIC)

scheme, this list can be documented on a flowsheet to indicate planned care; it can be checked off or initialed to indicate care given. One intervention label in this scheme can represent as many as 30 related nursing activities that together compose the intervention. Policy and procedure in the health care organization will establish if and how specific nursing activities need to be defined and documented as a component of the nursing intervention.

Case Management Plans: Integrating Pathways into Documentation Systems

Some health care organizations are introducing and incorporating critical pathways into their documentation systems, replacing the care plan or sometimes replacing the nursing notes. In addition, many health care facilities are developing their critical pathways to include multidisciplinary interventions and outcomes so that the entire course of treatment for a patient can be predetermined at admission and can be coordinated to control costs.

Health care organizations coordinate the critical pathway into their documentation system in various ways. Some administrators refer to standard guidelines or protocols or standing orders as pathways. The critical pathway can replace care plans or can be used in conjunction with care plans. The critical pathway can replace the care plan when the format allows enough room to make revisions for individualizing patient care and enough detail can be added to clarify interventions and outcomes.

When critical pathways are used instead of the care plan, care plan revisions can be made by circling the intervention that was not performed or short-term outcome that was not achieved and writing that intervention or outcome in the appropriate box within the format's time frame (day, shift, or hour). The variance explaining why the element was not accomplished and plans to resolve the problem are written on the variance report, which can be included with the care plan or can be used to replace progress notes.

There are a number of ways to accomplish this integration or replacement of notes:

- variance charting by charting by exception (CBE)
- variance charting by problem-oriented progress notes
- variance charting by Focus notes (DAR)
- daily documentation by flowsheet

Daily documentation by flowsheet may also include elements from the critical pathway on the flowsheet. Or the critical pathway itself can be in a flowsheet format for documentation normally written on nursing notes.

Critical Pathway Use for the Multidisciplinary Team. Since development of the pathway is done by multidisciplinary teams, the monitoring of care is a shared responsibility of the entire team. An individual primary nurse or nurse manager can be the key evaluator, but all are monitor participants. Team monitoring is facilitated and most effective when the critical pathway is incorporated into medical or interdisciplinary (health team) rounds, nursing rounds, and shift reports. Interventions completed and current outcomes achieved give an immediate report of where the patient is in the timeline and progress toward discharge from service. It is especially helpful during these reports to discuss concurrent variances and what is planned or being implemented to resolve the variance and get the patient back on track.

Systematic Evaluation of Case Management Plans*

Evaluating the effectiveness of critical path and case management plans is as important as their development and implementation. Data collection and analysis are imperative in any process used to demonstrate the effectiveness of case management plans. The accumulated variations from any plan then can be analyzed and used to improve the systems and processes around patient care.

Source: Hussein A. Tahan, "Evaluating the Effectiveness of Care Management Plans," *Journal of Nursing Administration*, Vol. 25, No. 9, September 1995, J.B. Lippincott.

Table 14–8 Checklist Review—Does the Documentation Reflect the Nursing Process?

ASSESSMENT

____ The nursing history and physical assessment are completed within 24 hours of patient admission to service.

____ The nursing history and physical assessment are completed by a registered nurse.

____ Data for inclusion in the history and assessment are taken from the patient/family interview and the patient's previous medical record.

____ The nursing history and physical assessment should include information on the following topics:

___ patient's chief complaint

___ patient's primary and secondary medical diagnoses

___ past major illnesses and surgeries

___ caregiver support if patient unable to give self-care and perform activities of daily living independently

___ learning needs and identified barriers to learning

___ environment and safety needs

___ psychosocial needs

___ current medications and treatments discharge planning

PLANNING

____ Problems for planned intervention are identified and supported in the nursing assessment.

____ The plan of care is reviewed and updated every seven days (or more often as needed).

____ The plan of care reflects the status of weekly goals.

____ The patient is involved in and agrees with the plan of care.

INTERVENTION

____ Responses to nursing interventions ordered on care plan are documented in nursing notes.

____ Documentation reflects patient's response to therapy, medication, procedures, and other nursing interventions.

____ Resolved problems on care plan are substantiated in nurses' notes.

____ Documentation of patient response to teaching efforts appears in nurses' notes.

EVALUATION

____ Discharge summary is completed on discharge.

____ Discharge summary reflects patient condition and patient progress toward goals.

____ Discharge summary reflects unmet needs with reasons and subsequent referrals for further care.

____ Documentation indicates the patient/caregiver has learned skills and rationale for care and is able to provide care.

Source: Ellen Thomas Eggland, *Nursing Documentation Resource Guide*, Aspen Publishers, Inc., © 1993.

Variance Analysis

A variance is defined as anything that is not achieved within the predetermined time frame on the case management plan, such as any patient care activity or outcome that is not performed or achieved as preplanned or expected. Variances can be identified either on admission or during the health care facility stay.

Variance data are of two types. The *first type* includes deviations from the case management plan. This kind of variance occurs when a pa-

tient care activity is not performed by the health care provider, as specified on the case management plan. To be considered a variance (deviation), the activity is purposely (intentionally) canceled, omitted, or delayed. The *second type* of variance data involves issues associated with achieving the expected outcomes of care. This kind of variance occurs when an expected outcome of care is not met for whatever reason. This variance usually results in altering the sequence of patient care activities on the case management plan to meet the expected outcome.

Figure 14–6 Steps in Developing Critical Pathways: Nursing Care

1. Identify patient population (case type).

    ↓

2. Recruit consultants.

    ↓

3. Collaborate with physicians.

    ↓

4. Collect data:
    - LOS
    - nursing diagnoses
    - patient-centered outcomes
    - critical events
    - sequencing of critical events

    ↓

5. Incorporate data into critical pathway format.

    ↓

6. Submit draft of critical pathway to consultants for review.

    ↓

7. Revise critical pathway until accepted by all consultants.

    ↓

8. Present critical pathway to appropriate committee for content and format approval.

    ↓

9. Incorporate any committee-mandated changes to final product.

    ↓

10. Pilot new critical pathway for three months.

Source: Laura E. Ferguson, "Steps to Developing a Critical Pathway," *Nursing Administration Quarterly*, Vol. 17, No. 3, Aspen Publishers, Inc., © Spring 1993.

Table 14–9 Examples of Variance

Operational Variance
- Machine breakdown
- Delay in test or procedure
- Lost laboratory requisition or specimen
- No rehabilitation technician on weekends

Community Variance
- No nursing home bed available
- No visiting nurse service available
- No family available to accompany the patient on discharge
- Wheelchair cannot be delivered home until four days after discharge

Practitioner Variance
- Ordering unnecessary test or procedure
- Medication error
- No consent obtained
- Omission of a test or procedure

Patient Variance
- Test refusal
- Change in condition
- Patient allergy
- Sign out against medical advice

Variance Based on Care Activity. Deviations from the case management plans due to delays can be classified by cause into operational, community, practitioner, or patient variances (see Table 14–9).

Variances in care are evaluated based on the time frames used in the case management plan. These time frames are studied closely while developing a case management plan and are based on the clinical area or service. For example, an emergency department case management plan is developed based on time frames of minutes, which means that treatments or activities are rendered within time intervals of minutes. If a treatment is not provided within the time frame specified on the plan, it is considered a variance. Every time an activity is not accomplished during the time frame specified on the case management plan, it is considered a negative variance.

Most of the time, negative variances result in a delay in the care and an increase in length of stay. They are best prevented through better management of care. If a patient's recovery progresses faster than the plan specifies or if a desired outcome is achieved before it is expected to happen, it is considered a positive variance.

Variances Based on Outcomes of Care. Clinical quality indicators usually identify the expected outcomes of care. By indicating these prospectively, quality is identified and maintained. These outcomes are either intermediate or discharge indicators.

Intermediate patient outcomes are triggerpoints or milestones established on the case management plan to alert the health care provider to implement certain actions. They are intended to denote a needed change in the course of care or therapy. These outcomes are to be achieved during the patient's stay.

Discharge patient outcomes, on the other hand, are the preestablished criteria for discharge. These outcomes should always be met before or at the time of discharge. They are developed based on the patient's diagnosis or reason for admission to the health care facility.

Variances are documented daily as they occur. Variances related to outcome indicators are classified as unmet clinical indicators or outcomes. Variance analysis and trending of the data collected are invaluable in determining the reason(s) an expected patient outcome or clinical quality indicator has not been met.

Evaluation of the intermediate indicators and instituting the necessary changes to meet these indicators help ensure that the patient is progressing toward the desired outcomes in a timely fashion. Whenever a problem or a variance is identified, that is, when a desired outcome is not met, the nurse case manager will determine why the problem arose and try to correct it. He or she may institute some changes in the case management plan that are thought to impact positively on the patient's condition, and correct the problem.

Using an Outcomes Management System

An outcomes management system is one means by which to demonstrate the effectiveness of care. Before the implementation of any outcomes management system, it is important to define the goals. Some of these goals as they relate to case management are:

* to determine if health care providers follow the case management plans consistently
* to determine if the planned results (expected outcomes) are met
* to identify the problems in the processes that need to be changed or revised if planned results are not met
* to analyze and trend the data and design a mechanism for feedback and corrective actions

This approach to outcomes management systems consists of four core components.

1. Tool Development. Data collection tools should be developed before starting the data collection process. Tools help focus on the type of data to be collected, streamline the process, and should be designed in a way that meets the goals of the outcomes management system.

2. Outcomes Measurement. Outcomes measurement is defined as the systematic quantitative observation of variances and outcome indicators, at one point in time, using the data collection tools that are developed based on the case management plan. This approach provides a one-time assessment of the provision and outcome of patient care. It also provides nursing administrators with a mechanism for identifying any gaps in patient care and deficient areas or areas of nonconformity with the standards of care that are established by regulatory agencies. Outcomes measurement also may serve as a baseline assessment of patient care that is an essential step when developing action plans for improving patient care processes and care outcomes.

3. Outcomes Monitoring. Outcomes monitoring is the ongoing/repeated measurement of variances and outcome indicators, with close attention to what might have caused the observed outcomes. The care processes should be studied very carefully so that inferential causes can be determined. Assessment, reassessment, and evaluation of patient care processes are necessary every time that action plans for improving patient care delivery are constructed. Outcomes monitoring usually provides nursing and health care administrators with the data needed to examine what is working of the recommended action plans. It also helps administrators make better decisions when evaluating the impact of these action plans on patient care activities and processes.

4. Outcomes Management. Outcomes management is the analysis and trending of the information collected through outcomes measurement and monitoring. Decision making is done, based on the analysis, to improve the effectiveness of the case management plans and the quality of care. Data obtained can be used in a quality improvement framework.

Data can be brought back to administration for administrative intervention or to the attention of the multidisciplinary team that developed the case management plan. Providing feedback to all the key personnel involved in the provision of care is an important factor in the success of outcomes management.

Chapter 15

Patient-Centered Care and Relations

THE PATIENT AS CUSTOMER

There is little argument that in health care today, the patient is the primary customer in a complex web of interrelationships. It is commonly affirmed that health care must be of the highest quality, as perceived by the patient and the provider, that the opinions of the patient are important, and that serving the patient is the primary focus of the organization. Whatever "quality" means to consumers, their perceptions of quality affect their choices among health care alternatives (see Table 15–1). Word-of-mouth recommendations are the most important marketing influence on health care buying decisions.

Customer commitment to the organization can be built by creating an environment where the needs of patients are understood, where mistakes are recognized or anticipated and prevented, where all errors or complaints are treated as useful sources of knowledge, and where mistakes are redressed sufficiently well to recover customer confidence. On the other hand, disappointing patients can be extremely costly. For example, the estimated cost to a health care facility of recapturing a dissatisfied customer, in terms of future encounters over that customer's lifetime and word-of-mouth effects, can range from a conservative estimate of $8,000 per patient to a less conservative estimate of approximately

$400,000. Even the most conservative cost estimates of losing a patient through dissatisfaction make managing customer loyalty and expectations an essential part of the management process.*

Assessing Congruence of Nursing Practice with Consumer Expectations**

Patient satisfaction depends on the extent to which there is a match between consumer expectations and the reality of nursing practice (see Table 15–2). The nurse manager can take action to assess unit congruence with consumer expectations.

Step 1: Assess Unit Values and Behavioral Norms. Discussing incidents with unit personnel will allow the nurse manager to analyze common elements of patient dissatisfaction. What types of patient expectations are not being met? The nurse manager also must determine how patient conflict is handled by the unit staff. Does

---

*Source: Kate Macintyre and Carolyn Cable Kleman, "Measuring Customer Satisfaction," Curtis P. McLaughlin and Arnold D. Kaluzny, eds., in *Continuous Quality Improvement in Health Care*, Aspen Publishers, Inc., © 1994.

**Source: Diane Greeneich, "Developing a Consumer-Focused Unit Culture," *Aspen's Advisor for Nurse Executives*, Vol. 9:7, Aspen Publishers, Inc., © April 1994.

Table 15–1 Expectation for Health Care Services: The Consumer's Point of View

- Consideration of the *total being* of the consumer
- Significant improvement in communications between care providers and consumers
- Health care professionals as models for health
- A focus on health promotion and health education
- Health care professionals as collaborators—comfortable with shared leadership for consumer health benefits
- Affordable health care

Source: Helen Yura-Petro and Brenda R. Scanelli, "The Education of Health Care Professionals in the Year 2000 and Beyond: Part I: The Consumer's View," *Health Care Supervisor*, Vol. 10, No. 3, Aspen Publishers, Inc., © March 1992.

Table 15–2 Consumer Satisfaction with Nursing Care

Factors That Influence the Consumer's Satisfaction with Nursing Care

- *Nursing personality characteristics:* sensitivity, friendliness, social courtesy, helpfulness, and kindness
- *Nurse caring behaviors:* empathy, compassion, communication, and comfort measures
- *Nursing proficiency:* nursing knowledge, demonstrated technical proficiency, and organizational skills

Factors over Which Nurses Have a Degree of Control

- Organizational environment
- Nursing service: staffing, visiting policies, control over practice
- Physical environment: noise level, lighting, food service, and housekeeping

These factors are important to the patient's level of contentment as well.

the unit culture support the intervention of the charge nurse as the only way to manage patient dissatisfaction, or are all the nurses given autonomy in managing such incidents?

Step 2: Analyze Information for Patterns. Quality-of-care values focus on concern for the patient, solving the problem, and preventing future similar incidents. An individual unit's interpretation of what constitutes quality care may be specialty specific.

A speedy response to complaints is the key to patient satisfaction. Behaviors displayed by unit staff in responding to patient dissatisfaction reflect unit rules for interpreting and handling patient complaints. For example, timeliness of response is tied to the group's perception of the expected level of performance. Are patient complaints construed as necessitating immediate intervention, or are they addressed only if the caregivers have time? Does the speed of the intervention depend on the type of patient satisfaction issue?

Step 3: Identify Behaviors That Reflect or Do Not Reflect a Consumer-Focused Unit Culture. The unit culture influences how caregivers interact with patients by establishing unit norms of behavior. Caring, communication, and walk-

ing that extra mile to accommodate patient requests are consumer-focused characteristics. Avoidance, abruptness, or lack of empathy reflect limited value for the customer. Social courtesy and explanation during incidents of angry patient behavior or family dissatisfaction also reflect a positive customer orientation.

How the staff describe their perceptions of the outcomes of incidents of patient dissatisfaction tells a lot about the priorities of the unit. Outcomes that reflect nursing standards for what should and ought to be done for the patient advance nursing priorities over customer priorities. Unit staff priorities may override patient expectations when time constraints are put on certain patient actions, when limited patient choices are presented among viable care alternatives, and when the caregiver focuses on the task rather than the person. On the other hand, enhanced communication, timely problem solving, and the promotion of patient requests for education are key consumer-focused behaviors.

DATA ON PATIENT ATTITUDES

Survey research can be obtained through one of four common forms: (1) telephone interviews, (2) personal interviews, (3) focus groups, and (4) mail. Table 15–3 lists some of the trade-offs to consider in the use of the four survey research methods.

Distinctions Between Survey Methods*

Telephone interviews are a quick way to acquire information. Using multiple interviewers in a telephone interview bank, data can be acquired in a short time frame. When the questionnaire is short, trained interviewers can usually be successful in obtaining a high completion rate from respondents. Telephone interviewing also allows for the targeting of responses. Using qualifying questions, a telephone interviewer can target the profile of respondent desired.

Personal interviews consist of one-to-one interviewing between interviewer and respondent. An individual interview is a valuable way to collect data when the respondent must be probed regarding his or her answers. Personal interviews are the preferred method when the survey requires the presentation of visual cues or a product demonstration.

The *focus group* is a version of the personal interview conducted with a group of consumers simultaneously by a trained moderator following an interview guide. The focus group moderator is a trained professional who uses this guide to generate discussion among the group's members. Focus groups are often used early in the research process when the researcher is not sure of the correct or exact questions to ask in a survey. An analysis of the focus group response can reveal issues that the researcher should explore quantitatively to determine how extensive they are in the general population. Data from focus groups consist of transcripts of the discussions and often videotapes.

Mail surveys have the advantage of being a relatively inexpensive way to collect data. Typically, costs involve the reproduction of the survey and postage to send and return it. A major advantage of mail surveys is that they provide anonymity to the respondent. Mail is also an inexpensive, efficient way to contact individuals who are dispersed over a large geographic area. In health care, mail surveys have often been used to collect patient satisfaction data. Another advantage to mail surveys is the elimination of interviewer bias.

Using Patient Satisfaction Findings*

An important aspect of using patient satisfaction findings in practice is to reinforce positive staff behaviors. Personal and public recognition of nurses mentioned by patients reinforces these behaviors and, thus, increases patient and family satisfaction. For example, nurse managers could individually recognize the many staff nurses who were identified by patients and family members as providing outstanding care. The entire nursing staff could also be given recognition for the positive feedback that was received from patients related to pain management, or from family members in regard to family support group meetings. Accumulated data can be presented at the divisional quality improvement meeting so that nurse managers can share the results with their staff at unit meetings, in performance appraisals or newsletters, and on unit bulletin boards.

Negative comments, on the other hand, should also be analyzed and communicated with the nursing staff as a cue to identify opportunities to prevent similar problems in the future. Generalizing the complaint at staff meetings and addressing the issues and alternatives in a problem-solving manner may serve as a useful means to handle negative comments. For instance, the nurse man-

---

Source: Eric N. Berkowitz, *Essentials of Health Care Marketing*, Aspen Publishers, Inc., © 1996.

Source: Karen Megivern, Margo A. Halm, and Gerry Jones, "Measuring Patient Satisfaction as an Outcome of Nursing Care," *Journal of Nursing Care Quality*, Vol. 6:4, Aspen Publishers, Inc., © July 1992.

Table 15–3 Survey of Marketing Research Methodologies

Approach Criteria	Personal Interview	Telephone Survey	Mail Survey	Focus Groups
Economy	Most expensive.	Avoids interviewer travel, relatively expensive. Trained interviewers needed.	Potentially lowest costs (if response rate sufficient).	Relatively expensive.
Interviewer bias	High likelihood of bias. Trust. Appearance.	Less than personal interviewer. No face-to-face contact. Suspicion of phone call.	Interviewer bias eliminated. Anonymity provided.	Need trained moderator.
Flexibility	Most flexible method. Responses can be probed. Assistance can be provided in completing forms. Observations can be made.	Cannot make observations. Probing possible to a degree.	Least flexible method.	Very flexible.
Sampling and respondent cooperation	Most complete sample possible, with sufficient call-back strategy.	Limited to people with telephone. No answers. Refusals are common.	Mailing list problem. Nonresponse a major problem.	Need close selection.

Source: Reprinted from S.G. Hillestad and E.N. Berkowitz, *Health Care Marketing Plans: From Strategy to Action*, ed 2, Aspen Publishers, Inc., © 1991.

Table 15–4 Steps for Performing Content Analysis of Patient Comments

1. Identify a source of patient comments (e.g., letters to the administrator, responses to open-ended surveys).
2. Read the comments to obtain a sense of their scope and nature.
3. Identify and list the major themes, topics, and dimensions that are raised by the comments to ensure that there is no overlap and that each major theme is represented.
4. Read through the comments a second time and classify them according to the major themes.
5. Construct a histogram or Pareto chart to display the number of comments that are related to each major theme.
6. Identify the top-ranked themes and place them in the major subcategories (e.g., three or four) that appear most frequently within each theme.
7. Read through the comments in the top-ranked themes a third time and classify them by the subcategories represented by the comment.
8. Display the subcategory results in a histogram or Pareto chart, and summarize the results and lessons learned.

Source: Eugene Nelson, Chip Cauldwell, Doris Quinn, and Robin Rose, "Gaining Customer Knowledge: Obtaining and Using Customer Judgments for Hospitalwide Quality Improvement," *Topics in Health Record Management*, Vol. 11, No. 3, Aspen Publishers, Inc., © March 1991.

ager could open discussion on the noise or privacy issues identified by patients and families. Patient complaints can also be shared with particular nurses as a red flag to watch this type of situation more closely. Such sharing opens communication and facilitates constructive problem solving and decision making for the provision of higher quality nursing care.

Poor ratings on aspects of nursing care may indicate the need for patient teaching to encourage more realistic expectations and, thus, promote greater satisfaction with nursing care and overall satisfaction with health care. Nurses have a great opportunity to shape the patient's expectations given that these perceptions are often not well formed before hospitalization.

Patient satisfaction studies may also assist nurses in identification of areas of practice that warrant further investigation, as well as to justify changes in care delivery systems.

Measuring satisfaction after a planned change in clinical practice may help evaluate its effectiveness. As an outcome indicator, patient satisfaction measures can assist nurses to evaluate the effectiveness of other structure and process changes or improvements in nursing practice, such as unit and waiting room design, patient teaching, staffing patterns, visitation policies, and family-focused interventions such as support groups or volunteer programs.

PATIENTS AND DELIVERY OF CARE

Respecting the Rights of Patients*

Patients are persons with whom negotiations are required. When patients are treated as objects, there is no need for collateral relations; objects are to be manipulated and used. To say that such manipulations are carried out "for the patient's own good" is not enough to justify ignoring the personhood of the patient. The growing sensitivity of both patients and nursing staff to this problem is manifested in what is termed the Patient's Bill of Rights (see Table 15–5).

Source: Adapted from Barbara J. Stevens, *First-Line Patient Care Management*, Aspen Publishers, Inc., © 1983.

Communicating with Patients

Obtaining consent for treatment requires communicating at several levels. At *the first level*, it simply involves a choice between giving and withholding information from the patient. Sometimes a patient is not told that he or she has options. Many patients are bullied into accepting a given treatment without prior discussion.

At *the second level*, communication requires that the treatment be described in terms intelligible to the patient. Few patients are familiar with medical terminology, and the first-line manager must forsake terminology for simpler descriptive language. The first-line manager must go beyond clear description and make an effort to be sure that the patient understands what he or she is saying.

The *third level of communication* involves informing the patient of the full implications of a treatment choice. Knowledge of the implications may evoke an emotional response as well as a cognitive one. It is one thing for a patient to know that part of his or her mandible will be removed; it is another thing to know the impact of that surgery on his or her speech, ability to eat, and appearance. Nurses may shrink back from trying to communicate the full impact of treatment to patients, for conveying this information often requires the nurse to inflict pain. Yet patients and their families may feel deceived if the full impact of a treatment is not known prior to its inception.

Sharing the Nursing Process: Supporting a Patient-Provider Partnership

The role of the patient as recipient of care given by the provider can evolve into a partnership in which patients, as consumers, and care providers share responsibilities in the development of desired outcomes and implementation of appropriate interventions.

In the past, nurses and patients depended on physicians for direction and information about expectations. The physician as paternalistic benevolent director of patient care was rarely questioned. Consumers are now wiser, smarter, and more assertive. Information about health care

Table 15–5 Patients' Rights Regarding Treatment

THE BASIC RIGHTS

☐ The right to reasonable informed participation in decisions involving one's own health care

☐ The right to receive a clear, concise explanation of one's condition and of all proposed technical procedures, including
  – the possibilities of any risk of mortality or serious side effects
  – problems related to recuperation
  – the probability of success

☐ The right not to be subjected to any procedure without one's voluntary, competent, and understanding consent or the consent of one's legally authorized representative

☐ The right to be informed where medically significant alternatives for care or treatment exist

☐ The right to know who is responsible for authorizing and performing the procedures or treatment

☐ The right to be informed if the health care facility proposes to engage in or perform human experimentation or other research/educational projects that would affect one's care or treatment

☐ The right to refuse to participate in any such experimental activity

THE RIGHT TO REFUSAL OF TREATMENT (NONCONSENT)

☐ The patient may refuse treatment to the extent permitted by law.

☐ However, when refusal of treatment by the patient or his or her legally authorized representative prevents the provision of appropriate care in accordance with professional standards, the relationship with the patient may be terminated upon reasonable notice.

Source: Cheryl K. Smith, "Legal Review: Informed Consent—A Shift from Paternalism to Self-Determination?" *Topics in Health Record Management*, Vol. 11, No. 1, Aspen Publishers, Inc., © September 1990.

cost, quality, treatments, and options is readily available from newspapers, an assortment of magazines, television, and the much-touted information superhighway of computerdom. Patients question the rationale for interventions and cost of services. They come to the physician expecting help to achieve outcomes on which they have already decided and are not hesitant to exercise their right to a second opinion. The physician role has changed through education and consumer demand. Physicians have become increasingly collaborative, cooperative, and willing to share more information and decision-making responsibility with other health care disciplines and the patient. The patient has become the center of attention; meeting consumer-identified needs has become the focus of physician-directed care.

Using a Patient Partnership System*

At many health care facilities, the nurse is a care manager, responsible for implementation of the nursing process in the clinical setting. Patients are assessed by a registered nurse, outcomes are jointly planned, interventions to support the care plan are implemented, and evaluation of progress toward outcome achievement and patient response to interventions completes the cycle. However, to support and contribute toward a patient-partnership, one medical center has initiated the use of patient versions of standards of care (SOCs). The patient copy, entitled *Information about Your Plan of Care*, states in lay terms what the patient can anticipate and use as a measuring stick. It includes basic unit care standards (BUCS), what to expect during the health care facility stay, and continued care considerations. Also included are statements that describe what the health care team will do, responsibilities of the patient as an active participant in care planning, and expected outcomes. The patient information sheets are one part of the care planning process specifically designed to encourage and

Source: Donna Cramer and Susan M. Tucker, "The Consumer's Role in Quality: Partnering for Quality Outcomes," *Journal of Nursing Care Quality*, Vol. 9, No. 2, Aspen Publishers, Inc., © January 1995.

support patient-provider partnership in achievement of quality outcomes for patients.

The BUCS, which are generic SOCs that are applicable to all patients in each clinical service area, address the biophysical, psychosocial, environmental, educational, self-care, and discharge-planning needs of the patient population. The BUCS are the first step.

In additional to the BUCS, there are SOCs that have been developed for the top 40 diagnosis-related groups (DRGs). A patient learning checklist is part of the SOC but is a separate document with preprinted educational directives and knowledge that patients will need based on their diagnoses.

Care paths are also provided for some conditions that require special coordination among multiple interdisciplinary providers. They have been developed for condition-specific populations and lengths of stay and are time and outcome oriented. The patient is given a copy with lay terminology, and the format and sequence parallels that used by the health care provider team. The care paths show the patient and family the expected sequence of care activities.

The challenge was to find a customer-focused tool that would communicate expected outcomes, health team interventions, and patient responsibilities in a manner that would be easily understandable for the majority of patients as well as easy and convenient for use by nursing staff.

The concepts of BUCS and the care path patient version provided the foundation for the solution. Using the basic SOC format, a template was developed for the patient SOC information sheet that includes columns for "Patient Care Issues" (problem statements), "What We Will Do" (health team interventions), "What You Can Do" (patient responsibilities), and "Expectations" (outcomes). See Table 15–6.

The patient SOC information sheet facilitates patient and family participation in development and implementation of the plan of care. In this capacity, the information sheet is used as an educational tool to inform the patient and family about the diagnosis-specific expected course of care; what to expect in terms of patient care procedures; and what changes, signs, and symptoms they should report to the health care team. Second, it supports the concept of partnership by promotion of an interactive process in which the patient and health care providers jointly agree upon outcomes. The patient care team members work together to achieve or modify outcomes. Third, it supports a customer-service orientation by encouragement of open communication between the patient and health care team. Interventions are modified based on patient response; outcomes are adjusted based on patient input and desires.

Cooperative Care System*

Cooperative care is a method of delivering nursing care to patients who require hospitalization but not necessarily intensive, 24-hour-a-day nursing observation. A self-care philosophy, intensive patient education, and a wellness-oriented atmosphere are crucial to a cooperative care center's operation. Cooperative care centers require involvement of the patient and family as active participants in the care during the hospitalization. Nursing interventions are provided, but the patient maintains a more proactive role in seeking the assistance and guidance of health care professionals.

The cooperative care concept is grounded in self-care principles in the belief that patients wish to be active participants in their care. This assumption may or may not reflect reality. The patient's initial response may be one of "culture shock," since expectations regarding traditional hospital services are contradicted.

Second, the model assumes that individuals have the capacity to learn. Patient education is a primary therapeutic tool in the cooperative care system. Theoretically, those persons with mental disabilities, sensory deficits, and age limitations should be excluded from the center. Any patient who is alert, oriented, and clinically stable and has a care partner could conceivably be a candidate for this unit.

Source: Sandra W. Murabito, "Cooperative Care: A Common-Sense Approach for Patient Care Delivery Systems," in *Patient Care Delivery Models*, Gloria Gilbert Mayer, Mary Jane Madden, and Eunice Lawrenz, eds., Aspen Publishers, Inc., © 1990.

Table 15–6 Sample Patient Standard of Care Information Sheet

INFORMATION ABOUT YOUR PLAN OF CARE
Compromised Respiratory Status (BREATHING PROBLEMS)

---

1. We will make a plan of care to meet your basic care needs.
2. It is important that you and your family let us know about any questions or concerns.
3. We will provide a safe and clean environment.
4. We will help you understand your condition and treatments.
5. You will be asked to participate in your care.
6. We will help you plan for your continued care.

Patient Care Issues	What We Will Do	What You Can Do	Expectations
You need information about your condition.	Health care team members will provide you with information about your condition. We will tell you about treatments, medicines you receive, and follow-up care.	Please ask any questions about your treatment and follow-up care. Let us know if you do not understand something we say.	You will have information you need and want about your treatment plan.
What will happen to you during your stay?	We will take your temperature, pulse, and blood pressure as needed. We may need to wake you at night.		You will understand the treatments and activities you experience during your stay.
	We may weigh you every day and keep track of how much you eat and drink and how much you urinate.	Help us keep track of what you eat, drink, and urinate.	
	You may be on a special diet.	Ask us any questions you have about your diet.	
	We will give you medications as your physician orders. Most medicines are given by mouth or through a needle in one of your veins.	If you have a needle in your vein, tell the nurse right away if you feel any burning or discomfort when medicine is going through the needle or if you see any swelling around the needle.	

continues

Table 15–6 continued

Patient Care Issues	What We Will Do	What You Can Do	Expectations
You may have shortness of breath or feel extremely tired.	The physician may ask us to give you respiratory treatments, oxygen, and medicines to help your body get rid of extra fluid.	Let us know if your shortness of breath gets worse or you have chest pain.	Our goal is for you to become less short of breath and be able to resume your normal activity gradually without feeling tired.
You may experience discomfort.	We will ask you if you are having discomfort. We will give you medication for your discomfort as you request and as your physician has ordered.	If you start to have discomfort, tell the nurse before it becomes too severe. If you feel no relief 30 minutes after you have received medication, tell the nurse.	Your discomfort will be controlled or relieved at a level acceptable to you.
Planning for your continued care.	We will ask you about any special needs you have at home. We will give you written instructions about medications, diet, activity, and things you need to report to your physician. We will assist you to schedule your follow-up visits with your physician.	Tell us about any concerns or needs you have. Review the instructions we give you; ask about anything that is unclear before you leave. Follow instructions about diet closely. Take your medicines as directed. Avoid smoking, alcohol intake, and stressful situations.	You will be able to care for yourself at home and gradually increase your activity. You will know who to call for questions and concerns.

Source: Donna Cramer and Susan M. Tucker, "The Consumer's Role in Quality: Partnering for Quality Outcomes," *Journal of Nursing Care Quarterly*, Vol. 9, No. 2, Aspen Publishers, Inc., © January 1995.

Third, the model suggests that a homelike environment is therapeutic to a patient's convalescence. Through simulation of a more familiar atmosphere, the negative connotations of hospitalization are expected to decrease. This is achieved through room decor, provision of privacy, and reduction of restricted patient areas on the unit.

Evaluation. Drawbacks depend on the setting, implementation, and emphasis of each individual center. Perhaps the major drawback is the need for total project support from the unit level to the top ranks of administration. Lack of understanding or commitment at any level can sabotage efforts. Staff nurses must be able to communicate and practice within the model's assumptions and concepts. Nursing administrators are essential in providing support to the staff and marketing the unit concept to the institution and throughout the community.

PATIENT EDUCATION

Setting Up a Patient Education Program*

The Joint Commission on Accreditation of Healthcare Organizations made patient and family education into an important function with the *1994 Accreditation Manual for Hospitals*. The standards focus on making patients and their significant others knowledgeable, competent, and active participants in the care process.

Determining the Programs Needed

There are several ways to go about deciding which patient programs to develop first.

- If reviews of the large specific-diagnosis populations included in the outcome criteria a criterion relating to knowledge, the need for a patient education program may have already been identified.
- Patients can be surveyed, either by a questionnaire, skills inventory, interview, or a combination of these three. For example, when a diabetic patient is admitted to a hospital, he or she could be given a skills inventory to complete. When it is completed, the nurse would have the necessary data to set up an individualized program for the patient. Also, if inventories were collected over a period of time, they could be correlated into the foundations of a patient education program.
- Another area to examine is the rate of readmissions to the health care facility, particularly of the patients with chronic conditions. If there is a high frequency of readmission, a specific group of patients may need instruction on how to care for themselves at home.
- Interviewing key medical and nursing staff is perhaps the most subjective way to deter-

mine the need for specific patient education, but it is one way to assist in determining patient education needs.

What Will the Program Cost?

The second step in identifying specific program needs is to determine what the cost will be. At this stage of the program development, the determination will have to be a somewhat tentative figure, but it must be examined at this point in order to realistically venture into the project. If it will be unfeasible for the institution to implement the program because of cost, some other decisions will need to be made (i.e., forget the program, modify it to reduce cost, or possibly charge the patient for that particular program). One cannot make the above decisions without knowing what cost is involved.

Some factors to consider in determining the cost of an educational program include the following:

- What audiovisuals are needed: movies, filmstrips, charts?
- What will duplicating cost: patient information booklets, pamphlets?
- What system will be used: closed circuit television, small groups, one-to-one basis?
- How much staff time will be involved: to design the program, for any staff training, and for the implementation on a day-by-day basis?
- Will the patient education program increase the budgeted nursing care hours?
- Will it entail a change in the number or mix of nursing personnel on any specific unit?
- If other departments become involved, how would it affect cost?

Who Will the Teachers Be?

Most nurses in an institution should be involved in patient teaching, some more directly than others. The specific organization implemented will vary from institution to institution, but there are definite responsibilities to be considered.

Source: Adapted from Lilah Harper, "Developing and Evaluating a Patient Education Program," *Patient Education,* National League for Nursing, Pub. No. 20-1633, 1976. Reprinted with permission.

Someone in the institution needs to be assigned specific responsibility for determining what programs are needed and for coordinating the development and implementation of the programs. This step will provide accountability and avoid unnecessary duplication (this person may logically be someone in inservice, staff development, or education).

Designing the programs should be a group activity, involving persons who will probably be doing some, if not all, of the teaching. Also, someone with a background in methods of teaching, change theory, and evaluation will be extremely helpful, perhaps again someone from staff development or education.

In determining which staff nurses to involve, the following groups should be considered:

- nurses who already include patient teaching as part of their professional practice
- nurses who have indicated an interest in teaching, such as teaching inservice classes, participating in nursing grand rounds, teaching in the community, assisting with the orientation of new personnel on the unit, or working actively with students

The first programs to be developed will run more smoothly if the planning group is interested, involved, and committed.

What Will the Teachers Need To Know?

Assuming that only a portion of the teachers will be on the patient education committee, once the program is developed there will need to be inservice sessions with all of the teaching staff. Also, other nursing department staff will need information sessions so that they can actively support those staff members who are teaching.

Included in the inservice sessions for the teaching staff should be:

- purpose of the patient education program
- objectives
- content
- methods of conveying the content (which will be determined by the patient education committee, but the staff nurses will need inservice training on methods in conduct-

ing discussions with small and large groups and in teaching on a one-to-one basis)
- how to measure if the patient is learning
- how to document the teaching-learning process
- how to use audiovisual equipment if it is to be used in the presentation

Funding Patient Education Programs*

There are three basic ways of financing patient education programs. Each has potential and is being used satisfactorily. Similarly, each has its drawbacks.

First, costs may be billed to *third-party payers.* (Most often in acute care hospitals, third-party reimbursement comes from private insurance companies and the government's Medicaid and Medicare programs.) Third-party reimbursement for patient education is considered important because most health care facility bills are paid by someone other than the patient. Theoretically, if third-party payers are willing to cover health education, ample funds would become available to fund such services.

Some services currently are routinely covered by third-party payers. If the education is directly related to the intake diagnosis and is essential to home care, then reimbursement can occur. If, however, the education deals with other health problems or with prevention in general, reimbursement does not occur under most plans. When such coverage does occur, it is usually simply included in the room and board rates.

Second, the *indirect costs* mechanism for financing patient education is that by which the health care providers conduct educational programs for patients, but do not separately identify this expenditure on the patient's bill. Such costs are integrated into the patient's daily room rate and consequently are indirectly reimbursed by the third-party payers.

Actually, the daily room rate includes charges covering many services, such as three meals a

---

**Source:* Donald J. Breckon, *Hospital Health Education: A Guide to Program Development*, Aspen Publishers, Inc., © 1982.

day, 24-hour-a-day nursing care, clean sheets and towels, clean and sanitary facilities, and record-keeping. Including patient education under this heading is an appropriate way for health care facilities to receive reimbursement for a service patients would not receive if identified separately. It is especially appropriate in that patient education has been identified as an integral part of high-quality health care.

Third, *direct billing* is a payment mechanism whereby funds are generated either by directly collecting from the patient receiving the services or from a separate funding agency or a private source. In most facilities, a fee for each service is usually charged.

Patient education can be billed at the same rates as other clinical services, or even at lower rates, because physicians often are not involved. Where groups are involved, even smaller fees can be charged. The rates should be set to recover actual costs. If staff time is covered in the fixed rates for comprehensive service, it may be appropriate for only an additional charge to be made for educational materials used. If the patient is to be billed, the patient should have previously agreed to both receive and pay for the educational service. This is usually facilitated by having physicians issue an educational prescription which the patients voluntarily fill, as they would a prescription for medicine.

CONTINUING CARE AND THE DISCHARGE PROCESS

Owing to more rigorous monitoring of health care by regulatory agencies and third-party payers, there has been a tremendous increase in the attention given to discharge planning and continuity of care. Shorter stays mean patients have less recuperative time in the health care facility, and thus greater demands are placed on patients, families, staff, and community resources.

The terms *discharge planning, continuing care*, and *continuity of care*, although frequently used interchangeably, are defined somewhat differently and should be clearly delineated.

Continuing care has been defined as a health care facility–based program that coordinates assessment, planning, and follow-up procedures by providing a multidisciplinary team approach to patients with postdischarge needs. *Discharge planning* is frequently used synonymously and has been defined as a centralized, coordinated program developed by a health care facility to ensure that each patient has a planned program for needed continuing or follow-up care.

Continuity of care is the term applied to the coordinated delivery of health services on a continuum. The *continuum* includes the delivery of health care services in the home through self-care or with the assistance of families or home health agencies. It includes ambulatory settings, such as neighborhood clinics, private practices, and emergency departments, and extends to inpatient hospital care, rehabilitation, or chronic care facilities as well as hospices. The patients' needs and desires for health services will vary considerably, depending on where they are on the continuum at any given time.

To achieve the goal of continuity of care, the patient and health care professionals from various disciplines and health care settings work together in a coordinated effort to achieve mutually agreed-upon goals. This involves a multidisciplinary approach to individualized assessment of the patient's health care needs as well as patient involvement in the decision-making process. It is the responsibility of each health care professional involved in the provision of the patient's care to participate in the discharge planning process.*

*Nursing Administrator's Role***

The nursing service director should promote an understanding of the needs of the discharged patient.

- Budget time and money for implementation of a discharge planning program.

---

*Source: Sally Anne McCarthy, "The Process of Discharge Planning," in Patricia A. O'Hare and Margaret A. Terry, *Discharge Planning: Strategies for Assuring Continuity of Care*, eds., Aspen Publishers, Inc., © 1988.

**Source: Opal Bristow, Carol Stickey, and Shirley Thompson, *Discharge Planning for Continuity of Care*, National League for Nursing, Pub. No. 21-1604, 1976. Reprinted with permission.

- Provide nursing leadership and involvement to ensure continuity of patient care. Problems and procedures should be standard items on the staff conference agenda.
- Require that discharge planning procedures be written and included in a procedure or policy book.

A manual should be on every unit. Specifically, information on the mechanics of making a referral, an outline of suggested nursing information to complete a referral, and a list of available nursing agencies with their services, addresses, and telephone numbers should be in this manual. A list of potential candidates for referral should also be included. The nursing policies must remain flexible enough to provide for the special needs of a patient. They should also reflect the attitude of the general program objectives.

Discharge planning, an important component of total patient care, should be part of every nurse's patient care plan. It must begin at the time of admission and follow the patient through the progression of his or her illness. Nurses must evaluate each patient's total situation. Merely considering a patient's diagnosis and the related discharge needs as a basis for referral is insufficient.

Structures for Discharge Planning

Discharge planning programs in health care facilities come in many shapes and forms. Some facilities choose to assign the functioning role to the primary nurse at the bedside, others choose to make this the sole responsibility of the social work department, while others have an elaborate structure of team participation with shared responsibilities.

There are several types of models. The first model is the most structured and involves a designated discharge planner (usually a nurse), who has clear responsibility to determine what services the patient may need after discharge. This person is an independent agent, selecting and assessing patient needs. A second model is a variation on the first, in which the nursing and

medical staffs identify patients with needs and then consult the discharge planner for assistance in determining appropriate services. A third model designates discharge planning activities to specific people. Nurses and social workers assigned to units collaborate on a day-to-day basis and screen patients for postdischarge needs. Then discharge planning activities are divided between nursing and social services, according to whether home care or nursing home placement referral is needed. In the fourth model the social service department receives requests for patient assistance from medicine and nursing and coordinates all discharge planning activities.*

The Multidisciplinary Discharge Team**

Postdischarge planning is more significant today than ever before because more patients are discharged in very serious phases of illness— frequently into home care situations, requiring high-tech home care services. A multidisciplinary team with the patient as the central focus permits a more comprehensive and viable postdischarge plan. The process involved in developing a cohesive discharge planning team is not an easy one, nor should it be taken lightly. The roles and responsibilities of team members can sometimes overlap and could lead to turf issues and conflict. Careful screening of all discharge planning team members will help mold a network of professionals capable of synchronizing a multifaceted, individualized plan for every patient it encounters.

The *social worker* is one of the main professionals involved with discharge planning. The social worker is the master of counseling, evaluation, and development of the social support sys-

---

Source: Margaret A. Terry, "Essential Considerations in Setting Up a Discharge Planning Program," in Patricia A. O'Hare and Margaret A. Terry, eds., *Discharge Planning: Strategies for Continuity of Care*, Aspen Publishers, Inc., © 1988.

**Source:* Deborah Anne Ondeck and Barbara Stover Gingerich, "Discharge Planning: An Act of Caring, *Journal of Home Health Care Practice*, Vol. 5:4, Aspen Publishers, Inc., © August 1993.

Table 15–7 Components of a Comprehensive Discharge Planning Program

____ A *multidisciplinary* health care team approach to work with patient and family

____ Centralized discharge planning and assessment, preferably under one person or department, such as social work, nursing, or quality assurance

____ Early initiative with or without a physician's order

____ Collecting all clinical and social patient information and documents and communicating their content internally and externally to ensure continuity of care

____ Evaluating and ensuring that adequate community resources reach the patient

____ Fully informing patient and family of available health benefits and subsequent reimbursement

____ Ensuring patients discharged to nursing homes are fully informed and adequately prepared for placement

____ Conferences with providers, family, and, when possible, the patient to break down barriers to effective discharge planning

____ Equal opportunity for all inpatients and outpatients to receive appropriate and timely discharge planning

____ Regular evaluation of discharge planning programs for effectiveness, efficiency, and compliance with established standards through use of monitoring techniques such as

___ direct patient contact

___ telephone surveys

___ questionnaires

___ written follow up from referral agencies

____ Medical staff involvement in all phases of discharge planning programs

____ Early family and patient participation in discharge planning problems such as nursing home evaluation and selection

____ Development and use of assessment criteria for initiating early discharge planning

____ Thorough patient and family awareness of differences between hospital and alternative care settings

____ A predischarge checklist to become a permanent part of the record

Source: Professional Practices Committee of the Maryland Hospital Association, *Good Discharge Planning: Patient Advocacy at Its Best*, The Maryland Hospital Association, Inc.

---

tem for the patient. It is often the social worker who is consulted to establish the most appropriate disposition for the patient after completely evaluating his or her physical, emotional, social, and financial needs.

A *home care coordinator* position is essential. Incorporation of an experienced home care nurse into this role enhances the planning team's effectiveness. The clinical expertise of an experienced home care nurse is essential today in coordinating the clinical needs of the patient. Working collaboratively with home care providers, the coordinator performs preliminary insurance verifications; seeks able, capable, and willing caregivers; and ensures that vital discharge patient instructions are provided to the patient before discharge. The referral is made days in advance of the actual discharge and allows the patient and family to become aware of their rights, knowledgeable about what to expect from the agency of their choice, and fully cognizant of their responsibilities for care.

The home care coordinator functions as the in-house expert on home care. Staff look to this position as a resource and seek out the coordinator for information that assists with optimal disposition planning.

This individual is knowledgeable about home care admission criteria, reimbursement criteria, roles and expectations of the patient and family, technical needs of the patient, and availability of providers in the area.

Just as home care coordinators are masters of skilled home care clinical needs, the *therapist* is the master of the muscle-strengthening program, and the physician is the master of the medical regime. The *physician* often has known the patient for a number of years and can verify the accuracy of the patient's report of available home support. Therapists provide invaluable wisdom, such as when the patient can become more independent, how safe the patient will be if left alone, how much assistance will be required for activities of daily living, and so forth.

The *pastoral care worker* assists patients with acceptance of the disease process and helps them attend to their spiritual needs.

The *respiratory department* can provide essential information regarding oxygen needs or ventilator support needs. *Dietary personnel* collaborate with the *pharmacy* and physician to establish patient-specific nutritional requirements for patients on total parenteral nutrition.

All these roles are vitally important aspects of the patient's care, and each of these disciplines is vitally important to the discharge planning team's cohesiveness.

The interdependent functioning of these roles results in intricate, comprehensive, multidisciplinary postdischarge plans.

Coordination with the Managed Care Company. Proactive communications with managed care companies are often necessary to establish the collaborative roles of the company and the health care facility discharge planning team. Some managed care companies want to do their own discharge planning. Although there are many well-qualified and committed planners working for managed care companies, to offset the health care facility's risk and liability it would be wise to explain to the patient that his or her insurance company is requesting the authority to plan his or her postdischarge care. Patients need to be made aware of the health care facility's planning process and offered this process as an option for the development of their postdischarge plan of care. Documentation of the discussion and the choice made by the patient for discharge planning as well as any communications is required. This documentation can avoid future confusion during the planning process. Ultimately, the manner in which the facility and planners represent the planning process will determine the impact and use of the services.

Coordination: From Hospital to External Agency. Coordination tools can be created to meet the specific needs of an external agency and the health care organization and to facilitate an efficient approach to discharge planning. To assist with home care planning, a preprinted index card can be placed on the unit's Kardex to inform all caregivers of the status of home care

Regardless of the situation, the postdischarge plan requires input from the patient, significant others, physician, nurse, social worker, therapists, and home care coordinator. Patients have a right to informed decision making and therefore have a right to be fully informed of all options. For more complex situations, family meetings are valuable because they pull all the key team members into one room to discuss thoroughly the pros and cons of available options.

plans (see the box entitled "Home Care Planning"). The home care referral should contain all demographic and medical information, including the physician's orders for home care. Referral worksheets can be used to transfer any vitally important information from the patient's medical record to the home care nurse, which enhances continuity of care. To complete the information exchange process, a postdischarge questionnaire can be completed at the time of home care admission and returned to the nursing unit. This form bridges the communication gap and increases the health care facility staff's awareness of postdischarge care needs.

Home Care Planning

____In progress. Refer to chart for details.
____Patient is a current patient of _____ (agency).
____Patient choice of provider is _____
____Home care referral is on chart. Please have it signed.
____Home care referral is signed. Refer to copy as needed.
____At the time of discharge, please ask the physician:

____Contact extension 0000 when patient is discharged.

Thank you for your help in planning _____'s discharge.

CONTINUANCE OF CARE PROCESS

Preadmission Planning*

Preadmission planning can assist in the continuing care planning process and in the use of outpatient preadmission testing programs. Preadmission planning is intended to be a resource for the physician, the physician's office personnel, the primary nurse, and the social worker as they help to plan for the patient's health care facility stay and discharge. A program such as this can assist the patient—and the family—in making an easier transition from home and community into the facility. The medical staff should view this program, however, as a resource they can use to get the patient through the system in the most cost-effective way, not as an intrusion on their right to practice medicine.

The advantage of a preadmission planning program are as follows:

- to identify before admission the expected postdischarge care needs of patients using admission and preadmission screening programs
- to identify early those patients whose postdischarge needs are expected to be complex so that the necessary postdischarge resources can be secured in a timely fashion
- to familiarize patients and their families with the available community resources
- to coordinate all bookings with physicians and to screen them for appropriateness of admissions, using preestablished admission review criteria
- to increase efficiency in the scheduling of diagnostic procedures on an outpatient basis
- to support quality assurance, utilization review, and risk management efforts by involving patients and families in long-term planning

- to initiate patient education and preoperative teaching before admission for elective surgical patients with a selected diagnosis
- to help the continuing care primary team to begin the discharge planning process sooner and to alert them to those patients with complex discharge needs
- to help decrease the length of stay and to prevent unnecessary admissions

Reorganizing To Meet Continuum of Care Needs*

Contemporary nurse executives are continually challenged to find ways to piece together the continuum of care to integrate inpatient and outpatient care. One option, available since many hospitals have expanded into on-site ambulatory clinics, is to create a merged nursing management for the inpatient unit and the corresponding outpatient clinic (see Figure 15–2). This works particularly well with clinical specialties requiring follow up to inpatient care, such as oncology or orthopaedics. The integration coordinates care and improves communication, continuity, and cost-effectiveness due to more efficient utilization of resources.

*Source: Mary Lou Holle, "A Prescription for Success: Integrating 12 Inpatient and 17 Outpatient Programs," Aspen's Advisor for Nurse Executives, Vol. 10, No. 4, Aspen Publishers, Inc., © January 1995.

Table 15–8 Discharge Planning Variables

- Degree of illness (or health)
- Expected outcome of care
- Duration or length of care needed
- Types of services required
- Addition of complications
- Resources available

Source: Opal Bristow, Carol Stickey, and Shirley Thompson, Discharge Planning for Continuity of Care, National League for Nursing, Pub. No. 21-1604, 1976. Reprinted with permission.

*Source: Nancy C. Zarle, Continuing Care: The Process and Practice of Discharge Planning, Aspen Publishers, Inc., © 1987.

Table 15–9 A Discharge Planning Screening Tool

**High-Risk Factors for Identifying Patients
Who May Need Discharge Planning
(Patients are often Type III or IV on
patient classification system.)**

- Activities of daily living (ADL) dependent (those who cannot manage self-care safely on their own)
- Comatose, semicomatose
- Disoriented, confused, forgetful
- Dressings and wound care (patients with complicated dressings; patients who cannot do the dressing themselves; patients who will probably not do the dressing unless supervised)
- Equipment and transportation (this function shared with social services)
- Medications schedules (patients with complex schedules, injections; patients who are noncompliant)
- Ostomies (colostomy, ileostomy)
- Social problems (patients who live alone and could manage with some assistance; those who do not live alone but live with someone who cannot provide adequate care; those who have no home to go to or whose present home is no longer adequate)

- Special teaching needs (e.g., new diabetic, complex diet, injections)
- Terminal, preterminal
- Therapies (occupational therapy, physical therapy, speech therapy)
- Tubes (Foley, gastrostomy, suprapubic, nasogastric, tracheostomy)
- Transfers (transferred here from another facility; patients who will be transferred to another facility)

Note: Following are the most commonly seen diagnoses of patients who need discharge planning on an acute medical unit:

Arthritis	Diabetes mellitus
Cancer	Emphysema
Cerebral vascular accident	Hypertension
Chronic renal failure	Myocardial infarction
Congestive heart failure	Patients on respirator

Source: Linda A. Rasmusen, "A Screening Tool Promotes Early Discharge Planning," *Nursing Management*, May 1984. Reprinted with permission.

Reorganization for the purpose of enhancing efficiency and effectiveness of nursing care across the continuum of care begins by examining reporting relationships for inpatient and outpatient nursing services. In one successful venture, a transition team was created as a steering committee for the project, and initial efforts focused on identifying clinics and inpatient units serving like patient populations and analyzing potential benefits to be gained by integrating these areas under the responsibility of the same nurse manager. The transition team concentrated efforts on gathering input from all areas and responding to concerns about reporting relationships and staff schedules and general concerns related to the evolving change.

Clinics and inpatient areas formed transition project teams comprising staff members from each area and the nursing manager. Project coordinators from the transition team steering committee were assigned to each project team to facilitate the work. Each project team was given the set of implementation guidelines shown in Table 15–10.

In the final structure (see Figure 15–2), one nurse manager assumes accountability for a care delivery continuum and full control over use of human resources. Customer expectations are met through achievement of the clinical outcomes specified in coordinated care plans. The coordinated care plan is an interdisciplinary treatment plan correlated with a time frame for a specific

Figure 15–1 Discharge Planning Process

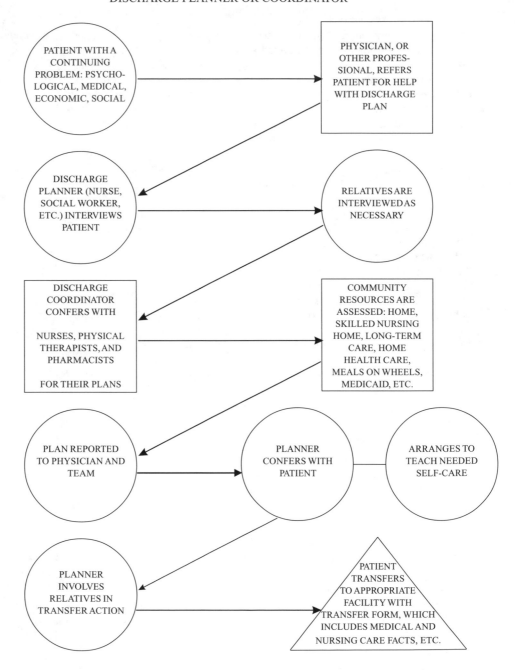

DISCHARGE PLANNING PROCESS
FOR THE
DISCHARGE PLANNER OR COORDINATOR

Source: Opal Bristow, Carol Stickey, and Shirley Thompson, *Discharge Planning for Continuity of Care*, National League for Nursing, Pub. No. 21-1604, 1976. Reprinted with permission.

Figure 15–2 Integrating Inpatient and Outpatient Nursing Service Organizational Structure

Separated structure   Integrated structure

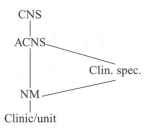

Table 15–10 Implementation Guidelines: Integrating Inpatient and Outpatient Services

- Identify patient populations that receive care across the continuum of outpatient and inpatient services, including home care, nursing home care, and referrals to external health care providers.
- Identify patient self-care and compliance issues (both inpatient and outpatient).
- Outline discharge planning issues that affect follow-up care.
- Indicate factors that influence quality of care (patient outcomes) and length of stay.
- Consider space and staffing and cross-training issues.
- Evaluate the roles of registered nurses, licensed practical nurses, nursing assistants, clinical nurse specialists, nurse practitioners, and nurse managers as they influence efficiency and effectiveness of patient care delivery.
- Identify workload data.
- Develop and review evaluation methodology to be used to measure overall goals.
- Review the process of referrals to outpatient services (both medical and nursing referrals).
- Conduct a literature review of pertinent trends in coordinating and integrating care. (Coordinators can be given packets of reference articles.)

---

patient type. The plan begins with the clinic visit and ends with a postdischarge telephone interview.

When integrating services, it is critical to involve other appropriate disciplines. There is a need for coordination between services and for coordinated patient education. One solution is to develop a critical path that all disciplines support. Improved coordination of patient education also can be addressed through the creation of a seamless outpatient-inpatient teaching program, supported by all disciplines.

Chapter 16

Information Management and Technology

OVERVIEW

The issue of information management and control is increasingly important, particularly with health care reform recommendations. In the contemporary health care environment, controlling and managing information play a critical role in the delivery of all health care services. With these trends in mind, it is advisable for nurse managers and leaders to review and strengthen their knowledge of nursing informatics. Managing nursing informatics is all about controlling information—clinical information, financial information, patient information, and more.

Information Technology*

A well-designed nursing information system performs nursing service administration research on all sorts of questions. Also, it suggests cures for identified deficiencies. For example, if staffing ratios are found to correlate with quality assurance reports, falling scores in the latter would indicate a need for more nurses.

It is important that the nursing management system be able to correlate managerial and clinical data. It is also useful if the nursing computerized system interfaces with the other systems of the institution. These systems, depending on their capacity, may hold patient data for orders and billing, personnel management systems, inventories of various sorts, and clinical data. Obviously, the more interactions that are possible, the more useful the system is to the nurse executive.

One problem with a sophisticated computerized system may be that it is capable of delivering information overload. The nurse executive may receive so many reports on so many aspects of institutional and divisional operations that it is difficult to get to them all, let alone make appropriate interpretations. When the system produces this sort of overload, the nurse executive will be wise to arrange for data to be processed for her consumption, with summative data, important correlations, and unusual data (management-by-exception) brought to her attention.

When the nursing division lacks its own systems specialist, it is useful to appoint a managerial communications committee to determine answers to the following questions:

*Source: Barbara Stevens Barnum and Karlene M. Kerfoot, The Nurse as Executive, Aspen Publishers, Inc., © 1995.

- What information do we need?
- How can it be programmed into the computerized systems? If it can't be computerized, how else can it be gathered?
- How should it be processed? Who should get what reports? At what intervals?
- How should the data be summarized?
- What evaluations should be made in relation to the data?

Another major problem with a computerized information system is control of access. The system must be designed so that only those who have a right to have the information are able to retrieve it. Issues of patient confidentiality (and staff record confidentiality) are of major concern in designing a system.

The nurse executive will need expert help in learning what can and what cannot be performed by computerized information systems. Essentially, they can handle and correlate easily quantifiable variables of the nurse executive's choosing. Not all computer systems have similar capabilities, so the nurse executive will have to have generalized knowledge about computer systems and also information concerning the specific capabilities of the system in her institution.

If installation of a new computer system is being planned, it is imperative that the nursing division be part of the planning. Otherwise, it is unlikely that anyone will consider the nursing needs that can be served by the system. A computer system is a good example of a sunk cost; once a given system is installed, it is often too late to get services that were not considered when the system was selected. Nursing must plan for its needs and make its requests long before computer purchases or leases are finalized.

Information Management: The Joint Commission's View*

The Joint Commission considers information management (IM) to be one of the four critical

Source: Jana Bradley, "Management of Information: Analysis of the Joint Commission's Standards for Information Management," *Topics in Health Information Management*, Vol. 16, No. 2, Aspen Publishers, Inc., © November 1995.

organizational functions. The Joint Commission has set forth 10 standards that represent a major departure from its previous approach to IM activities. Because of the importance of the Joint Commission accreditation of health care facilities, the new IM standards can be expected to have a substantial impact on management of information.

The standards describe information as vital to the Joint Commission's overall approach to quality health care. The elements of this concept are summarized in the following narrative paraphrased from the preamble (see Table 16–1 also).

- Health care is highly dependent on information and the need to coordinate and integrate the work of many individuals, departments, and services. Therefore, information is a resource and must be actively managed.
- The organization's leaders have overall responsibility for this activity. Staff at many levels must be educated and trained in the management and use of information.
- Information management is a function—a set of processes—focused on meeting the organization's information needs. These processes include:
  - identification of the organization's information needs

Table 16–1 Summary of Joint Commission's IM Standards

IM 1: Assessment of information needs

IM 2: Confidentiality, security, and integrity of information

IM 3: Uniformity and, through that, continuity and compatibility of information

IM 4: Education/training in principles of IM

IM 5: Timeliness and accuracy of information

IM 6: Linkages within and beyond the organization

IM 7: Patient-specific knowledge and information

IM 8: Aggregate data/information

IM 9: Knowledge-based information (recorded knowledge)

IM 10: Comparative data/information

– structural design of the information management system
– definition and capture of data/information
– data analysis and transformation of data into information
– assimilation and use of information

- Four types of information are identified: patient-specific data/information, aggregate data/information, expert knowledge–based information, and comparative performance data/information.

The following objectives are listed for improving IM in organizations:

- more timely and easier access to complete information throughout the organization
- improved data accuracy
- balance of security and access
- use of compiled data and expert knowledge–based information
- comparative data for performance improvement
- redesign of information-related processes to improve efficiency
- greater collaboration and information sharing to enhance patient care

The description of this concept of what IM is and why it is important is, in itself, a significant addition to the standards. First, this view of IM makes it an organizationwide priority, responsibility, and activity involving staff at all levels. This priority is reinforced by the requirement that individuals who generate, collect, and analyze data/information be trained in principles of IM. Second, the concept emphasizes continuous improvement in IM through the use of multiple types of information. Third, it identifies collaboration and information sharing as important for patient care.

For successful IM, collaborative agreement among clinical, administrative, and other staffs must be reached in many areas, including agreement on information needs, the purposes and uses of systems, the national indicators or local adaptations that will be used as indicators, other

definitions of key data and information, relevant expert knowledge and information, and so forth. Because of the importance of collaborative agreement among staff across boundaries in almost all aspects of IM, collaboration can be viewed as the invisible 11th IM standard: the component necessary for successful achievement of the other standards and of the intent of the preamble.

INFORMATION AS A RESOURCE

Internal Management Information System Technologies

Technology is going to become the essential tool for all health service professionals in the near future. Computer-based information systems (CBISs) in the health service field improve health service management decision making and are beginning to play an increasingly important role in organizational control, clinical decision making, and strategic planning. For a health care facility, there are three primary reasons for developing CBISs. First, they improve operational efficiency so that inadequacies in the operation of administrative systems (e.g., medical record processing, patient administration, and financial accounting management) can be detected and analyzed. Second, they promote organizational innovations by allowing new ways of doing old things. Finally, they build strategic resources that will give broad access to timely and relevant data.*

Computer Support for Health Managers*

As part of their job, health managers collect, use, and develop information of all types for the primary purposes of decision making, information dissemination, and redistribution. There is no question that the capacity to manipulate information as a resource and to manage it for decision making and communication is of great importance to the nurse manager. An automated

---

*Source: Joseph K.H. Tan, *Health Management Information Systems*, Aspen Publishers, Inc., © 1995.

management information system (MIS) provides managers with tools for fulfilling their functions.

MIS for Interpersonal Roles. A combination of advancing office and telecommunication technologies has provided management with new ways of keeping in close contact and maintaining an "electronic presence" with others. The office information system (OIS), which includes electronic mail, facsimile, voice mail, audio conferencing, computer conferencing, desktop publishing, groupware, presentation graphics, and video teleconferencing, provides effective mechanisms for managers to plan, organize, direct, control, and coordinate even when they are unable to be physically and interpersonally present.

Apart from reducing intraorganizational and extraorganizational communication costs, an OIS can greatly enhance managerial capabilities in capturing and transferring large volumes of information quickly through telecommuting. In effect, these technologies allow health service managers to continue their work outside the normal organizational confines of time and space, thus increasing their productivity.

MIS for Informational Roles. Middle and higher management in many health service organizations have over the years shifted their attention gradually from traditional data processing systems to management reporting systems and more recently to strategic information systems. Therefore, systems that will help serve and fulfill their informational roles include utilization management reporting systems, forecasting support systems, case-mix information systems, and other telecommunication systems (e.g., electronic mailing and networking).

Utilization management reporting systems will provide managers with insights about the appropriate or inappropriate use of health resources and assist them to stimulate continuous quality improvements throughout the organization. Case-mix applications are capable of identifying, segregating, and describing the organizational product, service, and patient characteristics. Strategic information system applications can assist the managers to solve a range of ad hoc managerial and policy decision-mak-

ing problems such as the need to plan strategically, to monitor environmental trends, to scan market opportunities, and to simulate various what-if scenarios.

MIS for Decisional Roles. The general goal of MIS technologies and applications in health care facilities is to assist health service managers in the fulfillment of their roles. These automated systems not only facilitate more efficient and cost-effective managerial performance but, more important, provide more effective means of information gathering, information interpretation, and information dissemination, thus enhancing health managerial service excellence.

Several MIS applications exist to aid health service executives and managers in their decisional roles. These systems range from simple management reporting systems to systems with advanced capabilities for structuring and analyzing relevant data and transforming them into timely and meaningful information for managerial decision making.

Presenting Data as Useful Information*

With the accumulation of data comes the obligatory administrative function of communicating the data, that is, conveying the information by packaging it into an insightful report.

When and What To Communicate. These are no straightforward steps that can be taken to select a "right" time for when an audience is ready to receive data. The nurse manager should consider what the benefits and consequences would be if the data are or are not communicated today, tomorrow, or next week. Prepare data to be translated and presented by going back to the intent, or why the data are collected: What message is the audience interested in? What does (or should) the audience want to know? Select the data organized and analyzed and compose the message content. Be careful to select only the "need to know" data. Hold additional or "nice to

---

*Source: Adapted from Betty Fuchs, "Translating Data into Information: A Primer of Preparatory Concepts and Skills," *Topics in Health Record Management*, Vol. 12, No. 4, Aspen Publishers, Inc., © May 1992.

know" data in reserve to be called on if and when desired.

What Can Be Communicated, If Needed? Removing mysteries about data often allows better communication. The audience may want to "interview" the data, to learn more about the origins, background, qualifications, and other specifics of the data. Prepare a data résumé that responds to questions such as those in the following box.

- How and where did the data originate? (reliability issues)
- Were the data collected in a standard, uniform manner? (reliability issues)
- What are the meanings and definitions of the data terms? (accuracy issues)
- How have the data been objectively and fairly evaluated? (analysis, design, and organization issues)
- How was it determined what data were and were not included? (population analysis and sample issues)
- Are there possible shortcomings, and what is the magnitude? (raw versus adjusted data analysis issues)
- What was the need for these data? (questions and assumptions of the data study)
- How were the findings reached? (analysis techniques used to assess time frames, patterns, fluctuations, trends, variations issues)
- What happens if the data are ignored? (risks and benefits of data-use issues)
- Why are these data important now? (timeliness of data-reporting issues)
- Who has access to these data? (security and confidentiality of data issues)
- What will these data do for me? (costs and benefits issues)

How To Communicate. Some individuals are well versed in specific "sublanguages" or jargon.

- Determine which language or sublanguages the audience is most comfortable with and uses frequently.
- Use their language when translating data into information.

It may mean that presentation of the data must take on a different structure, that of words rather than of numerical data, a written report as opposed to a graphic demonstration. Analyses prepared should be reviewed for information and context that can be used to build brief descriptor sentences and paragraphs.

A *visual presentation* makes use of tables and graphics. If data are presented in the format of a data table (lots of rows and columns of numbers covering most of the paper), do not be surprised if the data, while seen, are not understood. Formats that "overpresent" data can be distracting.

When translating data, consider whether there is a style of visual communication that is comfortable for the audience. For example, consider pie charts, histograms, or frequency polygons. Ascertain whether the audience's communication methods include a commonly used "picture" of data. If so, try applying it to the data at hand.

Access to External Health Care Information*

Internal and external data comparisons are important to validate the organization's level of quality and marketability. Comparisons with external health care organizations are assuming greater importance for employers, payers, and the organization itself. Indeed, the Joint Commission standards mandate the use of external databases.

In 1995, the standards related to organizational improvement suggested mechanisms for interpreting quality improvement data, including

---

Source: Dian I. Johnson, "Using External Data and Databases: Issues and Sources," *Journal of Nursing Care Quality*, Vol. 10, No. 1, Aspen Publishers, Inc., © October 1995.

comparisons of the organization with current information sources such as the Joint Commission's aggregate data or the Agency for Health Care Policy and Research (AHCPR) guidelines plus recent clinical or research literature, and comparisons with outside organizations. In fact, the organization's use of external data sources will be an assessment issue for accreditation.

The standards define external comparisons in terms of a reference database (i.e., data from many organizations that are organized and similar in nature). Another term for this comparative process is *benchmarking*, whereby the organization measures its performance in the specified area against the performance of a similar organization. With this mandate clearly in mind, health care organizations that have not already done so must set up processes to compare their organizational performance externally.

Searching for External Data

Health care databases related to outcomes are in their infancy, and herein lies a major stumbling block. The Joint Commission recently released 1994 performance results from 394 health care organizations across the United States that may serve as a source of external comparison. On the other hand, many index-type databases, such as *Index Medicus* and MEDLINE, are available to find clinical and research data from other organizations for the purpose of comparisons. The user can conduct a search using CD-ROMs (compact disks-read only memory) on a personal computer (PC). The compact disk (CD) contains a database with bibliographic references, abstracts, and/or full text of articles. Databases are also available on magnetic tape. Last, some on-line databases, such as MEDLINE, have software programs, such as *GRATEFUL MED*, that provide easier and cost-effective searches.

Now, anyone with a PC, a modem (a device to communicate with other computers over telephone lines), communications or on-line software, and/or a CD-ROM drive can conduct searches for comparative data without leaving the office or home. The user dials into an on-

Examples of CDs that may be helpful include the following:

- the National Center for Health Statistics National Health Survey CD-ROM: a database of health statistics available from the Government Printing Office (GPO)
- the National Institutes of Health (NIH) Computerized Retrieval of Information on Scientific Projects: a database of research projects
- Macmillan New Media Physicians MEDLINE: clinical data geared to physicians in office practice
- Compton's New Media Information USA: a federal information database with health clearinghouse, sources for clinical studies, statistical information, and other federal information
- Statistics, Inc. FedStat: a database of statistics
- GPO on Silver Platter: a database of federal publications
- Mecklermedia CD-ROMs in Print 1996: a database of currently available CDs

line service (a large commercial service with files, electronic mail exchange, and special interest groups) to access search facilities.

CompuServe is one of the largest on-line services with an extensive array of databases. Generally, databases fall into the categories of bibliographic references, bibliographic references and abstracts, or the full text of articles. The category type is included in the database description. Some of the databases available on CompuServe are the following:

- Health Database Plus: with full-text articles and abstracts at $1.50 per article
- Knowledge Index: with full-text drug information from the American Hospital Formu-

lary, a government publications reference list, MEDLINE citations, cancer literature, nursing and allied health citations, mental health abstracts, demographic information, and dissertation abstracts

- Paper Chase: for access to MEDLINE as well as CINDHAL
- IQuest: with access to more than 850 databases

Another source for comparative data is the Internet. The Internet is a loose network of computers from all over the world. The Internet may be accessed through direct connections; through a local, regional, or national provider; and indirectly through some of the large on-line services or bulletin board services (BBSs), which provide electronic mail, message capabilities, and access to files.

The strong presence of academic and government agencies as well as the Internet's roots in exchange of research information clearly make the Internet a potentially rich source of information. Examples of organizations available on the Internet either directly or indirectly include the following:

- U.S. government: NIH, Census Bureau, National Institute of Allergy and Infectious Disease, Department of Health and Human Services, National Library of Medicine, Economic Bulletin Board, Electronic Government Information Service, Food and Drug Administration, National Science Foundation, and Library of Congress
- academic: Johns Hopkins University, Harvard Medical School, Duke University, Cornell Medical College, Dana Farber Cancer Institute, Medical College of Georgia, and Albert Einstein College of Medicine
- health care organizations: Boston Beth Israel, Louisiana State University Medical Center, New York University Medical Center, and Stanford University Medical Center
- state and local government agencies, particularly those related to education and research

Mailing lists are another potential source of data. Users subscribe to the mailing list and receive via e-mail any information or messages posted at the subscription site. Nursing and medical mailing lists, such as Gradnurse, Mednews, Nurseres (nursing research), and Nursenet, are available.

The government has several BBSs that may be of interest to those searching for health-related data. Examples include the Office of the Assistant Secretary of Health, the Food and Drug Administration Electronic Bulletin Board, and the Economic Bulletin Board, which is a fee-based service containing statistical data. The latter two are accessible through the Internet as well as directly by modem. The Office of the Assistant Secretary of Health is accessible directly by modem.

UNDERSTANDING INFORMATION SYSTEMS AND APPLICATIONS

Health care providers need a conceptual framework that helps define, plan, and structure the work cycles, management processes, and information technology on which patient care depends. In this information-intensive era, when work is highly dependent on information flow and when information flow sometimes is the work, the fragmented approaches of the past have proved woefully inadequate.*

Classifying Information Systems*

To lay the foundation for a new conceptual framework, health care executives must resist the temptation to continue to define information systems by the different departments they serve. Instead, information systems can be classified based on the types of work that they handle. From this perspective, three classifications describe most health care computer systems:

---

*Source: Bernie Minard, "The Search for a Competitive Edge: Building a New Framework for Health Care Information," *Topics in Health Information Management*, Vol. 14, No. 1, Aspen Publishers, Inc., © August 1993.

- data collection and recording transactions, such as those that capture information about patients during registration or record a charge for some service
- data access transactions, such as those that retrieve patient data or managerial statistics
- directed data transactions or message transactions, such as orders from a nursing department to a diagnostic department, simple e-mail information messages, or computer faxes to physicians' offices

Data Collection and Recording. Modern computer systems possess the ability to collect a great deal of real-time or up-to-the-minute data. Still, few systems successfully collect data within a real-time data cycle because actual work cycles and established manual data entry cycles seldom coincide. Consequently, these on-line systems often are used only to perform batch data entry, usually by transcribing from worksheets manually prepared.

Although the potential availability of real-time data could enable computer systems capabilities to leap forward, use of such information requires that painstaking attention be paid to accuracy during data collection and recording. Moreover, adding a time notation as an integral part of the collected data could allow precise tracking and comprehensive evaluation of the medical activities being recorded.

Data Access Capability. As data access advances continue, and as access to relevant information becomes more critical to workflow, health care executives must face emerging issues involving the many methods by which workers search for, retrieve, and use information. For example, workers may peruse available data or they may study it intently. They may scan data for general information or search for specific critical indicators. Once they locate key data, they may want to drill down, gaining background and supporting information. They may retrieve and print data for review and study only to return subsequently in search of additional, amplifying data. These wide variations in data access methods and strategies require a corresponding variety of capabilities in evolving information systems.

Directed Data (Messaging) Transactions. A computer system can examine data fields of a message and take special action, such as displaying messages in some preferential order. It can monitor the work progress represented by directed data transactions and, according to set rules and depending on conditions, route future messages (work) in different ways. Such systems also can merge data messages from several sources, check for some parameter, and, when the parameter is identified, alert the appropriate worker.

Directed data transactions can trigger special action regardless of whether the information flows in batches or as individual messages. When data flow on request, such as when test results are passed to a physician's office, the fairly serial nature of the workflow makes it relatively simple to scan transactions and to invoke and manage priorities. Work collaboration and exchange of information among workers in this setting usually are direct and focused on the information and the work it represents, from the issue that initially caused the transaction through its step-by-step resolution.

On the other hand, many directed data transactions occur without requests. The information may be transmitted as soon as it becomes available, such as the results of stat orders for diagnostic tests. The messages may flow in batches with similar data, grouped so that office workers more easily can manage tasks such as compiling results of routine orders for diagnostic tests or generating monthly departmental financial reports. In these cases, directed data transactions essentially operate as buck slips to transfer work individually or in batches among people.

Nursing and Patient Care Applications*

Clinical support systems involve the organized processing, storage, and retrieval of information to support patient care activities. Many of these systems interface with other parts of the health

---

Source: Joseph K.H. Tan, *Health Management Information Systems,* Aspen Publishers, Inc., © 1995.

care facility's information system (e.g., admission, billing, etc.) Patient management systems (PMS) are the chief source of personal and clinical information on a patient.

(*Note:* Computer applications for specific functions on the nursing service, such as staffing, scheduling, quality management, and data analysis, are discussed in the chapters associated with those topics.)

The use of the computer-based utilization plan (UCP) follows protocol-based nursing care guidelines to assist in the planning and administration of patient care. The use of a UCP-based system in nursing is expected to result in a reduction of documentation time that will lead to an improvement in the quality of patient care as well as increased efficiency in the time spent on the wards. Charting and reporting will be enhanced. End-of-shift reports can be generated, promoting continuity of care between shifts, and exception reports can be produced indicating outstanding clinical interventions according to the nursing care plan. The UCP and other similar systems are defined as standardized patient guidelines that reside in a computer database to support comprehensive and high-quality patient care. They provide health practitioners with reminders, alerts, and clinical decision support and can be linked to bodies of medical literature and other medical aids.

Patient monitoring systems use computer technology to monitor vital signs continuously and physiological data periodically. Most modern medical devices are used in critical care units; they include vital sign monitors, ventilators, and infusion pumps. These machines are designed to allow digital communication of information. Some monitoring systems use microcomputers built into individual patient bedside monitoring units. Results are displayed on monitors at the bedside and at a central monitor display unit at the nursing station.

Computer systems also have been designed to process and interpret data from various diagnostic devices. Much of the work in signal processing has been done in the interpretation of electrocardiograms (ECGs) and the analysis of electroencephalograms. Pulmonary function testing also makes use of computerized analysis. To improve the decision-making abilities of all health professionals, point-of-care access allows patient data to be entered at the bedside as care is being provided.

The Clinical Information System (CIS)*

The medical records department has evolved to the clinical information department over the past decade in particular. It will continue to evolve substantially as integrated delivery systems create greater need for uniform and timely information. The department has changed from being the depository of medical information, to a vital source of data to support continuity of care, statistical information for reimbursement, utilization and peer review, legal issues, and similar clinical care and administrative demands. Manual processes in the department have been replaced in many cases by automated ones, such as computer-assisted diagnostic-related group (DRG) reimbursement calculations, chart tracking systems, and optical disc storage. A major shift in the method of entering and accessing the patient data is reflecting in the rapid change from hard copy records to the computer-based patient record. The activity level of the department has grown substantially, and, consistent with the changed functioning of the department, the roles and functions of the clinical information specialists have evolved to encompass greater responsibility.

It is desirable to place the functional responsibility for all aspects of clinical information processing in a central, comprehensive unit under the direct management authority of a specialist in health information management. In this way, continuity of care is more easily supported through continuous and coordinated documen-

---

*Source: Joan Gratto Liebler, "Clinical Information Services," in Lawrence F. Wolper, ed., Health Care Administration, ed 2, Aspen Publishers, Inc., © 1995.

tation processes. This comprehensive, centralized service has as its usual functions these specific activities:

- patient/client identification and numbering system
- creation and monitoring of clinical information documentation
- quality assurance/clinical studies for continuous quality improvement
- utilization review studies
- risk management review and studies
- word processing/dictation-transcription system
- statistical abstracts and indexes
- special studies for medical, professional, and administrative staff reviews
- financial reimbursement support data, including diagnostic and procedural coding
- storage and retrieval system, including chart tracking system
- assistance in complying with legal and regulatory provisions and accrediting agency standards concerning health care data
- data security, privacy protection, and confidentiality provisions
- in-service education and training for professional and support staff
- educational programs for students under contractual and/or affiliation agreements
- assistance in research studies

Requirements for a CIS*

Today's clinical information systems have to be different because today's clinical environment is different. For example, the introduction of new patient care delivery models has contributed to making the clinical information system a neces-

sity, for the models require clinical access to information not traditionally within the purview of the clinician and access to information in new formats and displays (see Table 16–2). Thus, not only can transactions be processed and care documented but, with the incorporation of "expert" or rules-based technology, the planning and delivery of care can be affected positively. The power of today's clinical systems should also allow health care professionals to collect and analyze the information needed to identify "best practices" medicine. Current systems enable providers to determine the appropriate allocation of resources and treatments that will lead to optimal outcomes within specific lengths of stay. With the emergence of managed care and capitation to control health care costs, the ability to effectively manage resource utilization and track outcomes is paramount. For a clinical information system to truly support the clinician (physi-

Table 16–2 Needs of Contemporary Patient Care Delivery Models

To support patient centered care and the case management model, the clinical information system must offer the following:

- electronically retrievable, integrated patient information
- longitudinal patient information
- clinical discipline-specific display of information (e.g., displaying different information for the renal clinic compared to the information for the diabetes clinic)
- integrated resource, patient, and staff scheduling
- automated clinical protocols
- clinical reminders and alerts
- concurrent quality management
- integrated orders and results management
- automated critical paths
- access to financial information
- patient-specific and aggregate variance reporting capabilities
- concurrent quality and utilization management

Source: Mark S. Gross, Barbara J. Hoehn, and Carolyn S. Rooks, "Clinical Information Systems: Why Now?" *Topics in Health Information Management*, Vol. 14, No. 1, Aspen Publishers, Inc., © August 1993.

cian, nurse, or therapist), it must meet a few basic requirements:

Support clinicians' specific automation requirements. The objective is to provide a system specifically designed to support clinical functions (progress notes, charting, results reporting, etc.) and to enhance clinicians' productivity. To be used actively in the clinical process, the system's functions and screen flow must follow a clinician's work logic.

Provide systems integration and easy universal system access. The primary issue is to cross departmental system boundaries and to access other systems' data. The overall objective is that a clinician be able to access any system from any terminal throughout the institution, including off-site physician offices.

Provide easy access to all databases. Clinical users typically have significant reporting requirements from a variety of internal and external entities, such as government agencies, insurance companies, and the like. The information system must provide easy access to these databases.

Be user friendly. Clinicians typically have a low tolerance for interacting with computers. The objective is to provide user-friendly systems (e.g., graphics, touch screens, help screens, point-of-care terminals, and handheld terminals). It is important that the system be flexible enough to provide specialty-specific clinical views of the patient information. For example, a cardiovascular surgeon requires a different set of information from that of a neurologist.

Provide excellent system performance. A clinical information system must offer 24-hour availability, have tremendous speed (subsecond response time), and provide "unlimited" on-line storage capability.

Support a continuum of care to the patient. The clinical information system must give clinicians access to life span patient data, regardless of when or where the patient was treated. Clinicians need to be able to access specific information rapidly, and so the system must provide logical, concise subsets of information.

Protect patient data confidentiality. Clinical information systems must include multilevel security systems that protect patient confidentiality.

IMPLEMENTATION OF AUTOMATED SYSTEMS

Determining a Unit's Nursing Information Needs*

By linking information requirements to organizational objectives, a model for determining nursing information needs can facilitate congruence of objectives and consistency of action by nurse managers. The model can also provide information tailored to a nurse manager's need in a concise, systematic manner that expedites and improves decision making. The process of determining information needs places nurse managers in a position to analyze their jobs, which provides structure, a change of focus, and a better understanding of the job.

Success Factors

- Determining how clinical information systems will improve operations, not just automate them

- Managing the information as a resource, not as a technology

- Treating information as an asset (for it will become even more of an asset in the future)

- Involving clinicians from the beginning in the planning process as well as in the implementation process

- Developing a long-term relationship with an information system vendor (for information systems are dynamic and will have to evolve with the organization)

The model will guide the interview between the computer analyst and the nurse manager, thereby ensuring uniform results and good utilization of time; no time is wasted deciding how or what to do. Finally, the model is good for all

---

Source: Alice M. Thomas, "Determining Nurse Manager Requirements," *Nursing Management*, Vol. 17, No. 7, July 1986. Reprinted with permission.

levels of nurse managers, which is ideal, since the information requirements will be uniform and gaps in information assimilation and responsibilities may be identified in the interview process.

An Eight-Step Process

1. Understand department objectives. The nurse manager must have a good understanding of the organization's goals and objectives and the objectives of the manager's unit. An example of a unit objective is "to maintain a level of staffing to meet patients' needs."

2. Identify critical success factors (CSFs). The nurse manager determines the CSFs for each objective. These are the few key areas where things must go right for the organization to flourish, tasks that must be accomplished successfully for the unit to achieve its objectives. Each CSF should be written as a short expression (e.g., "scheduling"). The number of CSFs varies for each objective and for each nurse manager but will generally number three to five. Examples of CSFs include a regular staff complement, a relief staff complement, qualified staff, scheduling, and performance appraisals.

3. Identify specific performance measures. The nurse manager must identify the specific performance measures for each CSF. The performance measures should be expressed in quantitative terms if possible. The dimensions of quantity, quality, cost, and time may prove useful as a starting point for generating performance measures.

4. Identify information required to measure performance. The information required must relate to the performance measure. If the performance measure is "actual-to-budgeted staffing patterns," the information required would be summaries of actual versus budgeted staffing for each unit and for the entire area of responsibility.

5. Identify major decision responsibilities. This step involves determining the major decision responsibilities of the nurse manager in order for the manager to achieve the unit's objectives. It is important here to eliminate any decisions of a minor nature to ensure that the manager does not become inundated with information.

6. Determine the specific steps required to complete each major decision. The nurse man-

ager articulates the various decision steps for each decision. A decision flowchart may be developed at this time to represent the decision process. This step may be difficult for decision situations that are poorly understood. However, this exercise may result in an improved understanding of the decision process and the information requirements.

7. Determine the information requirements for each decision. Keeping in mind the unit objectives, the nurse manager indicates to the analyst the information that is most supportive of each activity involved.

8. Verify the information requirements. This is done jointly by the analyst and the nurse manager (see box). Any revisions that are deemed necessary are made at this time. The nurse manager must be confident that the identified information requirements are complete and accurate.

Selecting the Information Services Consultant

Because of the high value placed on professional knowledge, the use of an outside consultant must be carefully approached. Key nursing groups will need to be involved in consultant selection, perhaps through informal interviews, in order that uncertainty about expertise is dispelled at the beginning. Otherwise, a tendency to distrust outsiders will limit the nursing organization's ability to apply the information provided by such experts.

The more sophisticated the actual technology associated with a new structure, the greater the need for support personnel. The presence of technology introduces complex and numerous line-staff relationships. Therefore, the time needed for successful change is increased as well as the complexity of the change process itself.

Source: Cathleen Krueger Wilson, *Building New Nursing Organizations*, Aspen Publishers, Inc., © 1992.

Key Issues in Preliminary Planning for an Overall System*

Key issues that will create the basic foundation for the design of the system must be considered and decisions made before developing a detailed implementation plan. These include the following:

- consistency of the nursing process and documentation practices across all units to determine which units should be automated and/or will require unique treatment and/or training
- existing knowledge and familiarity of automated software within the nursing staff to determine whether functionality can be implemented all at once or whether only basic use is to be initially implemented
- current status of policies and procedures, that is, whether they are developed for all documentation practices and are on a word processing system to allow easy revision
- results of prior accreditation reviews to identify areas that are known to require improvement
- the format and definition of standards of care and whether they can be automated or consolidated within the care plan format or whether critical pathways or critical pathway plans will be developed
- consistency of diagnoses/problem statements, expected outcomes, and interventions across all locations
- consistency and validity of the acuity system for medical-surgical and specialty units regarding skill-mix ratios, direct and indirect hour standards, and criteria; expectation regarding staffing levels and skill-mix ratios based on a new acuity system
- interaction with medical staff and other health care team members

- use of system by specialty areas such as emergency department, operating room, and critical care unit

The process of selecting a system and the most efficient utilization of a system involve other issues.

- selection and role of the committee that will serve as the implementation team
- responsibilities for approval of new documentation that will determine use of the new system
- communications tools to inform all users of project status
- security and access to the system, for example, whether unit secretaries and/or aides will be able to document on-line
- hardware requirements and placement of terminals (varies based on physical layouts, skill mix, and nursing process philosophy)
- interface capability among modules and to admission, discharge, transfer, patient accounting, and payroll systems

THE NEAR FUTURE: AUTOMATION REQUIRED FOR COLLABORATIVE/ CONTINUUM PRACTICE*

The models of collaborative practice commonly discussed in nursing practice include patient-focused care, case management, and managed care. Each of these models can be reviewed in terms of the technological tools required for achieving its goals of collaborative practice.

Information System Design and Patient-Focused Care

Patient-focused care is basically a method of delivering care that organizes diagnostic activi-

---

*Source: Mary Jean Barrett, "Optimizing Nursing Information Systems," *Journal of Nursing Administration*, Vol. 22:10, October 1992.

*Source: Roy L. Simpson, "Nursing Informatics," *Nursing Administration Quarterly*, Vol. 18, No. 4, Aspen Publishers, Inc., © Summer 1994.

Figure 16–1 Planning Steps in Designing and Implementing a Management Information System

1. Formulate System Requirements

Formulate system requirements based on findings and conclusions of evaluation and analysis
of information needs and existing MIS.
(1) Describe data and information to be provided
for operations personnel by department and functional unit, together with required accessibility
and timeliness.
(2) Describe information to be provided to top
executives and all managers, by department and
functional unit, together with required accessibility and timeliness, in the areas of strategic planning, financial management, human resource
management, organizational planning, controlling
and management of work processes.

2. Establish Development Priorities

Establish priorities for system development, by
department and functional unit and within each
department and functional unit.
(1) Consider operational processes.
(2) Consider management functions.

3. Select a Design Approach

Consider these options:
(1) Expand or alter the existing system.
Consider
    (a) further mechanization
(2) Install a new system. Consider
    (a) a customized system
    (b) a packaged system
    (c) acquisition of a transportable system
Start cost benefit analysis

4. Select Equipment System

Evaluate and determine equipment to implement
selected design approach. Make selection on basis of preliminary cost benefit analysis. Consider
all systems development costs, and both operational and maintenance costs.

5. Design the System

Reconcile system requirements (step 1) with
equipment capabilities (step 4). Prepare system
specifications to include (1) acquiring source
data; (2) flow charting data through the system;
(3) designing master files and preparing record
layouts; (4) preparing program specifications;
(5) developing procedures for report distribution;
(6) assuring error control, and (7) using complete
cost benefit analysis.

6. Develop Committee Recommendations

Review of system design documentations by MIS
planning and development committee.
Develop committee recommendations to implement based on requirements (step 1); priorities
(step 2); and cost benefit analysis (step 5). Submit recommendations to CEO for final approval.

7. Prepare an Implementation Plan

Prepare scheduled implementation plan after CEO
approval in terms of who, when, what, where, how
and expenditures as required. Plan authority delegations and responsibility assignments related
to creation of an information systems department;
equipment acquisition and installation; programming; training and orientation; file conversion;
systems testing and system documentations.

Implement the plan and maintain and upgrade
system as required.

Source: Owen B. Hardy and Clayton McWhorter, *Management Dimensions: New Challenges of the Mind*, Aspen Publishers, Inc., © 1988.

ties and care protocols around the individual patient's needs. The idea is to provide routine services by multidisciplinary, cross-trained caregivers—all at the patient's bedside. As a result, nursing units surrounding the patient act as "minihospitals," creating aggregate patient populations around similarity of needs, streamlining and simplifying documentation requirements, simplifying processes, and broadening caregiver autonomy.

The information system design also must change to accommodate patient-focused care. In other words, traditional departmentally focused systems must be replaced with patient-focused, integrated systems that emphasize the communication and decentralization characteristics of this new environment. Advanced information technology would support patient-focused care in the following ways.

1. *A longitudinal computerized patient record* would provide the long-term, holistic view of the patient's health required for improved patient care delivery. The Institute of Medicine (IOM) is creating standards for the ideal computerized patient record, which it estimates will not be available until the end of this decade.

2. *Distributed or client/server technology* would be required to provide clinicians with updated clinical and patient information at the patient's bedside. Client/server technology or distributed computing refers to putting more power in the hands of users rather than in the grips of a centralized (IS) department. This means each "patient server" or "substation" would be equipped with a fast, powerful (though relatively low cost) microcomputer or personal computer that could access a vast database of patient and clinical information quickly and easily. Most client/server models function over local area networks (LANSs), linking several workstations with a "file server"—a minicomputer that houses the database of information required by the user.

3. *Clinical systems* will likely be shored up and redesigned so that clinicians can track the progress of patients against the protocol or critical path initially specified.

4. *Instructional and reference systems* will be needed to support multiskilled, cross-trained care teams.

Finally, patent-focused care would require that technology be "open"—in other words, that whatever system is put in place could easily and immediately accept data from different software systems and hardware platforms.

Information Technology Design and Case Managed Care

Case management, an increasingly popular strategy for coordinating health care, can also be defined as a clinical system that focuses on the accountability of an identified individual or group for coordinating patient care across a continuum of care. It is also a model of collaborative care because it brings together primary and secondary health caregivers in a network designed to care for patients outside of acute care settings.

However, most information technology in use today is episodic oriented or transactional based. In other words, it takes a "snapshot" of what is going on, or reports on a specific transaction, but it does not provide a longitudinal view of patient care over time. For technology to support collaborative practice in the guise of case management, the following three components need to be in place.

A Longitudinal Computerized Patient Record. Once again, a computerized patient medical record that could provide a fluid, comprehensive, and time-sensitive view of the patient's changing health care status would greatly enhance the case manager's ability to provide holistic, preventive care.

Nursing Minimum Data Set. Probably the single, most effective barrier to true collaborative practice—whether it be in the guise of case managed care or any other model—is the lack of a common nursing language. Nursing must move swiftly to adopt a universally accepted nursing minimum data set so that computers can codify this knowledge for access by all nursing providers across the continuum of care.

Widespread Information Networks. For care to be effectively managed outside the walls of the institution and across the continuum, there needs to be an "electronic superhighway"—a vast network over telephone and cable lines that would connect (ideally) almost all citizens, corporations, and institutions, similar to the way telephones connect individuals today. It is envisioned that this network would be accessed either by personal computers or "smart" televisions. For case management purposes, a network of this magnitude would allow nurse case managers to communicate with patents on a regular basis for reminders, educational purposes, and "touching base" via exchanged messages or conversations over the computer.

This scenario is not too far off in the future; small-scale trials with network-based nurse–patient relationships have proved very successful already.

Information Design in a Managed Care Environment

Most clinical professionals today understand managed care as the most viable proposal for reforming the health care system. Managed care integrates information mainly at the administrative level, where health care financing is integrated with health care delivery. However, clinical information will also be integrated and shared as treatment protocols and clinical guidelines are put in place, preventive care is emphasized, and comprehensive services are established to support patients throughout the complete continuum of care.

To use technology for this clinical level (beyond the administrative management of benefits, contracts, and reimbursement issues), several technological advancements must be readily available: artificial intelligence systems, knowledge bases with inference "engines," client-server technology, and computer to computer interchanges.

Chapter 17

Staffing

PLANNING FOR STAFFING

When making plans for staffing the department, the director of nursing service must utilize and interpret the health care facility statistics that are available in annual reports and other published and unpublished records. Based on these data, the anticipated daily average patient census, seasonal variations, types of patients admitted, acuity of illness, and characteristics of medical treatment rendered by the medical staff may be forecast. Staffing needs are usually projected for the fiscal year ahead and often for a longer period.

On a broader level, staff planning must take into account future needs and prepare by cross-training and "grooming," candidates for positions with increasing responsibility. Anticipating resignations and selecting replacements in advance, from inside or outside the facility, are imperative to provide continuity in the exigency of turnover.

Other variables that influence the number and variety of staff must be given full weight. Among these are the facility's human resource policies and practices, its operating policies and practices, its physical facilities and resources, the method of assignment, and the efficiency of the entire management.*

Overview**

Staffing is the process of determining and providing the acceptable number and mix of nursing personnel to produce a desired level of care to meet the patient's demand for care.

A staffing program consists of four phases.

1. a precise statement of the purpose of the institution and the services a patient can expect from it, including the standard and characteristics of the care
2. the application of a specific method to determine the number and kinds of staff required to provide the care

---

*Source: Barbara Brown and Beverly Henry, "Nursing Administration: Practice, Education and Research," in *Health Care Administration: Principles, Practices, Structure, and Delivery*, ed 2, Lawrence F. Wolper, ed., Aspen Publishers, Inc., © 1995.
**Source: *A Review and Evaluation of Nursing Productivity*, DHHS, Pub. No. (HRA) 77-15, 1977.

3. the development of assignment patterns for staff from the application of human resource guidelines, policy statements, and procedures
4. an evaluation of the product provided and judgment reflecting the impact of the staff on quality

Staffing methods attempt to establish a set of patterns for supplying nurses to patient areas based on some predicted average workload conditions. Then, when patient demands increase or decrease on a unit during a particular period, it is necessary to reassign on-duty personnel to balance the staff to patient needs. This dynamic staffing or allocation process makes use of a number of adjustment techniques (see Chapter 19). Whichever method is used, it is important to base decisions on some workload measuring system.

In adopting patent classification and workload systems, the determination of patient need becomes more objective and the allocation process simpler. Reassignment remains a judgmental process based on supervisory decisions to move personnel between units to balance demand.

It should be noted that even though staffing processes tend to be effective, the system of providing nursing care also relies heavily on proper scheduling practices. Scheduling is an important factor in providing sufficient staff to meet patient demands. Therefore, any staffing appraisal should include a reassessment of the institution's nurse scheduling policies and practices as well.

Before any attempt is made at restaffing a nursing service area, it is recommended that a proven workload measuring system be adopted and the data be collected over a sufficient period to understand the patient demand. Also, when collecting workload data, it is recommended that all scheduling policies and practices be reviewed and some effort be made to predict future scheduling criteria. Finally, it is recommended that based on the workload measurement system and the scheduling policies and procedures, the institution attempt to devise an allocation process that balances patient need with available person-

nel while maintaining personal fairness and consideration without affecting patient care. For an explanation of the elements needed to establish a staffing system, see Tables 17–1 and 17–2.

Staffing Today*

In the current health care environment, in attempts to minimize expensive hospitalization costs, clients are not admitted promptly to a hospital once they become ill. They are often treated at home and seen at their physician's office. Therefore, once it has been identified that the individual needs to be hospitalized, he or she often has a higher acuity rating than was traditionally seen.

Because clients have higher acuity ratings while they are hospitalized, the hours of nursing care necessary to meet the client's needs have also increased. As more complex nursing care is required, nursing contact hours must also increase. This results in more money being spent to deliver the client care. Since the diagnosis-related group (DRG) system has limited financial reimbursement to hospitals, it becomes increasingly important for hospitals to be certain that the client care being provided is cost effective with acceptable levels of quality.

To ensure quality nursing care, the Joint Commission on Accreditation of Health Care Facilities requires that a hospital provide a sufficient number of nurses on each shift to meet the clients' needs. Generally, facilities within a local area tend to maintain similar *nurse-to-patient ratios*, so that community standards are fairly uniform. The ratios, however, must be based upon the nursing care needs of the clients, and a patient classification system (PCS) can be used to determine how much staff is necessary to meet the clients' nursing care needs.

Source: Catherine E. Loveridge and Susan H. Cummings, *Nursing Management in the New Paradigm*, Aspen Publishers, Inc., © 1996.

Table 17–1 The Staffing System

Process	Focus	Description	Used for/Purpose	Decision Based on	Method Used
Staffing	On long-range unit needs	Supplies the average numerical assessment of staff needed to service a unit 1. by skill position level 2. on each shift	Annual budget	Historical data or previous documented experience of patient census and nursing hours required (level of patient demand)	Census forecast; by assessment of previous year's collection of unit census reports
Measurements	On patient needs	Determines level of care and requirements of staff performance to meet that level	Supply of data		
Nurse Activity Study	On actual performance of nursing function	Observes a comprehensive list of nursing tasks performed on the unit; assessed for time standards and skill levels (a one-time study)	Calculation of standard nursing hours for delivery of patient care per day	Analysis of time study	Work sampling Self-reporting
Patient Classification	On patient needs	Identifies degree of nursing care needed by the patient population in a given type unit (from minimal to maximum)	*Short Range* Actual census of patients and need levels for the day to determine staff readjustment *Long Range* Provides, at end of month and year, data on level of patient occupancy to be used for forecast of future needs on the unit	Assessment of the intensity of patient needs for nursing care on any given shift or day	To construct classification system; application of standards for nursing care To use classification system: daily census report and assessment by delegated nurse

continues

Process	Focus	Description	Used for/Purpose	Decision Based on	Method Used
Workload Index	On daily patient needs and available scheduled staff	Quantifies the amount of care needed to be given, and identifies the number of personnel required to meet that need	Daily estimations of under- or overstaffing on the unit for short-range a locations	Comparison of the unit's actual census (patient count and degree of need) and the current on-duty staff, with the assessed standard number of personnel needed to give that level of patient care	Workload index: formula or workload tables
Scheduling	On nurse worker as well as unit needs	Aligns the work-hour conditions of the nurse worker (40-hour week, vacations, etc.) into a unit staffing pattern to provide for the requisite 24-hour-a-day patient coverage	Distribution of budgeted nursing personnel to meet unit's anticipated staffing needs on three shifts a day and weekends	1. Unit staffing positions 2. Required unit coverage 3. Facility policies (unit organization shift hours, on weekends, vacations, etc.)	Variety of methods are used, the most innovative being cyclical scheduling or block patterns. Can be calculated manually or with computer assistance
Daily Adjustments (or allocations)	On short-range unit needs	Provides for an increased or decreased supply of nursing personnel if the unit's actual working load on any given day is above or below the average need anticipated	Correction on a daily basis of any imbalance between the regularly scheduled staff and the actual patient workload	Short range: daily census reports of workload and data on scheduled staff. Long range: census forecast of seasonal peaks and lags in patient admissions	Imbalances corrected by a variety of methods: floats, nursing pools, transfers between units, temporary help from agencies, part-time employees, controlled admission

Table 17–2 Staffing Policy Checklist

The following list provides a convenient outline for evaluating the nursing department's staffing policies.

Employee Categories
1. Full-time
    1.1 Hours Worked per Week
    1.2 Weekends Worked per Schedule
    1.3 Benefits Calculation
2. Part-Time
    2.1 Hours Worked per Week
    2.2 Weekends Worked per Schedule
    2.3 Benefits Calculation
3. Float Pool
    3.1 Hours Worked Status
    3.2 Weekends Worked per Schedule
    3.3 Scheduling Pattern
    3.4 Assignment Method
    3.5 Line of Authority
    3.6 Salary and Benefits Paid
    3.7 Differentials Paid
    3.8 Orientation Provided
4. On-Call Pool
    4.1 Availability Requirements
    4.2 Weekends Worked per Schedule
    4.3 Assignment Method
    4.4 Line of Authority
    4.5 Compensation Calculation
    4.6 Orientation Provided
Scheduling
1. Authority and Responsibility
2. Length of Cycle Rotation
3. Posting Time
4. Reporting Responsibility
Assignments
1. Placement Determination
2. Basic Care Requirements
Days Off
1. Rotation Pattern/Service
2. Weekend Rotation
3. Special Requests
    3.1 School Schedules
    3.2 Change Status
Weekends
1. Definition
2. Family Member Schedules
Scheduling Requests
1. Request/Response Procedure
2. Weekend Requests
3. Educational Days
4. Emergency Leave
5. Failure To Report When Scheduled

Trade Procedure
1. Acceptable Trades
2. Request/Response Procedure
Vacations
1. Request/Response Procedure
    1.1 Time to Submit
    1.2 Place to Submit
2. Approval Guidelines
    2.1 Seniority Preference
    2.2 Who Decides
    2.3 Number Limitations
3. Change Request
4. Extended Vacations
Holidays
1. Paid Holidays
2. Request/Response Procedure
3. Approval Guidelines
    3.1 Granting Criteria
    3.2 Number Limitations
4. Unexcused Absence on a Holiday
5. Vacation during Holiday Period
Illness
1. Notification Procedure
2. Extended Days
3. Illness on Duty
Leave of Absence (LOA)
1. Request/Response Procedure
2. Paid Leave Time Interface
Failure To Report to Work
1. Consequences
Transfers
1. Request/Response Procedure
2. Approval Guidelines
Temporary Reassignment
1. Who Will Float
2. Refusal Consequences
3. Equitability
Absenteeism
1. Percentage Acceptable
2. Days Absent Patterns
3. Disciplinary Action
Tardiness
1. Percentage Acceptable
2. Disciplinary Action
Irregular Hours Worked
1. Report/Return Home
2. Called after Shift Begins
3. On-Call Availability

continues

Table 17–2 *continued*

Low-Census Procedures
1. Selection Process
    1.1 Sequence Followed
    1.2 Patient Care Safety Levels
2. Benefits Accrued
3. Paid Hours

Overtime
1. Payment Guidelines
2. Availability
Family Policy
1. Family Member Assignment
2. Time Off Policy

Source: West Coast Medical Management Associates, Inc., Westlake Village, Calif., 1980. Adapted with permission.

Factors Influencing Staffing*

A number of factors affect staffing—among them are the number of patients, the acuity of the individual patients (patient classification), the need for time standards for some of the more repetitive tasks, provision for type of nursing practiced, and the need to provide allowances for other professional aspects of nursing. The list of factors influencing staffing includes the following.

Characteristics of Staff. What is the mix of skill levels? Are many on the staff young and inexperienced or is the group more settled, not out to "remake nursing"? What are the levels of educational and experiential preparation? How many are there in total numbers and by position? What are the head nurses' orientations to nursing care? To what extent are registry nurses used for unit staffing (and how are the decisions made as to the number of registry nurses needed)? What is their general social and ethnic background? Are many of them graduates of foreign schools?

Domain and Boundaries of Nursing Services. What services is the nursing department responsible for? Do these include, for example, the operating room, errand and escort service, outpatient department, emergency services, special research or treatment units? Is the nursing department "extensible" according to the time of day and weekend, for example, are dietary and pharmacy services on evenings and nights the

responsibility of nursing? Are ward clerks or unit managers responsible to nursing administration?

Place in Formal and Informal Authority Structure. Is the informal authority of the nursing department congruent with its place in the formal structure? What actual power does it have?

Latitude for Flexibility. Is the prevailing consensus one of "doing things alike," or is there flexibility for delivery of care by different methods? Can, for example, primary care be used on one unit and team nursing on another?

Administration. What is the degree of centralization and general organization? Are many persons in middle management or supervisory positions? What is the prevailing management style? Is it, for example, organization or person oriented?

Teaching Programs. Is the health care facility associated with a school of nursing? If so, are there joint appointments? How extensive is staff involvement with student teaching?

Turnover. Are nursing staff attracted to the area for limited times such as for recreational or education purposes? Do new graduates of area schools tend to stay short periods and then move on? What is the turnover rate for differing skill levels?

Group Cohesiveness. How closely knit are the unit staff? Are they small work groups or a collective of persons?

Resources Available within the Department. Are there persons skilled in staff development or inservice education? Are there certain indi-

---

Source: Methods for Studying Nurse Staffing in a Patient Unit, DHHS, Pub. No. (HRA) 78-3, May 1978.

viduals with particular clinical skills, research skills, language facility?

Standards of Care. Are the standards clearly spelled out and available to all staff? How many standards are informal, unwritten ones? Do the nursing units set their own objectives and, if so, are they reviewed and revised on a routine basis? Are standards of care fairly uniform across the nursing areas?

Priorities in Non–Patient Care Activities. How much emphasis is placed on formal educational development, participation in research activities, inservice, and staff development?

Professional Activity. How much active involvement is there with professional organizations?

Presence of Unionization. Are either nonprofessional or professional staff unionized? If so, what do the contracts cover? What is the resultant climate within the nursing department after election or nonelection of union representation?

Traditions and History. Although linked with institutional traditions and history, the nursing department may have its own unique blend of traditions and past events that are informally influential in the organization of services and espirit de corps.

Trends in Nursing Care Delivery. To what extent are emerging and/or unclear roles in existence? Decisions, for example, relative to having clinical specialists in an organizational staff versus line relationship will prompt critical examination of traditional supervisory roles.

Interrelationship of Factors at the Unit Level

All the foregoing factors, as noted, may be seen as having variable influences on the total plan of services to be given in the institution. To get at the overall plan of nursing services and a staffing program that results in individual unit staffing plans and organization of care, however, attention must be focused on what goes on at the

unit level in determining the actual care given and the evaluation of nursing care and patient outcomes.

The right side of Figure 17–1 makes more specific the various kinds of daily events and crises that may arise to cause discrepancies between the staffing plan and organization of care and the actual care given to and received by the patient. They include changes in census, patient needs, physicians' schedules, and supporting services available, as well as staff fluctuations due to illness, emergencies, days off, vacations, and so forth, and the variabilities in the capabilities of total staff on duty because of these unplanned fluctuations. Because very little can be done to alter the occurrence of these types of changes and crises, their influence is depicted as operating in one direction. Personnel needs for satisfaction and demands for organizational maintenance (represented by its subelement: "Demands for Input into Informational and Record System" in the diagram), however, are subject to alteration by "what's going on" and may have a definite influence on the outcome. Thus, they are depicted as having a two-way, or interactive, relationship with the system.

The left side of Figure 17–1 depicts the interdependency of all groups within the health care facility in the process of evaluation of the actual nursing care given. As indicated, no one measure of "care" is, or probably could be, employed exclusively (e.g., expected patient outcomes by medical standards may or may not be accompanied by patient satisfaction). Similarly, the level of personnel satisfaction is involved in the process, as are the congruences and coordination with the services of medicine and of other departments. Actual care is always evaluated against certain nursing standards, and, finally, cost of providing the nursing care is a critical factor in the evaluative process. As with the other components, the open system features of the framework allow for the evaluation of the nursing care to feed back into planning for future nursing services, the staffing program, the overall plan of nursing services, and the "negotiated agreement." The open system features also make it clear that the system of events recycles and is repeated continuously.

Figure 17–1 Relationship of Factors Entering into Provision of Nursing Care at the Unit Level

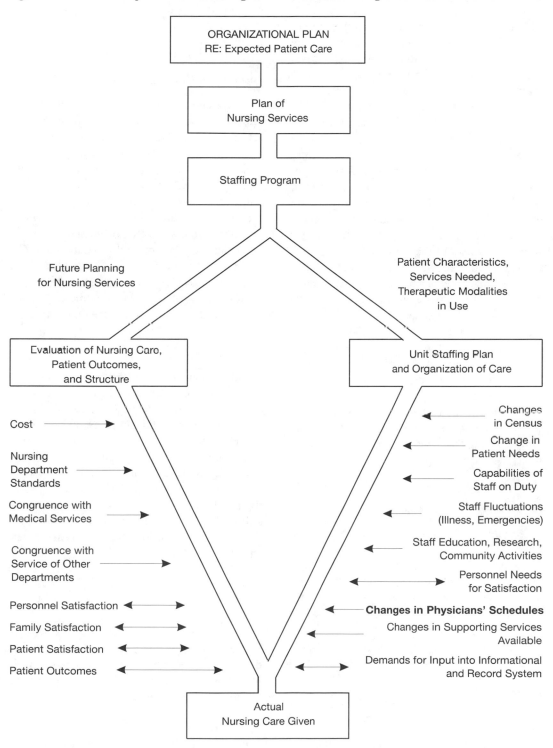

Source: Methods for Studying Nurse Staffing in a Patient Unit, DHHS, Pub. No. (HRA) 78-3, May 1978.

Difficulty in Assessing Staff Requirements*

There is absolutely no doubt that there are resource management problems in nursing at all levels, and nurses need appropriate tools and approaches to assist in their decision making. Every day, head nurses and unit leaders make assessments of patient needs and staff capabilities and, using some model, create assignments to ensure that appropriate care services are delivered. This process may be repeated several times during each shift as the situation changes. Also, each day, decisions are made at an administrative level about how many nursing personnel at each level of skill should be assigned to each patient care unit. Such allocation of personnel to units and the subsequent assignment each individual receives can vary widely in terms of workload. Thus, a huge process of resource management, occurring at several levels in the nursing hierarchy, happens each day in each institution. Throughout the nation, the vast majority of decision making in this process is based on the experience of those involved and their abilities to mentally juggle many complex factors to predict care workload and determine staffing requirements. This feat becomes monumental when one considers the fact that there are nonpredictable occurrences and variation in patients' needs and nurses' skill levels and competencies.

Nonroutine, Nonpredictable Occurrences

Nursing units, as a rule, experience more than their share of unexpected events, which drain staff time. Unexpected physicians' visits and orders, patients going "sour," interruptions from support departments and other nursing personnel, observation of previously unidentified patient needs, and visits from friends and family members are among the many occurrences that the nursing staff must cope with each day. In addition, some "routine" things can quickly take on an air of uniqueness. Answering call lights,

admitting and transferring patients, and preparing patients for surgery or diagnostic tests all tend to confound traditional resource management techniques.

Variation of Patients' Needs

One necessary component for human resource allocation is an adequate description of the total set of objectives that must be accomplished. On a patient unit, patients' needs represent this component and categorization schemes exist today that effectively divide patients into groups according to their self-sufficiency. Although research has documented that nursing personnel spend less time with self-sufficient patients than with total care patients and that patient classification schemes are important to the staffing function, the implementation of these schemes has been widely avoided due to the time-consuming process of obtaining the information required.

Overlapping Skill Levels

There is no longer any doubt that tremendous overlap exists, in terms of capability for meeting certain patient needs, between registered nurses, licensed practical nurses, and aides. Resource allocation models have great difficulty in accepting and dealing with this fact, while practicing nurses know it as reality and must deal with it in decision making. Complicating this is the additional problem of role definition. It is still difficult to point to any single concept of the role of the registered nurse, licensed practical nurse, and aide that can be translated into concepts describing their capacity to accomplish patient care activities.

Varying Individual Competencies

A great deal of the adequacy of a patient's care depends on the individual competencies of the nursing staff; and nursing personnel categories are neither equal nor uniform. Differences are due to factors such as educational programs (there are several different types of programs which prepare the registered nurse), experience, motivation, and other individual factors. For

*Source: Louis Freund and Ronald Norby, "A Model for Staffing and Analysis," *Nursing Administration Quarterly*, Vol. 1, No. 4, Aspen Publishers, Inc., © 1977.

those addressing the resource allocation problem, this knowledge creates special difficulties. Personnel at each skill level should not be considered equal, yet most models require this assumption and leave sensitivity to differences up to the implementer. In practice, however, these individual differences in competency are extremely important variables, and hence models that cannot accommodate them are largely ignored by nurses.

What is needed are methodologies and techniques particularly responsive to nursing resource management that are acceptable to the nurses involved, actually obtain better solutions to problems than nurses can achieve without assistance, and have a foundation in theory that enables administration to understand more fully how this multifaceted resource is used at every level.

Perhaps of equal importance is that such methodologies not function in isolation but become an integral part of a larger analytical model. Too often, nurse staffing is considered as an end in itself. That is, efforts are directed solely at readjusting or otherwise providing individuals to cover workload. While important, this must be accomplished with consideration directed toward many other factors, such as desired quality levels; goals related to allocation of responsibility for care delivery; the effect of staffing on morale, turnover, and absenteeism; personnel cost; actual ability to meet workload, recruitment, and so forth.

Forecasting Personnel Needs*

Personnel forecasting is the prediction of needed health care and the availability of staff to perform the needed health care functions for some future time period. Each department is expected to forecast future supply and demand, areas of expected operations and staff needed taking into consideration expected turnover, retirements, vacation benefits, and so forth, by training and utilizing their personnel. The main

steps in the personnel planning process are as follows:

1. *Analyze the present supply situation by making an inventory of the work force.*
   - Determine how many employees there are by unit, skill, age, sex, education, classification, career interest, and length of service.
   - Analyze present work force trends and problems: absences, turnover, vacancies, recruiting problems, numbers in training, standards, and wage/salary distribution.
   - Analyze organizational structure and personnel policies: duplications, underutilizations, supervision ratio, and policy problems.
2. *Analyze the demand situation—short and long term.*
   - Analyze organization plans and future priorities: activity changes, types of work, needs forecast, and budget forecast.
3. *Analyze productivity trends and review technological changes, productivity experiences of the past, and governmental/environmental changes.*
4. *Evaluate and update the forecast.*
   - Analyze the flows and trends in the supply of personnel in relation to future needs.
   - Prepare tentative personnel forecast.
5. *Evaluate and update the forecast periodically.*
   - Inaugurate and evaluate related processes of recruitment, selection, training, career planning, and organizational development.

Centralization versus Decentralization in Staffing*

A division is highly centralized if major decision-making power and responsibility for key

---

Source: Joan Holland, "Workshop: Manpower Planning To Meet Needs," *Health Care Management Review*, Vol. 1, No. 4, Aspen Publishers, Inc., © 1976.

Source: B.S. Barnum and K.M. Kerfoot, *The Nurse as Executive*, ed. 4, Aspen Publishers, Inc., © 1995.

functions are concentrated in the top levels of that division. A division is highly decentralized if decision making and responsibility for key functions are delegated to the lowest possible managerial level in the division. Thus, a centralized nursing division might have major decisions made by a council of the nurse executive and his or her associate directors. Such a division would be likely to have many major functions (e.g., budgeting, staff education, quality assurance, and nursing research) in separate departments reporting directly to the nurse executive or his associates.

In contrast, a decentralized division might place most decision making at the head nurse level, with each head nurse running his or her unit independent of the decisions of peer head nurses. Unlike a head nurse in a centralized division, the head nurse in a decentralized division would provide for budgeting, staff education, quality assurance, nursing research, and staffing of the unit with his or her own personnel and unit resources.

Nursing organizations vary greatly in their degree of centralization. The degree may differ for different tasks and responsibilities. There are general advantages and limitations to each mode of departmentalization. A highly centralized division, for example, usually commands considerable power, achieves economies of scale, and develops expertise in the specialized functions that are served by discrete departments. A limitation of a highly centralized operation is that it may not attract ambitious first-line and middle managers who are looking for authority and control over their own units.

A highly decentralized division has the advantage of placing the decision making near the action; it also allows for diverse responses from managerial unit to managerial unit. Limitations of the decentralized form are that it loses economies of scale and that it sometimes shifts responsibility and authority to managers unprepared for them. For example, a head nurse who is responsible for providing inservice education for his or her own staff may not have the educational expertise required for the job.

Today, most nursing services claim to be decentralized because it is highly recommended by the experts. But one must look closely to see what is actually decentralized and what is not. In some cases, decentralization becomes a ploy for weakening and breaking a united nursing service. If a strong nurse leader gives up a centralized role to become a staff consultant to decentralized subordinates, those subordinates (each weaker than the centralized leader) may be vulnerable to separate power plays.

Decentralization has another limitation when functions are decentralized to the level of incompetency. Here, a unit is given responsibility for a function it is unprepared to carry out. Usually that function falls through the cracks and is forgotten. The nurse executive must always ensure that a unit develops competency in the functions that are being decentralized before this reorganization takes place.

The nurse executive cannot delegate to someone who is unprepared to handle the function. Therefore, it is imperative that he or she not decentralize functions until competency has been established and the function can be performed at the appropriate level of quality.

Decentralization also is an error if too many tasks and responsibilities are decentralized to someone already suffering from role overload. This is a frequent occurrence in today's cost-conscious management. Functions and responsibilities must be sent down the line to persons prepared to do them and having enough time to absorb them into their role functions.

Because decentralization is seen generally as a good thing and centralization as suspect, most errors are made in decentralizing rather than centralizing. Decentralization is often a risky tactic in an environment in which the nursing division is under threat from powerful, competitive organizational components. See Table 17–3 for a comparison of centralized and decentralized staffing.

Table 17–3 Comparison of Two Methods of Staffing

Decentralization

- Maximizes unit staffing

- Minimizes or eliminates a centralized float pool
- Gives head nurse accountability for the entire staffing budget
- Gives head nurse responsibility for 24-hour staffing and scheduling
- Provides for contingency staff backup from companion or sister units, per diem (on-call) staff, increased hours of part-time staff, or overtime when shortages occur
- Assigns selection of all unit staff members to head nurse
- Provides that head nurse keeps updated record of current staff skills
- Puts decision making at the unit level
- Promotes relationships among sister units

- Commits staff to making method successful

Centralization

- Manages staffing of nursing departments as a whole
- Maximizes utilization of float pool

- Gives head nurse accountability for staffing budget on the unit
- Gives head nurse responsibility for 24-hour patient care
- Permits reassigning float personnel when shortages occur

- Assigns core unit staff selection to the head nurse
- Centralizes updated record of skills required

- Puts decision making in the central office
- Does not emphasize relationships between like specialties
- Depends more on central office management for success

Source: Joyce Rhodes, "Staffing and Resource Development," in *Managing for Productivity in Nursing*, Barbara Rutkowski, ed., Aspen Publishers, Inc., © 1987.

STAFFING SYSTEMS

Guidelines for Establishing a Staffing Program*

To initiate a staffing program, which includes as its purpose the projection of the amount of staff needed, and to begin the educational program associated with building understanding of the comprehensiveness and complexity of staffing, *a nursing service administrator* is advised to employ the following steps:

1. Organize a committee of the nursing staff for purposes of becoming informed about

---

*Source: Nursing Staff Requirements for Inpatient Health Care Services, American Nurses' Association, Pub. No. NS-20, 1977. Reprinted with permission.

staffing—its purpose, philosophy underlying the concepts, objectives, methodology—and to gather information about the populations of patients being served.
2. Appoint an individual to assume responsibility for the program.
3. Collect data about personnel needed to predict the requirements.
   - personnel policies
   - personnel statistics: average number of workdays; average number of holidays, vacation, illness, leave of absence for various purposes; turnover rates; supply; and so forth
   - current number of personnel, by category, in the department and individual nursing units
   - cost

4. Collect data about patients.
   - by individual nursing unit—admission and discharge rates or visits to clinics; average length of stay; occupancy or turnover rate; and any other type of data that will be useful
   - consideration of use of a classification scheme and methodology
5. Review staffing patterns currently used by nursing unit, and document rationale employed.
6. Involve the committee in the selection of a staffing methodology and staffing policies and patterns desired and feasible; recognize constraints that exist in the adoption of the ideal.
7. Introduce the methodology to collect data regarding patients, and state why it was selected (the rationale).
8. Write staffing policies that will be generally applied.
   - the placement of holidays (attached to weekends or not)
   - the type of work assignment adopted
   - the maximum and minimum number of consecutive days to be worked before a day off
   - the number of weekends off per month (or unit of time)
   - the number of shifts to be worked by each classification (whether all are straight shifts, or two-shift rotation, or three-shift rotation)
   - the number of weeks per shift, if rotation shifts are used
   - placement of vacation (distributed over the year or not)
9. calculate the number of personnel required, by shift, by type of nursing personnel, through use of the methodology adopted.
10. Adjust the number to provide leadership and coverage to plan for implementation of staffing policies.
11. Plan for how the evaluation of the staffing and scheduling will be made.
12. Implement the staffing program.
13. Evaluate the program.

Using a Staffing Study Committee

Once it has been determined that a study will be done, a study committee consisting primarily of members of the nursing service administrative group and the health care facility administrative staff should be designated. In addition to specifying the number and types of units, the desired schedule, and the nature and scope of the final report, the study committee is responsible for appointing a study coordinator and assigning the necessary supporting people as observers, data clerks, and assistants.*

Committee Members*

Study Coordinator. The coordinator is the key person in the conduct of the study and should be selected from the nursing service staff.

Since the position of coordinator may require full-time activity, the coordinator's release from regular duties is essential during the time the study is being made and the report written. Some health care facilities may want to have the study coordinator continue in a position that will provide continuity for the initiation and supervision of any reorganization decided upon. It is the responsibility of the coordinator to supervise the training of the observers and other members of the study team.

The coordinator carries out the following activities:

- instructs and supervises the study team
- assigns and trains observers
- orients other staff and patients
- prepares study materials and data collection forms
- selects the patient samples
- monitors and edits observers' record taking
- assists with the analysis, interpretation, and evaluation of the data
- prepares the study report

---

*Source: *Methods for Studying Nurse Staffing in a Patient Unit*, DHHS, Pub. No. (HRA) 78-3, May 1978.

Other Members. The other members of the study team, including data clerk and typist, are selected by the study committee. The data clerk will be needed to assist in preparing statistical tables and is usually chosen from the business office because of experience with business machines and data computation.

Head Nurses or Charge Nurses. The head nurses or charge nurses of the unit or units selected for study are vital members of the study team. They are directly responsible for categorizing patients according to nursing care requirements. They use their nursing judgment to assess the adequacy or inadequacy of the staffing on their unit, and they also assist the study coordinator. Their importance in providing complete support to the study project cannot be overestimated. These nurse leaders set the tone of the units on which the studies are carried out.

Their activities, in brief, are to:

- Classify patients according to indicators and guidelines for nursing care requirements.
- Record their perceptions of the adequacy or inadequacy of staffing on their units for the periods studied.
- Assist the study coordinator in checking observer reports.
- Orient patients to the study.

Observers. If the observers are to be selected from the nursing service staff, the study committee appoints the observers. Nurses selected to be observers should carry out their observations on units other than their own.

Responsibilities of Committee*

The function of the staffing study committee is to produce a set of staffing policies and procedures that satisfy the unique needs of the nursing service.

---

*Source: Nursing Staff Requirements for Inpatient Health Care Services, American Nurses' Association, Pub. No. NS-20, 1977. Reprinted with permission.

Among the policies and procedures that they would be responsible for creating are

- a written statement of the purpose, philosophy, and objectives of the nursing program of care
- a written statement of the purpose, philosophy, and objectives of staffing
- an identification of the database (i.e., the information regarding patients, staff, and costs)
- a written statement of the rationale for the selection of the staffing methodology employed
- a coherent set of personnel policies and procedures related to scheduling and plans for implementation
- a statement of basic staffing patterns for each nursing unit
- a set of performance standards for the nursing staff
- a plan for supplementing staff at times of staff illness, emergency leave, and prolonged heavy workloads and for reducing the staff when prolonged light workloads occur
- a quality assurance program to measure quality of care
- a written plan for evaluating the staffing program that includes identification of a system for monitoring the success of the program, for examining the staffing patterns at regular intervals in light of changing conditions, and for initiating appropriate changes

Selecting a Staffing System

While it may be tempting to select a staffing system successfully used in another health care facility, the nurse manager should be forewarned that what is appropriate for one facility is rarely appropriate—without modification—for another.

The difficulty lies in the range of variable factors: organizational systems, patient unit arrangements, nurse-support systems, levels of technology, employment policies, facility architecture, and so on.

Essentially the parameters of what is being measured in one health care facility are different from those being measured in another. These parameters affect the end figures on which staffing calculations are based—that is, the time standards for nursing activities, the total available nursing hours, the actual workload, the proportionate distribution of nursing hours and work among staff skill levels, the decision rules for patient classification, and so on.

The process of gathering information to arrive at these figures is called data collection. It is a process that each nursing service unit should employ, using techniques of measurement that are generally applicable and valid in order to produce the unique figures for particular departments and units. Once these base figures have been established, they can then be adjusted to accommodate new conditions or new standards and thus satisfy the changing as well as the continuing needs of the nursing service.

Criteria*

The following criteria could be used in selecting the best staffing system for a nursing unit or department:

- It encompasses enough pertinent variables in its application to produce valid results.
- It uses measurement devices that produce reliable and valid data about these variables.
- It is simple, in that it is not time consuming and can be applied by the personnel within the institution with a minimum of consultant specialized personnel in its application.
- It provides baseline data that can be used in comparative studies within the institution or within a set of similar institutions in the delivery system.
- The cost benefit can be predicted and is worthwhile. A more costly methodology

may in the long run be less expensive in terms of benefit.

- It is responsive to changes in the delivery system, such as the introduction of new positions or elimination of old and the creation of new supporting systems to the nursing care delivery system.

Staffing: Model System 1*
(Emphasis on Utilization Control)

The "Staff Utilization Control System" provides a means for predicting nursing requirements so that available personnel can be assigned to the nursing units where they are most needed. In addition, the reporting system provides data that can be used in a variety of ways to manage more effectively.

The control system described here is one that is currently being used in several Texas hospitals. It is intended to provide a typical example, since many variations are possible. The procedures and reports would have to be adapted to a facility's special requirements and conditions.

Nurse Staff Table

The first step in implementation of the control system is to develop the nurse staff table. Figure 17–2 provides an example of a nurse staff table for one hospital. This table is developed directly from study results, so requirements can reflect the nursing philosophy and procedures in your hospital. The required hours of care determined for each patient classification and shift are converted to equivalent nursing personnel and arranged in tabular form to simplify estimating personnel requirements.

When the nurse staff table is complete, all of the basic information necessary for implementing a staff utilization control system is available. The patient classification plan used during the

*Source: Nurse Staffing Methodology, DHEW, Pub. No. (NIH) 73-433, 1973.

*Source: SMS Nursing Service Study Guide: Staff Utilization (A Project of The Texas Hospital Education and Research Foundation), Shared Management Systems for the Texas Hospital Association. Reprinted with permission.

Figure 17–2 Nurse Staff Table

Personnel Required, Including Both Direct and Indirect Care/Administrative Activities

No. Patients	Admit		Disch.		Min. Care			Par. Care			Tot. Care		
	D	E	D	E	D	E	N	D	E	N	D	E	N
1	.16	.16	.14	.11	.16	.12	.07	.25	.15	.10	.33	.31	.22
2	.32	.32	.28	.22	.32	.24	.14	.50	.30	.20	.66	.62	.44
3	.48	.48	.42	.33	.48	.36	.21	.75	.45	.30	.99	.93	.66
4	.64	.64	.56	.44	.64	.48	.28	1.00	.60	.40	1.32	1.24	.88
5	.80	.80	.70	.55	.80	.60	.35	1.25	.75	.50	1.65	1.55	1.10
6	.96	.96	.84	.66	.96	.72	.42	1.50	.90	.60	1.98	1.86	1.32
7	1.12	1.12	.98	.77	1.12	.84	.49	1.75	1.05	.70	2.31	2.17	1.54
8	1.28	1.28	1.12	.88	1.28	.96	.56	2.00	1.20	.80	2.64	2.48	1.76
9	1.44	1.44	1.26	.99	1.44	1.08	.63	2.25	1.35	.90	2.97	2.79	1.98
10	1.60	1.60	1.40	1.10	1.60	1.20	.70	2.50	1.50	1.00	3.30	3.10	2.20
11	1.76	1.76	1.54	1.21	1.76	1.32	.77	2.75	1.65	1.10	3.63	3.41	2.42
12	1.92	1.92	1.68	1.32	1.92	1.44	.84	3.00	1.80	1.20	3.96	3.72	2.64
13	2.08	2.08	1.82	1.43	2.08	1.56	.91	3.25	1.95	1.30	4.29	4.03	2.86
14	2.24	2.24	1.96	1.54	2.24	1.68	.98	3.50	2.10	1.40	4.62	4.34	3.08
15	2.40	2.40	2.10	1.65	2.40	1.80	1.05	3.75	2.25	1.50	4.95	4.65	3.30
16					2.56	1.92	1.12	4.00	2.40	1.60			
17					2.72	2.04	1.19	4.25	2.55	1.70			
18					2.88	2.16	1.26	4.50	2.70	1.80			
19					3.04	2.28	1.33	4.75	2.85	1.90			
20					3.20	2.40	1.40	5.00	3.00	2.00			
21					3.36	2.52	1.47	5.25	3.15	2.10			
22					3.52	2.64	1.54	5.50	3.30	2.20			
23					3.68	2.76	1.61	5.75	3.45	2.30			
24					3.84	2.88	1.68	6.00	3.60	2.40			
25					4.00	3.00	1.75	6.25	3.75	2.50			
26					4.16	3.12	1.82	6.50	3.90	2.60			
27					4.32	3.24	1.89	6.75	4.05	2.70			
28					4.48	3.36	1.96	7.00	4.20	2.80			
29					4.64	3.48	2.03	7.25	4.35	2.90			
30					4.80	3.60	2.10	7.50	4.50	3.00			

study now becomes an integral part of the system for predicting nursing requirements. The only change in this procedure results from the fact that it is necessary to *predict* patient classification rather than record it during the shift, as was done during the study. If patient classification and nursing care plans are incorporated into a single procedure, a simple one-step planning process is provided that results in the patient classification.

Patient Classification Procedure

Eight criteria for measuring the intensity of care to be provided have been established. (See Figure 17–3.) These are elements of physical care and comprise a high percentage of the nursing care that requires the greatest amount of time. They are Diet, Vital Signs, Respiratory Aids, Suction, Cleanliness, Toileting/Output, Turning/Assisted Activity, and Isolation.

This measurement is used to assess the classification of each patient and determine if he or she is to be considered total, partial, or minimal.

Total the number of points in all elements of physical care. Compare the total number of points with the conversion table. Place the patient in the appropriate classification.

Staffing Requirements Report

The following is a typical procedure for predicting nursing staffing requirements and preparing a staffing requirements report. (See Figure 17–4.)

The staffing requirements report is prepared by the head nurse each day, covering a 24-hour period beginning at 7 AM.

- Determine patient classification for each patient on the unit (check appropriate blanks). Check "Discg." blank for patients expected to be discharged that day and no other classification is required.
- When a patient is admitted to the unit during the day, initiate a patient classification plan. The patient should be classified as an admit during the first shift he or she is on the unit. Enter the number 1 after "Admission" at the bottom of the staffing requirements report. Check the appropriate blanks to indicate the patient classification for the remaining shifts of the 24-hour period.

The staffing requirements report is revised as necessary at 7:00 AM the next day. Significant changes are recorded and totals entered to indicate the correct number of patients in each classification and for each shift during the preceding 24-hour period.

The information provided on the staffing requirements report serves two general purposes.

- It predicts nursing requirements for each unit so that immediate action can be taken for optimum use of available staff.
- It provides historical information for evaluating utilization and planning changes to improve use of personnel in the future.

Although nursing administration can start using this information to allocate personnel as soon as the staffing requirements report has been implemented, substantial improvement in staff utilization should be expected to require long-range projects to develop and test alternative approaches to staff planning and control. The implementation of a simple and effective system of utilization reports will ensure that the information necessary to support these improvement projects is available.

The original copy of the staffing requirements report provides the correct number of patients in each patient classification and the required hours for each nursing unit. Provisions should be made for maintaining a record of the number of patients in each classification since this patient mix will become an important factor in any system for planning future nursing staff requirements and budgets. The required hours, or staffing table hours, for each unit are recorded daily on the weekly nursing utilization report.

Weekly Nursing Utilization Report

The weekly nursing utilization report (Figure 17–5) will become the central document in the staff utilization control system. The information related to actual hours used and census is required from the beginning of the study to provide for evaluation of current staffing patterns.

The weekly nursing utilization report is prepared for each nursing unit. Actual hours worked for each personnel skill are also recorded daily and totaled. The utilization percentage is calculated for each day and shift by dividing the staffing table hours by total hours used. The midnight census is recorded and the average hours per

Figure 17–3 Patient Classification Plan

PATIENT CLASSIFICATION PLAN

A. RESPIRATION AIDS AND SUCTION
1 point— bedside humidifier ____
     — standby routine suction ____
2 point— cough and deep breath q 2 hrs. ____
     — oral suction prn ____
     — NASAL—pharnygeal suction prn ____
3 point— continuous O_2 ____
     — cough & deep breath q 1 hr. ____
     — TRACH suction q 1 hr. ____
4 point— TRACH suction q 30 min. c̄ pt. responsive ____
5 point— TRACH suction q 30 min. c̄ pt. unresponsive ____

B. CLEANLINESS
1 point— self bath, bed change ____
2 point— assist bath, bed change ____
     — sitz bath ____
3 point— assist bath, occupied bed ____
     — partial bath given, bed change ____
     — bathed & dressed by personnel (peds), bed change ____
4 point— bathed & dressed by personnel, special skin care, occupied bed ____

C. ACTIVITY
1 point up in chair c̄ help once in 8 hrs. ____
2 point— up in chair c̄ help twice in 8 hrs. ____
     — walk c̄ assist. ____
3 point— walk c̄ assist. of 2 personnel ____
     — turn q 2 hrs., bed fast ____
4 point— turn q 1 hr., bed fast ____

D. DIET
1 point— feed self, or family feeds ____
2 point— feed self c̄ supervision ____
3 point— feed self c̄ constant staff presence ____
4 point— feed patient totally by personnel ____

E. TOILET
1 point— toilet c̄ supervision ____
     — specimen collection ____
2 point— toilet c̄ supervision ____
     — uses bed pan ____
3 point— toilet c̄ stand-by supervision ____
     — daily colostomy irrigation ____
4 point— incont. average output ____
5 point— incont. c̄ diarrhea ____

F. VITAL SIGNS
1 point— TPR routine ____
2 point— V.S. q 4 hrs. ____
     — night check q 1 hr. ____
3 point— V.S. & observation q 4 hrs. ____
     — V.S. q 2 hrs.—vital signs monitored ____
4 point— V.S. & observation q 1 hr. ____
5 point— BP-pulse-respiration & neurological evaluation q 30 min. ____

G. INTAKE & OUTPUT
1 point— routine I&O ____
     — strain all urine ____
2 point— Clinitest and Acetest ____
     — IV push medications ____
3 point— gastrostomy feeding q 4 hrs. ____
     — N/G tube irrig q 2 hrs. ____
4 point— continuous IV ____
     — blood transfusion ____
     — hourly output ____
5 point— tube feeding more frequently than q 4 hrs. ____
     — drainage c̄ frequent dressing changes ____

H. MISCELLANEOUS
1 point— modified isolation ____
2 point— strict isolation ____
3 point— pt. pre-op (for OR in 24 hrs. or less) ____
     — pt. post op (had surgery in past 24 hrs.) ____
     — pt. on continuous monitor ____
4 point— patient instruction ____
     — patient markedly disturbed ____

Conversion Table
1–9   minimal
10–21   Partial
22–30   Total
31   Transfer to ICU

POINTS
A____
B____
C____
D____
E____
F____
G____
H____

TOTAL
Classification

Figure 17–4 Staffing Requirements Report

STAFFING REQUIREMENTS REPORT
EXAMPLE
For 24-Hour Period Beginning 7 AM–## (DATE:) 4/30

Room/Bed	Rev. ✔	Discg.	Min. Care D	Min. Care E	Min. Care N	Par. Care D	Par. Care E	Par. Care N	Tot. Care D	Tot. Care E	Tot. Care N	Room/Bed	Rev. ✔	Discg.	Min. Care D	Min. Care E	Min. Care N	Par. Care D	Par. Care E	Par. Care N	Tot. Care D	Tot. Care E	Tot. Care N
101-A						X	X	X				115-A			X	X	X						
102-A			X	X	X							115-B			X	X	X						
103-A						X	X	X				116-A											
104-A						X	X	X				116-B						X	X	X			
105-A						X	X	X				117-A			X	X	X						
105-B						X	X	X				117-B											
105-C												118-A			X	X	X						
106-A						X	X	X				118-B			X	X	X						
106-B			X	X	X							119-A						X	X	X			
106-C									X	X	X	119-B											
109-A												120-A						X	X	X			
109-B												120-B						X	X	X			
109-C			X	X	X							121-A			X	X	X						
109-D												121-B		X									
110-A		X										122-A											
110-B			X	X	X							122-B						X	X	X			
111-A			X	X	X							123-A			X	X	X						
111-B			X	X	X							123-B			X	X	X						
112-A			X	X	X							124-A						X	X	X			
112-B			X	X	X							124-B						X	X	X			
113-A			X	X	X							125-A			X	X	X						
113-B			X	X	X							126-A						X	X	X			
114-A			X	X	X							127-A			X	X	X						
114-B			X	X	X							128-A			X	X	X						
Subtotals			12	12	12	6	6	6	1	1	1	Subtotals			11	11	11	8	8	8			
Subtotals			11	11	11	8	8	8															
TOTALS			23	23	23	14	14	14	1	1	1												

STAFFING GUIDE HOURS

	Day	Eve	Night
Admissions			
Discharges	2) .28		
Minimum Care	23) 3.68	23) 2.76	23) 1.61
Partial Care	14) 3.50	14) 2.10	14) 1.40
Total Care	1) .33	1) .31	1) .22
PREDICTED STAFF REQUIRED	40) 7.79	38) 5.17	38) 3.23

Figure 17–5 Weekly Nursing Utilization Report

WEEKLY NURSING UTILIZATION REPORT
EXAMPLE

UNIT: I   WEEK OF: 7-15

DAY	7-15	7-16	7-17	7-18	7-19	7-20	7-21		TOTAL WEEK
				------DAY------					**TOTAL WEEK**
Staffing Table Hours	46	41	31	44	44	37	53		296
Hours Used RN	16	16	8	16	16	8	16		96
LPN	9	16	16	8	8	8	20		85
AUX	48	39	32	56	56	32	48		311
Total Hours Used	73	71	56	80	80	48	84		492
Utilization %	63	58	55	55	55	77	63		60

				------EVENING------					
Staffing Table Hours	33	28	23	30	29	25	49		217
Hours Used RN	10	8	8	8	8	8	8		58
LPN	16	16	18	16	16	18	16		116
AUX	24	24	16	24	24	24	24		160
Total Hours Used	50	48	42	48	48	50	48		334
Utilization %	66	58	55	63	60	50	102		65

				------NIGHT------					
Staffing Table Hours	16	14	16	14	14	13	20		107
Hours Used RN	8	8	8	8	8	8	8		56
LPN	8	8	8	8	8	8	8		56
AUX	32	16	—	16	24	8	24		120
Total Hours Used	48	32	16	32	40	24	40		232
Utilization %	33	44	100	44	35	54	50		46

				------TOTAL------					
Staffing Table Hours	95	83	70	88	87	75	122		620
Hours Used RN	34	32	24	32	32	24	32		210
LPN	33	40	42	32	32	34	44		257
AUX	104	79	48	96	104	64	96		591
Total Hours Used	171	151	114	160	168	122	172		1,058
Utilization %	56	55	61	55	52	61	71		59
Midnight Census	23	21	18	23	24	19	27		155
Hours/Patient Day	7.4	7.2	6.3	7.0	7.0	6.4	6.4		6.8

Skills Mix %			20	24	56
			RN	LPN	AUX

Activity   *------UNMEASURED HOURS-------*

patient day calculated to provide additional information for analysis.

The staffing table hours and hours used are totaled at the end of the week and weekly utilization calculated for each shift. The average hours per patient day are also calculated on a weekly basis.

"Skills Mix %" reflects the percentage of total hours used by each of the major personnel skills. This relationship of skill hours to total hours can be effectively used to ensure staffing patterns that are compatible with nursing objectives.

One copy of the weekly nursing utilization report should be returned to the appropriate head nurse, with the original filed in nursing administration. Graphs of utilization for each unit can be used to illustrate improvement trends and point out the need for corrective action.

Goals for Skills-Mix Ratio

The skills-mix ratio provides one simple way to express the relationship of registered nurse (RN) hours to licensed practical nurse (LPN) hours to auxiliary personnel (AUX) hours on a nursing unit. For example, if 120 hours were worked on a nursing unit, including 30 RN hours, 60 LPN hours, and 30 AUX hours, the skills-mix ratio would be 25%–50%–25%.

RN	30 Hours	25%
LPN	60 Hours	50%
AUX	30 Hours	25%
	120 Hours	100%

Nursing administration is responsible for determining the proper skills mix for each unit. The skills-mix ratio provides a means of expressing the plan so that a goal can be established for each unit that is compatible with both quality and economic objectives for that unit. No guidelines have been developed for this ratio, although the example used (25%–50%–25%) is typical of ratios in existing programs.

An example of how the skills-mix ratio is determined is provided in Figure 17–6.

Improvement Projects

After studying the staffing patterns that emerge from these staff utilization reports, the nurse manager may want to initiate improvement projects appropriate for the department or a particular unit. Among such projects might be the following.

Relative Staff Utilization Percentage. Review current staffing patterns and correct any obvious inequities that result in consistently high or low utilization percentages for a specific unit or shift.

Skills Utilization. A considerable amount of data are available concerning activities of personnel in each skills classification. Consistently low or high utilization of personnel in a specific skills classification suggests an adjustment in staffing patterns to correct inequities in distribution of work.

There are many factors to be considered when evaluating skills utilization in relation to determining the desired or optimum skills-mix ratio (RN hours–LPN hours–AUX hours).

- services or tasks that actually create workload
- policy that determines who can perform a specific task or service
- skills that will provide best or better patient care in the performance of a specific task
- availability of personnel in any one skills classification in relation to workload
- job enlargement—increasing the responsibilities for personnel in each classification, which results in more interesting work for all employees
- economics—using lowest skill acceptable in order to minimize overall cost

The information necessary for reviewing current staffing patterns and assignment policies and practices is now available. The best time to review skills utilization is when these data are current.

Figure 17–6 Nursing Care Hours and Utilization Report

NURSING CARE HOURS AND UTILIZATION REPORT
MONTH: FEBRUARY
EXAMPLE

Unit	Current Month								Year to Date					
	Pt. Days	*% Occup.*	*Care Hours*	*% Util.*	*% RN*	*% LPN*	*% AUX*	*Hrs. Per Pt. Day*	*% Occup.*	*% Util.*	*% RN*	*% LPN*	*% AUX*	*Hrs. Per Pt. Day*
1 East	1405	97	5881	97	32	41	27	4.2	87	93	32	42	26	4.4
1 West	1265	89	5207	92	29	42	29	4.1	82	91	30	43	27	4.2
2 East	1031	83	5046	88	33	44	23	4.9	73	84	32	40	28	5.3
2 West	1234	85	5343	98	32	43	25	4.3	77	89	30	46	24	4.6
3rd.	1285	89	5661	92	28	45	27	4.4	82	89	32	45	23	4.4
SUBTOTAL	6220	89	27138	94	31	43	26	4.4	80	89	31	43	25	4.5
CCU	163	—	2132	—	55	45	0	13.1	—	—	56	44	0	14.6
ICU	4	—	88	—	55	45	0	22.0	—	—	55	45	0	22.0
SUBTOTAL	6387		29358		33	43	24	4.6			33	43	24	4.8
Adm. & Supv. Hours Worked	6387		1576					.25						.26
Hours Paid Not Worked	6387		1670					.26						.28
Orientation Inservice, Etc.	6387		293					.05						.04
DEPT. TOTAL	6387		32897					5.15						5.38

Personnel Interunit Transfer and Nursing Pool. The accomplishment of high average staff utilization is often dependent on development of more effective procedures related to transfer of personnel from one unit to another based on workload. Charts illustrating the variations in daily workloads and actual hours worked for each nursing unit will normally show considerable potential for improvement in matching hours worked to estimated requirements. The implementation of a better system for interunit transfer will often improve this condition.

The determination of optimum staffing for each unit at some point below the peak requirements and the assignment of part-time nursing personnel to units when peak periods are predicted have proven effective in increasing average utilization. The nursing pool is also often used as a means of providing personnel for units when peak workloads occur.

Work Distribution. Projects that result in action to shift nursing workload from one period of the day to another and reduce extreme variations in workload during the day offer opportunities for improving utilization.

Scheduling Innovations. Scheduling changes and use of part-time personnel to provide supplementary staffing during certain days or periods of the day can result in better matching of hours worked to estimated requirements.

Development of Part-Time Nursing Resources. Any use of part-time work schedules normally requires action to develop sources for qualified part-time nursing personnel. A specific project designed to make these schedules desirable and develop sources may yield significant results.

Cyclic Scheduling. Often, development of a cyclic scheduling system that improves the distribution of hours worked in relation to requirements will improve average utilization, as well as eliminate inequities in existing scheduling systems.

Off-Unit Activities. If the study indicates a relatively high occurrence of off-unit activities (errands), it suggests the possibility of an analysis to determine if other alternatives (errand service) should be considered. Improvements might be limited to specific assignments on the nursing unit to ensure the most economical performance of these activities.

Methods Improvement. The completed study provides detailed information concerning both direct care and indirect care/administrative activities, including identification of the specific services/procedures that require the most time. Opportunities for improving services and reducing the time required are present and the lists of tasks developed provide an important source of projects. Generally speaking, the tasks that require the most time will have the highest potential for improvement.

The assignment of small task-analysis teams of nursing personnel to investigate specific tasks and recommend improvements is an essential part of an ongoing improvement program. This activity will help to create and maintain interest in effective nursing care as well as result in tangible savings.

Nurse Staff Planning. The staff utilization control system provides data that can be used for more effective staff planning and budgeting. A project to develop a formal staff planning system for budgetary control based on these data can result in better communications between nursing and health care facility administration concerning nursing requirements.

The basic system, which is simple, uses historical data concerning census, patient mix, and the actual staff utilization percentages experienced on each unit to forecast the same factors or quantities during the following weeks or months.

Staffing: Model System 2*
(Emphasis on Budget Control)

Overview

The nurse staffing system is composed of five major components: staffing standards, annual budgeting, schedule planning, daily assignment, and management reporting and control.

The staffing standards portion of the system establishes the critical workload-to-staff relationships that are used in each of the three planning cycles, and consequently is the key feature of the total system. The annual budgeting, schedule planning, and daily assignment sections represent the staff planning activities that take place yearly, every three to seven weeks, and on a daily basis, respectively. The effectiveness of planning efforts is then measured and reported by the management reporting and control section, which provides feedback on a periodic basis.

There are several assumptions inherent in this staffing system.

- There is a small group of float or prn nursing personnel who are not permanently assigned to a specific unit.
- Nurses who are normally assigned to nursing units must expect limited reassignment to similar units.
- The nurse staffing function is consolidated in a central staffing office with overall responsibility for nurse staffing, including the establishment of time schedules, authorization of overtime, assignment of float personnel, and reassignment of unit staff.

Classifications of patients are not intended to directly relate to the medical conditions of the

---

*Source: Thomas F. Kelley and W. Andrew McKenna, "An Integrated Nursing Staffing System" (paper presented at the Seventh National Conference, AHE, Hospital and Health Services Division, February 1976). Partners, Touche Ross & Company, Atlanta, GA. Reprinted with permission.

patients; rather, they are indicative of the time requirements for providing nursing care. The staffing standards used in this system are designed for use with established classifications, providing a more accurate determination of staffing needs.

Step 1: Developing Classification Criteria. In developing staffing standards by patient classification, implement the patient classification process first. This involves a number of time-consuming steps, including definition of classification criteria, testing of criteria for validity, and training of nursing personnel to use the classification scheme. Once the patients are routinely classified by degree of care required, it becomes an easier task to develop staffing standards for each classification.

Step 2: Determining the Workload Index. The actual determination of staffing standards is accomplished using a variety of input sources. Available historical data on actual nursing hours per patient day are analyzed for determination of past performance and comparison with data from similar health care facilities. The primary data for the staffing standards come from direct time study and random sampling of unit operations. In addition, head nurses can provide a valuable source of information on appropriate staffing levels. The results of the work measurement activities and discussions with nursing personnel are summarized by patient type, employee type, and shift to establish "goal" nurse hours per patient day for each patient type. (See Table 17–4.) A reasonableness test is performed by using each unit's actual distribution of census by patient type to calculate a weighted average of total hours per patient day using the developed standards. These results can then be compared to historical data and similar data from other facilities.

The Annual Budget and Staffing

The preparation of an annual budget for nursing is the first step in the overall staff planning cycle. The budgeting process uses a forecast of

Table 17–4 Goal Distribution of Nursing Hours by Patient Type for General Medical-Surgical Units

	Patient Type				Weighted Total
	A	B	C	D	
7–3 Shift:					
RN	.74	.53	.37	.24	.48
LPN	1.39	.99	.69	.45	.89
Tech/Aide	.95	.68	.48	.30	.61
	3.08	2.20	1.54	.99	1.98
3–11 Shift:					
RN	.55	.40	.28	.18	.36
LPN	1.04	.74	.51	.33	.67
Tech/Aide	.72	.51	.36	.23	.48
	2.31	1.65	1.15	.74	1.51
11–7 Shift:					
RN	.39	.28	.19	.12	.25
LPN	.72	.52	.37	.23	.46
Tech/Aide	.50	.35	.25	.17	.32
	1.61	1.15	.81	.52	1.03
Total	7.00	5.00	3.50	2.25	4.52
Expected Distribution of Patient Type	15%	40%	35%	10%	

A: maximum care; B: complete care; C: partial care; D: self-care.

census by unit and data from the staffing standards table to establish unit staffing levels. The census forecast is prepared for each unit on a monthly basis and is based on past trends and projections of future changes in patient load. Of course, the census forecast by unit must tie directly to other organizational forecasts used for budgeting. The usual approach to budgeting is to have one source in the facility for all volume forecasts to ensure consistency in all revenue/expense projections.

After completion of the forecast, unit staffing requirements by month are established using a standard staff budgeting form. The next section provides a detailed procedure for completion of the form. The budgeting form (Figure 17–7) uses the appropriate goal hours per patient day and the projected average daily census (ADC) to compute required full-time equivalents (FTEs) by employee type and shift. Note that there is a provision for five day per week coverage for one head nurse and two unit secretaries that are not part of the census-related staffing. No relief coverage is provided for the head nurse, and relief for the unit secretaries is provided from the float pool.

Procedure for Completion of Staff Budgeting Form

Following is an outline of the process for completion of the staff budgeting form (Figure 17–7). There will be 12 monthly forms completed for each unit and the float pool.

1. Using the appropriate staff budgeting form for the unit, enter the projected ADC for the unit and period on line 2 of the form. Also complete lines 1, 3, 4, and 5.
2. Multiply the *goal hours* (7) for each position by the ADC to obtain *daily hours* (8).
3. Enter the number of days covered in the period (e.g., 30 for the month of September) in the fourth column (9) and multiply by *daily hours* in the third column (8) to obtain *planned hours* (10). Note that the number of days covered in the period has been preentered for head nurse and unit secretary positions.
4. Enter the planned *cost per hour* for each position for the time period in the sixth column (11). This dollar per hour figure should include the impact of shift differentials, charge pay, and planned merit increases. Multiply the fifth column by the sixth to obtain *total cost* (12).
5. Obtain the required *FTEs* (13) for each position by dividing *planned hours* (10) by the *work hours in the time period* (5).
6. Compute totals for *planned hours, total cost,* and *FTEs* for the entire unit.
7. Calculations can be cross-checked by the following:

- Divide the total of the *planned hours* column by line 5. The result should equal the total of the *FTE* column.
- Multiply the total goal hours by line (2), then by .175. The result should approximate total FTEs excluding the unit secretary and head nurse positions.
- Obtain the average unit rate by dividing total cost by total FTEs. Compare this number to other units as a reasonableness test.

The staff scheduling process matches the working hours of budgeted personnel to provide 24-hour-a-day patient coverage. The staff schedule should be developed based on a repeated pattern for each cycle. For further information, see "Approaches to Scheduling" in Chapter 18.

Daily Staffing Assignments or Adjustments

This procedure is performed daily for each shift and unit by the central staffing office. The purpose and objectives of the daily staffing procedure are

- to alter the scheduled staff complement based on the *actual* census and patient mix by unit
- to react to unplanned absences due to illness, etc.
- to assign "float" or prn nurses to a unit and to effect transfers of staff nurses between units if needed

The adjustments are based on reported census by patient classification for each unit. Each nursing station prepares a shift report that includes a summary of current census by classification. A copy of this report goes to the staffing office. The staffing coordinator then calculates the required nursing coverage based on unit census and patient mix using a table of staffing (Table 17–5) prepared from the staffing standards and a shift staffing report (Figure 17–8). The end result of the calculation is the required staffing by employee type and by unit for the upcoming shift.

Once the staffing requirements are established, the staffing coordinator assigns float personnel

Figure 17–7 Staff Budgeting Form—General Medical-Surgical/OB-GYN Units

Unit:_____ (1)   Time Period: _____ (4)

Projected Average Daily Census: _____(2)   Work Hours in Time Period: _____ (5)

Beds Available: _____ (3)

(6) Position Title	(7) Goal Hours	(8) Daily Hours (7) × (2)	(9) Days Covered in Period	(10) Planned Hours (8) × (9)	(11) Cost per Hour	(12) Total Cost (10) × (11)	(13) FTEs (10) ÷ (5)
7–3 Shift							
Head Nurse		8.0	21.6				
RN*	.48						
LPN	.89						
Tech./Aide	.61						
Unit Sec.†		8.0	21.6				
Total	1.98						
						7–3	☐
3–11 Shift							
RN							
LPN	.36						
Tech./Aide	.67						
Unit Sec.	.46	8.0	21.6				
Total	1.49						
						3–11	☐
11–7 Shift							
RN	.25						
LPN	.46						
Tech./Aide	.32						
Unit Sec.							
Total	1.03						
						11–7	☐

			Hours		Cost	FTE
Total	4.50		☐		☐	☐
					(A)	(B)

☐   Unit Avg. Rate
(A) ÷ (B)

*Total RNs including charge nurses and staff nurses.
†Day off for unit secretaries will be staffed from the float pool.

Table 17–5 Table of Staffing Requirements for 7–3 Shift (All Units Except Intensive Care and Nursery)

	Type A				Type B				Type C				Type D		
Census	RN	LPN	T/A	Census	RN	LPN	T/A	Census	RN	LPN	T/A	Census	RN	LPN	T/A
1	.00	.25	.25	1	.00	.25	.00	1	.00	.25	.00	1	.00	.25	.00
2	.25	.25	.25	2	.25	.25	.25	2	.00	.25	.25	2	.00	.25	.00
3	.25	.50	.50	3	.25	.50	.25	3	.25	.25	.25	3	.00	.25	.00
4	.25	.75	.50	4	.25	.50	.25	4	.25	.25	.25	4	.00	.25	.25
5	.50	.75	.50	5	.25	.50	.50	5	.25	.50	.25	5	.25	.25	.25
6	.50	1.00	.75	6	.50	.75	.50	6	.25	.50	.25	6	.25	.25	.25
7	.75	1.25	.75	7	.50	1.00	.50	7	.25	.50	.50	7	.25	.50	.25
8	.75	1.50	1.00	8	.50	1.00	.75	8	.50	.75	.50	8	.25	.50	.25
9	.75	1.50	1.00	9	.50	1.00	.75	9	.50	.75	.50	9	.25	.50	.25
10	1.00	1.75	1.25	10	.50	1.25	.75	10	.50	.75	.50	10	.25	.50	.50
11	1.00	2.00	1.25	11	.75	1.25	1.00	11	.50	1.00	.75	11	.25	.50	.50
12	1.00	2.00	1.50	12	.75	1.50	1.00	12	.50	1.00	.75	12	.25	.75	.50
13	1.25	2.25	1.50	13	.75	1.50	1.00	13	.50	1.25	.75	13	.50	.75	.50
14	1.25	2.50	1.50	14	1.00	1.75	1.25	14	.50	1.25	.75	14	.50	.75	.50
15	1.50	2.50	1.75	15	1.00	1.75	1.25	15	.75	1.25	1.00	15	.50	.75	.50
16	1.50	2.75	2.00	16	1.00	2.00	1.25	16	.75	1.50	1.00	16	.50	1.00	.50
17	1.50	3.00	2.00	17	1.00	2.00	1.50	17	.75	1.50	1.00	17	.50	1.00	.50
18	1.50	3.25	2.25	18	1.25	2.25	1.50	18	.75	1.50	1.00	18	.50	1.00	.75
19	1.75	3.25	2.25	19	1.25	2.25	1.50	19	1.00	1.50	1.25	19	.50	1.00	.75
20	1.75	3.50	2.50	20	1.25	2.50	1.75	20	1.00	1.75	1.25	20	.50	1.25	.75

to units requiring additional staffing and reassigns other unit personnel if required. An important consideration in the quality of patient care is to control the mix of regular, full-time staff in a unit relative to float and part-time staff in that unit, making sure that continuity of care is achieved through the full-time staff.

Reporting System

A series of management reports is produced to control the effectiveness of the staffing system. These reports measure the difference between

- planned and actual census by unit for the period
- expected and actual mix of patients by acuity of care classification
- planned, required, and actual staffing hours and cost

The reports are produced on a daily basis and summarized upward for different management levels at weekly and monthly intervals.

- Daily reports are used by assistant directors of nursing to identify problem units on a current basis, in terms of:
  - unusual census fluctuations
  - patient classification problems
  - inappropriate staffing levels or mix
- Weekly reports are reviewed by the director of nursing to assess the overall department performance and to analyze trends for discussion in weekly staff meetings, and so on.
- Monthly reports are reviewed by facility administration to ensure adherence to overall organizational financial plans and objectives.

The key to effective management control lies in a detailed analysis of variances. Therefore, the reporting system must isolate the following types of variances in terms of both hours and dollars:

- *Planning variance.* This is the difference between budgeted staffing and required

Figure 17–8 Shift Staffing Report (Excerpt)

Sample Units

7–3 Shift
Date:

	Census	RN	LPN	T/A		
A	5	.50	.75	.50		
B	15	1.00	1.75	1.25	2 North	
C	12	.50	1.00	.75		
D	3	—	.25	—	U.S.	Total
Req.	2.00	3.75	2.5	1	9.25	
Act.	2	3	3	1	9.00	
				Variance	(1.75)	

	Census	RN	LPN	T/A		
A	2	.25	.25	.25		
B	11	.75	1.25	1.00	3 North	
C	12	.50	1.00	.75		
D	3	—	.25	—	U.S.	Total
Req.	1.50	2.75	2.00	1	7.25	
Act.	2	3	3	1	9.00	
				Variance	(1.75)	

Shift Summary of All Units

	RN	LPN	T/A	U.S.	Total
Req.	13.25	21.00	13.25	8	55.5
Act.	15.00	18.00	14.00	7	54.0
Var.	1.75	(3.00)	.75	(1)	(1.5)

staffing. It measures the effectiveness of the utilization forecast procedure.

- *Efficiency variance.* This is the difference between the required staffing and the actual staffing. It reflects the effectiveness of the staffing office in matching daily patient care needs with the available nursing resources.

The management reporting system must also include reporting on quality of care and monitoring of patient classification. Quality-of-care monitoring through nursing audits and other tools is used to relate quality of nursing care to productivity changes, since productivity increases at the expense of patient care quality are usually unacceptable. In addition, staffing by patient classification requires a method of auditing classifications to discourage misuse of the system.

Staffing with Acuity Systems

Because patient acuity can change quickly and the number of patients on the unit varies during a 24-hour day, an acuity rating should be done every shift on each patient. When the amount of time needed to provide the nursing care per shift is known, the required staffing can be determined by shift instead of for the 24-hour period.

When the prototype evaluation or a checklist factor evaluation PCS is utilized, the clients are categorized by classes. Additional studies are then required to identify the average amount of time spent providing nursing care to patients of the different classes. Time and motion studies can be conducted to obtain this information. For in-house time and motion studies, the specific amount of time spent providing nursing care is carefully recorded by an independent observer. Over time, the average amount of time spent by nurses for each class of patients can be computed.

Once it is known how much time is spent, on the average, for each class of patients, the number of clients per class can be multiplied by the average number of hours needed for that specific classification rating. This reflects the amount of time needed to provide services to the patients in that category. This is then repeated for each class on the unit. When the numbers of hours for all the classes have been computed, they can be summed to identify the total hours needed to provide nursing care to that group of clients.

To show how staffing can be done with the PCS, Table 17–6 displays classifications for the day shift for all the clients on 2 North using a prototype evaluation or a checklist factor evaluation PCS. The PCS shows that there are currently 3 class II, 14 class III, and 3 class IV patients. It should be noted that there are no class I clients listed using the PCS. Class I clients are considered to be stable since they need only a minimal amount of nursing care within a 24-hour period. Therefore, to contain costs these clients are discharged as soon as possible. Based upon a hypothetical time and motion study conducted for 1 year on the unit, it has been determined that the following average times per class are reasonable:

- class I = 2 hours of nursing care/24-hour shift
- class II = 3 hours of nursing care/24-hour shift
- class III = 4.5 hours of nursing care/24-hour shift
- class IV = 6 hours of nursing care/24-hour shift

To identify the staff needed for a 24-hour period, it is necessary to assume that the client will basically maintain the same classification during that time period. Because the clients are rated every shift, staffing can be recalculated as their condition changes. The next step in determining the number of staff needed is to multiply the

number of hours per class by the number of patients currently in each class. For Table 17–6, the day shift on 2 North, the hours of care required are as follows:

- class II = 3 hours × 3 patients = 9 hours of care
- class III = 4.5 hours × 14 patients = 63 hours of care
- class IV = 6 hours × 3 patients = 18 hours of care
- Total hours of care needed for the 24-hour period = 90 hours

Once the hours of care for the day are known, that value must be multiplied by the percentage of the staff allocated to each shift. For example, 35% of the staff are allotted to days and to evenings:

$$90 \text{ hours of care} \times 0.35 = 31.5 \text{ hours of care}$$

In addition, 30% of the staff are allocated to nights:

$$90 \text{ hours of care} \times 0.3 = 27 \text{ hours of care}$$

Now the hours of care for the shift are divided by the number of hours in the shift to identify the number of employees needed to staff the unit. With 8 hours per shift, the following calculation applies:

$$\frac{31.5 \text{ hours of care}}{8 \text{ hours of time/shift}} = 3.94, \text{ or } 4 \text{ employees}$$

$$\frac{27 \text{ hours of care}}{8 \text{ hours of time/shift}} = 3.37, \text{ or } 3 \text{ employees}$$

Table 17–6 Classification Ratings per Bed on 2 North for Day Shift

Room 201, Bed A—empty Bed B—class III
Room 202, Bed A—class III Bed B—class II
Room 203, Bed A—class IV Bed B—class IV
Room 204, Bed A—class III Bed B—class III
Room 205, Bed A—class II Bed B—class III
Room 206, Bed A—class III Bed B—class III

Room 207, Bed A—class III Bed B—class IV
Room 208, Bed A—class III Bed B—empty
Room 209, Bed A—class III Bed B—class III
Room 210, Bed A—class II Bed B—class III
Room 211, Bed A—empty Bed B—class III
Room 212, Bed A—empty Bed B—class III

Therefore, based upon the prototype evaluation or a checklist factor evaluation PCS for 2 North with 3 class II, 14 class III, and 3 class IV patients, four employees are needed to provide the current nursing care needs for day and evening shifts. For the night shift, three employees are needed. As the levels of the patients change, the amount of staff required may also vary. That is one of the reasons why the PCS must be updated each shift.

When staffing is determined using a relative value unit (RVU) method of the factor evaluation PCS, the calculations vary to some extent. Since each task reflects a predetermined time allotment, the staffing is only calculated on a per-shift basis, not for a 24-hour period. Time and motion studies are conducted before the RVU methodology is utilized to verify the average amount of time spent for each RVU. In the example of 2 North, the amount of time was determined to be 3 minutes per RVU. Table 17–7 reveals the number of RVUs assigned to each client for the day shift based upon the PCS.

On the day shift, 2 North currently has 645 RVUs of care to provide. The number of RVUs can be multiplied by the minutes per RVU to obtain the number of minutes of care required for the shift. The minutes of care per shift, 1,935 minutes, can then be converted to the hours of care required for the shift, or 32.25 hours. That value is then divided by the hours per shift to identify the number of employees. For example:

$$645 \text{ RVU} \times 3 \text{ minutes/RVU} = 1,935 \text{ minutes of care}$$

$$\frac{1,935 \text{ minutes of care}}{60 \text{ minutes/hour}} = 32.25 \text{ hours of care}$$

$$\frac{32.25 \text{ hours of care}}{8 \text{ hours/employee}} = 4.03 \text{ employees}$$

The value of 4.03 employees per shift is slightly higher than the 3.94 employees identified by the PCS methods using class ratings. With the RVU system, the numerical values assigned to each patient are more exact than the class ratings, and that can alter the number of staff. If more class III patients are at the high end of the rating scale, the RVU system will reflect more points. This will generally result in the RVU system showing a larger number of staff. The same is true when the patients are at the low end of the class rating scale; the RVU method will then give them fewer points, and usually the staffing values will be smaller.

Maintaining accurate, up-to-date information about the acuity levels on each unit allows for appropriate but not excessive staffing patterns to meet the clients' needs. This minimal staffing pattern helps keep the cost of delivering nursing care at the most cost-effective level possible. The Joint Commission stipulates that clients must have adequate staff to provide the care and that the care must be implemented in accordance with the qualifications of the nursing staff (i.e., within their scope of practice). An objective and reliable PCS is one methodology that can be used to

Table 17–7 RVU Assignments per Bed on 2 North for Day Shift

RVU (Class)	RVU (Class)
Room 201, Bed A—empty Bed B—35 (III)	Room 207, Bed A—26 (III) Bed B—43 (IV)
Room 202, Bed A—27 (III) Bed B—12 (II)	Room 208, Bed A—28 (III) Bed B—empty
Room 203, Bed A—45 (IV) Bed B—47 (IV)	Room 209, Bed A—31 (III) Bed B—29 (III)
Room 204, Bed A—26 (III) Bed B—35 (III)	Room 210, Bed A—20 (II) Bed B—38 (III)
Room 205, Bed A—18 (II) Bed B—34 (III)	Room 211, Bed A—empty Bed B—36 (III)
Room 206, Bed A—38 (III) Bed B—40 (III)	Room 212, Bed A—empty Bed B—37 (III)

Total RVU for this specific shift = 645 RVUs

allocate patient assignments. Once the number of staff needed for the shift has been determined, the acuity system can also be used to assign the staff in an equitable manner.

PATIENT CLASSIFICATION SYSTEMS

Overview*

The primary objective of the first generation of patient classification systems was to predict nurse staffing levels from shift to shift. Today, the objectives have greatly expanded. Information related to productivity monitoring, long-range planning, budgeted staff tracking, trend analysis, costing, and charging and the linking of patient classification information to a wide variety of pertinent data such as quality criteria, length of stay, nursing diagnoses, and medical care data are among the frequent demands. Nursing executives now use workload information for negotiating contracts with health maintenance organizations, evaluating trends in patient care demands, and generally minimizing economic risks.

With these and other expanded requirements of patient classification data comes the added pressure to repeatedly demonstrate the accuracy of the information. The methods traditionally employed for maintaining and monitoring the reliability and validity of patient classification systems are increasingly being recognized as inadequate for the complexity and sophistication of the expanded objectives.

With the advent of microcomputers and relational database software, nursing executives are now able to track reliability and validity on an ongoing basis. Because patient classification data are retained, they can be used to provide more accurate workload predictions and descriptions. Further, the ability to identify the source of prob-

lems with unit-specific instruments or nurse classifiers leads to the required corrective mechanism. Increased confidence in the reliability and validity of the workload data provides the staff nurse with direct evidence of the accuracy of the patient classification instrument and provides the nursing executive with a significantly stronger tool in budget planning and tracking, contract negotiations, and financial risk reduction.

Types of Patient Classification Systems*

Patient classification systems (PCS) provide a method to classify patients according to a specific group of tasks, acuity of illness, degree of nursing dependency, and/or risks and to predict the amount of nursing time that will be required to care for the patients on the unit. A nurse manager can predict the staffing needs fairly accurately with a subjective assessment, but it is essential to have objective data to support staffing and budgetary needs. It is important to assign staff based on the actual need rather than on the amount of care actually provided. There are many different types of patient classification systems that are being utilized today, but what is most important is that whatever system is used must demonstrate validity and reliability in accurately predicting nursing care hours. Hospitals have developed PCS to reflect the severity of the client's condition known as *acuity systems*.

An acuity system can be used with any nursing care delivery system. The way the nursing care is delivered is not directly related to how sick the clients are or their acuity rating. The PCS identifies the amount of nursing care required for each patient and how many nurses are needed on each shift to provide adequate nursing care. It has been determined that acuity systems can

*Source: Phyllis Giovannetti and Judith Moore Johnson, "A New Generation Patient Classification System," *Journal of Nursing Quality Assurance*, Vol. 20, No. 5, Aspen Publishers, Inc., © 1990.

*Source: Adapted from Catherine E. Loveridge and Susan H. Cummings, *Nursing Management in the New Paradigm*, Aspen Publishers, Inc., © 1996.

also be used to identify the cost of the nursing care services being provided.

Because each hospital provides health care services to a local population, an acuity system needs to be site specific. There is no single format for a PCS that can be applied to all organizations. Therefore, each facility must develop or adapt a PCS that appropriately suits the needs of its institution.

There are numerous acuity systems that have been developed commercially and adopted by hospital facilities. These systems may be loosely grouped into two basic formats, as prototype evaluation and factor evaluation rating methods. Both types of PCSs are developed from critical indicators or descriptors reflecting common types of nursing care provided to clients.

A *critical indicator* is a specific task that is commonly needed for the clients on that unit. Indicators vary, some depending upon the type of unit and some on the type of patient being treated. For example, on an obstetrics unit a critical indicator could include changing a sanitary napkin or checking a client's fundus. In an intensive care unit, however, few patients would require those services, so that a more appropriate critical indicator might be monitoring a Swan-Ganz catheter or an arterial line.

Prototype evaluation systems rate a client simultaneously on the specific critical indicators listed on the PCS. The critical indicators are used to separate clients into categories requiring more or less nursing care. Each category is designed to be broad but mutually exclusive. Table 17–8 shows an example of a prototype evaluation PCS (this is a generic example and is not intended to be comprehensive enough to apply to all hospital units).

The nurse using the prototype evaluation PCS rates the client simultaneously on a variety of patient care needs. The category that best describes the amount of nursing care needed by the client at the time of the rating determines the patient's classification. If a client can fit into two categories at the same time, the nurse makes a subjective decision and assigns the level that he or she believes is the most appropriate.

A prototype evaluation PCS is a way to rate clients simultaneously in several related aspects of their nursing care. These rating systems are usually easy to implement and do not require extensive training to be understood. They can be subjective, however, and it may be difficult for two independent raters to consistently produce the same rating on the same patient. Once the clients on a unit are rated and classified, the information can be used to determine the number of nurses needed to care for the group of clients.

The second format that can be utilized in an acuity or PCS system is known as the *factor evaluation* method. This methodology rates the client separately on various critical indicators instead of simultaneously, as seen with the prototype evaluation method. Each category of client needs (i.e., assessment, mobility, hygiene, etc.) is given a separate score. A total overall rating or score is then computed. Although this method is more time consuming to complete, it is less ambiguous and more objective than the prototype evaluation method. Table 17–9 is an example of a generic factor evaluation PCS and, like Table 17–8, is not intended to be comprehensive.

For Table 17–9, the items that pertain to the patient are identified, and the point value for each item is recorded under the appropriate shift. The numerical values assigned to each section of the acuity tool can then be summed and utilized in one of two methodologies: in a checklist format or as *relative value units* (RVUs).

When the factor evaluation acuity tool is used as a checklist, the items relevant to the client are checked off, and the total points assigned to each item are added. This method requires prior analysis of the unit to determine the range of points applicable to each acuity classification. For example, assume that Mrs. A and Mr. B are patients on the 2 North unit. Studies on 2 North have determined that clients can be categorized into classes based upon the following point system:

- class I, 0–10 total points
- class II, 11–25 total points

Table 17–8 Generic Prototype Evaluation Acuity System

Category	Class I	Class II	Class III	Class IV
Assessments	VS q shift, self-care	VS qid, daily standing wt., no tubes	VS q4h, bed scale wt., neuro checks q2–4h, 1–2 tubes	VS q2h, neuro checks q1h, 3 or more tubes
Mobility	Up ad lib	Ambulates or chair with one-person assistance	Ambulates or chair with two-person assistance	Ambulates or chair with three-person assistance, two- to three-person assist on and off gurney
Hygiene and elimination	Self-care	BSC or bedpan with one-person assist, partial bath, Foley care, Fleets enema	BSC or bedpan with two-person assist, complete bath, SSE, complete linen change with two people	Incontinent care, complete bed bath, enemas til clear, several linen changes per shift
Diet	Feeds self, NPO	Positioning by one person for meal, set up tray	Positioning by two persons for meals, assist with feeding	Feeder, tube feeding, high risk of aspiration
Medications and tubes	Meds 1–2 trips/shift	Meds 3–5 trips/shift, IV or HL with 1 IVPB/shift	Meds 6–7 trips/shift, IV or HL with 2 IVPB/shift, hang 1 U of blood	Meds 8 or more trips/shift, IV Hyperal or heparin, 3 or more IVPB/shift, hand 2 U of blood or more
Treatments	Simple dsg change qd	Simple dsg change q8h, assist with simple procedure	Complex dsg change q4h, empty colostomy bag, assist with 2 procedures	Colostomy irrigation, assist with complex procedure, more than 1 complex dsg change q4h, suction q1–4h
Teaching and emotional	A&O × 3, simple teaching	Anxious, reinforced teaching, Posey vest or wrist restraints, some family interaction	Disoriented or hostile, some language barrier, Posey and wrist restraints, frequent interaction with family, teaching new material or discharge instruction	Needs constant monitoring, major language barrier, teaching complex procedures, extensive family interaction
Other	None	Telemetry monitoring	Blood and body fluid precautions	Code, postmortem care

Total score

Table 17–9 Generic Factor Evaluation Acuity System

D	E	N	Client Care Categories
			Assessments
			1 VS q shift
			2 VS QID
			2 VS q4h
			3 VS q2h
			1 neuro check q8h
			2 neuro check q2–4h
			3 neuro check q1h
			1 daily standing wt
			2 daily bed scale wt
			1 1–2 tubes
			2 3 or more tubes
			Mobility
			1 up ad lib
			2 up only BID or TID with 1 person assist
			3 up QID with 1 person assist
			3 up only BID with 2–3 person assist
			4 up TID or QID with 2–3 person assist
			2 assist pt. on & off the gurney
			Hygiene & Elimination
			1 self care
			2 partial bath
			3 complete bath
			5 multiple baths per shift—incontinent
			2 BSC or bedpan with 1 person assist
			3 BSC or bedpan with 2 person assist
			1 Foley cath care
			1 Fleets enema
			2 SSE enema
			3 enemas til clear
			Diet
			1 NPO
			1 feeds self, able to position self
			2 feeds self, 1 person assist for positioning
			3 assist feed, 2 person assist for position
			4 feeder or tube feeding, aspiration risk
			Medications & Tubes
			1 1–2 med trips/shift
			2 3–5 med trips/shift

continues

Table 17-9 continued

D	E	N	Client Care Categories
			3 6–7 med trips/shift
			4 8 or more med trips/shift
			2 IV or HL with 1 IVPB/shift
			3 IV or HL with 2 IVPB/shift
			4 IV of Hyperal or Heparin
			4 3 or more IVPB/shift
			3 hang 1 unit of blood/shift
			4 hang 2 or more units of blood/shift
			Treatments
			1 simple dsg change qd
			2 simple dsg change q8h
			3 complex dsg change q4h
			3 more than 1 complex dsg change q4h
			2 assist with simple procedure
			3 assist with 2 simple procedures
			4 assist with complex procedure
			3 empty colostomy bag
			4 colostomy irrigation
			4 suction q1–4h
			Teaching & Emotional
			1 simple teaching (5 min)
			2 continual reinforcement teaching (10 min)
			3 teaching new material or discharge instruction
			4 complex teaching, multiple parts (20 min)
			3 some language barrier
			4 major language barrier
			1 alert & oriented × 3
			2 very anxious and agitated
			3 disoriented or hostile
			4 needs constant monitoring
			2 some general family interaction
			3 frequent family interaction
			4 extensive family interaction
			2 Posey vest or wrist restraints
			3 Posey vest and wrist restraints
			Other
			2 telemetry monitoring
			3 blood & bodily fluids precautions
			4 code or postmortem care
			Total Score

- class III, 26–40 total points
- class IV, 41 total points or more

In addition to using the factor evaluation PCS as a checklist, the numerical values can also be treated as RVUs. With an RVU system, the numbers assigned to each item or each critical indicator are equated to the amount of time required to do the various tasks. The time allotments are identified from time and motion studies done on the unit. During time and motion studies, an independent observer carefully times and records the time spent by each caregiver in performing various nursing care services. The amount of time required to chart each task is included in the time calculation for the study.

In summary, clients can be categorized in terms of their acuity rating, or the amount of nursing care they require, by using either a prototype evaluation or a factor evaluation PCS. The ratings received with the prototype evaluation format and the checklist method of the factor evaluation system should be the same. The RVU format of the factor evaluation PCS provides a direct comparison of the amount of time required to provide nursing care for different clients.

The advantage of the prototype evaluation method is that it is quick to complete, but it allows for a more subjective rating. The factor evaluation acuity system requires more time to complete and more extensive training for the staff. The major advantage of the factor evaluation PCS is that it is more objective in determining the amount of time or assistance required by the patient.

Both types of PCS meet the Joint Commission's requirement that patients be classified according to the severity of their condition or the amount of nursing care required. As mentioned earlier, either method can be employed regardless of the type of NCDS used. Whether the delivery of patient care is being done with case management, primary nursing, team nursing, or some variation of these, the classification system still reflects the amount of nursing care required.

Components of an Effective PCS for the Nurse Manager*

For the nurse manager the ideal PCS would project staffing needs for the nursing budget; measure efficiency of nurse managers in matching workload requirements on a daily, monthly, and annual basis; justify temporary and permanent changes in staffing; and provide a basis for nursing changes.

In conjunction with a quality assurance program, nursing administration can use a PCS as a tool to assess quality and quantity of care provided and establish priorities for improvement.

Finally, a PCS may be used to justify staffing ratios to third-party payors and funding agencies, as well as provide a vehicle for nursing reimbursement based on the complexity of care delivered.

Developing a Patient Classification System**

The development of an appropriate patient classification system should be based on an objective approach. There are essential characteristics of such a system that are important in establishing a base for the development of a patient data monitoring mechanism. Patient classification should relate not only to the level of staffing but also to the impact of acuity on the processes of delivering nursing care.

All patient classification systems must meet some basic criteria.

- They must identify patients in conjunction with each other so that they can be classified into relatively clear categories of care.

---

*Source: Rebecca K. Donohue, "Patient Care Classification Systems: A Study in Home Care," *Journal of Home Health Care Practice,* Vol. 5, no. 2, pp. 20–37, Aspen Publishers, Inc., © 1993.

**Source: Copyright © 1988, Katherine H. West.

- There must be a systematic and organized approach to the classification and integration of various patient types and components.
- The timing of each classification must be identified so that the numbers of classifications and the time it takes to deliver care can be consistent with the service offered.
- The calculation must make provision for the utilization of human resources and their application to the requirements for patient care.

There are almost as many patient classification systems available as there are institutions using them (see Table 17–10 for an example). The elements listed should be consistent within almost any such system.

The nurse manager must be careful to conduct a balanced and systematic assessment of the variables that go into the design of the classification system. Following are some key questions to be addressed.

Are objective processes being used to determine the relationship between nursing staffing needs and patient acuity levels?

Is the financial framework that provides the resources for nursing care flexible in responding to changes in acuity?

What do acuity and patient classification measures indicate when correlated with financial, standards, and quality indexes that define the nursing care expectations on an individual unit, department, or service?

How deeply is the nursing staff involved in the process of classifying and using the data for determining patient care needs and staffing levels?

Does the patient classification system serve as a component of the database that assists the manager in making decisions on allocation and utilization of human resources for delivering standard-based nursing care, meeting the predefined levels of quality, and operating within the prescribed financial limits?

MEASURING NURSE ACTIVITY*

Criticism of Measuring Techniques

The criticisms leveled at the various techniques for quantitatively measuring nursing activities are important to note.

- A narrow view of nursing practice results from the use of work measurement techniques. Their use implies that nursing work is distinctly procedural in character: task-oriented with specific beginnings and endings.
- There is a lack of precision in the results of these sampling methods. One can raise questions about whether the nursing practice observed is the most effective that *can* be provided. Omissions of care are not identified. So too, in many reports using these techniques, evidence is markedly lacking that the data presented are objective, reliable, and accurate. The reliability of raters and the problems of error in recording or reporting data are seriously ignored.
- The result is that patient classification schemes reflect specific nursing tasks, a number of which arise because of medical order and acuteness of illness. The schemes do not reflect emotional needs, orientation of the patient, instruction needs, and comfort other than through the process of providing physical care. Few have even attempted to include these items.

Techniques of Measuring Nurse Activity

Four techniques are used to measure the work of nurses; all of these involve the concept of time

---

*Source: This section consists of material adapted from *Nurse Staffing Methodology*, DHHS, 1973, Pub. No. (NIH) 73-433, and Chapter IV of *Development of Methods for Determining Use and Effectiveness of Nursing Service Personnel*, San Joaquin Hospital, 1976. [PHS No. 1-NU-34038, Laurel N. Murphy, Project Director.]

Table 17–10 Patient Needs Classification System

I. (65%) A PATIENT WHO REQUIRES ONLY MINIMAL AMOUNT OF NURSING CARE (An average of 2.8 nursing hours per 24 hours)

Examples

- A patient who is mildly ill (generally termed convalescent)
- A patient who requires little treatment and/or observation and/or instruction
- A patient who is up and about as desired; takes his or her own bath or shower
- A patient who does not exhibit any unusual behavior patterns
- A patient without intravenous therapy or many medications

II. (100%) A PATIENT WHO REQUIRES AN AVERAGE AMOUNT OF NURSING CARE (An average of 4.3 nursing hours per 24 hours)

Examples

- A patient whose extreme symptoms have subsided or not yet appeared
- A patient who requires periodic treatments and/or observations and/or instructions
- A patient who is up and about with help for limited periods; partial bed rest required
- A patient who exhibits some psychological or social problems
- A patient with intravenous therapy with medications such as IV piggybacks every six hours
- A newly admitted patient, either surgical or medical, who is a routine admission and not necessarily acutely ill

III. (135%) A PATIENT WHO REQUIRES ABOVE AVERAGE NURSING CARE (An average of 5.8 nursing hours per 24 hours)

Examples

- A moderately ill patient
- A patient who requires treatments or observations as frequently as every two to four hours
- A patient with significant changes in treatment or medication orders more than four times a day
- An uncomplicated patient with IV medications every four hours and/or hyperalimentation
- A patient on complete bed rest

IV. (200%) A PATIENT WHO REQUIRES MAXIMUM NURSING CARE (An average of 8.6 nursing hours per 24 hours)

This classification is most often used in intensive care areas.

Examples

- A patient who exhibits extreme symptoms (usually termed acutely ill)
- A patient whose activity must be rigidly controlled
- A patient who requires continuous treatment and/or observations and/or instructions
- A patient with significant changes in physician's orders more than six times a day
- A patient with many medications, IV piggybacks, and vital signs every hour and/or hourly output

The total amount of time required to care for each patient determines his or her classification.

Note: The percentage figure is the relation of care in the category to the daily standard of 4.3 hours. For example, Category I requires only 65% of the standard daily hours, or 2.8 hours. This four class system is patterned after Joint Commission guidelines. To acquire a nursing hours baseline, use was made of historical data. The number of hours per patient day was derived by taking the previous year's number of patient days divided by the number of paid nursing hours; the quotient was 4.2. Since nursing and fiscal affairs both wanted to increase patient care hours, the figure was adjusted to a baseline of 4.3 hours. Other estimates of nursing hours can be calculated from nurse activity studies.

Source: E.A. Schmied, "Nurse Staffing after Hospitals Merge," *Nursing Administration Quarterly*, Vol. 2, No. 1, Aspen Publishers, Inc., © 1977.

required for performance. Differences in techniques reside in how data are collected, how they are categorized, how amounts of time are estimated, and how minutely nursing work is described. The four techniques are

- time study and task frequency
- work sampling of nurse activity
- continuous observation of nurses performing activities
- self-report of nurse activity

Time Study and Task Frequency

The time study and task frequency technique involves analyzing nursing work into specific tasks and task elements. A decision is made regarding the points at which a task (procedure) begins and ends. Individuals are then timed as they perform the task (procedures). The total number of timings (sampling) depends on the degree of confidence one wishes to place in the average time obtained for the task (procedure). An allowance is made for fatigue, personal variation, and unavoidable standby. The average time plus the allowed time gives a *standard time* for the procedure (task). The measurement of nursing activity is made by multiplying the *frequency of task* by the *standard time*. The total of all tasks multiplied by their standard times equals the volume of nursing work. The basic documentation in staffing approaches using this technique includes a manual of hundreds of "standard procedures" and a standard time for each. The frequency of task performance is usually obtained by a checklist, with the individual reporting his or her performance of the task, his or her skill level (defined by position classification), and the place of performance.

Work Sampling

In work sampling technique (a procedure also used to measure productivity—see Chapter 21) nursing work is identified by major and minor categories of nursing activities. Through random sampling of nursing personnel as they perform their work, observers obtain observations of nursing personnel performing various activities. The total number of observations divided by the frequency occurring in a specific category yields the percentage of total time (during which observations were collected) spent in the performance of that activity. The total number of observations to be made is determined in advance and is based on the amount of sampling required for confidence in the data sampled.

The categories that occur most frequently are *direct care* and *indirect care*, indicating that most individuals studying the problem of utilization are interested in the amount of time spent by the nursing personnel with the patient in direct care as opposed to the time away from the patient. (See Table 17–11.)

The observer also records the skill level of the person performing the activity. One can then project the direct care hours per shift as compared with time for other activities. These values can be used to determine the amount of service being provided by the nursing staff for that particular census and mix of patients.

Early studies indicate that a five-day work-sample study generally yields sufficient data for most evaluations.

Work sampling has the advantage of not having to depend on staff memory (and time to record). Its primary disadvantage is that short observations do not depict the whole complex of an activity sequence. Also, observers need to be trained, supervised, and tested for reliability.

Although work sampling is a relatively nonintrusive procedure, having observations made of their activities every 10 or 15 minutes can be irksome to staff, though there is a tendency to ignore the observer after the first several rounds of observations. Observing personnel when they are in a patient's room may also be an irritant to the patient. A brief explanation by staff or observers before observational rounds begin that a nursing activity study is taking place will usually be adequate.

In the work sampling form (Table 17–11), *direct care* refers to any nursing activity that is patient centered; *indirect care* refers to activities that are away from the patient but are in preparation for or in completion of direct nursing care; *unit care* refers to activities necessary

Table 17-11 Work Sampling Form

Facility _____ Unit _____ Shift _____ Observer _____ Day of Study _____ Date _____

Time:

#	Description of Activity	HN, CN	RN	LPN	NA, Ord.	Stu.	WC	HN, CN	RN	LPN	NA, Ord.	Stu.	WC	HN, CN	RN	LPN	NA, Ord.	Stu.	WC	HN, CN	RN	LPN	NA, Ord.	Stu.	WC
1	Communication with Patient/Family																								
2	Medications, I.V. (administering)																								
3	Nutrition & Elimination																								
4	Patient Hygiene																								
5	Patient Movement																								
6	Positioning, Exercising																								
7	Rounds or Assist MD or Other with Pt.																								
8	Routine Checks, Patient Rounds, Symptom Observations—Nursing Personnel Only																								
9	Specimen Gathering and Testing																								
10	Treatments and Procedures—Nursing Only																								
11	Vital Signs																								

Direct Care #1–11

continues

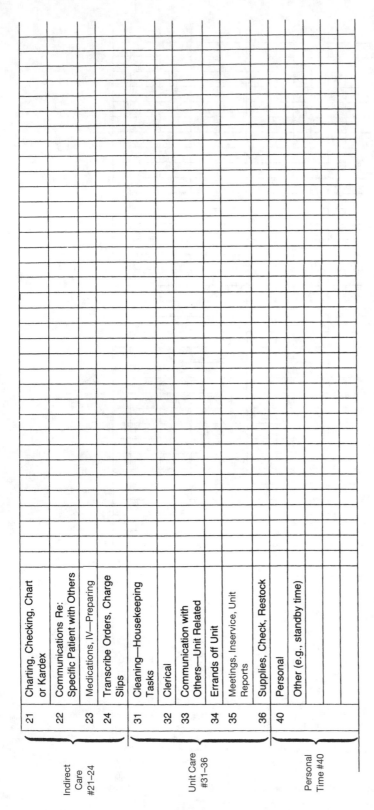

Source: Laurel Murphy, Development of Methods for Determining Use and Effectiveness of Nursing Service Personnel, San Joaquin General Hospital, © 1976.

for the general coordination of the unit or well-being of the patient population—not for a specific patient. *Personal time* includes meals, breaks, standby, and socializing with other personnel.

A category for "other" activities was also provided on the recording form; observers were instructed to check this space and describe the activity when they were unsure how to code it. It was found that almost all "other" activities could be coded under the 22 categories provided.

Continuous Sampling

Continuous sampling follows the same general pattern of categorization in work sampling except that an observer follows or accompanies only one individual for an extended period of time in the performance of his or her job. The observer may also observe the nursing work performed for one patient or for more if they are in the same room or if they can be observed concurrently (usually called *direct patient care sampling*).

Continuous observation of all personnel on a unit, with recording made in detail of all activities performed, is not justified or feasible. One observer can usually follow only one other person—an exorbitantly expensive and slow way to gather data if many personnel are involved.

Direct Patient Care Sampling. The purpose of direct patient care sampling is to determine the amount and source of direct care to patients by

- determining the amount of direct nursing care provided to each category of patient (patient categories are discussed in "Patient Classification Systems," above)
- determining who provides the direct nursing care

The direct care sampling procedure consists of making observations of the services received by patients. A set of patients is selected and at specified intervals of time the direct care activities taking place are recorded. Here, too, the observer also records the level (e.g., RN, LPN, aide, or student) of the person performing the

activity. This information can then be used to determine the number of hours of direct patient care provided for the existing patient population and mix from the amount of time spent with individual patients.[1]

Self-Reporting

In self-reporting, the individual checks a predetermined list or logs in diary form the tasks he or she has performed. The entries in the diary or log may be made at time intervals or may be made at the close of a major category of work or a specific task assignment. The self-reports are analyzed by sorting the entries into categories or classes of tasks similar to those for work sampling or by the development of themes or problems describing the activity.

When conscientiously carried out, a large amount of data can be collected. Observers do not have to be hired and/or trained. The method may thus be seen as less costly, but this may not be true. A thorough orientation of all staff members must be done, and when all shifts are involved and when one takes into account days off, float persons, and part-time persons, the problem of orientation is considerable. And even with a complete orientation, constant monitoring is necessary. Initial "best of intentions" can wear off rather rapidly and individuals may simply forget to record. Without a strong commitment to the study, resistance can develop. Recording *is* tiresome and staff can easily begin to see it as an additional burden in an already busy day. Much depends, too, on the complexity of forms used and the time required to mark them. The method is commonly used, however, and many find that the results are accurate enough for their needs.

THE WORKLOAD INDEX

Patient classification does not measure the amount of care required by patients. However, the category a patient falls within can be correlated with the total amount of nursing care re-

[1]*Methods for Studying Nurse Staffing in a Patient Unit*, DHHS, Pub. No. (HRA) 78-3, May 1978.

quired by that patient. Patients within the more acute categories will have to be allotted more nursing time than patients in the less acute categories. When these correlations are formalized, it is called a workload index.

Briefly, here is how a workload index is created. The results of patient classification and measurements of nursing services provided are combined to obtain the hours or minutes of direct patient care for each class of patient for each shift during the period of observation. The total minutes or hours of care, then, for any population of patients in a unit can be estimated and so give an objective basis for arriving at the services required for the given mix and census of patients.

The estimated workload is presented in terms of the total amount of care required of the staff.*

How To Calculate Required Nursing Hours**

The workload worksheet is used to calculate the mean number of nursing hours required on the unit (see Table 17–12).

---

*Source: R.K. Dieter Haussman, Sue T. Hegyvary, and John F. Newman, *Monitoring Quality of Nursing Care—Part II*, DHHS, Pub. No. (HRA) 76-7, Appendix 6, July 1976.
**Source: Ibid., Appendix 4.

Table 17–12 Workload Worksheet

1. Unit: _____

2. Find the daily average number of patient types 1–4 on the unit. (To do so, add the number of type 1 patients each day in the month and divide by the number of days in the month. Do the same calculation for types 2, 3, and 4.) Enter the number of each type in Column A.

		A	B†	C
Average number	Type 1 =	01		
	Type 2 =	03		
	Type 3 =	07		
	Type 4 =	14		

3. Multiply each number of Column A by the number in Column B. Write the product in Column C. (Column B is the mean hours required for each patient type, based on pre-

†Column B lists the mean hours required for each patient type. In this example the ratios are 1:3:7:14. Each hospital unit must establish its own ratio according to need and available resources.

vious study; C is the number of nursing hours required per type in 24 hours.)

4. Add the four numbers in Column C. Enter the number in the blank at the right.

_____

5. Divide the total of Column C by the sum of the daily average number of patients on the unit (from step 2 above). This figure tells you the number of hours per patient day required. Enter the answer in the blank at right.

_____

Example: Patient unit 3 West
(Steps 2–4) Average patient mix:

		A	B	C
T1	=	08	01	08
T2	=	10	03	30
T3	=	15	07	105
T4	=	02	14	28
		35		171 hours

(Step 5) $\dfrac{171}{35} = 4.9$ hours per patient day required

Chapter 18

Scheduling

OVERVIEW

The basic problem of scheduling is to provide patient care every day around the clock using nurses who generally work five days a week, one shift per day, and prefer to have weekends off. Scheduling is usually done by nurse managers for the units or floors for which they are responsible. They estimate patient care requirements and allocate the available nursing staff to the days of the week so that these requirements are approximately satisfied and human resource regulations observed. They try to schedule the nursing staff so that each nurse gets his or her share of weekends off and none of the nurses is rotated to evenings or night shifts for an unduly long time, and they also try to accommodate individual nurses' requests for specific days off. Often a schedule is prepared every other week, specifying workdays and days off for each member of the nursing staff over the ensuing two weeks.

Preparation of the schedule is a time-consuming task for the nurse manager and there is usually dissatisfaction with the results. Problems probably arise because coverage tends to fluctuate widely, particularly in the case of registered nurses (RNs); the number of registered nurses assigned to a given unit on a given shift may vary from day to day by a factor of two or more. The attempt to resolve scheduling and allocation problems can result in excessive use of overtime. In addition, schedules frequently have to be changed on short notice because of changes in patient care requirements, illness of a nurse, and so on. This leads to last-minute informal choices that might reflect favoritism.*

Objectives

- Adequate patient care is ensured while overstaffing is avoided.
- A desirable distribution of days off is achieved.
- Individual members of the nursing staff are treated fairly.
- Individuals know well in advance what their schedules are.

---

*Source: Reprinted with permission from *Socio-Economic Planning Sciences*, Vol. 7, Christopher Maier-Rothe and Harry B. Wolfe, "Cyclical Scheduling and Allocation of Nursing Staff." Copyright 1973, Pergamon Press, Ltd.

Factors in Scheduling Decisions*

The different skill levels of nursing staff—registered nurses, licensed practical nurses, and nurses' aides—have different capabilities. Licensed practical nurses (LPNs) and aides are legally allowed to perform only certain functions. Even within these categories, individuals can be classified by degree of experience and by the amount of responsibility they are able to assume.

Nursing coverage must, of course, be provided 24 hours a day, seven days a week. Nursing requirements are typically lower during the evening and night shifts than during the day shift. Saturday and Sunday requirements tend to be 20–30 percent lower than weekday requirements, depending on the medical service, due to a lower patient census, fewer new physician orders, or both.

Vacations and time off for holidays must be staggered to ensure continued patient coverage and equitable treatment for nurses.

Weekend days off are highly prized by the nursing staff, preferably both days in a row. Next in preference is two or more days off in a row in the middle of the week. Long stretches of consecutive working days (usually defined as more than five in a row) are undesirable.

Shift preference is a factor. Despite a salary differential, the evening and night shifts are more difficult to staff than the day shift. As a result, schedules must provide for rotation; daytime staff must work on the other two shifts from time to time. Also, staff on evening and night shifts may sometimes have to work on the day shift in order to attend special programs, training courses, and so on.

Unit preference is also a factor. Most nurses prefer to remain on one nursing unit rather than being floated or shifted from one unit to another, partly because of the competence and expertise they are able to develop in a particular unit and partly because of the camaraderie of continued association with the same group. However, there are some nurses who do not mind, and in fact prefer, floating because of the variety of experience it gives them.

Criteria for Evaluation*

Coverage. The number of nurses (by skill class) assigned to be on duty is in relation to some minimum number of nurses required.

Quality. Quality is a measure of a schedule's desirability as judged by the nurse who will have to work it. This measure includes weekends off, work stretches, single days on, split days off, and certain rotation patterns in addition to how a schedule conforms to the nurse's requests for days off for a particular scheduling period.

Stability. This is a measure of the extent to which nurses know their future days off and on duty and the extent to which they feel that their schedules are generated consistent with a set of stable policies (e.g., weekend policy, rotation policy).

Flexibility. This is the ability of a scheduling system to handle changes, such as from full time to part time, from rotation to working only one shift, and special requirements—class schedules of nurses, requests for days off, vacation, leaves of absence, and so on.

Fairness. This is a measure of the extent to which each nurse perceives that he or she exerts the same amount of influence on the scheduling system as other nurses.

Cost. The resources consumed in making the scheduling decision are the cost.

Guidelines

- Schedules should represent a balance between the needs of the employee and the

---

Source: Reprinted with permission from *Socio-Economic Planning Sciences*, Vol. 7, Christopher Maier-Rothe and Harry B. Wolfe, "Cyclical Scheduling and Allocation of Nursing Staff." Copyright 1973, Pergamon Press, Ltd.

Source: D. Michael Warner, "Computer-Aided System for Nurse Scheduling," *Cost Controls in Hospitals*, edited by J.R. Griffith, W.M. Hancock, and F.C. Munson, Health Administration Press. Reprinted with permission.

employer (patient care). When conflicts arise, patient care should have priority.

- Schedules should distribute fairly the "good" and "bad" days off among all employees.
- All employees should adhere to the established rotation. Exceptions should be rare and granted only if the employee is requesting two weekdays off (working every weekend). All requests and exceptions should be in writing and should specify the period of time off requested.
- Advance posting of time schedules allows employees to plan their personal lives. Therefore, absenteeism and requests for changes are reduced.
- Time schedules should not be a mystery nor a tool of control or discipline.
- There should be a mechanism for emergency changes to accommodate both employee and employer.
- Schedules must conform with all labor laws and organizational and departmental policies.
- Schedules should be established to provide correct numbers and mix of personnel, allowing continuity, which is essential for quality care.
- Schedules should be consistent, enabling work groups to develop teamwork, another contributor to quality care.*

*Constraints**

- Number of weekends off—one in four, one in three, every other weekend
- Maximum length of consecutive days worked—for example, no more than six
- Whether the days off should be together or split
- Payroll and overtime considerations (i.e., 5 workdays per week, 10 days per pay period)*

*Cautions**

- Giving more or less of one variable affects the ability to give more or less of the others.
- There is no one schedule that will work for all health care facilities and all departments.
- Select several different schedules that complement each other and develop the best cyclical schedule for the department.
- Experiment with combinations of different schedules.

CENTRALIZED, DECENTRALIZED, AND SELF-SCHEDULING

Centralized Scheduling**

Under centralized scheduling, one person in the nursing administration office plans coverage for all nursing units. A master staffing pattern is developed for these units and staffing is based on a preestablished standard. This staffing coordinator has access to clerical help to type, process, and distribute the master plan to the units. The coordinator knows the number and availability of staff on any given day and therefore is able to make the necessary day-to-day changes when sickness or other emergencies occur. The coordinator is able to do this by rotating nurses from one floor to another to achieve the best coverage throughout the health care facility. Such a person is important in keeping nurses involved in nursing rather than non-nursing functions.

The pitfalls of centralized scheduling are many. The staffing coordinator, unaware of the implications of clinical problems, may not understand that nurses need certain clinical expertise if they are rotated to more specialized units. Nurses are often placed into regimented schedules and offered no choices and few

Source: Thomas Kliber, *Modes of Scheduling*, Blue Cross of Western Pennsylvania, 1978.

**Source:* Gloria Swanberg and Eunice L. Smith, "Centralized Scheduling: Is It Worth the Effort?" *Nursing Administration Quarterly*, Vol. 1, No. 4, Aspen Publishers, Inc., © 1977.

Source: Patricia L. Eusanio, "Effective Scheduling— The Foundation for Quality Care," *Journal of Nursing Administration*, January 1978. Reprinted with permission.

options for change. They are not included in the decision-making process, which leads them to frustration and feelings of helplessness and insignificance.

Policies for Centralized Scheduling

Without specific policies for scheduling employees, consistent and equitable treatment of nursing staff is impossible. Typically, policies relate to approved shifts, number of weekends off, identification of weekend days for the night shift, minimum and maximum consecutive workdays, time lapse between shifts if personnel rotate, and the scheduling of holidays and vacations. Policies for both full-time and part-time employees should be delineated.

Head Nurse Participation. Head nurses should be held accountable for personnel expenditures over which they have control. This requires that they *participate actively* in determining the staffing needs for their individual units and *understand fully* the method of projecting full-time equivalents and calculating nursing hours per patient day (actual hours worked and total paid). Employees in staff departments with expertise in collecting and reporting statistics should furnish regular, timely, brief reports to their head nurses for quick reference in monitoring actual hours compared to budgeted hours.

Head nurses who have participated actively in determining the staffing needs, have projected the personnel budget for their units, and have meaningful, timely information regarding achievement of budgetary goals can and will be accountable for personnel expenditures over which they have control. If they have the authority to prepare and control their budgets, understand and support the scheduling policies, and have an opportunity for effective communication with the scheduler for their units, they will have little hesitancy to relinquish responsibility for scheduling personnel.

When the difference between line and staff functions is not understood, by both head nurses and employees in the scheduling office, conflict may arise. The head nurses may feel they have lost authority, particularly when a question arises regarding the adequacy of the staff on their units

to meet current needs. When employees in the scheduling office are not clear regarding their responsibilities and authority, they may feel totally responsible for controlling the budget, and their reactions may be extreme—either too rigid, alienating line personnel and impeding effective nursing, or too accommodating, attempting to do everything anyone requests.

Line versus Staff Responsibilities under Centralized Scheduling

Confusion in responsibility and authority may result in staff personnel making decisions in areas where line managers are accountable.

Line positions in the nursing department are supervisory (management positions at the level of head nurse and above); these nurses are accountable for nursing care of patients on specified units or services. When scheduling is centralized, the employees in the scheduling office are in a staff relationship with management personnel in the nursing department.

The *line* functions for which the nurses in management positions should be responsible are the following:

- establishing and controlling the personnel budget
- developing a master staffing pattern based on patient needs and the methods of assignment
- developing procedures for adjustment of staff on a daily basis
- establishing requirements for each position on the staff (such as assignment to an intensive care unit or charge responsibility)
- developing employees to meet requirements of their positions and evaluating their performance
- hiring, promoting, disciplining, and discharging employees

The *staff* functions for which the central scheduling office is responsible are the following:

- gathering facts and preparing reports for line personnel to facilitate budgeting

- scheduling employees according to policies in staffing patterns established by line personnel
- implementing procedures for reallocation of staff to meet daily needs; consulting with immediate superior when demand exceeds supply
- implementing procedures for position control
- maintaining records needed by line managers for evaluation (regarding absenteeism, for example)
- maintaining effective communications with appropriate departments, such as payroll and human resources

Decentralized Scheduling

Decentralized scheduling has helped to solve some frustrations. Nurses have more input into staffing patterns because the responsibility for staffing is entrusted to the unit nurse manager, who is aware of the clinical needs and personal needs of the staff nurses. However, because the nurse manager is not an expert in staffing methods and does not have access to clerical help, long tedious hours are spent in non-nursing functions. The schedule remains confusing and inconsistent in spite of sincere efforts.

Self-Scheduling*

Self-scheduling is the process by which staff nurses on a unit collectively decide and implement the monthly work schedule. Given the criteria for adequate unit staffing for each 24-hour period by the head nurse, each staff nurse chooses which day and shift he or she will work.

To implement a self-scheduling system, the head nurse sets up a series of meetings to:

- Identify problems with the existing scheduling system.
- Present self-scheduling as an alternative system.
- Establish a few practice sessions with self-scheduling.

Then, if the staff agree to pursue self-scheduling as an alternative form of scheduling, the head nurse posts large signs containing specific criteria the staff must follow in filling out their monthly schedules. The criteria must indicate the number and mix of registered nurses, licensed practical nurses, and nursing assistants (NAs) needed to give quality nursing care to the patients for all shifts each day of the week.

After the criteria are posted, the staff nurses are obligated to fill in their schedules and to check the schedule periodically for conflicts that result from over- or understaffing. When these situations occur, and they will, the staff nurses must negotiate with one another to meet their scheduling needs and the needs of the unit.

Generally, it is helpful if the night and evening nursing staff fill in their schedules first, so that day staff can determine when they must rotate. The head nurse must emphasize to the night and evening staff, however, that they must cover their shifts as evenly as possible to be fair to the rotating day staff. Also, the rotating staff should be given criteria as to the expected frequency of rotations per month (Table 18–1).

Additional signs should remind the nursing staff of their own professional scheduling obligations. For example, preceptors should plan their schedules to coincide with their preceptees. Primary nurses and associate nurses should coordinate their schedules to provide for maximum continuity in their patients' care. Nurses also must remember to plan their schedules to include committee meetings, classes, and seminars they must attend.

Usually, vacations and holidays are handled through a sign-up sheet at the beginning of the calendar year and are supervised by the head nurse according to nursing department policy. For example, if there is a nursing department policy that no more than two nurses from the same unit can be on vacation simultaneously,

---

*Source: Michelle Luckhardt Miller, "Implementing Self-Scheduling," *Journal of Nursing Administration*, March 1984. Reprinted with permission.

Table 18–1 Monthly Rotation Schedule

Rotation	Frequency (per month)
RNs to nights	3 nights
RNs to evenings	3 evenings
LPNs to nights	2 nights
LPNs to evenings	3 evenings
NAs to evenings	4 evenings

then the group must adhere to this policy in negotiating their vacations. Holidays may be handled in various ways. There might be a sign-up sheet for the year's holidays to be negotiated at the beginning of the year or every staff nurse might agree to work every other holiday. This also might be decided either by the group or nursing administration. Special requests for days off are simply designated by writing an "R" in the appropriate space.

Most important, the nursing staff must understand that it is their obligation to switch with a nurse of the same professional level (e.g., an RN switches with an RN, etc.) unless otherwise approved by the head nurse. It is not the responsibility of the head nurse to switch individual nurses to obtain adequate staffing. That is the responsibility of the nursing staff.

The head nurse will need to monitor the process occasionally for irregularities (e.g., paying overtime to an overzealous staff nurse), ensure fairness for the less assertive staff members, and nudge the process along if enthusiasm wanes.

Eliminating Obstacles to Self-Scheduling

Any dramatic change, such as self-scheduling, will meet with some degree of resistance. Staff nurses must either have or acquire appropriate interpersonal skills with which to negotiate their schedules with one another and develop the maturity to accept responsibility for adequately staffing the unit. These interpersonal skills do not develop overnight.

Specifically, the greatest resistance to this change will stem from the disruption of the staff's routine. Success with self-scheduling depends on the staff's ability and motivation to check and revise the monthly schedule periodically to en-

sure that the guidelines for adequate staffing for their unit are followed.

Flextime and Job Sharing*

Total Flextime. Under a total flextime arrangement, employees may come and go as they please; they need only put in whatever total hours are required of them for the workweek (usually 35 to 40). They are of course required to accomplish the work expected of them.

Total flextime is impractical for all employees except for those rare individuals whose work is so totally independent of the work of others as to be appropriately accomplished at any time at all. Also, even when total flextime may appear appropriate within a work group, it can present problems or at least perceptions of problems in that it is vulnerable enough to potential abuses to appear to be uncontrollable.

Limited Flextime. Limited flextime allows workers the option of establishing their own starting and quitting times on the condition that they be present for a specified block of time that may be relatively broad or narrow.

Team Flextime. Under the team flextime concept, all employees of a department or clearly designated team agree on their starting and quitting times as a group. This arrangement has been particularly popular with tightly unified work groups, such as operating room teams who may choose to arrange their schedule around surgeons' operating practices.

Job Sharing. Job sharing consists of two or more people working part time and mutually arranging their schedules to fill one single position. The most common job-sharing situations involve two part-time employees filling one full-time position. One pertinent example would be the position of department secretary in the department of surgery in a particular facility; this

---

Source: Charles R. McConnell, *The Health Care Supervisor's Guide to Cost Control and Productivity Improvement*. Aspen Publishers, Inc., © 1986.

position is filled by two half-time employees who each work alternating weeks of three days and two days.

APPROACHES TO SCHEDULING*

Nurse scheduling is defined as determining when each member of the nursing staff will be on duty and on which shift each will work. Scheduling should take into account weekends, length of an individual's work stretches, and nursing requests for vacation and time off. Scheduling is typically done for a period of four or six weeks, and the scheduling is frequently tailored to each individual nursing unit. There are three commonly used approaches to nurse scheduling: the traditional, the cyclical, and the computer-aided traditional approaches.

Traditional Scheduling. In traditional scheduling, the nurse schedulers start from scratch each period (week, month). Generally, the head nurse makes the scheduling decisions by taking pencil and paper in hand and looking at the roster of personnel who are available to work on specified dates and for certain durations. This places in the head nurse's hands a great deal of responsibility for the quality and quantity of coverage on the nursing unit. The major advantage of this traditional approach is its flexibility. Since nurses begin essentially from scratch each period, they are able to adjust to changes of environment on the nursing unit quite quickly. Some of traditional scheduling's disadvantages include spottiness in coverage at times and uneven quality of coverage. Unless policies in the nursing administration leave some flexibility in the process, uneven staffing could also lead to higher personnel cost.

Cyclical Scheduling. Cyclical scheduling is a system that covers a certain period of time, perhaps one or three months. This block of time is the cycle or scheduling period. Once having agreed on a definite period, the scheduling in the cycle simply repeats itself period after period. The advantage of cyclical scheduling is that

it provides even coverage with a higher quality of coverage determined for each nursing unit. Special requests would interfere with the coverage, which could impact the quality of staffing. The major disadvantage to cyclical scheduling is that it is inflexible compared to the traditional system and is not able to adjust rapidly to changes in the nursing unit environment. The ability to adjust is important, since change characterizes so many nursing units. The environment in which cyclical scheduling seems to work best is one in which the number of patients and their needs are fairly constant and the nurses are stable and do not rotate between shifts. New nurses can be hired into any open cyclical slot with very little difficulty.

Computer-Aided Traditional Scheduling. The third approach to scheduling uses the computer to help the traditional method of scheduling. This permits mathematical programming to be applied to traditional nurse scheduling. This system provides the traditional approach with more flexibility, and it also reduces the operating costs involved in calculating and in working with the schedule. To some extent, the computer centralizes the scheduling process. If mathematical models are properly used, the computer can produce high-quality schedules. The system will also facilitate the incorporation of standard personnel policies into the schedule, and the policies can be applied uniformly over all nursing units. It will also add more stability to the entire nursing department. The advantages of computerized scheduling are most dramatically apparent in situations where nurses rotate frequently among shifts and where nursing environments are subject to chronic change. Computer-aided, centralized schedules minimize the time spent on preparing and maintaining schedules.

Scheduling Formats*

Several basic types of scheduling ease the complexity of the process, including block scheduling, cyclical scheduling, and computer sched-

*Source: I. Donald Snook, *Hospitals: What They Are and How They Work*, Aspen Publishers, Inc., © 1992.

*Source: Barbara Stevens Barnum and Karlene M. Kerfoot, *The Nurse as Executive*, ed 4, Aspen Publishers, Inc., © 1995.

uling. Each of these represents an improvement on the preceding form, but examples of all three still are in effect today.

In block scheduling, the work schedule for a unit is planned in a block of weeks. The term *block* originally was applied to this scheduling because days to be worked often were blocked together, forming patterns such as that illustrated in Figure 18–1.

Block scheduling often is done for 4 to 8 weeks at a time. It can be calculated without great difficulty and has flexibility in that the next block of time need not necessarily follow the pattern of the preceding block.

Cyclical scheduling is an improvement on block scheduling in that it has repetitive work patterns assigned to personnel. Because each employee has a permanent pattern, he can calculate even months in advance when he will be on duty. A cyclical schedule has a repeated pattern of interweaving schedules.

These interlinking parts are a permanent plan, a fixed cycle of, usually, 4 to 6 weeks. The employee may have a different schedule for each of the weeks contained in the cycle, but the pattern repeats without change. Some assignment slots within a cycle may be perceived by employees as more desirable than others. Typically, the choice of assignment slots is handled on a seniority basis. Figure 18–2 illustrates a cyclical schedule.

Several things should be noted in this cycle. First, the employee schedules have been meshed so that (1) there are never less than two RNs on duty, (2) there are never more than two persons (RNs and LPNs considered together) off on the same day, and (3) there is never a day without at least one LPN on duty. These are the factors that dominated the interlinkages of these employee schedules.

Also, the cycles consider the individual employees insofar as each employee has at least one full weekend off per 4-week cycle. Beyond this general principle, it is obvious that some cycles would be preferred over others. For example, RN 2 actually has two weekends per period (as one cycle joins the next with Saturday and Sunday off). Also, this schedule never has the nurse working more than 5 consecutive days. In contrast, RN 4 usually has split days off, and she has one period in which she works 8 days in a row. (The only appealing component in this schedule is the 3-day weekend between weeks II and III.) A nurse new to the unit would probably be given the fourth rotation pattern. She would probably bid for a change of schedule if another RN were to leave the unit.

Even though some cycles are less than perfect, nevertheless the employee can plan ahead because the pattern (in this case a 4-week pattern) keeps repeating. Moreover, a schedule need only be developed once per staffing pattern. Because it repeats without change, the only schedules that need attention are those in which exceptions occur, as in a week containing a holiday.

Computerized scheduling enables the user to devise a plan that considers more variables than would be possible for hand calculations. For example, one might design a computer program for scheduling with the following dictates:

- patterns that must be maintained
    1. Miss G goes to school every Friday; she must have that day off.
    2. Mrs. T's religion will not allow her to work on Saturdays; she must have that day off.
- first-priority options when possible
    1. Mr. F must hire a babysitter if he works Tuesday or Wednesday; he would prefer to have these as his days off.
    2. Give every employee one weekend off per 4-week period if possible.

Figure 18–1 Three Nurses Filling Three Staffing Positions

X = days worked in the week

Week	RN	M	T	W	Th	F	Sa	Su
I	A			X	X	X	X	X
	B	X	X			X	X	X
	C	X	X	X	X			X
II	A	X	X			X	X	X
	B	X	X	X	X			X
	C			X	X	X	X	X

Figure 18–2 Cyclical Staffing Pattern

X = days worked in the week

Staff	Week I							Week II							Week III							Week IV						
	S	M	T	W	T	F	S	S	M	T	W	T	F	S	S	M	T	W	T	F	S	S	M	T	W	T	F	S
RN 1	X		X	X	X		X	X	X	X			X	X	X	X	X		X	X			X	X	X	X	X	
RN 2		X	X		X	X	X	X	X			X	X	X		X	X	X		X	X	X	X		X	X	X	
RN 3	X	X		X	X	X			X	X	X	X		X	X	X		X	X		X	X	X	X	X			X
RN 4	X		X	X		X	X	X		X	X	X	X			X	X	X	X	X		X	X	X			X	X
LPN 1		X	X	X	X	X			X	X	X		X	X	X		X	X	X	X		X		X	X		X	X
LPN 2	X	X	X		X		X	X	X	X		X		X	X	X	X		X	X			X	X	X	X		X

3. Where possible, give an employee 2 days off together instead of split.

- secondary priorities (to be followed if they do not interfere with priority options above)
  1. Preferably, do not have an employee work more than 6 days in a row.
  2. Schedule holiday time off within 10 days of the occurrence of the holiday.

These variables are only a sample of the constraints that may be incorporated into a computer program for scheduling. Most computer programs can combine general directives applicable to all staff with other variables applicable only to individual staff members. Also, a good program can handle those rules that must be applied in addition to rules that are assigned different priorities.

There are instances when staff complain that the computer is less successful than a human scheduler. Usually, this reflects not so much a computer deficiency as a failure to update the program or make it comprehensive. A computer will consider only those elements that are programmed into its circuits. A poor computer scheduling system indicates a poor program.

Advantages of Cyclical Scheduling*

Cyclical scheduling, once established, provides all of the following advantages.

The amount of highly skilled professional time spent on scheduling functions is reduced. Once a master rotation plan has been developed, trained clerical personnel can prepare and maintain schedules—freeing nursing time for more direct patient care functions.

The "good" and "bad" days off are spread equitably among all employees. The premises of cyclical scheduling require standard rotation of days off—distributing "good" days, such as weekends, fairly among all.

Schedules can be known in advance (almost ad infinitum) by each employee. This contributes to personnel satisfaction by making it easier for employees to plan their personal lives. It also reduces the number of absences that occur because of social events. By knowing their time schedule far in advance, nurses can plan many of their social events to occur on their scheduled days off.

The scheduling of correct numbers and mixes of personnel on duty each day is simplified. Once a master schedule has been developed that provides the correct number and mix of personnel, it can be virtually recopied each time period. The need to continuously count and adjust while developing a schedule is abolished.

Continuity of care is provided by minimizing floating. With the correct number and mix scheduled each day for each unit, the "plug-the-holes" process is virtually eliminated.

Work groups develop team synergy by stabilizing scheduled days off and lessening floating. A master schedule provides coverage for days

*Source: Patricia L. Eusanio, "Effective Scheduling— The Foundation for Quality Care," *Journal of Nursing Administration*, January 1978. Reprinted with permission.

off by the same part-time or full-time personnel—allowing the advantages of stabilized work groups to evolve. This aspect of scheduling is frequently overlooked, resulting in a helter-skelter selection of nurses who must work with great disadvantages.

Automated Scheduling Systems

There is an ever-increasing demand by multiple "customers" for health care provider–related information. This calls for increasing expertise in responding promptly to the many requests for staffing/scheduling data associated with assessing unit coverage: excessive or insufficient staff appropriateness of skill level and so on. Managers of clinical areas must possess the ability to analyze staffing-related needs and respond to them. Nursing administrators should be aware of the extent of the information available to them and how it may be used. The various types of information produced by a staffing and scheduling system can be used to facilitate change at these diverse organizational levels.

Checklist for Choosing an Automated Scheduling System*

Computer logic and speed must balance with nursing judgment and nursing service preferences. A schedule that identifies both minimum and maximum staff for the average care delivery needs of a unit, as well as the personal needs of each staff member, is the primary goal.

The final posted schedule must meet everyone's standards for clarity, logic, accuracy, fairness, aesthetics, and usefulness. Schedulers should not force nurses to learn another language or to build schedules around complicated translation tables. Instead, nurses should be able to substitute the computerized schedule for the handwritten schedule, with a minimum of confusion and "getting used to it."

Flexibility. Schedules should reflect any type of staffing assignment currently used in professional practice. These assignments must include

- floating to another unit or facility
- rotating to any shift
- working any combination of shifts, of different lengths, including 4, 8, 10, or 12 hours within one period
- accommodating individual preferences, including work stretch, weekend assignment, rotation assignment, primary shift, and fixed or cyclical patterns
- differing length cycles for days on/off during each period
- changing names, titles, work status, or full-time employment in the middle of a period

Efficiency. The scheduler must be efficient in its ability to manage large amounts of changing data and must produce a schedule more quickly than doing so by hand. Efficiency variables include the following:

- maintains overall speed of both data entry and schedule production
- posts vacation time and special requests (but should take into account that vacation time can be only 40 hours per week, or some fraction of 40 if part-time, and should not assign the vacation symbol on all seven days)
- updates schedules and staffing decisions and enters them in as few places as possible, thus eliminating data entry time
- provides on-line warnings when minimum coverage is scheduled
- creates warnings that prevent employees from receiving too many or too few days off
- incorporates additions into, or deletes staff from, preexisting schedules rather than forces the creation and generation of new schedules
- generates a schedule, after all data entry, within two minutes
- inserts birthdays, holidays, workshops, meetings, and classes automatically
- decreases the time required to generate, maintain, and edit schedules manually

---

*Source: Kathryn K. St. Morris, "Criteria for Selection of an Automated 'Intelligent' Scheduling System," *Nursing Administration Quarterly,* Vol. 16, No. 4, Aspen Publishers, Inc., © Summer 1992.

- displays schedules on screen for quick review
- contains master patterns of rotation that cover several periods and then recycles automatically
- removes staff in orientation or other categories of paid status, such as jury duty, who are not providing direct care
- generates rotation patterns that distribute staff to off-shifts fairly and in sequence
- produces schedule templates to serve as unit worksheets, with all fixed weekends and rotation patterns already delineated

Degree of Customization and Editing. The ability to customize the schedule's format and content to resemble more closely what a service already has in place could make the difference between success and failure of the scheduler. Therefore, some of the criteria to be examined should include the scheduler's ability to:

- Accept organizationwide rules.
- Adhere to unit-specific rules.
- Integrate employee-specific rules.
- Accept an unlimited number of rules.
- Prioritize rules in a user-defined sequence, for example, employee rules could overrule the unit rules that, in turn, take precedence over the organization rules.
- Provide enough dictionary files to capture all the variations in job titles, shifts, holidays, employee groupings, unit titles, and special designations.
- Establish the "clock" for the start of the next 24 hours; for example, the organization can start the day at 12 AM or 7 AM.

Note: To efficiently edit the schedule after it has been posted on the unit, managers should be able to make changes to the schedule as they occur. Sick calls, floated staff, emergency leave, and so forth, should all be manually entered and stored in the main computer. The final schedule, then, is certified by the manager and could be used for time card preparation.

SHIFTS

Overview*

There has been much discussion of the benefits of altering the traditional patterns in scheduling, the standard eight-hour shifts, to new and different configurations.

Labor Laws and Unusual Shifts

The Fair Labor Standards Act supplies the basic provisions governing hour and wage regulations and determines the conditions under which overtime pay is allocated. Two conditions are set for employees working in the health care services industry:

- In a one-week period, overtime is paid for time in excess of 40 hours in the weekly period.
- In a 14-day period, overtime is paid for time in excess of 8 hours in any day or 80 hours for the 14-day period.

These conditions permit a freedom in scheduling arrangements without incurring high additional costs for overtime wages. Depending on which base is chosen and the designated start of the workweek, little or no extra expense is incurred with a 10-hour shift for four days a week, a 12-hour shift for three days one week and four days the next, or a 9-hour shift for seven consecutive days on and seven off. Two daily meal periods, 30 minutes each, are disallowed from the hour count on the longer shifts.

Various configurations can be worked out to meet special demands of the nursing units and health care facility departments. However, employees must agree in advance to the work-hour arrangements. Statements of the work arrangements should be added as an item of the facility's preemployment policy.

Source: "Review and Analysis of Changed Work Schedules in Hospitals," William Clint Johnson, Manpower Administration, Department of Labor, May 1975. (Unpublished Contract Grant DL 91-48-72-37.)

Cost Analysis of Proposed Nursing Schedule

When the nurse manager considers an alternative scheduling package or other work redesign as part of the approach to dealing with staffing problems, he or she should conduct an analysis of the baseline cost of the new schedule before implementation.

The cost of the schedule or other structural work change can then be used as a baseline for a projected cost benefit analysis. This type of cost benefit examination gives a preimplementation estimate of the potential success of the change being considered.

Benefits other than financial should also be considered when evaluating a new schedule innovation. Evaluation of nonfinancial benefits may initially require the collection of data not usually considered for a cost benefit analysis, such as quality-of-care scores and surveys of staff nurses' work attitudes. At a later time, however, it may well be possible to use such data to derive financial information.

Source: Paul A. Reichelt and Patricia A. Larson, "Preimplementation Financial Evaluation of a Structural Work Change: Cost Analysis of an Innovative Staffing Schedule," *Nursing Administration Quarterly*, Vol. 18, No. 3, Aspen Publishers, Inc., © Spring 1994.

Shift Options*

It is important for staff nurses and nursing administrators to be aware of the various options in work schedules, as well as the advantages and disadvantages of each. The staff nurse will then be able to select the scheduling pattern best suited to meet his or her need. The nurse administrators will be able to select the scheduling pattern

---

Source: Except where noted, material on shift options is from Sherri R. Rasmussen, "Staffing and Scheduling Options," *Critical Care Quarterly*, Vol. 5, No. 1, Aspen Publishers, Inc., © 1982.

best suited to meet the staffing needs of their floor or unit.

Eight-Hour Shifts

Planning staffing for employees on the eight-hour shift includes arranging for staffing for three shifts—days, evenings, and nights. The day shift begins at 7 AM and ends at 3:30 PM, the evening shift begins at 3 PM and ends at 11:30 PM, and the night shift begins at 11 PM and ends at 7:30 AM. Full-time employees on the 8-hour shifts work five days a week for a total of 40 hours per week. Staff may work permanent days, evenings, or nights, or they may rotate to different shifts.

Advantages of the 8-hour shift may include these.

- The traditional workday is 8 hours. Therefore the body does not have to adjust to an extended workday.
- Staff may have the option of selecting from three shifts the shift they prefer to work.

Disadvantages of the 8-hour shift may include these.

- The 8-hour shift schedule does not allow staff to have every other weekend off.
- It does not permit the employee to have several consecutive days off.
- The 8-hour shift results in unsafe traveling times. Individuals on the evening shift leave work at 11:30 PM and individuals on the night shift come to work at 11 PM.
- Nurse administrators must plan staffing for three different shifts.

Ten-Hour Shifts

The most popular configuration for the 10-hour shift is the 10-hour day, four days a week (the 4/40 workweek). (See Table 18–2.) Various other configurations include two days of 12-hour shifts followed by two days of 8-hour shifts, or seven days of 12-hour shifts followed by seven days off. Other institutions have used 10-hour days on either one or two shifts. Some have used a 10-hour shift, 5-hour shift, 10-hour shift for

Table 18-2 Personnel Staffing Schedule: Ten-Hour Shift

No.	NAME	1ST WEEK							2ND WEEK							3RD WEEK							4TH WEEK						
		S	M	T	W	T	F	S	S	M	T	W	T	F	S	S	M	T	W	T	F	S	S	M	T	W	T	F	S
A-1				X	X			X			X	X			X			X	X			X			X	X			X
B-1		X				X	X		X				X	X		X				X	X		X				X	X	
		1	2	1	1	1	1	1	1	2	1	1	1	1	1	1	2	1	1	1	1	1	1	2	1	1	1	1	1

LONG WEEKENDS

No.	NAME	1ST WEEK							2ND WEEK							3RD WEEK							4TH WEEK						
		S	M	T	W	T	F	S	S	M	T	W	T	F	S	S	M	T	W	T	F	S	S	M	T	W	T	F	S
A-2		X	X					X	X	X					X	X	X					X	X	X					X
B-2					X	X	X					X	X	X					X	X	X					X	X	X	
		1	1	2	1	1	1	1	1	1	2	1	1	1	1	1	1	2	1	1	1	1	1	1	2	1	1	1	1
		2	3	2	2	2	2	2	2	3	2	2	2	2	2	2	3	2	2	2	2	2	2	3	2	2	2	2	2

Source: Thomas Kilber, *Modes of Scheduling,* Blue Cross of Western Pennsylvania, 1978. Reprinted with permission.

days, evenings, and nights, respectively, in order to recruit more part-time nurses for the evening shift.*

Advantages of the 10-hour shift may include these.

- It allows for several consecutive days off.
- Employees can have more weekends off.
- Individuals on different shifts have an opportunity to work together, improving staff interpersonal relationships.
- The overlap of shifts allows for more personnel at busy times and for lunch and dinner coverage.
- Staff members are able to take advantage of unit classes, facility inservices, patient care conferences, staff meetings, and interdisciplinary conferences occurring during the overlap of shifts.
- During overlap of shifts, staff may have the opportunity to work on unit and facility projects and committees.

Disadvantages of the 10-hour shift may include these.

- The longer work hours may lead to fatigue of staff.
- With the prolonged shift, the workdays seem to be all work, with little time for relaxation.
- The 10-hour shift also results in unsafe traveling times for the evening and night shift staff.
- It requires more employees than the 8- and 12-hour shift schedules.
- Nurse administrators must plan staffing for three different shifts.

To implement such a shift, changes, such as the following, would be necessary:**

- establishment of a new system of priorities (e.g., baths no longer given in the morning)
- holidays and vacations scheduled in terms of hours rather than days, for example:

*Source: DHHS, Pub. No. (HRA) 77-15, 1977.
**Source: Thomas Kliber, *Modes of Scheduling*, Blue Cross of Western Pennsylvania, 1978.

5-day week: 10 holidays × 8 hours = 80 hours
4-day week: 8 holidays × 10 hours = 80 hours

*Seven on—Seven off.** The longer shift of 10 hours, combined with a pattern of seven days of work followed by seven consecutive days off, creates a 7/70 schedule, a radical departure from traditional schedules.

At Mercy Medical Center in Dubuque, Louisiana, the same number and mixture of personnel is on duty seven days a week, with each employee given every other weekend off. The staff is split into two groups, each nurse working 70 hours in a two-week period (there are two 10-hour shifts and one 5-hour shift each day). Other changes include standard extra pay for working holidays and the scheduling of inservice and educational programs during the employees' time off. Among the administrative benefits of the new schedule have been a reduction (by 26 percent) in employee turnover, nursing care hours, and overtime hours. Results of a survey conducted by an independent research group showed that RN satisfaction was 6 percent above industry norms and 8 percent above the hospital employee norm, but less for part-time employees.

Following are the principal benefits of the seven on—seven off shift:

- increased utilization of space and equipment
- improved service to patients
- increased morale and efficiency
- greatly reduced absenteeism
- reduced personnel costs

Twelve-Hour Shifts

Planning staffing for employees on the 12-hour shift includes arranging for staffing for only two shifts—day and night. The day shift begins at 7 AM and ends at 7:30 PM; the night shift begins at 7 PM and ends at 7:30 AM. Full-time employees on the 12-hour shift may work three days for two weeks and four days a third week; in other words, 36 hours per week for two weeks and 48 hours per week for one week. This averages 40 hours per week. Staff may work per-

*Source: DHHS, Pub. No. (HRA) 77-15, 1977.

manent days or nights or they may rotate from one shift to the other.

Instead of head nurse and assistant head nurse being assigned to evening shifts and no night shifts, it is possible to have the busy part of the evening shift covered by supervisory personnel and the slow part relegated to limited coverage—a savings for the facility of at least half of supervisory salaries used formerly for the evening shift. Other advantages of the 12-hour shift may include these.

- Twelve-hour shifts provide for several consecutive days off.
- Employees can have more weekends off (e.g., every other weekend).
- Employees have more time to pursue recreation and leisure interests.
- Twelve-hour shifts allow safe traveling hours.
- Employees have fewer days on duty, therefore decreasing traveling time to and from work.
- Twelve-hour shifts decrease the time spent in change-of-shift reports—two per 24 hours compared with three for the 8- and 10-hour shifts. This provides more time for patient care, patient teaching, or staff education.
- The same nurse is caring for a patient when physicians make morning and afternoon rounds. Thus, the nurse is able to describe to physicians the patient changes and treatment effectiveness.
- Fewer staff positions are needed.
- Twelve-hour shifts seem to be a drawing card for recruitment.

Disadvantages of the 12-hour shift may include these.

- The longer working hours may lead to fatigue of staff.
- The half-hour allotted for change-of-shift report may not be sufficient time.
- Attendance at inservice education programs, staff meetings, and nursing care conferences may be reduced because nurses work fewer days.

How does one bring about an organized schedule change? As with all changes, it requires in-depth planning, supervised implementation, and evaluation.

A proposal for implementation of the shift should include the following:

- The floors or units that will be involved in the schedule pattern change.
- When the schedule change will be implemented and how long the trial period will be (usually three to six months).
- Specification of shift hours. Usually the first or day shift is from 7 AM to 7:30 PM, and the second or night shift is from 7 PM to 7:30 AM.
- A discussion of meals and coffee breaks during a 12-hour shift. Breaks include one 30-minute meal period and two or three 15-minute coffee breaks or rest periods.
- The schedule pattern for full-time and part-time staff. Full-time employees work three days for two weeks and four days a third week.
- Discussion of holiday, vacation, and sick time. These benefits are usually unchanged and are the same as for full-time staff on an 8-hour shift.
- Payroll considerations. Shift differential and overtime pay must be addressed; overtime pay is usually paid for any hours in excess of 40 hours per week.
- Time for staff development classes. Most classes are only 8 hours long; therefore, the other 4 hours of the shift are either spent working or taken as vacation or leave of absence.
- Advantages and disadvantages plus strategies to minimize the disadvantages.
- Plans for evaluation.
- A breakdown of the duties for the day shift and night shift for each floor or unit.

During implementation it is crucial for head nurses, nurse managers, and staff nurses to assess how the new shifts are working out. Nursing administrators should be available to answer questions staff may have regarding the shifts and to identify problems, develop strategies to solve the problems, and communicate these strategies to the involved staff.

Chapter 19

Adjustment Techniques for Staffing

In the 1990s' meaner and leaner health care environment, staff adjustments have taken on more complex and serious overtones. The last-minute daily scramble to cope with an unexpected surge in the patient population or an intensification of patient care needs has always been considered part of the job. Harried and over-wrought, the nurse manager, over the years, has developed a number of techniques to control the daily crisis situation. These are discussed below, with special emphasis given to the handling of understaffing, the most common of problems.

The real difficulty today lies in the cost-containment need to terminate staff, which can result in an insufficient number of employees. To soften the harsh reality of the staff reduction trend, several terms have been adopted to indicate different levels of termination and the motivation behind them. *Layoff* traditionally refers to letting go of employees until conditions get better. This may be optimistic thinking, although staff members may get rehired on a part-time basis if the cuts were too drastic. *Reductions in force* is more definitive, referring to a permanent termination of employees due to required staffing changes. The term *downsizing* may be used as a euphemism, as it suggests streamlining operations and readjusting positions. Frequently, however, staff cannot be relocated and are let go. As a result, some procedures are made more efficient, others more narrow in scope or discarded.

Whichever term is used, the nurse manager must plan ahead, exercise tact, and be aware of the constraints and ramifications of the manner in which staff reduction is performed.

DAILY STAFF ADJUSTMENTS

Staffing adjustments should not be confused with regular scheduling. Scheduling is concerned with planning for personnel usage throughout the year—taking into account the changing needs due to shifts, seasons, holidays, vacations, and the full range of predictable factors.

Staff adjustments, on the other hand, are concerned with unexpected conditions, the day-to-day variations in need or situation that result in overstaffing or understaffing.

Unfortunately, such variations cannot be accurately forecast. Adjustments must be made not only if supply is to be matched with demand but also if the amount of absenteeism on any given day is to be reckoned with.

Staff adjustment can be called reallocation, and it is done centrally (or decentrally, among divisions of the health care facility) each shift, with the assignment of the float nurses and/or the "pulling" of nurses from the units to which they were originally scheduled.[1]

The process is in two phases. First, the demand for nursing care services must be measured on each unit, taking into account the current number, type, and condition of patients.

The second stage is to adjust such demand to the supply, which includes the "core" staff (permanent staff scheduled to a particular unit), the float and/or "pull" staff, and outside resources.

There are a wide range of techniques available for making adjustments for both under-staffing and overstaffing.

Methods for Handling Understaffing

If a specific station is understaffed while another is overstaffed, a nurse may be floated (i.e., reassigned to another station). Pool personnel can also be used to cover shortages on specific stations. If it becomes apparent that the nursing stations in total will be understaffed for a given shift, several steps can be taken. Part-time employees assigned to nursing units and assigned to the nursing pool can be contacted and requested to work an extra shift. In addition, an "on-call" pool should be developed to cover in such situations; these people can also be contacted. Another mechanism to add needed personnel is to use temporary professional nurse agencies. Basically, the system has been constructed so as to be able to expand on short-term notice; however, anticipation of and planning for these situations are of key importance.[2]

One considerable concern when using any short-term adjustment technique is the adequacy of preparation of nurse replacements in a practice arena that is becoming more and more clinically specialized. To combat this problem, some nurse managers are using a preparatory system called *cross-training*.

Cross-training is the preparation of individuals to function effectively in more than one area of professional responsibility. Within nursing, cross-training involves the preparation of registered nurses for delivery of patient care in more than one clinical specialty at an institution.

Nurses cannot be expected to maintain competency in specialties that are not similar. Therefore, nursing departments should establish companion or "sister" units—cross-training groups that are comparable and related. Examples of cross-training groups include

- labor, delivery, and postpartum care nurses, newborn nursery, pediatrics
- neonatal intensive care unit and pediatric intensive care unit
- intensive care unit, coronary care unit, emergency care nurses
- medical-surgical preoperative and postoperative units, medical units
- mental health units, substance abuse units, eating disorder units
- day surgery and recovery nurses

The cross training program should provide for the same orientation to the unit as is provided all new employees. Inservice education and staff development activities are shared between nursing and education departments. Skill checklists for all specialty orientations should be completed, kept available for reference, and filed according to the facility procedure.[1]

Advantages of cross-training for the manager include increased ability to deal with changes in census and acuity and greater availability of qualified nursing personnel. Apparently, for the staff member, the process heightens professional satisfaction, providing increased stimulation as a result of exposure to more than one unit.

[1]D. Michael Warner, "Nurse Staffing, Scheduling and Reallocation in the Hospital," *Hospital & Health Services Administration*, Summer 1976.

[2]Merrill Lehman and Q.J. Friesen, *A Centralized Position and Staffing Control Administered by Non-Nursing Personnel*, Methodist Hospital, St. Louis Park, Minnesota, 1975.

[1]Joyce Rhodes, "Staffing and Resource Development," in *Managing for Productivity in Nursing*, Barbara Rutkowski, ed., Aspen Publishers, Inc., © 1987.

Note: A more recent development that extends the cross-training concept is *clustering*. Clustering refers to using multiunit-trained staff interchangably in two or more related units on any given day. This system maximizes the resource pool for each of the clustered units.

Floating Nurses

Few nursing administrators like the idea of using floating nurses, yet running a nursing department would often prove unmanageable without them. A national survey of *Nursing '75* discovered that 54 percent of all nurses have to float; 42 percent said they are often pulled from one unit to another. Many of them are unhappy doing it; most of those who were against floating felt that nurses could not provide quality of care in a variety of units. Others clearly indicated that they liked familiar surroundings and wanted to feel that they were part of a group. Obviously, the use of floating nurses should be minimized. But when they are used, here are some suggestions for making them more comfortable and effective.

- Conduct an inservice program where head nurses of different units explain the special demands and procedures of their units. Have nurses take notes or distribute summaries that can be used as a reference guide during the float assignment.

- Allocate assignments that a float can perform with confidence. Ask nurses to list unit preferences and keep a file of potential float nurses for each unit. This also builds a corps of float nurses who become familiar with particular units.

- Delegate a "float-orientation nurse" in each unit who will give the floater a 15-minute introduction to unit needs and arrangements as well as answer questions.

- Inquire of the float nurse, after the shift is over, what aspects on the unit were most difficult. Include explanations of these matters in the next orientation.

- Remember courtesies; thank both the float nurse and the head nurse from whose unit he or she was released.

Flying Squad*

An added "wrinkle" to the system normally not seen in many health care facilities is the use of a "flying squad." The flying squad, normally consisting of two nurses, is not assigned to any specific station, but moves from station to station throughout the shift based on varying needs of the stations during the shift. The flying squad members carry pocket pagers so that head nurses in need of additional help can easily reach them. The flying squad will actually work on several different stations during each shift, thus often overcoming the necessity of providing extra staff on several stations just for the purpose of meeting peak activity times. Again, flexibility is added to the system.

Controlled Admissions*

The first day of patient stay, particularly for nonelective admissions, imposes more than twice the demand on nurse staff than do subsequent days. Given some choice in placing a new admission, plus knowledge of the number of intensive and first-day patients on each unit, there is a potential for stabilizing workloads by selective admission to units.

Nursing Pools—Permanent*

A nursing pool can be of key importance to the staffing system, as it provides needed flexibility. The size of the pool can be varied by the staffing coordinator to meet projected patient care needs. For example, in the Methodist Hospital in St. Louis Park, Minnesota, there are three separate area pools—a medical-surgical pool, a pediatrics-OB/GYN pool, and an intensive care pool. Nurses who are recruited for each of the pools receive orientation to all stations within their respective areas and to each nursing station in the hospital. While they may float to any station in the hospital, the nurses in the pools normally float only within their area of training. Each nurse reports to the assistant staffing coordinator before each scheduled shift to receive his or her station assignment.

*Source: Merrill Lehman and Q.J. Friesen, *A Centralized Position and Staffing Control Administered by Non-Nursing Personnel*, Methodist Hospital, St. Louis Park, Minnesota, 1975.

*Source: Merrill Lehman and Q.J. Friesen, *A Centralized Position and Staffing Control Administered by Non-Nursing Personnel*, Methodist Hospital, St. Louis Park, Minnesota, 1975.

Pool nurses are scheduled on a monthly basis, as are all employees in the hospital. As permanent vacancies occur on nurses' stations, pool employees transfer to a nurses' station, thus providing the hospital with a reservoir of trained employees who can fill permanent station assignments. (For a sample nursing pool structure, see Table 19–1.)

Per Diem Employees*

Per diem (or prn) nurses are hired by the health care facility to work as needed. Per diem nurses plan their schedules with the facility. Then if the facility finds that on a given day it does not need the per diem nurse's help, the per diem nurse is canceled for that day. Per diem employees may work whatever schedules the facility offers. Advantages of per diem employment include these.

- Per diem nurses usually are allowed to make their own work schedules, except that a set number of weekends and nights must be scheduled.
- Per diem nurses receive more money per hour than do career or part-time nurses.
- Out of desire to keep the job, prn nurses are more apt to fill in when staff are needed to work.
- Per diem nurses are frequently required to work a set percentage of weekends and nights, which may decrease the friction between career and per diem employees.
- Per diem nurses are interviewed and hired by nursing service. Therefore, nursing service is aware of the educational and experiential level of each per diem nurse. With this information, their assignments can be made so that they work on the floors or units where they have experience.
- Per diem nurses work at the same facility consistently. Therefore, they are better informed about the unit and floor environments and about the facility's policies and procedures.

Disadvantages of per diem work may include the absence of benefits such as sick pay, vacation and holiday pay, and insurance. Usually, per diem nurses are employed by facilities only when temporary staffing is needed. Per diem nurses therefore do not have job security.

Shared Services Pool*

One shared services organization, composed of seven member health care facilities, implemented a program to provide nursing personnel on an on-call or as-needed basis to its member facilities. The organization itself employs nursing personnel who are sent into the member facilities on request to compensate for census peaks, vacations, and employee absenteeism. Three individuals manage the nursing personnel department: a director, a scheduling coordinator, and an RN consultant.

With few exceptions, utilization on a day-to-day basis does not vary significantly. Requests for personnel usually decrease beginning Friday before any three-day weekend or holiday and are usually higher on days that facility employees are paid. Requests by shifts also remain fairly constant in distribution. Fifty-nine percent of the total requests are for the 7–3 shift, 29 percent for the 3–11 shift, and 12 percent for the 11–7 shift.

Requests for nurses are received by telephone and logged on scheduling sheets by the department coordinator. Requests are received from as little as one hour to up to several weeks before the shift to be filled begins. Although nursing personnel call in for scheduled work at weekly intervals, they are called by the coordinator for last-minute requests.

Nursing personnel are oriented in each facility in which they decide to work. The length and type of orientation depend on the institution's needs.

A cost formula has been developed to compute the actual cost of personnel on the basis of current and projected salary levels, shift differentials, and taxes.

Source: Sherri R. Rasmussen, "Staffing and Scheduling Options," *Critical Care Quarterly*, Vol. 5, No. 1, Aspen Publishers, Inc., © 1982.

Source: Excerpted from *Hospitals*, Vol. 50, No. 10, by permission, May 16, 1976, Copyright 1976, American Hospital Publishing, Inc.

Table 19–1 Sample Nursing Pool Structure

Topic	Unit-Based Pool	Divisional Pool	Special Staffing Team
Employee status	Pool	Pool	Permanent; full-time
Hours worked per week	Flexible, no hours guaranteed	Flexible, no hours guaranteed	Work 40 hours per week
Cancellation	Facility can cancel up to two before start of shift	Facility can cancel up to two before start of shift	Not canceled
Order of cancellation/ reassignment	Canceled/reassigned after divisional pool	Canceled/reassigned first	Assigned to an area, not canceled
Manager	Unit nurse manager	Staffing coordinator	Staffing coordinator
Scheduling requirements	Same as unit staff	16 hours of weekend time per month; one major holiday	40 hours per week including every other weekend
Number of positions available	Based on unit vacancies	Not limited; based on supplemental staffing needs	Four
Benefits	FICA; Florida retirement (by law)	FICA; Florida retirement if and when eligible	All benefits awarded to permanent employees
Required experience	One year of recent experience in clinical area	One year of recent experience in clinical area	Five years of recent critical care experience
Employee types	RN, LPN, paramedic, mental health technician, surgical technician, emergency medical technician, obstetrician, ultrasound technician	RN, LPN, paramedic, mental health technician, surgical technician, emergency medical technician, obstetrician, ultrasound technician	RN only

Source: Mary Bogos Kutash and Deana Nelson, "Optimizing the Use of Nursing Pool Resources," *Journal of Nursing Administration*, Vol. 23:1, January 1993. J.B. Lippincott.

Facilities are charged a flat hourly rate for each classification of personnel regardless of the individual's salary level or the shift worked. However, a shift differential is paid. The rates are calculated to cover personnel costs and program overhead and include a 4 percent contingency factor.

A break-even point was reached after the program had been operative for about 12 months and a sufficient volume had been attained. The current rates for the shared services personnel are about 12 percent lower than those of area commercial pools.

Temporary (Supplemental) Agencies*

What has been known as "pools" in earlier stages of growth have actually evolved into full-scale nursing service organizations. Because of agency competition, voluntary certification, state-imposed licensing (in some states), consumer demands, and professional standards, these private corporations seem to have peaked

*Source: T.F. Moore and E.A. Simendinger, *Managing the Nursing Shortage: A Guide to Recruitment and Retention*, Aspen Publishers, Inc., © 1989.

in proliferation and are currently being sifted out by quality control utilization.

These supplemental services are independently owned or are part of a national or regional organization in which they are structured as a branch (company-owned) office, a "licensed" office, or a proprietor franchise.

Services include almost any level of nursing care around the clock for private duty in facilities, supplemental staffing in facilities, and discharge planning assistant and home care. Supplemental agencies provide adequate insurance for their employees. Supervision of agency employees is provided by their own nursing/administrative staff. A round-the-clock communication by nursing supervisors to facilities and by nursing supervisors to employees assures prompt response to staffing needs and/or problem solving.

Because they are a full-service nursing agency, you should expect that

- Employees are screened and hired according to standard employment practices, including personal interview.
- Assignments are made according to the nurse's past experience and individual training and capabilities.
- Documentation, including complete employee files and client files, is maintained according to established policies and procedures on standard forms.
- Physicians' orders are obtained and kept current, and collaboration with all team members is orchestrated by the nursing supervisor who is the case manager.
- On-site, routine (RN) supervisory visits are made for the purpose of assessment, supervision, problem solving, teaching, and coordination of health resources for home health. The necessary frequency of visits is initially established, then later reevaluated, but ongoing frequency should never be less than every few weeks.

Advantages of Temporary Staff

Predictable and adequately staffed units definitely contribute greatly to the recruitment and retention of a nursing staff. When patient census or acuity level fluctuates, supplemental staff can be used or not used, with no carryover of people or benefits when they are not needed.

Illness such as rampant flu can understaff a unit as quickly as seasonable and unplanned vacancies during vacation season.

When new positions or units open, supplemental agencies can provide the necessary human resources to adequately accommodate planned, timely, and beneficial growth (see Table 19–2).

Unpopular shifts, weekends or nights, may always remain the nemesis of the schedule. Supplemental nurses can help fill those voids. To this advantage, add caution. It is important to learn from the agency their policy toward how often and under what conditions their supplemental nurses can work these shifts. An important restraint here is a policy of limiting shift hours or consecutive double shifts worked by supplemental staff nurses. An advantage of covering difficult shifts with a nurse's prolonged compressed schedule is quickly offset if fatigue hinders or threatens the quality of patient care. Care may also be hindered if, after a supplemental nurse is assigned, a unit is still short-staffed and/or a strong staff person is not also assigned.

Disadvantages of Temporary Staff

Some administrators try to avoid the use of supplemental nurses or other levels of caregivers because of the lack of continuity they have experienced with some agencies. They say that the staff nurses then seem to spend their time constantly orienting, directing, and guiding supplemental staff nurses, which takes away from their own activities and responsibilities.

Other disadvantages are that the facility staff is discontent if salaries are compared; and the facility does not "know" the supplemental nurse because the employee file, including references and evaluations, is in the employer's (supplemental agency) office. Some nursing supervisors also feel that supplemental nurses are not as committed to the facility's patient care as staff nurses are, because chances are the supplemental staff nurse may or may not return. Other nursing administrators feel that the commitment and performance toward quality care is determined by

Table 19–2 Supplemental Staff Agency and Health Care Facility Interactions

AGREEMENT*

Agency Agrees To:

- Screen nurse to verify qualification (license) and competence (previous experience) (records available to health care facility on demand).
- Pay nurses—including responsibility for taxes, FICA, etc.
- Assume responsibility for workers' compensation and general liability.
- Require employees to work within health care facility policies and procedures.
- Pay for one-day orientation for each nurse.
- Release agency nurse for permanent facility employment after 14 days' written notification from the nurse, upon mutual agreement between the nurse and the facility.
- Maintain shift rates for one year, amended only by mutual agreement.

Health Care Facility Agrees To:

- Use contracted agencies exclusively, if they can meet the facility's needs.
- Notify the agency of cancellations more than one hour before the shift or pay for four hours (facility reserves the right to then employ the nurse for four hours).
- Authorize the director of nursing designee to ask any agency nurse deemed incompetent, negligent, or engaged in misconduct to leave with payment only for hours worked.
- Provide a one-day orientation for each nurse.
- Maintain the shift rates for one year, amended only by mutual agreement.

DOCUMENTATION FOLLOW UP**

External

To familiarize the agency with the nursing department, the health care facility should:

- Provide position descriptions and applicable policies to the agencies.
- Provide written evaluations on each agency employee assigned to the facility.
- Provide copies of applicable nursing policies and procedures on each nursing unit.
- Provide all positive and negative observations regarding agency employees functioning at the facility as well as all incidents involving the agency nurses.

Internal

The health care facility should maintain a file of agency employees who are preferable, to include:

- Verification of license and renewals
- Evidence of preemployment physical examination
- Evaluation, following 10 shifts, and annually thereafter
- Documentation of inservices, annual CPR certification, and safety and infection control reviews
- Skills checklist

Source: Donna R. Sheridan, Jean E. Bronstein, and Duane Walker, "Using Registry Nurses: Coping with Cost and Quality Issues," *Journal of Nursing Administration*, October 1982. Reprinted with permission.

**Source:* Adapted from "Agency Nurse Guidelines," *Help News*, Vol. 4:6, June 1981, Alexander & Alexander.

---

the personal integrity and professional competence of the individual nurse, not his or her employment choice.

The quality of supplemental nurses is sometimes criticized. Be assured that a nonregulated

(or even a regulated) supplemental agency can be a haven for nurses who have been "let go" from facilities for quality of care or personal impairment reasons. Choosing an agency is comparable to making a major investment. All avenues and all aspects should be investigated as such with emphasis on the local agency office and its administration.

Short-Term Overstaffing*

A technique to contract staffing was developed by one hospital to meet short-term decreased patient care requirements. This is done by means of a requested absence (RA). If it is found that the nursing stations in general will be overstaffed on a given shift or during a given period, the assistant staffing coordinator will contract scheduled nursing employees and ask if they would prefer not to work. Often nursing employees are willing to comply with the request. Since this method is mutually agreeable to both the nursing service and the employee, an efficient means of dealing with temporary overstaffing is created. During the employment interview and the staffing orientation session, employees are notified of this option. The option has proved to be quite popular.

Policies for Implementation

- The staffing office may request that an employee take an RA day or the staff member may initiate the request for an RA day by notifying the staffing office. The RA must be mutually agreeable to both the employee and the staffing office.
- Employees contacted to take an RA day are responsible for notifying the staffing persons if they are to work charge or have other responsibilities on the proposed RA day.
- The total RAs taken by one employee may not exceed 20 days (160 hours) for one year.
- There will be no loss of time in calculating benefits during a requested absence.
- RA days may not be used in lieu of leave of absence days.

Source: Merrill Lehman and Q.J. Friesen, *A Centralized Position and Staffing Control Administered by Non-Nursing Personnel*, Methodist Hospital, St. Louis Park, Minnesota, 1975. Reprinted with permission.

HANDLING STAFF REDUCTIONS

Developing a Staff Reduction Plan*

It is imperative that a staff reduction plan for nursing be developed in advance of the need for it so that a thorough and objective system can be designed. Last-minute plans for a layoff are invariably ill conceived and implemented and result in more organizational chaos than is necessary. The time to plan for a staff reduction is before a crisis occurs, when there is time to think clearly and objectively about the staff reduction process.

This plan must be designed to include issues related to not only the employees being laid off, but also the employees who remain. The remaining employees represent a far larger group and require careful reassurance about the organization and their own job security.

Basic areas that should be addressed are the following.

Indicators for Decisions Regarding Staff Reduction. At what point, financially or otherwise, will the decision be made to reduce staff? What criteria will be used to determine the number of positions to be abolished? Which positions will be eliminated? What will be the target staff mix and numbers be?

Options and Alternative Plans. What options, long- or short-term, will be considered? What are the criteria to determine if long- or short-term problems exist? What are the advantages and disadvantages of each option?

Criteria for Determining Employees To Be Reduced. What policies on staff reduction exist? Are the criteria clearly spelled out (e.g., seniority, job performance, etc.)? Are there union contracts prescribing layoff procedures? Are data available on each employee to assist in ranking (e.g., length of employment, special qualifications, age, race, education, sex, job performance evaluations)?

Source: Katherine W. Vestal, "Staff Reduction: The Nursing Administrator's Role," *Nursing Administration Quarterly*, Vol. 8, No. 2, Aspen Publishers, Inc., © 1984.

Implementation Plan. Has a timetable been developed that allows time for the reduction process to be conducted smoothly? Who and what will the reduction affect, and where and when will the effects occur? Have all managers been thoroughly educated in the process? Have employees been informed of the deteriorating financial state of the institution? Is the plan workable and reasonable?

Evaluation Plan. Is there a plan to evaluate the staff reduction process? Are mechanisms for communicating with staff in place? Could the process have been handled better in any manner?

The Value of a Plan

The value of a cohesive, well-designed, and well-written plan cannot be underestimated. In fact, such a plan actually allows the nursing administrator to be more sensitive to the staff during difficult times, rather than be sequestered in a room, initiating a crisis plan. A nursing plan, coordinated with the human resources department, allows nursing to be at the forefront in policymaking and to protect essential positions as difficult decisions are made.

General Approach to Limiting or Reducing Staff*

Staff reduction is never popular no matter where it takes place, be it in industry or the health care field. However, there are times when circumstances make it necessary.

Some general points should be kept in mind by nurse administrators when considering action leading to staff cuts.

- Staff adjustments should take into account activities and the corresponding skill level required. Wholesale and indiscriminate reductions could purge the nursing service of valuable people having important talents. This should be avoided.

- The total staffing in an area should initially be adequate. A 5 or 10 percent across the board cut in all nursing unit rosters, while of minor consequence to overstaffed areas, can seriously hinder operations where units are already understaffed.

- The means of effecting the staffing reduction should be carefully weighed. Some causes of action have greater impact than others. If the same ends can be achieved through expected normal attrition or encouragement of early retirement, this is certainly a better approach than causing wholesale layoffs on an indiscriminate basis. While the latter is certainly quick and sure, the former, taking some amount of planning and work, would produce the more positive results from a personnel relations standpoint.

Long-Term Techniques for Downsizing*

In the following discussion of how to reduce staff, an attempt has been made to present the less extreme methods first and the more drastic measures last. The exact rank is open to individual preference. (Table 19–3 contains a different sequence of staff reduction measures.)

Attrition. If time permits, staffing can be adjusted on a long-term basis through attrition. Such action can be difficult if

- the rate of attrition, departmentwide, is low
- the rate of attrition in a given unit (because of size or type of work) is low
- the time to achieve reduction is short

While attrition is not necessarily the way to end up with optimum staffing in a department (it is possible that the most productive persons will leave), it is one of the most "painless" means of reducing staff.

Source: "Selected Procedures and Methods of Staff Reduction," Haricomp Guide Series Publication, Pub. No. 79a, 1975. Reprinted with permission.

Source: "Selected Procedures and Methods of Staff Reduction," Haricomp Guide Series Publication, Pub. No. 79a, 1975. Reprinted with permission.

Table 19–3 Sample Sequence for Downsizing

Step 1: Attrition—over the course of three months only essential vacancies are filled.

Step 2: Temporary early retirement—a temporary early retirement program is offered to all eligible employees.

Step 3: Elimination of management positions—the management structure is streamlined and positions are eliminated.

Step 4: Conversion of a number of full-time to part-time positions—to increase the percentage of variable staff, designated full-time staff become part time.

Step 5: Terminations—implemented as a last step to minimize actual numbers affected (depends on effectiveness of previous steps).

Source: April J. Rozboril, "Systematic Downsizing: An Experience," *Journal of Nursing Administration*, Vol. 17, No. 9, September 1987.

Overtime. Work should be planned so that it can be accomplished in a normal workweek. In cases where the workload varies because of sudden heavy inputs that cannot be normally handled or deferred, overtime can be authorized. The same argument holds for emergency work.

A review of overtime hours might point out the need for a revamping of personnel scheduling. Too often, inflexibility in scheduling can induce overtime where it could otherwise be avoided.

Transfers and Promotions. Where there are apparent cases of under- as well as overstaffing, efforts should be made to transfer employees within the organization and between nursing service units, keeping requirements in mind.

This can be encouraged by posting job openings for which any qualified employee can apply. Worker morale and loyalty can be significantly improved with this type of well-administered program. In other circumstances, the human resources department may have to act as the agency to match personnel from over- to understaffed departments.

Promotion from within is based on similar arguments and further encourages employee performance in the hope that when appropriate openings occur, they will be filled from within.

Leave of Absence (LOA). The department should encourage the taking of extended leaves of absence such as educational LOAs. The impact on the budget would not be major, since usually only the barest of benefits are carried in cases of authorized LOA.

Reemployment could be contingent on there being positions open at the time a person on leave would seek to return. The exception to such a policy would be with respect to military and family or medical leaves, for which the returning employee is guaranteed a position.

Retirement Phaseouts. Health care facilities have long kept employees on the payroll even though they have passed the widely recognized retirement age of 65. Following such a practice unfortunately may penalize the facility in many ways. Older employees may present a picture of marginal productivity (in labor-intensive, non-professional positions) and increased injury/illness days; yet often, because of seniority, they enjoy the largest salaries and the most vacation days in their job classification.

Replacement might be possible or a shift to a lower paid position as part of an evaluation of duties and/or a departmental organization.

Minimize Part-Time Staffing. An attempt should be made to minimize the use of part-time staff. This might be done through rescheduling existing full-time personnel or combining the workload of many part-timers to create a lesser number of positions.

Elimination or restriction of hiring of temporary or supplemental staff should be considered. Where the reason for using such personnel is uneven scheduling of workload, attempts should be made to balance the "peaks and valleys" with the resulting loss of need for temporary help. Another common situation that causes a "need" for staff is the failure to preplan vacation schedules. A disciplined policy for taking earned vacation time should cause few if any staff shortages during these times.

Interfacility Transfers. Where severe overstaffing exists, the human resource department might attempt to arrange employee transfers to other health care facilities in the area where appropriate positions are open. These workers would be considered as "new employees" in their new employment but would also enjoy relative job continuity.

Management Engineering. Management engineering can be of use to the department in indicating performance levels and improvement areas.

A review can be made to determine if, in fact, a valid need exists for the hiring of new personnel or replacing vacant positions in the department. A check could also be made to determine if positions could be reclassified to a lower level based on existing departmental requirements.

Usually, savings can be effected with the creation of a vacancy, since the new employee could be paid at the reclassified, lower rate.

Disciplinary Enforcement. In tight labor markets or when there is a high demand for personnel, enforcement of disciplinary policies tends to become relaxed. A problem worker will be tolerated because replacing him or her could be difficult. The reverse corollary is also true.

Incompetency and Probation Dismissals. In a somewhat similar vein, nurse managers and head nurses may have identified some of their staff as being incompetent in the work required of them. When faced with a staff cut, various means should be taken to encourage these employees to resign.

Also, as a prelude to a general layoff, consideration should be given to the dismissal of employees currently on a probationary status.

Layoff. A layoff of staff should be a last resort after all other attempts at trimming personnel have been exhausted.

People affected by the layoff should be given a thorough explanation of the circumstances and be informed of what efforts were made to find positions for them by the human resources department.

They should further be advised that as circumstances change, they will again be considered for employment, but this period of layoff could last for an extended number of months.

Finally, they should be fully informed of their unemployment status and told of their unemployment entitlements.

Preventing Labor Problems Stemming from a Reduction-in-Force Action

Responsible managers who want to avoid major labor-management problems will give careful consideration to the legal precepts and practical factors that should guide decisions about a reduction in force (RIF).

The RIF policy should be developed by the executive management team with the advice of the health care facility's labor relations consultant or labor attorney. All levels of management should be trained in the interpretation and application of the policy.

Fairness can be achieved by a RIF policy that is designed to treat similar cases alike, avoiding partiality, discrimination, or arbitrariness in selecting employees to be laid off. Ideally, the RIF policy should provide for psychological and vocational counseling, placement services, and severance pay.

In a unionized facility, the procedure for an RIF will be established by the contract. Deviation from the terms of the contract by either party will result in a labor dispute that will have to be resolved by arbitration or litigation. In health care facilities where union contracts do not exist, a RIF policy should be established to guide all levels of management in planning for and implementing employee reductions. A properly developed policy will reduce the risk of acting illegally and will greatly assist in the maintenance of constructive employee-management relationships during and following the RIF.

A RIF policy should be designed to provide the health care facility and nursing management with the greatest staffing flexibility possible while still being fair to the employees affected by its application.*

Source: Richard Ashton and JoAnne Ashton, "RIF: The Legal and Practical Considerations," *Aspen's Advisor for Nurse Executives*, Vol. 1, No. 2, Aspen Publishers, Inc., © 1985.

Minimizing the Risk of Discrimination*

The possibility that, in a layoff, the varying discrimination acts may come into play must also be examined. Strict seniority-based layoff procedures are the safest to use and easiest to implement. This, however, presupposes that the initial determinations as to which units will be subject to layoffs are based on objective criteria. An employer's decision to make reductions in a particular department or classification, although facially neutral, could have an adverse impact on protected groups if the chosen department or classification has a disproportionate number of protected employees. Thus, employers are well advised to review how the policy will work when applied during an actual layoff *before* a layoff is announced. If the "test run" results in a disproportionate impact on a particular protected group, the policy should be reexamined for hidden bias.

Helping Employees during Health Care Facility Closure**

Health care facility closings, acquisitions, and mergers have been a major concern of the health care industry in recent years. According to the American Hospital Association, 828 hospitals in the United States closed from 1980 through 1991, and 67 hospitals closed in 1991 alone. As health care facilities prepare to close, leaders are expected to provide direction that causes the least harm to the greatest number of employees. These leaders must be able to sustain themselves and help staff to keep their morale high, even though the organization's demise is imminent. Nurse executives may bear a disproportionate amount of responsibility for human resources, since their departments usually hold the largest number of employees. Therefore, nurse executives must be resilient, able to withstand the stress that comes

with the process of closure, and flexible enough to adjust to the many changes required during the phaseout period.

The following balancing factors are important: a realistic perception of the event, adequate situational support, and adequate coping mechanisms. With proper attention to these balancing factors, the nurse executive can assist staff to weather the crisis and can plan an effective strategy for leading a nursing organization through the closure process to acceptance of the loss.

For nurse executives, the following advice is recommended:

- Learn the signs of impending closure. Be alert so you can identify the presence of these signs should they occur in your organization.
- Prepare for impending closure by developing a written plan for phasing out your area of responsibility as soon as you see signs of possible closure. A facility that is operating in the red usually has a diminishing income from its client base, a sign of potential closure.
- Remember you are still the official leader of your department; staff will expect and need your direction.
- Get an outside mentor or consultant to help you, specifically. Preferably, this should be someone who is familiar with the various experiences you will be undergoing (e.g., an outplacement counselor or a nurse executive who has participated in closing a facility). The local organization of nurse executives might be able to provide leads to such resources. Remember, you too will need support to get through this experience without self-destructing.
- Keep a calendar of planned and projected events and dates for required follow up. This creates order for monitoring the performance of individuals and systems. Keep written notes. Do not rely on memory.
- Communicate! Communicate! Communicate! Have one-to-one conversations with staff often. This can be face to face or on the telephone. Hold frequent meetings with

**Source:* Skoler, Abbot & Presser, *Health Care Labor Manual*, Aspen Publishers, Inc., © January 1991.

***Source:* Naydja Domingue and Enrica Kinchen Singleton, "Hospital Closure: Reflections of a Former Nurse Executive," *Journal of Nursing Administration*, Vol. 23, No. 5, May 1993. J.B. Lippincott.

nursing managers to keep them abreast of activities. As necessary, follow oral messages with a written communique. Post information on bulletin boards when appropriate.

- Do not miss any of the meetings designed for the administrative team. Be sure that you provide input in decisions that affect your staff.

- Be flexible. Major plans may be altered without previous notice. You cannot afford to be too rigid in this changing emotional environment.

Note: Further assistance is available from the American Hospital Association (AHA) *Guidelines for Managing Hospital Closures* (1992).

Part IV

Operations

Chapter 20

Operational Reviews

THE COST- AND QUALITY-EFFECTIVE NURSING DEPARTMENT*

In 1988, the National Commission on Nursing Implementation Project identified four major characteristics of effective, high-quality, cost-effective nursing departments; delivery-related features, evaluation-related features, market-related features, and policy-related features.

Included among the *delivery-related features* are (1) working relationships among nurses, physicians, and other members of the health care team; (2) roles that incorporate authority, autonomy, and responsibility and offer appropriate compensation; (3) involvement of nurse managers in preparing the budget, managing resource utilization, and preserving a safe practice climate with acceptable outcomes; and (4) market knowledge concerning the ability to efficiently produce a service that will sell or draw consumers.

Evaluation-related features include (1) mechanisms for determining consumer satisfaction and providing feedback to the unit and to the practitioner, along with the monitoring of reten-

tion rates; (2) consumer feedback mechanisms; (3) manager and peer evaluation; and (4) a nursing quality assurance program. Additional components include an evaluation mechanism for assessing cost-effectiveness, quality standards, and productivity standards; a reliable and valid classification system; information systems with outcome measures; staff participation in designing cost accounting and reporting systems; and staff education about the systems.

Market-related features include features that affect the demand for nursing services, such as (1) the involvement of practicing nurses in the selection and evaluation of technology and programming used in the provision of client care, (2) information systems that track utilization patterns, (3) consumer input and regular program evaluation, and (4) involvement of nurses in public relation activities of the organization.

The *policy-related features* identified affect nursing's ability to influence overall policies in the organization. These include (1) the formal placement of nursing so as to allow it to influence policy formation and implementation relevant to the organization as a whole, (2) membership of middle-management and clinical nurses in institutional committees that set policies and procedures for patient care at the operational and patient unit levels, and (3) the possession by nursing of accountability and authority over the fiscal resources for nursing practice.

*Source: Virginia Del Togno-Armanasco, Susan Harter, Nannette L. Goddard, "Cost and Quality: Are They Compatible?" in *The Encyclopedia of Nursing Care Quality Volume I: Issues and Strategies for Nursing Care Quality,* Patricia Schroeder, ed., Aspen Publishers, Inc., © 1991.

Quality and Cost Indicators

To evaluate quality, each health care facility must first define and accept for itself a concept of quality. Second, it must identify all cost factors affecting the achievement of this quality. Once these concepts are defined and identified, they must be integrated into the facility's daily operational components. These actions result in the identification of patient care service as an essential indicator of the organization's overall performance.

Examples of *quality indicators* that can be used are the achievement level of nursing care standards, length of stay variances attributable to nursing actions, infection rates, and patient incidents attributable to nursing actions. *Cost indicators* affecting the achievement of quality that need to be evaluated are compliance with staffing standards, professional to nonprofessional personnel ratios, budgeted to filled position ratios, patient acuity, and compliance with salary and nonsalary budgets.

ORGANIZATIONAL AND MANAGEMENT EFFECTIVENESS

Essential Principles*

The Joint Commission on Accreditation of Healthcare Organizations distributed for review 12 key principles that are intended to characterize a health care organization's commitment to improve continuously its quality of care. These principles represent the first major step in the Joint Commission's plans to refocus and stream-

line its standards and to monitor organizational performance more effectively.

One of the prerequisites for improving an organization's clinical performance is organizational and management effectiveness. Therefore, the Joint Commission set out to identify those principles of organizational and management effectiveness that could serve as a basis for measurable indicators of effectiveness and for standards on which to base accreditation decisions.

1. Organizational Mission. The organizational mission statement clearly expresses the commitment to improve continuously the quality of patient care. The commitment is translated into measurable objectives and action plans through the organization's strategic, program, and resource planning processes. The mission statement and plans are mutually developed and regularly evaluated by the governing board and managerial and clinical leadership.

2. Organizational Culture. The organization fosters a culture that promotes a high degree of commitment to quality patient care. In promoting this culture, the organization seeks the involvement of all those who use or provide its services. The organization encourages self-assessment, open communication, appropriate participatory decision making, and fair conflict resolution among all levels of clinical and managerial personnel.

3. Organizational Strategic, Program, and Resource Plans. Strategic, program, and resource plans are based on a broad range of assessments pertaining to the external environment, access to care, adequacy of patient volume to support clinical competence, and quality-of-care judgments rendered by patients, their families, health care practitioners, other employees, payers, the community, and other organizational care providers. The planning process addresses the financial support needed to meet short- and long-term goals to improve the quality of patient care.

4. Organizational Change. The governing board and managerial and clinical leadership continuously assess the need and recognize opportunities for change prompted both internally

---

*Source: © Agenda for Change Update. Oakbrook Terrace, IL: Joint Commission on Accreditation of Healthcare Organizations, 1989, p. 1. Reprinted with permission.

and externally in order to plan and implement change in support of quality patient care.

5. Role of Governing Board and Managerial and Clinical Leadership. The organization's commitment to improve continuously the quality of patient care is reflected in the roles and performance of the organization's leaders. These expectations are translated into definitions of authority and responsibility and specific work objectives contained in written role/position descriptions. These leaders articulate the organization's values involving the continuous improvement of quality patient care, and they systematically seek, measure, and use the judgments and evaluations of patients, their families, health care practitioners, other employees, payers, the community, and other organizational care providers as an ongoing method of evaluating and improving the quality of patient care.

6. Leadership Qualification, Evaluation, and Development. The governing board and managerial and clinical leadership consist of well-qualified people who possess the knowledge, skills, attitudes, and vision for achieving the objective of measuring and continuously improving the quality of patient care. The leadership is regularly evaluated for its effectiveness in acquiring, utilizing, and coordinating resources and using information to promote the quality of patient care as delineated in their role expectations (e.g., job descriptions). In support of this effort, there is a well-conceived plan that addresses both internal and external opportunities for the growth and development of leaders to improve continuously the quality of patient care.

7. Clinical Competence of Independent Practitioners. Initial assessment and continued monitoring and evaluation of practitioners' clinical skills are intended to ensure that high-quality patient care is provided by each independent practitioner.

8. Human Resources. Recruitment, development, evaluation, and retention policies and practices are instituted to ensure that the health care practitioners and others who support patient care are competent and have appropriate skills, attitudes, and knowledge. Adequate staffing levels are maintained to meet the individual's role expectations as well as the organization's goals of continuously improving the quality of patient care.

9. Support Resources. Facilities, equipment, and technology will be acquired and maintained in accord with the mission statement and strategic, program, and resource plans. The decision-making process regarding facilities, equipment, and technology is characterized by broad-based participation among relevant parties.

10. Evaluation and Improvement of Patient Care. The monitoring, evaluation, and continuous improvement of patient care are overseen by the governing board and involve appropriate individuals and organizational units. This organizationwide assessment process integrates data from quality assurance, risk management, and utilization review and seeks ongoing feedback on the quality of care from patients, their families, health care practitioners, other employees, payers, the community, and other organizational care providers. The analysis of this information is used for short- and long-range planning decisions and is reflected in departmental objectives and job performance measures.

11. Organizational Integration and Coordination. To achieve continuous improvement of quality patient care, organizational leaders will ensure that there is appropriate communication, coordination, conflict management, and integration among relevant parties. Each department develops policies and procedures that recognize its responsibilities to other departments' efforts to improve the quality of patient care and explicitly delineate its responsibility for communicating and coordinating its patient care efforts with these departments.

12. Continuity and Comprehensiveness of Care. There are effective linkages developed and maintained with external care providers to ensure access, continuity, and comprehensiveness of care received by patients, including care before admission and after discharge.

Leverage Points for Increasing Organizational Effectiveness*

Leverage points are those few places where changes, often made with little intervention, within an underlying structure have pervasive results.

A key concern is how to find leverage points. How does one determine which structures to adopt? How does one know the operating forces and their strengths? Changes in seven primary leverage points can make a significant impact on patient care and nursing.

1. Leadership. Nursing leaders who make a difference stand for something, articulate a vision, and are committed, even under pressure. They empower themselves and others and create organizational structures that get results; they go beyond what seems ordinary to take risks. To redesign the work of nursing is to be vulnerable, because, in letting go of sacred cows, redefining quality, restructuring decision making, and offering incentive pay, leaders risk standing alone.

2. Governance. Governance defines power, reporting relationships, decision making, and access to information, and it is often the basis for managing conflict. Nurses, who make life and death decisions at the bedside, cannot be governed by a structure that renders them powerless in the organization. Shared governance offers one way to shift control and the power base. For organizations contemplating shared governance models, key considerations are the readiness of nurses and the potential for using the model organizationwide. Well-executed work redesign incorporates all departments, since shared governance by nursing alone risks "backlash."

3. Staffing and Scheduling. Clearly defining and coordinating centralized and decentralized functions and holding appropriate persons accountable can make significant differences in work and nurse-nurse relationships. Although

this sounds simple, it is not. The key is balance. Authority and accountability for staffing must be held by the nurse manager, with some scheduling responsibilities delegated to a centralized staffing office. This office functions in a staff or consultant relationship to the manager and not as a replacement.

Essential for well-managed scheduling are competent budgetary management and reporting systems that provide appropriate information when needed and in an understandable form consistent with reports used by the fiscal department. All players need to know what it costs to provide patient care and what revenues they generate to really share in the organization's work.

4. Rewards and Incentives. Organizations that have flexible plans (offering child care as well as tuition support), that pay on the basis of performance, that use a pay scale not capped prematurely for nurses, and that recognize and promote nurses can exploit the complex needs of employees for rewards and incentives.

5. Career Development. Career development, along with training, compensation, and supervisory practices, is part of supporting and managing work.

Typically, career development practices have been fragmented and have not been compatible with creating challenging work and motivating individuals to approach their potential. Mentorships and partnerships with other practitioners are steps in the right direction, but they need to be complemented by practices such as providing regular sabbatical leaves and giving rewards for doing things differently and by structures such as those supporting "think tanks" comprising those at the bedside as well as their leaders.

6. Connections between Nursing and Other Departments. Work sampling provides objective information about apparently subjective problems. Issues such as reducing the amount of time between an order for medication and its administration are examined, solved, and monitored by steering committee members from involved departments. The departments directly involved have the benefit of ideas from those that are not.

Keeping the connections in place after a work redesign project and spreading connections

Source: Gloria Gilbert Mayer, Mary Jane Madden, and Eunice Lawrenz, eds., *Patient Care Delivery Models,* Aspen Publishers, Inc., © 1990.

beyond the steering committee can be achieved in several ways. Organizationwide shared governance, multidisciplinary ad hoc groups for problem solving, and having people deal directly with those with whom they have a problem are examples of methods that have made a difference. Alignment of all disciplines toward organizational goals requires that changes made in the redesign process become part of the culture of the organization.

7. *Physician-Nurse Collaboration.* Work redesign offers a systemic way of resolving systemic problems. A multidisciplinary project requires the full participation of physicians who have organizational power or who provide informal leadership. As physicians and nurses share issues and "walk in each other's shoes," a foundation for mutual respect and trust is laid. Not surprisingly, nurses and physicians discover a strong, shared commitment to patient care. As the depth of the commitment to patients is uncovered and trust grows, nurses and physicians move from being adversaries to becoming *real* allies.

Collaboration between physicians and nurses requires negotiating roles. This can be done only by the physicians and nurses involved, and it necessitates a time commitment from each person. Once begun, the process becomes part of the cultural norm and is expected and rewarded. Organizations with a reputation for collaborative relationships between nurses and physicians hold a unique market position with respect to nurse recruitment and retention.

ASSESSMENT OF ORGANIZATIONAL PERFORMANCE

Overview*

When an examination of the organization's performance is undertaken, all of the indicators of productivity, costs, and quality are reviewed. To identify important trends, data are collected

Source: Vi Kunkle, *Marketing Strategies for Nurse Managers: A Guide for Developing and Implementing a Nursing Marketing Plan,* Aspen Publishers, Inc., © 1990.

retrospectively, preferably five years back. Budgeted data are compared to the actual by service or by unit. Some of the questions to be explored here are the following:

- How cost-efficient is the nursing department?
- How productive is the nursing department?
- What were the self-defined quality ratings by unit and service?
- Is there an inverse relation between quality and productivity?
- Are some services more efficient than others?
- Is overtime justifiable?
- Do salary cost increases exceed the consumer price indexes?
- Are there appropriate levels of professional care?
- Are negative trends sporadic or subtle indications of major problems?

To provide the highest quality for the best price (the best value), the nursing department monitors the cost, productivity, and quality indicators monthly and annually, plotting five-year trends. Financial, productivity, and quality problems are identified by service and unit. Other questions for analysis are as follows:

- If productivity is increasing and hours per patient day (HPPD) decreasing, is quality affected? In other words, has short staffing affected quality?
- If overtime is increasing, are the actual staff positions less than budgeted (acuity data included in budgeted staff)? What justifies the overtime?
- If productivity is low and productive HPPD high, is low census the problem? If not, are vacations being given properly, or are there orientees on the unit?

Most administrators make use of a reporting format that can be used on a monthly basis to monitor unit financial management, productivity, human resource management, quality of care, and organizational development.

An Operational Audit*

An *operational audit* is an independent appraisal of the adequacy, effectiveness, and efficiency of an operational process. It entails determining the following general objectives:

- What is the purpose of this operation? How effectively is the purpose being accomplished?
- Is the purpose of the operation in congruence with the overall philosophy and purpose of the organization of which it is a part?
- How effectively and how efficiently are the assets and resources (including personnel) utilized, accounted for, and safeguarded?
- How reliable and useful is the information system supporting the operation? How well controlled is it?
- What is the extent of compliance with outside contractual obligations, industry standards, and governmental laws and regulations?

Types of Questions in an Operational Audit

- What specific relationships exist with physicians, other departments, and external agencies, organizations, vendors, and so on?
- What credentials are necessary for the staff? How are they documented?
- What resource constraints exist in terms of staffing, equipment, space, supplies, and storage?
- What possibilities exist for marketing?
- Are departmental policies and procedures current?
- Is staff turnover a problem?
- Is recruitment difficult?
- Are any major projects planned or being implemented?

- Is the organizational chart in the department job description current and accurate?
- Does pricing adequately cover costs?
- What are the major problems the department faces?
- What sorts of routine analysis are performed?

The type of reviews conducted are listed in Table 20–1.

ORGANIZATIONAL CULTURE AND CLIMATE

Organizational Culture Models*

Organizational culture comprises broadly shared, deeply held values that are enacted by organizational members. Many models characterize organization culture as existing on several levels of accessibility. In one three-tiered model, for example, the upper layer represents the most concrete aspects of culture—creations and artifacts. Observables such as policies, practices, stories, ceremonies, work attire, and technologies make it the easiest layer to study, as researchers have demonstrated. Creations and artifacts can contribute to or diminish the stress experienced by organizational members through work schedules, conflict-handling techniques, degree of support given to managers and staff, working conditions, and the like.

The middle layer consists of values per se—esteemed ideals shared by managers and employees. While not observable, values can be reported and compared for consistency. At the value layer in health care institutions comes, among other things, attitudes toward helping others, the importance of individual growth and development, and stances toward being one's own person.

*Source: William L. Scheyer, eds., *Handbook of Health Care Materiel Management,* Aspen Publishers, Inc., © 1985.

Source: Jeanine M. Aurelio, "An Organizational Culture that Optimizes Stress: Acceptable Stress in Nursing," *Nursing Administration Quarterly*, Vol. 18, No. 1, pp. 1–10, Aspen Publishers, Inc., © 1993.

Table 20–1 Checklist of Audit Review

An auditor will want to use the following review process:

____ Review the organization's long-range plan for applicable goals. Determine the current status of goal implementation.

____ Review applicable corporate policies and procedures and check for compliance.

____ Review departmental goals and objectives. Are they consistent with the long-range plan? Are they measured?

____ Review the departmental policy and procedure manual. Verify that required policies are in place and followed. Comment on discrepancies between policy and practice.

____ Review the quality assurance plan. Check for compliance. Review any written quality assurance reports prepared.

____ Review pertinent compliance and regulatory requirements. Acquire evidence that each requirement is complied with. Comment on any deviation.

____ Review the department description. Verify its accuracy through interviews and personal observation.

____ Determine consistency of goals, objectives, and policies and procedures at the organizational and departmental levels.

____ Review the job descriptions for all department personnel. Determine their accuracy through interviews with department management and staff and personal observations. Note any discrepancies.

____ Review the staff files for
__proof of licensure
__discipline not in accordance with organizational policy
__excessive staff turnover

____ Review patient or other opinion poll responses and incident reports. Note any repetition of complaints or incidents that indicate areas of potential liability.

____ Prepare a flowchart of operations where applicable, based on your understanding of department operations gained through the above work. Submit the preliminary flowchart draft to the department director for review. Incorporate any revisions into the final copy. Analyze the flowchart for control strengths and weaknesses and consistency with external, organizational, and departmental dicta.

____ Review computer programming or systems requests and their current status. Evaluate the logic for acceptance or rejection of these.

____ Review the financial and utilization reports prepared by the accounting department. Analysis of these should give the auditor an understanding of department utilization of financial and personnel resources. Growth rates, seasonal variations in expenses and revenue, control of overtime, and so on, should become evident.

____ Review any formulas that compute departmental productivity standards. Determine whether or not these formulas are reasonable as a basis for standards.

____ Review past capital budget requests. Determine the reasonableness of the rationales for acceptance or rejection of these requests. Identify capital requests that may require construction work for installation. Is the construction costed and included in the cost of the capital request? If not, why?

____ Obtain a blueprint of the department floor plan. Evaluate how well the floor plan design accommodates the department's needs.

____ Review procedure manuals. Are they informative? Adequate? Understandable? Understood? Complied with? Consistent with organizational policies and procedures?

____ Conclude by referring to the audit objectives at the beginning of the program. Evaluate to what extent the questions raised in the objective statements can be satisfactorily answered. Be specific.

____ Draft a report. Include all noteworthy comments and recommendations.

____ Plan future review and follow up.

The lower layer of organizational culture is the most unconscious yet most essential tier of organizational culture—basic assumptions organizational members hold about life in general and their organization in particular, containing unconscious core beliefs about such facets of life as human nature and relationships, the environment, reality, and time. The lower layer is the most difficult to tap, yet researchers speculate that knowledge of it would enable the organization to sustain important changes. The contents of this layer are not observable, nor can cultural members accurately state their core beliefs because, given day-to-day concerns, they are not aware of them.

The Differentiation of Organizational Culture*

Organizational culture should be differentiated from other organizational forces with which it is sometimes confused. These forces include organizational climate and managerial control.

Climate reflects individual perceptions or feelings about an organization, whereas culture consists of common beliefs and expected behaviors. Social climate scales enable the manager to create environments that will increase social functioning, worker satisfaction, and productivity by identifying the problems contributing to worker dissatisfaction and poor performance. In contrast, cultural assessments focus on understanding and predicting how an organization will behave under differing circumstances.

In contrast with managerial control, culture is a form of *internal* group control based on what the group members believe is necessary for group survival. Managerial control is exerted *externally* through stated goals, consciously derived strategies, organizational charts, codified policies and procedures, and consistently applied sanctions. The more managerial directives propose to change cultural behaviors, the most external force will be needed to enact them.

The fit between activities imposed by management and those dictated by group culture varies within an organization. When these forces conflict, creative management is needed to bridge the gap. Over time, a change introduced by management will probably become part of the culture if the group sees it as facilitating group survival. The challenge to nursing unit managers, who are members of two organizational cultures, namely, that of their management group and that of their nursing unit, is to take an innovation initiated by upper levels of management and make it acceptable to their particular nursing unit while still meeting management's objectives for the innovation.

Creating the Organizational Culture*

The primary force in creating the optimum organizational culture for the changing health care environment is the nurse executive. By role modeling a positive attitude toward change and exhibiting high-quality leadership skills, the nurse executive guides the way to the desired organizational culture. This also becomes part of the vision communicated by the nurse executive.

It is important for all members of the organization to understand the expectations, values, and direction of the organization. The goals and objectives of the nursing department should be developed in accordance with the health care institution's goals and objectives. The mission, philosophy, and vision of the institution should be known and understood by all personnel. The nurse executive's global perspective helps integrate the nursing department into the health care institution, which is important in creating the desired organizational culture.

*Source: Harriet Van Ess Coeling and Lillian M. Simms, "Facilitating Innovation at the Nursing Unit Level through Cultural Assessment, Part I: How To Keep Management Ideas from Falling on Deaf Ears," *Journal of Nursing Administration,* Vol. 23, No. 4, April 1993, J.B. Lippincott Company.

*Source: Kristi Kawamoto, "Nursing Leadership: To Thrive in a World of Change," *Nursing Administration Quarterly*, Vol. 18, No. 3, pp. 1–6, Aspen Publishers, Inc., © 1994.

The nurse executive promotes a positive cultural environment by coaching and mentoring the next level of managers. In turn, these managers can mentor and coach the staff members who report to them. It is at this point that the nurse executive uses leadership skills for self-empowerment and thus is able to empower others.

One person alone does not create an environment or culture. Empowerment of staff allows the nurse executive to develop a team effort to accomplish the vision. There are a variety of methods that can be used to empower staff and meet the goals of a positive, innovative organizational culture. The concept of shared governance has become more popular in health care, and participatory management styles are common. The trend has been to put decision making at the level where the expertise resides. Decentralizing decision making promotes creativity and autonomy because staff are actively involved in achieving goals that are in line with the vision of nursing. Empowerment becomes part of the organizational culture.

Planning Change*

Before implementing a plan, a health care leader must first know what the perceptions are within the organizational climate. Achieving needed changes requires accurate identification of the positive as well as the negative perceptions that operate within the health care facility. Meaningful data are needed; diagnosis must precede the planning.

Identification. Identify what the staff are proud of and what makes the facility special. What are the positive, energizing sets of beliefs or emotional forces within the facility? List the positive attitudes and perceptions that knit the staff together.

Source: Mark B. Silver, "Success Strategies: Victor or Victim?" in *The Health Care Executive Search: A Guide to Recruiting and Job Seeking,* Earl A. Simendinger and Terence F. Moore, eds., Aspen Publishers, Inc., © 1989.

Correction. What does not need fixing? What is working well here and should not be changed? Internally, what is being done right and effectively? Where is cohesiveness and cooperation in meeting the external challenges evident?

Structure. How clear and effective are assignments, tasks, and the organizational charts? To what extent does the organization's structure facilitate or hinder the achievement of goals? How does its structure facilitate or hinder coordination in getting jobs done?

Systems. Where do the arteries of information flow or get clogged? Is there adequate and sufficient information downward or between departments? Identify where more reliable, faster, and more current communications are needed.

Symbolism. A culture rewards and reinforces acceptable behaviors; management pays attention and gives emphasis to what it considers important by rewarding different results. What symbolic behaviors signal what is acceptable and what is not acceptable? What symbolic behaviors are rewarded or punished? To what does management pay great and ongoing attention or pay little or inconsistent attention?

Shared Values. Cohesive and consistent beliefs provide pride and direction through visions. List positive values and visions of the facility. List negative values, which hide in the "little corners" among the employees.

Strategy. Key result areas and identified ways to achieve successful and sustainable effects are critical in competitive times. Identify where there are mixed signals (confusion) regarding strategy. What strategy targets of the facility need to be stated or clarified?

Barriers. "We versus they" barriers can paralyze action. Where is the administration enslaved and encumbered by bureaucratic habits, out-of-date systems, unnecessary rituals, and comfort? Identify ways to de-layer, de-value, and de-manualize. What rules, which interfere with relations, can be changed?

Trust. Describe the level of team interaction and trust in the facility. List adjectives staff use that reflect trust and openness between people. Identify situations or areas where there is organizational gridlock, lack of decision making because of artificial walls, broken trust, and poor communication.

MANAGEMENT OR OPERATIONAL CONTROL

The Distinction between Operational and Management Control System*

The purpose of operational control systems is to ensure that specific tasks are carried out in accordance with well-defined expectations. The performance of a task is monitored continuously, and whenever it is found not to be within the standard, prespecified corrective mechanisms are triggered so that the task is ultimately carried out satisfactorily.

Management control systems are typically based on retrospective assessments of trends and are more likely to require subjective judgments. In contrast to operational controls, the corrective action in a management control system can seldom be defined a priori and is designed to affect all instances of the future performance of a given task rather than merely correct, as operational controls do, each individual deviation as it is detected. For instance, in some institutions the management control system for the surgical operating room suite is based on regular reports that provide the percentage utilization of operating room capacity, number and type of procedures performed, length of waiting queue, and similar measures. If these measures show decreasing use of the operating room suite's capacity in the face of a lengthening queue for elective procedures, the control system triggers an investigation into the possibility of inefficient scheduling of the operating rooms and other operational problems, result-

*Source: Loen Wyszewianski, J. William Thomas, and Bruce Friedman, "Case-Based Payment and the Control of Quality and Efficiency in Hospitals," Inquiry 24, Spring 1987, © 1987 Blue Cross and Blue Shield Association.

ing in corrective actions to eliminate future underutilization of operating room capacity.

The differences between operational and management controls make them complements. Operational control systems are best for rectifying the occasional deviation from a specified standard—for example, a drug reaction—but they are not well suited for repeated, systematic deviations from the standard, such as a pattern of inappropriate prescribing of drugs by one or more physicians. Detecting and correcting such problems are much more the province of management controls. Accordingly, some management control systems monitor how frequently an operational control triggers corrective actions, and when an undesirably repetitive pattern of such corrections occurs, the management control system initiates changes in the appropriate administrative and organizational areas to eliminate the pattern.

Example: Controls in the Operating Room

Operational Controls. Characterized by routine application and well-defined, immediate corrective measures, operational controls are well suited to ensure compliance with many common requirements of operating room management. Such requirements include laboratory tests routinely ordered preoperatively to anticipate possible surgical complications or uncover contraindications for certain types of surgery: white blood cell count, hemoglobin concentration, chest film, and basic liver and kidney function tests.

Harm to the patient will be minimized and quality of care thereby safeguarded if operational controls ensure that no surgery is performed unless all applicable prerequisites have been satisfied. In addition, unnecessary preoperative stays as well as last-minute cancellations of the surgical procedure can be avoided— thereby also saving the consequent costs of idle operating rooms—if for elective cases a set of operational controls prevents scheduling of a time slot for the operating room unless all necessary tests have been ordered and the requested date allows sufficient time for the results to be received and evaluated before the operation. Additionally, other controls can monitor test results to make certain that all test results have been received and to flag any findings so outside the norm as to require cancellation of the procedure.

All such controls require linkages between the operating room scheduling system and the system for ordering tests and reporting their results. If the linkages are not already in place, establishing them is within the reach of the many organizations in which these separate functions are already computerized.

The process of developing operational controls may itself lead to an increase in efficiency. Once it becomes clear that surgical procedures will be canceled if certain test results are not available on time, the medical staff may review the need for all preoperative tests and conclude that some are altogether unnecessary whereas others ought to be required more selectively. The net result would be a gain in clinical efficiency from the reduction of preoperative testing costs and higher quality of care through elimination of the risks associated with unnecessary tests.

Management Controls. Management controls can similarly have a positive effect on quality and efficiency in the operating room. In the operating room suite, a management control system might monitor how often requests for scheduling operating room time are turned down by operational controls because the necessary prerequisites have not been satisfied and how often surgery is automatically canceled by the operational control system because test results are not available or the results are outside acceptable norms. These are costly and disruptive events that may indicate inadequate handling of cases. When such events occur too often, management controls can prompt the formulation of appropriate educational or administrative interventions to reduce their incidence.

Management control systems can also be used to monitor the quality and efficiency of the surgical care provided. For instance, length of operating room time can be monitored as an indicator of both the quality and efficiency of the surgeon's technique. If standard times are established for the most frequently performed procedures, a pattern of excessive departure from those times, in either direction, is cause for further investigation and possible remedial action. Although such a pattern sometimes reflects nothing more than differences among surgeons in the pace of work, it can also be an indication of hurried and poor surgical technique or a repetitive history of intraoperative complications. Similarly, unsatisfactory performance can be identified not only by monitoring reports of normal tissue removed but also by monitoring the amount of blood and blood components transfused intraoperatively and during the immediate postoperative recovery period for specific procedure groups.

Chapter 21

Productivity

OVERVIEW

Productivity Measurement*

As financial constraints continue to mount, productivity becomes an ever-increasing concern for health care organizations. The area of productivity measurement, however, remains somewhat of a mystery in many industries, not just health care. In health care, the difficulties are compounded by problems related to quality and output measurement. Productivity represents the measurement of inputs required to produce an output. However, outputs have always been difficult to define in health care. Proxies such as visits, treatments, patient days, and discharges have been used.

In many industries, the product being produced is made in a repeated process. The same product is made over and over, and it is relatively easy to identify which resources were used to make which products. For any given product, the total inputs and their cost can be accumulated for a period such as a month and divided by the total units produced to find the cost per unit. If

---

Source: Steven A. Finkler, *Essentials of Health Care Cost Accounting,* Aspen Publishers, Inc., © 1994.

394

the cost per unit can be reduced, productivity will rise.

In the health care field, there are several obvious limitations of that approach. First, the product varies considerably. A health care facility will likely treat patients from several hundred different diagnosis-related groups (DRGs), and within DRGs there is substantial variation among patients. Further, "production" is not continuous; a health care organization can only work with the patients it has. That sometimes means unavoidable down time (and lost resources) waiting for the next patient.

Additionally, it is difficult to assign costs of most departments directly to patients of any given type. Although cost accounting systems are moving in the direction of direct association of costs with patients, it is not clear that resource inputs will ever be assigned to patients with the same degree of accuracy and detail as is possible in a factory process that produces only one given type of product.

Thus the health care organization can run into problems of productivity measurement.

NURSING PRODUCTIVITY

Factors Affecting Staff Productivity*

Productivity can be defined as the ratio of output, in terms of products and services, to input, in terms of resources consumed. The productivity of the nursing staff is measured by the number of nursing hours (resource inputs) provided to meet the demands of the mix of patients (services output) on a nursing unit.

The primary inputs affecting nursing staff productivity are the characteristics of the staff, the patients, and the nursing unit itself. Staff characteristics include the level, mix, qualifications, experience, and stability of staff members. Ob-

viously, well-educated, experienced, highly motivated nurses will be more productive than those with less education, experience, and motivation. Patient characteristics include the number of patients to be cared for and their ages, diagnoses, and treatments. Many acutely ill patients with complicated diagnoses that require multiple treatments will make greater demands on the nursing staff than a few patients with less severe problems. Unit characteristics refer to the unit's size, layout, and location as well as the equipment and services available on the unit. A well-designed working area that is in close proximity to equipment and services used by the staff will greatly boost staff productivity compared to close, cramped quarters that are inconvenient to the services and equipment used.

The primary outputs of the staff are acuity-adjusted patient days, improved patient health, patient satisfaction with service, medical records, and patient education. Methods of assessing staff output and productivity include the patient classification system, cost accounting, budget and general ledger reports, position control, and quality monitoring.

The challenge to managers of nursing resources is to maximize the productivity of those resources to optimize costs and to preserve an appropriate quality level. Peter Drucker has said that productivity is *the* job of a manager, and the management of productivity is the true test of a competent manager.

There are many factors that bear upon nursing staff productivity. They do not affect all organizations equally, or in the same way, but must be considered when managing nursing staff productivity. Among these factors are

- a patient classification system that reflects resource consumption
- a nursing utilization system that prospectively allocates staff and retrospectively monitors productivity
- a scheduling system that allows for planning of nursing resource assignments, yet is sufficiently flexible to respond to changes in demand

Source: Charles C. Gabbert, "Nursing Staffing, Scheduling, and Productivity," in *Nursing Administration and Law Manual,* Karen Hawley Henry, ed., Aspen Publishers, Inc., © 1986.

- nursing staffing and personnel policies that support productive resource use (e.g., every third weekend off rather than every other weekend off, permitting "doubling back" with only eight hours off between shifts)
- an optimal mix of skills that allows individuals to do the jobs they are trained to do in response to demand
- an efficient interface between nursing and ancillary departments regarding patient access, with a master scheduling system in place for each patient
- a physical plant layout that minimizes unnecessary travel and activity on the part of nursing personnel
- flexible medication, meal serving, and shift reporting procedures that prevent peaking of workload
- an ability to forecast census and patient mix in order to plan resource allocation
- nursing managers who are constantly looking for better ways to do things with fewer resources

These are generalized factors that affect health care facilities in different ways. The important point to consider is that, if each element of this short list of factors were to be addressed, productivity in any nursing department would be positively affected to a substantial degree.

Approaches*

The study of nursing productivity is the study of how to deliver the best nursing care in the most appropriate manner at the lowest cost. In this sense, nursing productivity is a concept that ties together all the factors involved in the provision of quality nursing care.

Criteria frequently used in evaluating nursing productivity include nursing hours per patient day, ratios of staff to patients, cost per patient

*Source: A Review and Evaluation of Nursing Productivity, DHHS, Pub. No. (HRA 77-15), 1977.

day, numbers of encounters, and many more. Depending on the health care setting and the persons performing the evaluation, each of these items may represent a meaningful, if simplistic, measure. But even with these simple, often accepted performance indicators, there tend to be inconsistencies in the manner in which hours, dollars, numbers, and ratios are determined.

Following are some suggestions on specific approaches.

Measure of Nursing Productivity. Develop a measure of nursing productivity based on nursing outcomes, through the following steps:

1. Define nursing outcomes and determine how these should be measured. Include the following:
   - health status
   - patient knowledge
   - patient satisfaction (measured indirectly and directly)
2. Define patient-oriented goals based on these nursing outcomes.
3. Measure the extent to which these goals are achieved (this is a measure of nursing quality).
4. Use this nursing quality measure as a part of a nursing productivity measure (the other part being efficiency—use of resources to deliver the quality).

Role Definition. Improve the role definition of the nurse at all levels from director of nursing service to staff nurse, and do it both in leadership and clinical areas.

- Assign personnel at levels consistent with their competence and preparation.
- Provide management training for nurses at the master's level and through inservice education.
- Involve the nurse in the development of his or her own role.
- Study the disparity between nursing education and nursing practice and determine how to reduce or eliminate it.

Participative Management. Encourage experimentation with and research into participative nursing management.

Incentives. Develop and use quality, financial, and other incentives for both individuals and the institution. Determine through research the extent to which incentives can affect productivity.

Technological Factors. Investigate the interrelationship of various factors that affect nursing productivity, for example, the relationship between nursing care organization (team, functional, primary) and facility design.

Mechanization and Automation. Develop a model for nursing productivity that will:

- use quantified outputs and inputs
- fit into a model of health services evaluation
- use as inputs nursing personnel, facilities, equipment, supplies, and so on
- provide output measures of patient health status, knowledge, and satisfaction

Productivity System Issues*

When implementing a productivity system, the following issues must be considered.

Acceptable Range of Productivity. Because most employees in a nursing department work either 8- or 12-hour shifts, it is often difficult to arrive at 100 percent productivity. Because much of the care on a nursing unit is time sensitive (meaning it must be performed at specific moments), it is not always possible to have exactly the right staffing available at a given time. It is, therefore, essential that a reasonable range of productivity be established as a standard for comparison. This range is often between 85 percent and 115 percent.

Source: Letty R. Piper, "Patient Acuity Systems and Productivity," *Topics in Health Care Financing,* Vol. 15, No. 3, Aspen Publishers, Inc., © 1989.

Direct and Indirect Care. The care on a nursing unit can be described as direct, indirect, fixed, and variable. Direct care is the actual care provided to patients. Indirect care is the documentation, direction, and planning of the direct care. Fixed care is the minimal required staffing for a unit; this does not vary with the acuity. Variable care is the component of care that is directly driven by the acuity.

Most acuity systems are quite good at measuring direct care and often have additive factors that also account for the indirect time directly related to the direct care. However, in units such as the emergency department, delivery suites, and intensive care units, there is a larger component of indirect care due to the uneven flow of patients. For example, although a nurse may have the time to care for additional patients, there may not be any additional patients available.

Fixed and Variable Components. When establishing a productivity system, it is important to determine the variable portion of staffing. This component should be compared with the acuity standard, and the fixed portion should be compared with a per diem or per shift standard. On a nursing unit, the head nurse and clerk are often fixed and the staff registered nurses and nurses' aides are variable.

Updating and Validation. Systems are designed to be used for periods of years. Because the policies and procedures of the department are frequently altered by technology, physical layout changes, and practice pattern modifications, it is essential that the user understand how the time values assigned to indicators or descriptions were established so that the values can be modified or validated over time. Patient acuity systems must not remain stagnant but must have the flexibility to change with the practices that they measure.

In conjunction with validation, it is necessary to note that there are always differences in the amount of time various individuals need to perform a task. However, it is also important to note that, frequently, two tasks can be performed simultaneously or in an abbreviated fashion, thereby altering the productivity equation.

Work Distribution Chart*

There are many analytical techniques for implementing a work simplification program. Six of them are briefly described in Table 21–1. (Two are illustrated in Figures 21–1 and 21–2.)

The work distribution chart (Figure 21–2) is designed for analyzing the functions performed in a department or unit. When properly prepared, it enables managers to see clearly in one place

---

Source: Addison C. Bennet, *Methods Improvements in Hospitals,* J.B. Lippincott Company, © 1964.

- the work activities performed and the time it takes to perform them
- the individuals who are working on these activities
- the amount of time spent by each person on each activity

The work distribution charting technique can help in developing improvements in the way things are being done.

- It indicates what activities take the most time.
- It points out the unnecessary work that is being performed.
- It indicates whether or not skills are used properly.

Table 21–1 Analytical Techniques for Work Simplification

1. **The flow process chart** should be used in a work study situation in which it appears desirable to follow the actions pertaining to a *single* person, a *single* material, or a *single* form. This would include (a) the activities of a *person* who is involved in a straight sequence of events, with some movement from place to place; (b) the handling of any single *material* that flows through a connected series of events; (c) the flow of a single-copy or single-part *form.* (See Figure 21–1.) (Although this vertical type chart may be ideal for gathering and recording facts relating to a single item involving process, the procedure flowchart (a horizontal-type chart) is more adaptable to work procedures of a more complex nature.)
2. **The flow diagram** should be used in a work study situation in which it appears desirable to examine the *paths* of movement of people, paperwork, or materials. This form of analysis is particularly useful in work where (a) the distance traveled is excessive, (b) the flow is complicated, (c) the work area is congested, (d) backtracking is evidenced. The flow diagram in its simplest form is used to supplement the flow process chart.
3. **The organization chart** should be used in a work study situation in which it appears desirable to analyze and evaluate the present organizational structure of a department or unit. This chart can be helpful in providing a broad overall view of the department or unit as it now exists.
4. **The work distribution chart** should be used in a work study situation in which it appears desirable to examine in greater detail the work being done in a department or unit. This chart will present clearly in one place (a) the work activities performed by the department and the total time it takes to perform them, (b) the individuals who are working on each of these activities, (c) the amount of time spent by each person on each activity. (See Figure 21–2.)
5. **The procedure flow chart** should be used in a work study situation involving the performance of many different work routines by individuals in different capacities and, perhaps, in different departments. It is also recommended for charting the details of procedures that involve the flow of multicopy or multipart forms.
6. **Work sampling** should be used in work study situations in which the functions being investigated are nonrepetitive in nature. This technique makes it possible to gather detailed information that would be difficult to obtain by means of continuous observation.

Figure 21–1 Flow Process Chart

PRESENT METHOD ☑ PROPOSED METHOD ☐

FLOW PROCESS CHART

PAGE 1 OF 1

SUMMARY

1 TRIP:	PRESENT	PROPOSED	DIFFERENCE
○ OPERATIONS	7		
⇨ TRANSPORTATIONS	8		
□ INSPECTIONS	1		
D DELAYS	3		
▽ STORAGES	2		
DISTANCE TRAVELLED	740 FT	FT	FT
TIME MIN.	45		

JOB HANDLING VALUABLES OF PRIVATE AND SEMI-PRIVATE PATIENTS

Subject Charted NURSE

CHART BEGINS AT NURSE'S STATION

CHART ENDS AT NURSES STATION

CHARTED BY L. WEEKS DATE 10/25/61.

	DESCRIPTION OF EVENT	OPERATION / TRANSPORT / INSPECTION / DELAY / STORAGE	QUANTITY	DISTANCE IN FEET	MIN TIME	NOTES
1	AT NURSES' STATION	○⇨□D▽				3RD FLOOR
2	GETS ENVELOPE AND FORM	○⇨□D▽			1	
3	FILLS IN NECESSARY DATA	○⇨□D▽			2	
4	WALKS TO PATIENT'S ROOM	○⇨□D▽		30	½	
5	CHECKS VALUABLES WITH PATIENT	○⇨□D▽			5	
6	RECORDS AMOUNT & KIND OF VALUABLES ON ENVELOPE & FORM	○⇨□D▽			2	
7	SIGNS TEMPORARY RECEIPT	○⇨□D▽			½	
8	DETACHES TEMPORARY RECEIPT AND GIVES TO PATIENT	○⇨□D▽			½	
9	WALKS TO ELEVATOR	○⇨□D▽		180	3	
10	WAITS FOR ELEVATOR	○⇨□D▽			5	AVERAGE OF 6 TRIPS PER DAY
11	RIDES TO MAIN FLOOR	○⇨□D▽		35	1	
12	WALKS TO CASHIER	○⇨□D▽		125	2	
13	GIVES VALUABLES TO CASHIER	○⇨□D▽				
14	WAITS WHILE VALUABLES ARE CHECKED & PERMANENT RECEIPT OBTAINED	○⇨□D▽			10	
15	WALKS TO ELEVATOR	○⇨□D▽		125	2	
16	WAITS FOR ELEVATOR	○⇨□D▽			5	
17	RIDES TO NURSING FLOOR	○⇨□D▽		35	1	3RD FLOOR
18	WALKS TO PATIENT'S ROOM	○⇨□D▽		180	3	
19	GIVES PERMANENT RECEIPT TO PATIENT	○⇨□D▽			1	
20	RETURNS TO NURSES' STATION	○⇨□D▽		30	½	
21	AT NURSES STATION	○⇨□D▽				
22		○⇨□D▽				
23		○⇨□D▽				
24		○⇨□D▽				

Figure 21–2 Work Distribution Chart

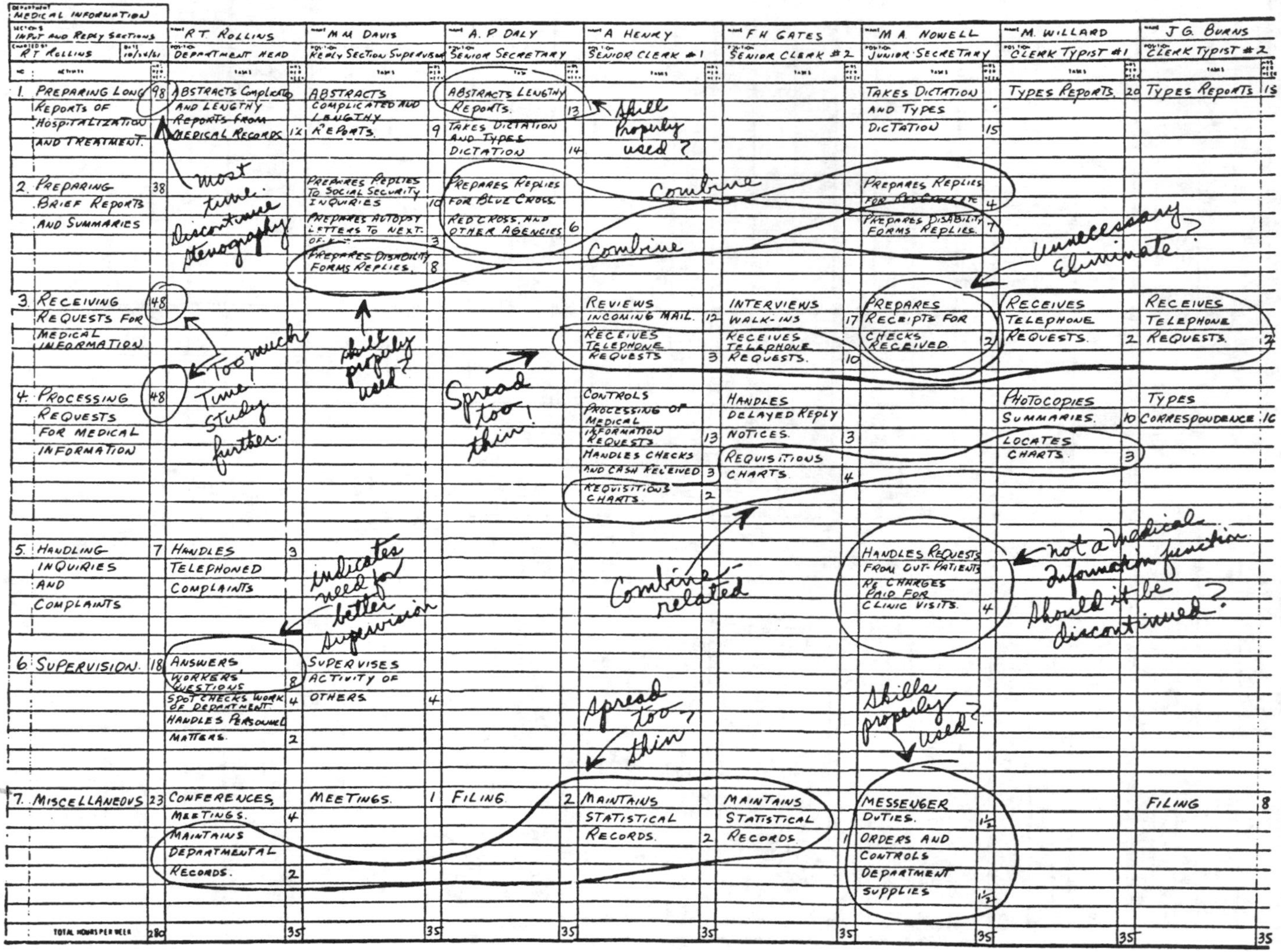

Department: Medical Information
Section: Input and Reply Sections
Charted by: R.T. Rollins Date: 10/24/61

Activity	Hrs. per week	R.T. Rollins, Department Head: Tasks	Hrs.	M.M. Davis, Reply Section Supervisor: Tasks	Hrs.	A.P. Daly, Senior Secretary: Tasks	Hrs.	A Henry, Senior Clerk #1: Tasks	Hrs.	F.H. Gates, Senior Clerk #2: Tasks	Hrs.	M.A. Nowell, Junior Secretary: Tasks	Hrs.	M. Willard, Clerk Typist #1: Tasks	Hrs.	J.G. Burns, Clerk Typist #2: Tasks	Hrs.
1. Preparing Long Reports of Hospitalization and Treatment	98	Abstracts Completed and Lengthy Reports from Medical Records	12	Abstracts Complicated and Lengthy Reports	9	Abstracts Lengthy Reports Takes Dictation and Types Dictation	13 14					Takes Dictation and Types Dictation	15	Types Reports	20	Types Reports	15
2. Preparing Brief Reports and Summaries	38			Prepares Replies to Social Security Inquiries Prepares Autopsy Letters to Next of Kin Prepares Disability Forms Replies	10 3 8	Prepares Replies for Blue Cross, Red Cross, and Other Agencies	6					Prepares Replies for [illegible] Prepares Disability Forms Replies	4 7				
3. Receiving Requests for Medical Information	48							Reviews Incoming Mail Receives Telephone Requests	12 3	Interviews Walk-ins Receives Telephone Requests	17 10	Prepares Receipts for Checks Received	2	Receives Telephone Requests	2	Receives Telephone Requests	2
4. Processing Requests for Medical Information	48							Controls Processing of Medical Information Requests Handles Checks and Cash Received Requisitions Charts	13 3 2	Handles Delayed Reply Notices Requisitions Charts	3 4			Photocopies Summaries Locates Charts	10 3	Types Correspondence	10
5. Handling Inquiries and Complaints	7	Handles Telephoned Complaints	3									Handles Requests from Out-Patients re Charges Paid for Clinic Visits	4				
6. Supervision	18	Answers Workers' Questions Spot Checks Work of Department Handles Personnel Matters	8 4 2	Supervises Activity of Others	4												
7. Miscellaneous	23	Conferences, Meetings Maintains Departmental Records	4 2	Meetings	1	Filing	2	Maintains Statistical Records	2	Maintains Statistical Records	1	Messenger Duties Orders and Controls Department Supplies	1½ 1½			Filing	8
Total hours per week	280		35		35		35		35		35		35		35		35

- It indicates whether or not any employees are doing too many unrelated tasks.
- It points out tasks that may be spread too thinly throughout the department or unit.
- It shows whether or not work in the unit is distributed evenly.

To begin with, the preparation of a work distribution chart is made possible through the use of a *task list* and an *activity list*. The information that is entered on these records is assembled subsequently onto a work distribution chart.

The task list is used to develop a listing of the duties actually being performed by each employee in the department or the unit, indicating the estimated number of hours spent per week on each duty. This listing of tasks should be made out for each position presently occupied in the organizational unit, including the department head and supervisory positions. If difficulty is encountered in estimating time spent on each task, it may be necessary for the employee to maintain a record of hours spent on each activity over a period of one or two weeks so as to establish a proper allocation of time.

The activity list is used to record the major activities that are performed or that should be performed to fulfill the objectives of the department or the unit. The list should be prepared by the manager of the organizational unit.

The next step is to assemble these data in such a way as to be able to analyze them conveniently. This is accomplished by transferring the information found on the activity list and the task lists onto a work distribution chart. First, rank each activity, assigning a number. Starting at the extreme left of the sheet, rule a column for activities, followed by a column for each employee in the unit. On the right side of each of these columns, allow space for the entry of hours per week. Review all task lists for the purpose of identifying each entry with an activity number appearing on the activity list. Enter in each appropriate employee column all the tasks that have been classified as number 1. At the same time, record the number of hours spent on activity 1 by each employee. When all information has been entered on the chart, total the time entries for all employees as well as for all activities. These totals should be the same. See Table 21–2 for a summary of the process involved in analyzing work distribution.

MEASURING PRODUCTIVITY

(*Note:* See Chapter 17, "Staffing," for a full discussion of work measurement techniques.) To achieve staff savings and to monitor labor productivity on a continuing basis, labor standards are essential. Their development requires not only technical expertise, but also the exercise of managerial judgment.

The techniques available for developing standards are varied, ranging from the simple use of historical data to highly refined, predetermined time systems. Three are adaptable for health care facility use: (1) estimating the time required to perform a given task, (2) the classical time and monitor study approach, and (3) the historical data evaluation approach.

Regardless of the method used to develop standards, if the standards are to be effective in improving productivity and reducing cost, managers must be held accountable for performance against these standards.

Process for Developing Productivity Standards*

A manager (or management engineer or other work analyst) will ordinarily begin the process of setting productivity standards for a department by assessing the department's work and identifying all tasks that are done. Standards are most frequently established in order of the proportion of the department's time that various tasks require; that is, the first tasks for which standards are set are usually those that consume the largest part of the employees' time.

Source: Charles R. McConnell, *The Health Care Supervisor's Guide to Cost Control and Productivity Improvement,* Aspen Publishers, Inc., © 1986.

Table 21–2 Analyzing Work Using a Work Distribution Chart

Step 1. Analyze All Activities

Taking each activity listed vertically in the column at the extreme left of the chart, ask questions, for example:

- *What* is the purpose of the activity?
- *Why* is it necessary?
- *Why* is this activity a function of this department?
- *What* activities take the most time? *Why*?
- *What* is a reasonable time for each activity?

These questions will help to determine the importance of each activity and whether any activity can be eliminated.

Step 2. Analyze Each Task of Each Activity

Taking one activity at a time, read horizontally across the chart and ask questions about each task assigned to it, for example:

- *What* is the purpose of the task?
- *Why* is it necessary?
- *Where* should the task be done?
- *When* should the task be done?
- *Who* should perform the task?
- *Who* duplicates or overlaps in performing the task?

These questions will help to determine whether each task is being done in the right place, at the right time, by the right person, and in the right way.

Step 3. Analyze Each Person's Tasks and Activities

Taking one person at a time, ask questions concerning each duty or task listed vertically in the assigned column, for example:

- *How* closely related are the duties?
- *How* are skills utilized?
- *How* heavy is the workload?
- *How* repetitive are the tasks?

These questions will help to uncover unrelated tasks, misuse of skills, uneven distribution of work, and tasks spread too thin.

Assuming that a particular task has been identified and that a productivity standard is to be set, the process may proceed as follows.

1. Identification of Steps. The content of the task is analyzed for the purpose of identifying all steps involved, all inputs required, and all supporting activities that may have to take place for completion of the task. Special attention is given to identifying clearly recognizable starting and ending points for the task.

2. Evaluation of Each Step. The content of every step is evaluated in detail, and every effort is made to alter the steps in the interest of improving productivity while not adversely affecting quality. Such evaluation will usually include attempts to reduce delays, reduce travel or handling, improve materials and equipment, and improve workplace layout.

3. Determination of Time. Using a method such as stopwatch time study, predetermined motion times, or work sampling, *normal time* for the task is determined. Normal time is the bare clock time, unaltered by allowances for performing the task.

4. Calculation of PFD Factor. An appropriate factor is applied to compensate for personal, fatigue, and minor delay time that may be experienced. Commonly referred to as a PFD (personal, fatigue, and delay) factor, this may be established for the institution as a whole or for a specific department by extensive work sampling study. Many health care facilities use institutionwide PFD factors, most of which fall in the range of 15 to 20 percent. If the organization's PFD factor is 17 percent, for example, the normal time referred to in the preceding step is multiplied by 1.17 to arrive at the *standard time,* the time required by a qualified and properly trained person working at a normal pace to complete the task.

5. Identification of Work Units. If not already accomplished, the department's *work units* should be clearly identified. These work units are the common units of service that constitute the department's output, such as admissions (the admitting department), discharges (the medical record department), square feet of building space service (the housekeeping department), bills rendered (the patient billing function), tests (laboratory), procedures (radiology), meals served or patient days (food service).

6. Final Calculations. Determine the *work unit time per occurrence* for each task. When such times for all tasks having a bearing on producing a unit of service are added together, the result will be the *standard time per unit of service.*

7. Establishing the Relationship of Indirect Tasks. It is next necessary to account for *indirect tasks* that are not accounted for in the standard thus far but nevertheless necessary to the production of the department's output. These can be handled in two ways.

In the first way, if there is a reasonable relationship between the indirect tasks and the units of service produced, that is, if the indirect

work varies up or down as the units of service vary up or down, the indirect tasks (at least some of them) can be added to the standard as an additional per-unit allowance. For example, obtaining supplies, cleaning up after working, and preparing certain reports might be includable in the standard.

Conversely, if there is no direct relationship between indirect tasks and amount of output, indirect time may be expressed as an amount of constant time per day. Certain supporting activities, foremost among them supervision, secretarial support, and attending meetings, are departmental activities that occur roughly to the same extent regardless of variations in levels of output. For example, a given department may function at all times using one manager and one secretary over a broad range of output levels. Thus, the resulting standard for an entire department is often a two-part expression—hours of constant time per day and time per unit of service.

8. Applying the Productivity Standard. The resulting *productivity standard* is applied in measuring and monitoring the department's productivity. Common forms of health care facility productivity standards include

- admitting: hours/calendar day, plus hours/ admission
- food service: hours/calendar day, plus hours/ patient day
- housekeeping: hours/calendar day (with staffing based on square feet of area)
- laboratory: hours/calendar day, plus hours/ test; or hours/calendar day, plus CAP units
- medical records: hours/calendar day, plus hours/discharge
- nursing (for specific nursing unit); hours/ patient day
- physical therapy: hours/calendar day, plus hours/modality

9. Setting Up a Target Utilization Factor. It may at times be necessary to alter a department's productivity standard further to account for interference factors referred to earlier. Interference factors result from forces beyond the control of the manager, such as sporadic workload arrival, the need for standby coverage, and problems with a physical layout. A *target utilization factor* may be established for this purpose. Usually based on a combination of measurement, observation, and judgment, a target utilization factor recognizes that practical productivity is often less than theoretical productivity. If a department's target utilization factor is 90 percent (an official recognition that 90 percent utilization is the maximum practical utilization for this department), the variable portion of the standard (the hours per unit of service) will be divided by 0.90 (inflated by 10 percent) to reflect this. (The constant portion of the standard, the hours per calendar day, remains unadjusted.)

10. Conclusion. With or without the necessary adjustment of a target utilization factor, the *productivity standard* for a department will be of the form—usually two-part, but occasionally a single expression—described above. This productivity standard makes it possible to value the department's output in terms of work time so output may be compared with work time applied as input.

Additional Factors To Consider in Setting a Productivity Standard

In addition to the essential work content of a job, a number of additional factors will have a bearing on the manner in which a productivity standard is set. The more significant factors include the following.

The Degree of Repetitiveness of the Task. A task that is performed only occasionally does not allow opportunity for the worker to get fully up to speed, unlike a task that is done over and over again. For many tasks, repetition builds familiarity, which in turn builds output efficiency.

The Fatigue Potential of the Job. Some tasks, through either physical or mental demands, induce fatigue to an extent that can markedly affect performance time. Virtually all tasks induce fatigue to some degree: A person who enters a job fresh and rested is capable of greater performance than one who is tired from hours of work. This must be recognized in the time standards.

Dependence on Other Employees. Many tasks are such that they cannot be completed alone; they require the accompanying efforts of other persons or they require related tasks to be accomplished first or perhaps between steps. This dependence, which is manifested in what may appear to be idle time, must be reflected in the time standard as long as it is valid.

Interference. Natural disruptions sometimes prevent a worker from seeing a task through to completion, or work does not arrive in a time sequence that matches the worker's capacity. An interrupted task, one that must be stopped and restarted several times (such as the typing of a report by a secretary who doubles as a receptionist and thus must stop frequently to answer inquiries), will take longer because of the stops and starts than would otherwise be required. As to the timing of work arrival, a worker may be available to work but have nothing to do at times because no work has arrived. Some emergency department staffs experience interference factors in this respect; because of the essentially random arrival of patients, they cannot always be gainfully occupied, but minimum staffing requirements dictate that staff must always be there.

Chapter 22

Quality Concepts

OVERVIEW

Management Principles for Quality*

The purpose of quality management is to establish a system that measures and manages patient care in a way that provides the best care for all patients. It identifies opportunities for improvement as well as system problems that require resolution. It ultimately fulfills a societal commitment of the health professions to the public.

- Quality of care is a responsibility owed by health care professionals to those served.
- A knowledge of organizational systems, clinical medicine, general management, and statistics is vital to the management of quality.
- Quality-of-care measurement and management is a distinct body of knowledge with its own theories, concepts, methods, and techniques.
- Quality is both objective and subjective.

- A thorough knowledge of the health care delivery system is essential for understanding quality.
- Quality of care is not solely the domain of clinicians. It results from an interrelated system of processes.
- Quality management is an important management function. Good management theory applies to clinical quality management in the same way it applies to fiscal management.
- There is no "one" or "best" way to measure or manage quality.
- Quality of care can be continuously improved.
- A good quality management system is vital to organizational survival.

It is expected that a variety of regulatory and voluntary approaches to quality management will develop. This blended approach will focus heavily on efficiency, effectiveness, and accountability. The trend toward outcome measurement and management will continue as total quality management and quality assurance become integrated and adopted as a "clinical quality improvement" system.

Quality measurement systems will evolve into integrated systems that track and monitor the

---

*Source: Daniel R. Longo and Donald W. Avant, "Managing Quality," in *Manual of Health Services Management*, Robert J. Taylor, ed., Aspen Publishers, Inc., © 1994.

processes and outcomes of care across settings and providers.

Evolution of the Quality Concept*

Historically, the quality of health care has been measured through analysis of mortality and morbidity records, improvements in professional education, and establishment of professional standards of care, credentialing, and reimbursement. In the last few decades, the thrust toward controlling quality and working toward quality health care has intensified. In response to public concern about escalating health care costs, the government has also enacted several legislative efforts to ensure cost-effective care. The Joint Commission on Accreditation of Healthcare Organizations (Joint Commission) continues to measure compliance to its standards but has changed its focus several times.

Quality control, a concept of the 1970s, examined the operational and structural requirements needed to keep a unit operational. It had little to do with the clinical processes related to patient care, but it supported clinical practice. (For information on quality control, which is once against considered significant as a part of total quality management, see Chapter 20, "Operational Reviews.")

The 1980s ushered in the concept of quality assurance at the departmental level (e.g., the nursing department), which was then brought to the unit level (e.g., the operating room). The 1970s short-term focus on a specific medical diagnosis or procedure has been replaced with a 10-step Joint Commission monitoring and evaluation process of high-risk, high-volume, and problem-prone aspects of care over a period of time.

Under this approach, care that is given is measured against predetermined standards. Problems and areas of noncompliance with standards are identified and resolved through appropriate

action. Evaluation of the effectiveness of corrective actions is accomplished by ongoing monitoring. Quality assurance in the 1980s focused on the identification and correction of problems.

In the 1990s the concept of quality is still evolving. The focus is now on total quality management (TQMs) and continuous quality improvement (CQI). CQI is not another model for conducting quality assurance activities; it is a management style that supports and enhances the efforts of quality. The focus is on improving care and service. CQI requires examination of the processes of care and service in order to improve outcomes.

Quality assurance activities such as monitoring and assessment enable identification and resolution of problems. Continuous quality improvement goes beyond the problem-oriented approach; the data derived from monitoring is used to continuously improve—*even in the absence of problems*.

For the CQI concept to succeed, quality must be a priority at all levels within the organization. Staff must be encouraged to improve care. There must be multidisciplinary and interdisciplinary reviews of systems and service with efforts focused on improvement of processes and systems.

THE SCOPE OF TOTAL QUALITY MANAGEMENT

TQM is both a management philosophy and a process. As a process, it focuses attention on organizational systems rather than individuals, and on continual improvement rather than inspection. In this regard, TQM is highly rational and entails following a well-defined and universal sequence of steps. TQM requires the adoption of a new philosophy. It is this philosophy that creates the context within which the processes occur, and which enables the organization to achieve quality as a normal and integrated activity within the organization.*

Source: Joanna Eisenberg, "Quality Assurance—Continuous Quality Improvement," in *The Manual of Operating Room Management: An Administrative Patient Care Resource*, Cynthia Spry, ed., Aspen Publishers, Inc., © 1990.

Source: Margarete Arndt and Barbara Bigelow, "The Implementation of Total Quality Management in Hospitals: How Good Is the Fit?" *Health Care Management Review*, Vol. 20, No. 4, Aspen Publishers, Inc., © Fall 1995.

Basic Elements*

1. TQM as a Philosophy: Setting the Context

The TQM philosophy encompasses both a commitment to a process as well as a set of beliefs about what quality is and management's role in inculcating those beliefs into the organization's culture. Among the essential beliefs are that the organization's quality is defined in terms of its customers, whether internal or external (see Table 22–1), and that quality is knowable and measurable.

In its role as a management philosophy, TQM requires a change in an organization's culture and lifestyle. Top managers, and the chief executive officer in particular, are charged with the responsibility of imbuing organizational members with a shared sense of purpose aimed at creating both value for the customer and the committed involvement of organizational members.

Management must accomplish several tasks if it is to meet its responsibility. First, management must focus on the inadequacies of the work process (not of the workers) as the source of error. Second, organizational members must be trained in the techniques of TQM. By starting with training at the upper-management level, top managers can set an example and take over the training of others. Third, an infrastructure is required that gives people access to the problem-solving process, removes barriers to quality, and offers freedom from fear of reprisal.

Finally, for the TQM philosophy to suffuse the organization, top management must provide leadership. The concept of leadership is central to all of the writing on TQM.

2. TQM as a Process: The Sequence of Steps

The specific steps in the TQM process encompass

- the selection of an improvement opportunity
- the definition of a specific problem

- the identification of the problem's root cause
- the choice, testing, and implementation of a remedy

Improvement opportunities are identified as those organizational processes that are known to be unsatisfactory or to harbor potential shortcomings. Improvement opportunities can result from, among others, a search for new topics, complaints from customers, or monitoring of work processes, and nominations should be addressed to all products and processes.

While there are suggestions for different criteria for selecting among alternative improvement opportunities, the Joint Commission's steps encompass the identification of "the most important aspects" of care or service and the development of performance indicators and triggers. Many agree that it is the responsibility of the organizational leadership and experts to make the selection. Similarly, it is the responsibility of management to appoint the project team that will tackle the improvement opportunity. Upper management involvement on teams is critical because it provides leadership by example as well as exposure of top management to the work that is involved.

The "diagnostic journey" begins at the next step, the development of the problem statement. At this stage, the team attempts to understand the symptoms and agrees on the reason for the undesirable situation. The problem statement is critical for the success of the endeavor since it ensures that all team members have the same understanding of the problem. The diagnostic tools associated with TQM play an important role in this task. These tools include the use of statistical methods to compare and assess processes. (These are discussed later in this chapter and also in the book's Appendix.)

The third stage includes those functions that make a distinction between "common" and "special" causes or "false alarms" and "real changes," and identify the "root cause" whose elimination will solve the problem. As with the previous stage, collection and presentation of objective data are the basis for this function.

Finally, the "remedial journey" involves the testing and selection of a solution, followed by

---

Source: Margarete Arndt and Barbara Bigelow, "The Implementation of Total Quality Management in Hospitals: How Good Is the Fit?" *Health Care Management Review*, Vol. 20, No. 4, Aspen Publishers, Inc., © Fall 1995.

Table 22–1 Customers and Suppliers Concept

The definitions here include the customers and suppliers that exist *within*, as well as *outside*, the organization (i.e., internal and external).

- *Customers* are the people or organizations who receive the product, service, or outcome.
- *Suppliers* are the people or organizations who contribute to the process, who share in performing the set of tasks that results in a product, service, or outcome.
- Every customer and supplier relationship should be viewed as reciprocal. For example:
  –External customers of the health care facility—patients, insurance carriers, and other third-party payers—purchase the health care services of the facility, thereby being both the customers of the institution and suppliers (financial).

–Within the health care facility setting, each health care professional/employee is both a supplier and a customer of other health care workers. Physicians write orders for the care of patients. Nursing staff, the supplier of care at the next level, responsibly carries out the orders they receive from their suppliers (physicians) to meet the objectives of the patient's care while making the experience as pleasant as possible for the patient/customer. Both nurses and physicians receive feedback from patients about each patient's condition, thus becoming customers of these patients.

- Difficulty in identifying the customer usually indicates a need to define precisely the process being studied.

Source: Adapted from Chapter 2 of *The Team Handbook: How To Use Teams To Improve Quality,* © 1988 Joiner Associates Inc. All rights reserved. Used with permission of the authors. For more information about *The Team Handbook*, please call Joiner Associates, Inc., at 1-800-669-8326.

---

monitoring for subsequent process control. The selection of corrective action provides closure to the process.

Distinguishing between QI and QA*

Quality improvement (QI) builds on the strengths of quality assurance (QA) and to many is the next logical step. Quality assurance refers to the internal and external methods of assessing the incidence and levels of quality problems and attempts to ensure that the problem is contained or resolved. QA methods have evolved over the years from implicit peer review to medical audits to monitoring and evaluation.

The health care facility conducts reviews based on definite criteria and reviews based on specific incidents. The orientation is to look for the "bad apples." This mode of inspection rarely motivates anyone to study systematically how to improve the quality of the entire group or process or "product." Most QA staff time is spent

meeting minimum external requirements. Thus, it can be said that quality assurance is motivated by external requirements, focusing on the "bad apple," and fosters a department-oriented approach to quality.

In contrast, quality improvement focuses on finding the root cause, and the importance of a cross-functional and multidisciplinary approach to process improvement. TQM recognizes that the entire organization must be committed to improvement (see Table 22–2). In essence, quality improvement involves a major cultural change in organization, plus management commitment and involvement, employee participation, and the use of scientific tools.

Supporting Quality Management with Information*

Quality management data are data generated and used internally by the organization to measure, analyze, and improve performance.

Source: Adapted from *Quality in Health Care: Theory, Application, and Evolution,* Nancy O. Graham, ed., Aspen Publishers, Inc., © 1995.

Source: Patrice L. Spath, "The Interface of Quality Management and the Hospital Information Department," *Topics in Health Information Management,* Vol. 13, No. 3, Aspen Publishers, Inc., © February 1993.

Table 22–2 The Components of TQM/CQI

Attitude +	*Method* +	*Tools* = *TQM/CQI*
Prevention versus detection	Process improvement	Flowchart
Customer centrality	Systems approach	Run chart
Do things right the first time	Team and teamwork	Scatter diagram
Top commitment	Decrease variation	Cause and effect
Empowerment		Pareto
		Histogram
		Control chart

Attitude + Method + Tools = TQM/CQI

The design of systems should support the activities of the quality management function by providing for the collection of data to assist in:

- monitoring customer expectations and satisfaction, processes and outcomes of care, and their variations
- evaluating the need for improvement and using the results for process improvement
- comparing the organization's performance with internal past performance, with that of other organizations, and with information from the literature
- evaluating the appropriateness of various technologies
- evaluating the costs of various technologies
- analyzing resource utilization for patients with particular clinical problems to enhance cost-effectiveness of care
- enhancing workflow activity
- supporting clinical and administrative decision making

The information management function should collect "performance indicators that can be used to maximize achievable clinical and operational benefits." A component of data capture is the development of minimum data sets, data definitions, codes, classifications, and terminology that are standardized within the organization and with other organizations. The function of data analysis and transformation into information includes the use of measurement instruments, statistical tools, and data analysis methods to provide for accurate, reliable, valid, and interpretable infor-

mation for quality management purposes. The desired attributes of quality management data are shown in Table 22–3.

QUALITY IMPROVEMENT PROJECT CONCEPT

A *quality improvement project* is a structured team effort to either address a problem, respond to an opportunity, or design a new process. The project is typically conducted by a multidisciplinary team, using the concepts of modern quality management and employing a set of simple process- and data-analysis tools. A quality improvement project (QIP) also typically follows a well-defined road map, called a "quality improvement project model," that everyone on the project team (and perhaps everyone in the organization) agrees to use as a unifying framework to guide the effort. While there are many, seemingly different, models to choose from, it turns out that all effective QIP models share a common conceptual and theoretical basis, an understanding of which enables one to work with and learn from these different models.*

Basic Concepts*

The elements of this common conceptual framework combine the principles that are the

Source: Adapted from Paul E. Plsek, "Tutorial: Quality Improvement Project Models," *Quality Management in Health Care*, Vol. 1, No. 2, Aspen Publishers, Inc., © Winter 1993.

Table 22–3 Objectives for Quality Management Data

- *Accurate:* Quality management data correctly describe the process or patient outcome that is being measured.
- *Complete:* Quality management data include all the patient and system characteristics necessary for analysis of the measurement result.
- *Reliable:* Quality management data are reproducible if the same information will be obtained when data are collected by others.
- *Valid:* Quality management data are a faithful descriptor of the processes or outcomes that are being measured.
- *Timely:* Quality management data are collected and reported as close to the time of the care or service episode as possible.
- *Usable:* Quality management data are presented in language and formats that allow for interpretation, analysis, and decision making.
- *Uniformly defined:* Quality management data element definitions have been standardized within the organization and are consistent with industrywide definitions, as appropriate.
- *Comparable:* Quality management data from individual institutions are evaluated, whenever possible, using relevant reference databases, research and literature sources, and other benchmarking opportunities.
- *Secure:* Quality management data are maintained in a manner to ensure the confidentiality of patient-specific information.
- *Procurable:* Quality management data can be easily obtained from direct communication with providers, patients, records, and other sources.

---

foundation of quality management and the basic principles for an effective project undertaking. A summary of these appears in Table 22–4. These concepts and their role in shaping an effective quality improvement project model are described below.

1. Principles of Quality Management

Effective quality improvement project models reflect the basic values and principles that underlie all of quality management science. The summary below presents these principles in generic language and describes how each should be reflected in an effective quality improvement project model.

Processes. All work involves the execution of processes. A process is a sequence of steps in which something is passed along and modified, producing some eventual output. The "something passed along" might be a patient (the admissions process), information (the lab results reporting process), materials (the process for stocking exam rooms), or thought (the process for clinical or administrative decision making). An ef-

---

Table 22–4 Key Concepts in Quality Improvement Project Models

Principles of Quality Management	Principles of Projects
<ul><li>Processes</li><li>Customers</li><li>Variation</li><li>Continuous improvement</li><li>Prevention</li><li>Scientific method (plan-do-check-act cycle)</li><li>Positive view of people</li><li>Leadership</li></ul>	<ul><li>Universal sequence of breakthroughs</li><li>Four phases of improvement</li><li>Pareto principle</li><li>Convergent/divergent thinking cycle</li><li>Creative/empirical thinking cycle</li></ul>

fective quality improvement project model guides the team to define explicitly the process under study and to identify and eliminate waste and unnecessary complexity in that process.

- *Customers.* Processes exist to produce outputs and services that provide a benefit to, or meet the needs of, someone. In quality management theory, these beneficiaries are called "customers." These customers can be external to the organization (e.g., the patient is the customer of the medication delivery process, and the payer is the customer of the billing process) or internal (e.g., the nurse who must administer the medication is also a customer of the medication delivery process, and the senior administrator who reviews accounts receivable reports is also a customer of the billing process). If a process does not produce a benefit or meet a need for someone, it is pointless and should not exist. It follows, therefore, that if an organization is going to carry out a process, then it should seek to provide the greatest benefit to the customers of that process. A good quality improvement project model encourages such "customer thinking" within the team.

- *Variation.* The outcomes of processes are naturally variable. For example, patients will not have exactly the same response to a given therapy, the time required to process a purchase order will not be precisely the same for all orders, and so forth. This variation in outcome is due to both the intended and unintended variation in the people, machines, materials, methods, and measurements that make up the process. An effective quality improvement project model guides the team to a deep and thorough understanding of this variation and all of its potential sources.

- *Continuous Improvement.* Organizations that implement modern quality management are seeking to push the performance of their processes beyond existing standards and industry norms. The goal is to achieve and maintain a never-before-achieved level of performance. This is typically accomplished through a series of incremental improvements. A good quality improvement project model should facilitate such continuous, iterative, incremental improvements by encouraging alternating cycles of change,

followed by stability, followed by more change, and so on.

- *Prevention.* A process is not fundamentally improved when steps are simply added to check for and screen out errors and problems after they occur. This only makes the process more complex, while leaving intact the underlying causes of inefficiency, waste, and dissatisfaction. An effective quality improvement project model will encourage a project team to find the root causes of problems and develop processes that prevent error, waste, and customer dissatisfaction from occurring again.

- *Scientific Method or the Plan-Do-Check-Act Cycle.* Fundamental to quality management is the commitment to using data and a logical process to build knowledge and make decisions. One popular adaptation of the scientific method, called the plan-do-check-act (PDCA) cycle,[1] is useful in quality improvement. It is suggested that knowledge can be systematically built by *planning* a change, *doing* it, *checking* to see its effect, and then *acting* on what is learned by either rejecting the change or making it a standard part of the process (see Table 22–5). The concept of systematically building knowledge through disciplined data collection and deliberate experimentation lies at the foundation of all effective quality improvement project models. During the course of a project, a team typically conducts multiple iterations of the PDCA cycle in building knowledge about the process and the actions necessary to improve it. The quality improvement project model should guide the team and remind the members about the importance of this disciplined and deliberate study.

- *Positive View of People.* Quality management theorists view the people who work in the process as the ultimate source of knowledge about how to improve it. The quality improvement project model should remind the organization and the project team about the importance of constructively involving the people who actually do the work in activities designed to improve that work.

---

[1]W.A. Shewhart, *Economic Control of Quality of Manufactured Product* (New York: Van Nostrand, 1987).

Table 22–5 FOCUS-PDCA

Find a process improvement opportunity.
Organize a team that understands the process.
Clarify the current knowledge of the process.
Uncover the root cause of variation and poor quality.
Start the "plan-do-check-act" cycle.

Plan the process improvement.
Do the improvement, data collection, and analysis.
Check the results and lessons learned.
Act by adopting, adjusting, or abandoning the change.

Source: Courtesy of Columbia/HCA Healthcare Corporation, 1992, Nashville, Tennessee.

Table 22–6 Process Design Project Model

Project Definition and Organization

- List and prioritize problems.
- Define project and team.

Conceptual Design

- Clarify customers and purpose.
- Develop process flows.
- Perform customer needs analysis.

Problem Prevention

- Consider potential problems.
- Consider potential causes.
- Develop prevention.
- Design control system.
- Implement new process.

Holding the Gains

- Check performance.
- Monitor control system.

Source: Reprinted with permission from Paul E. Plsek & Associates, Inc., 1005 Allenbrook Lane, Roswell, GA 30075. © 1989.

- *Leadership.* The need for effective leadership is a central theme in quality management theory. Without strong, effective leadership and an infrastructure to support quality management, improvement efforts may not happen or, if they do happen, may quickly dissipate because of neglect and lack of integration with other activities in the organization. The mere presence of an agreed-upon model supports this leadership principle because it provides a predictable path for improvement efforts. This path gives leaders the opportunity to become involved through initiation, review, and coaching of improvement efforts.

2. Principles of Projects

Quality improvement project models go beyond the general principles of quality management and incorporate other key concepts that address the different points of view and ways of thinking present in complex organizations. These additional principles are described below.

- *Universal Sequence of Breakthroughs.* Underlying all effective quality improvement project models is Juran's "universal sequence of breakthroughs." (Table 22–6.) First, Juran suggests that there must be a *breakthrough in attitude.* Here,

the team and the organization challenge the historical standard of performance and come to believe that there is both a need and a means to do better. Next, there is the need for a *breakthrough in organization.* Since most significant processes and problems involve multiple functions and departments within an institution, a representative quality improvement team must be created to provide a thorough understanding and analysis of the process. Achieving a new level of performance in a process also often requires a *breakthrough in knowledge.* Here, the team reaches new plateaus in its knowledge of how the process operates and what causes poor performance. Then, because the people who work in the process are accustomed to the historical level of performance and the traditional ways of doing things, Juran suggests the need for a *breakthrough in cultural patterns.* This involves such things as dealing with resistance to change and providing training in new methods. Finally, the changes need to be implemented and a *break-*

through in results verified. This includes setting up measurement systems to monitor and sustain the new level of performance.

• *Phases of Improvement.* The first phase of an improvement effort involves *identification and selection of improvement opportunities.* Most organizations can come up with a long list of problems and improvement opportunities based on consideration of customer feedback, imperfect outcomes, high costs, poor utilization, or waste in processes. But, in order to make effective use of the organization's limited improvement resources, a leadership group should take initial steps to set priorities among these opportunities, gather and publish data to show proof of the need for improvement and to stimulate breakthroughs in attitude, and establish a project team to generate a breakthrough in organization. Quality improvement project models typically reflect this early phase of activity through the use of key words like *focus, define, clarify, organize, charter*, and so forth, in the initial steps of the model.

Following this is the second phase of the project effort: *determination of the causes of the problem or barriers to improvement.* In this phase, breakthroughs in knowledge lead to identification of the underlying causes of poor process performance, or the conceptual barriers that stand in the way of realizing an improvement opportunity. The analysis work is done by the improvement team and typically involves repeated cycles of the scientific method or PDCA cycle (described above). Quality improvement project models typically use key words like *diagnose, analyze, understand, root cause, key factors*, and so forth, to describe activities in this phase of the effort.

Having identified the underlying causes or barriers, the team can now enter the third phase of the effort: *development and implementation of improvements.* Here, the team works together with the responsible departments and individuals to develop appropriate process changes, implement those changes, and achieve breakthroughs in cultural patterns. Effective project models use key words and phrases like *design, remedy, process change, countermeasure*, and so forth, to describe this third phase of the effort.

In the final phase of a quality improvement project, *establishment of ongoing control*, the operating departments and the quality improvement team collect and analyze data on the performance of the new process and confirm a breakthrough in results. The operating departments then continue to monitor the new control system in order to maintain the breakthrough in performance. The quality improvement project model might use words and phrases like *check, measure, monitor, stabilize, hold the gains, institutionalize*, and so forth, to indicate what needs to be done in this final phase of the improvement effort.

• *Pareto Principle.* The Pareto principle states that in any group of items that contribute to an effect, a relative few of the contributors will account for the majority of the effect. The key point here is that by isolating and focusing on these so-called vital few factors, a team or organization can make maximal use of its limited improvement resources. An effective quality improvement project model should, therefore, guide the team and the organization to identify and focus on the vital few problems, opportunities, customers, processes, causes, barriers, changes, and control variables.

• *The Divergent/Convergent Thinking Cycle.* The divergent/convergent thinking cycle refers to the cycle of first expanding the team's thinking (divergent thinking) and then narrowing it to a focus (convergent thinking). A quality improvement team might list various theories of cause in order to expand its knowledge and understanding of the problem. But following this, team members need to converge and focus their efforts on the major root causes.

Effective problem-solving teams are keenly aware of the need to balance between divergent and convergent thinking. They recognize the need to focus their attention and energies in order to move on after broad discussion of general facts and opinions. But they also recognize the need to spend time answering the "what else?" question before devoting their attention to a specific course of action. Therefore, an effective quality improvement project model should contain some steps that direct the team into divergent thinking

Table 22–7 Cut-the-Jargon Questions

Understanding the fundamental concepts behind the various quality improvement project models helps quality management practitioners to cut through the jargon and learn from the improvement projects of others, regardless of the model used. So, when reading a case study, hearing a conference presentation, or discussing efforts with colleagues in other organizations, concentrate on learning the answers to questions such as those listed below.

- How were customers and their needs identified and addressed?
- What did the team learn about the process?
- What key sources of variation did the team identify?
- What incremental improvements were made?
- What future improvement efforts are planned?
- What data did the team use in its decision making?

- How were both staff and leadership involved?
- How did the team use the scientific method to build knowledge?
- How did the team stay focused on the "vital few"?
- How were breakthroughs accomplished?
- Who was on the team?
- How did the team break through the prevailing attitude and cultural patterns?
- What results did the team achieve?
- What steps did the team undertake in analyzing the process?
- How did the team go about generating creative, effective, and acceptable recommendations?
- How did the team implement its recommendations?
- What ongoing monitors and controls did the team put in place?
- How did the team demonstrate and balance divergent, convergent, creative, and empirical thinking?

Source: Adapted from Paul E. Plsek, "Tutorial: Quality Improvement Project Models," *Quality Management in Health Care*, Vol. 1:2, Aspen Publishers, Inc., © Winter 1993.

---

and some steps that direct them into convergent thinking.

- *The Creative/Empirical Thinking Cycle.* A second, related thought cycle is that between creative and empirical thinking. This also is fundamental to an effective quality improvement project model. There are points during problem solving when the team needs hunches, guesses, and opinions. Creative (or intuition-driven) thinking is needed when listing problems, theories of cause, possible solutions, and potential barriers to change. But there is an equally important need to rely solely on the facts at other points in the improvement effort. Such empirical (or data-driven) thinking is mandatory when prioritizing problems, analyzing symptoms, testing theories of cause, checking performance, and monitoring the control system. As with divergent/convergent thinking, effective project teams are also keenly aware of the need to balance between creative and empirical thinking.

INSTITUTING TOTAL QUALITY MANAGEMENT: TRANSITIONS, TEAMS, AND TOOLS

Transitional Stages and Challenges*

The process of TQM adoption faces significant challenges at various stages that involve units of the organization and the organization as a whole, particularly regarding design issues related to the transitions that management must make.

TQM adoption requires multiple decisions and actions over time, involving various individuals and work units within the organization. Figure 22–1 presents the three stages of the basic

---

*Source: Arnold D. Kaluzny and Curtis P. McLaughlin, "Managing Transitions: Assuring the Adoption and Impact of TQM," © Quality Review Bulletin. Oakbrook Terrace, IL: Joint Commission on Accreditation of Healthcare Organizations, 1992. Reprinted with permission.

Figure 22–1 The TQM Adoption Process

The following presents the basic sequence in the adoption of total quality management. Each stage presents three challenges. If the last challenges are not successfully met, the process will have led to the institutionalization of TQM.

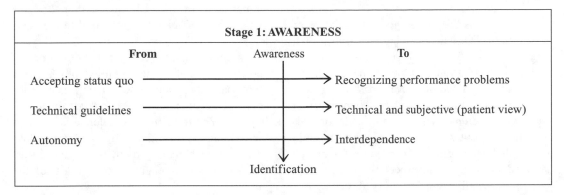

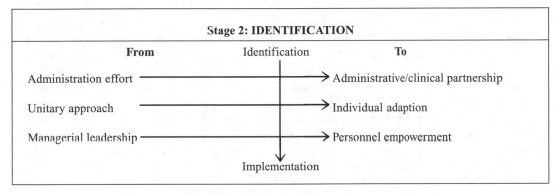

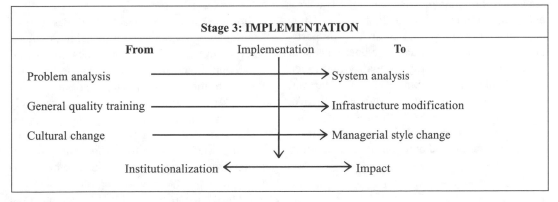

process: awareness of a problem, identification of a solution, and implementation.

Institutionalization and impact—the two end points—are highly interdependent. Impact is the difference that TQM makes in organizational or work group performance; institutionalization is the extent to which TQM is integrated into ongoing activities of the organization. Following are the stages of the process along with specific transition challenges that management faces during each stage.

Awareness

Awareness is the first stage in the process of adoption of TQM and includes three transitional challenges (see stage 1 in Figure 22–1). The first is the identification of a performance gap in which the organization moves from the acceptance of the status quo to the recognition that there is a discrepancy between how the organization is currently performing and how it could or should be performing. This awareness may be sparked internally by the expectations of employees or externally by community or regulatory pressures.

A second challenge occurs when management realizes that the existing definition of *quality* is no longer appropriate or adequate. The transition involves a shift from a technical definition of quality to the recognition that effective care requires a subjective as well as technical evaluation. Specifically, a definition of health care quality is inadequate if it does not include the customer.

A third challenge involves the transition from an emphasis on the autonomy of the provider to the recognition of interdependence of all personnel involved in providing quality of care. Thus, it is no longer appropriate to artificially partition issues of cost and quality, relegating cost to management and quality to quality assurance professionals. Instead, clinical care must be seen as a network of deep interdependencies involving other professionals, nonprofessional staff, information systems, policies and procedures, physical systems, and other influences affecting clinical care.

Identification

The second stage of the adoption process is the recognition that TQM is the appropriate solution to the performance problem. This awareness may come through passive activities such as quality seminars or more painful realizations such as the superior performance of competing

institutions. Several transition challenges are presented in stage 2 of Figure 22–1. Take, for example, the transition from strong managerial leadership to employee initiatives within the organization. Management must ask, and personnel have to be made aware that they are empowered sufficiently to respond to the challenge.

A second transition involves the development and adaptation of a guiding philosophy. TQM is more than a program of activities; it is a philosophical perspective about how organizations function. The transitional challenge is to adapt the approach to the organization and its employees. Moreover, management must give different work unit supervisors ownership of the initiative.

The transition challenge comes when TQM moves from being solely an administrative activity to one that involves administrative and clinical quality issues. Experience suggests that the process is highly idiosyncratic and that it involves a continuous transition depending on the readiness of these various groups. Most likely, the transition begins with focusing predominantly on administrative activities and moves incrementally to clinical issues.

Implementation

Implementation refers to the presence of TQM activity within the organization or among relevant groups within the organization. Institutionalization and impact occur, however, when these activities are truly integrated into the operations of the organization and substantively affect performance.

As presented in stage 3 of Figure 22–1, the transitional challenges focus on ensuring institutionalization and impact within the organization. A critical challenge is the transition from a voluntary, participatory, problem-oriented initial phase to one that focuses on major opportunities for change, requiring greater probabilities for conflict, and that is driven by external competitive forces, requiring a sense of competitive urgency. Employees must shift from targets of interest such as scheduling problems or equipment shortages to a systematic assessment of the

Figure 22–2 QI Structure Using a Team Quality Approach

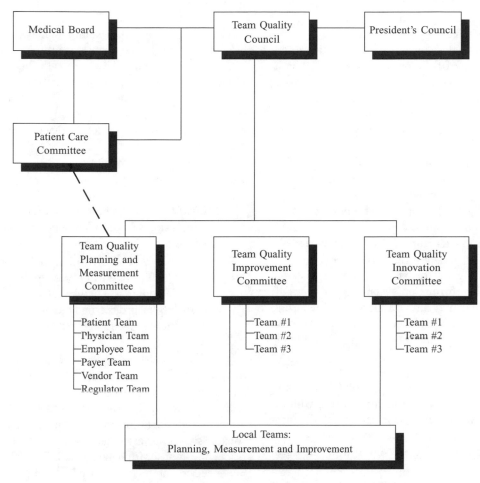

Source: Venetia Kudrle, "Making Payors Part of the Total Quality Management," *Managed Care Quarterly*, Vol. 1, No. 2, Aspen Publishers, Inc., © Spring 1993.

key success factors that would ensure organizational survival. The transition, however, must evolve over time. For example, although significant payoff to health care quality could be achieved through multidisciplinary efforts that focus on the total system delivering care to the patient with special attention on integrating the work of various components involved in the overall system, any attempt to deal with a problem of this size and scope would clearly overwhelm even the most enthusiastic group attempting to apply TQM. Experience suggests that it is easier to implement TQM within a more limited work group and methodically expand to systemwide problems.

Management must thus be prepared to guide the transitions from a focus on work units to more complex multidisciplinary issues as employees gain confidence and experience.

Another critical transition is training and mentoring to ensure the growth and development of work groups. This requires that a series of compromises be made to facilitate training and confidence building. The challenge is to manage the training program to meet the needs of various groups as they move through the adoption process. Management must ensure that work groups and various ad hoc groups are receiving the necessary skills and receiving "just-in-time" support to improve overall group effectiveness.

A final challenge involves a transition in the infrastructure of the organization as well as in cognitive structure at the level of top management. Given the complexity of TQM, as well as the adopting organization, other changes occur in administrative systems, many of them subtle, with profound consequences for both the process and ultimate impact of TQM adoption. Perhaps most critical is the recruitment, selection, and hiring of employees, since it is through this process that the long-term institutionalization of TQM can be ensured.

Other infrastructure challenges include modifications in job descriptions, reward systems, and existing performance appraisal systems. Moreover, information systems must be modified to focus not only on the vertical reporting relationships, but also on getting information to work laterally among groups within the organization.

The role of existing quality assurance personnel will also have to be redefined. Health care organizations are experimenting with alternative approaches, with some facilities retaining quality assurance as an independent activity but adopting TQM to deal with clinical issues. Other organizations have merged quality assurance into a larger quality management function. Finally, institutionalization and impact cannot be successful unless top management realizes that what is required is not the simple manipulation of a cultural change within the organization, but a fundamental change in management style. Specifically, managers must "walk the talk"; that is, they must change the way they use facts, delegate decisions, respond to recommendations, and view people. Consultants report that it is at this juncture that managers either provide true leadership or simply become part of the problem. This realization will facilitate the institutionalization of TQM and prevent the "solution of the month" syndrome that has characterized so much of management in general and health services management in particular.

Stages and Roles in the Formation of a QI Team*

The quality council, a senior management project sponsor, a team leader, team members, and a facilitator all play key roles in the success of the team. A team development model can be used as a framework to aid in identifying the role each of these groups plays in assisting the team with the critical tasks to be accomplished at each developmental stage.

Stage 1: Forming

- *Critical tasks:* team process—introduction and inclusion of team members, including the reason for their selection
- *Project/tool use:* clarification and understanding of the opportunity statement or charter, including why it was selected, general goal of the project, and the process improvement approach to be used

The *quality council* must be sure that improvement opportunities or projects are selected or approved with care. Projects should be aligned with core systems or processes, related to customer requirements, informed by data, given reasonable scope, and assigned an appropriate team leader and sponsor from the council. Team members need to commit to contribute their process expertise, accept the team leader and other team members, and ask questions to clarify the improvement opportunity, the approach to be used, and the composition of the team.

The key tasks of the *team leader* in this stage are planning with the facilitator and perhaps a quality council representative for the first meetings of the team; getting team members introduced (with an appropriate ice breaker or warm-up exercise); orienting the team to the improvement opportunity, the structure/format for meetings, and the process improvement model

*Source: Adapted from Doug Mosel and M. Johanna Shamp, "Enhancing Quality Improvement Team Effectiveness," *Quality Management in Health Care*, Vol. 1, No. 2, Aspen Publishers, Inc., © Winter 1993.

to be used; and helping the team with initial organization, such as ground rules, project timeline, and meeting time, length, and frequency.

The *facilitator*'s primary role is to assist the team leader with planning for the first meeting(s) of the team. This can include preliminary work on the road map/timeline and storyboard that will help the team leader and team as needed to include all team members, to develop ground rules, and to provide any just-in-time teaching that may be required.

Stage 2: Storming

- *Critical tasks:* team process—identifying and accepting different ways of thinking and learning
- *Project/tool use:* clarifying roles of members and agreeing on or clarifying the process improvement model and the meeting structures as methods of operating

The quality council must be sure that a project sponsor or "champion" is available to answer any questions during important meetings of the team. Team members should assist the team by listening to information provided by other members, suspending judgment as necessary. They share their own knowledge of the process and actively support the process improvement and team meeting methods.

The team leader's role in this stage is to lead discussion related to the opportunity statement; team member roles; the process improvement model; and team meeting format, timeline, or ground rules. The expression of feelings or opinions should be encouraged and assistance provided with consensus on key decisions.

The facilitator plans with the team leader for the management of any expected conflict; helps the leader and the team if they get stuck in conflict; and provides any necessary clarification or teaching on process improvement, team dynamics, or meeting methods and roles.

Stage 3: Norming

- *Critical tasks:* team process—the establishment of formal and informal team norms

related to interpersonal behavior, such as conflict management, respect, and shared responsibility
- *Project/tool use:* clarification and information sharing on key questions about the process being studied and methods being used

The quality council's role during this stage is to provide continuing support of the team as it works out its own norms and style. Team members need to continue active participation and support of other members, while avoiding groupthink in the form of unexamined ideas or hasty decisions. They should pay attention to the team's agenda in order to balance attention to the team and the project.

Here the team leader's tasks include leading the discussion of the team's dynamics in order to foster shared responsibilities for teamwork, perhaps initiating the completion of unfinished work on ground rules or norms, and, if necessary, refocusing the team on the agenda without squelching interpersonal caring.

The facilitator must plan with the team leader for the management of the team's dynamics, such as balancing participation, providing teaching and/or feedback to the leader and the team in relation to group dynamics, and supporting the leader in keeping the team's attention balanced.

Stage 4: Performing

- *Critical tasks:* team process—achieving functional interdependence and sharing leadership
- *Project/tool use:* effectively using the process improvement model, the related tools, and the meeting process, and ultimate completion of the project

At this important time in the team's development, the quality council's task is to review the team's progress at key points, such as when flow charting is complete, when root causes or key variables have been isolated through data collection, or when an improvement has been selected and a pilot plan developed. The special responsibility of the project sponsor is to assist the team in preparing for its review.

Team members must continue to contribute their process expertise and to accept that of other members, while insisting on data rather than opinions in the analysis of the process. The key roles of the team leader are to create opportunities for team members to begin sharing leadership by reducing the level of direction provided and by recognizing the contributions and leadership of others; to assist the team with the use of quality improvement tools; and to support the ongoing improvement of the team process.

The facilitator helps the team leader plan for turning more leadership over to the team and supports that leadership by recognizing the effectiveness of the leader and members when the team evaluates meetings. The facilitator also continues to assist as needed with the use of the process improvement model, the quality improvement tools, and meeting methods and advises the team as they prepare for review sessions.

Special Stage: Closing

- *Critical tasks:* team process—celebration or grieving and closure
- *Project/tool use:* establish and document evidence of outcomes and of lessons learned

The role of the quality council is to provide for a supportive final review of the project, with a focus on lessons learned as well as outcomes of the project. Team members help with this unique stage by accepting feelings of regret if there is reluctance to end the project, or of grief that may occur if the project has not been successfully concluded. They also must work together to plan for how to communicate lessons learned to the quality council and to others to enhance organizational learning.

The tasks of the team leader are to assist team members in dealing with feelings related to closing; help with identification of lessons learned; assist with planning for how gains can continue to be known to the team after it has disbanded; and structure or support the celebration of the team's work, regardless of outcome.

The facilitator's role is to help the leader and the team identify lessons learned and plan for how they will be communicated, provide special support for the team if the project has not resulted in the desired outcome, and help with the planning for celebration and closure.

Measurement Tools*

Measurement is a central element of any CQI effort. Health care institutions are full of data, but they are also full of "factoids"—opinions and anecdotes masquerading as facts. Adopting a scientific approach requires using data to evaluate the current situation, analyze and improve processes, and track progress. The methods used to analyze data include both those originally developed for industrial models of quality management and those developed in the specialties of biostatistics, economics, epidemiology, and health services research. They provide information on the consistency (or lack thereof) of the current process, point out sources of errors and variation, and indicate where improvements can be made most effectively.

There is no *one* specified point in the process of implementing CQI where one method of measurement and analysis should be used on a continuous basis. Different tools will be more helpful at different stages of each improvement project, from the initial analysis to the monitoring of changes that have already been instituted. It is essential to know what each statistical tool reveals about the process being improved, when to use it, and how to use it.

Tools of Data Analysis and How To Use Them for QI

The most popular tools used in QI process analysis are a set of data analysis tools seen as basic to the application of the approach. They include flowcharts or diagrams, cause-and-effect diagrams, checksheets, Pareto diagrams/charts, frequency distributions (histograms), run charts,

---

*Source: Susan Paul Johnson and Curtis P. McLaughlin, "Measurement and Statistical Analysis in CQI," in *Continuous Quality Improvement in Health Care*, Curtis P. McLaughlin and Arnold D. Kaluzny, eds., Aspen Publishers, Inc., © 1994.

regression analyses, and control charts. Although any pair of writers usually agree on at least six of the seven, eight items are commonly included in this famous set. The eight statistical methods are shown in Table 22–8 in relation to the QI stage at which they are most commonly used. (Brief descriptors and pictorial displays are available in the Appendix.)

MONITORING AND ASSESSING QUALITY CARE

The Measurement of Quality*

Three issues affect the current concepts of measuring quality.

First, *scientific methods of measurement* are increasingly necessary. Evaluation requires sound methods in order for the resulting data to be sound. Further, data from evaluations are being used to create significant change within organizations, so faulty data based on inaccurate measurement methods carry a great risk.

The *return to outcome measures* has been fostered by many outside of the care delivery setting. Consumers and third-party payers of health care are increasingly asking what outcomes they can expect from care received and money paid. The Agency for Health Care Policy and Research (AHCPR) is investigating and defining outcome measures of quality health care. In addition, research on patient outcomes is being carried out, and clinical practice guidelines are being developed by expert multidisciplinary teams. Further, the Joint Commission has moved boldly into the outcome arena, requiring that patient outcome indicators be used for monitoring and evaluating activities. It is developing outcome indicator sets for which mandatory data collection will eventually be necessary. The resulting data are to be used internally within the health care setting, by the Joint Commission on its periodic surveys, and for the development of a national database.

The third issue changing quality programs is the *shift to a quality improvement (QI) philosophy*. QI embodies the message that quality will not be improved simply as a result of inspection. It must be built into the people and the processes carrying out the work of the organization. QI uses workers at the point of service to define quality, measure its achievement, and create innovations to constantly improve. A QI program requires active involvement of all within the organization, from the mailroom to the boardroom. Visible, supportive leadership is essential.

Directions for Monitoring Quality*

The systematic review and evaluation of standards of care and practice will take place in an environment of multidisciplinary collaboration and with an emphasis on clinical research that will link nursing practice to patient outcomes.

Determination of the focal point for quality-related activities will be the caregiver–care receiver encounter and a results-oriented evaluation of patient outcomes. The purpose set forth by the Joint Commission is to foster an internalization of commitment to quality within the organization through an ongoing monitoring and feedback system. The institution will oversee the integration of quality control into every aspect of organizational life and will measure the quality of the practitioner by the quality of patient outcomes.

Standards of care and practice will be measured by generic, predetermined clinical indicators shared among all similar health care organizations. The indicators will not be the only determinants of quality, but they will serve as triggers for review and corrective action. The focus for institution-specific efforts to determine quality will continue to be on the development of indicators that address high-risk, high-volume, and problematic issues.

Source: Patricia Schroeder, "Improving Health Care Quality in the Nineties," in *The Encyclopedia of Nursing Care Quality Volume I: Issues and Strategies for Nursing Care Quality*, Patricia Schroeder, ed., Aspen Publishers, Inc., © 1991.

Source: Mary Ellen Connington and Pamela Dupuis, *Unit-Based Nursing Quality Assurance: A Patient-Centered Approach*, Aspen Publishers, Inc., © 1990.

Table 22–8 CQI Process Stages and Quality Tools

	CQI Process Stages			
Tools	1. Describe process and identify sources of variation	2. Do in-depth analyses to clarify knowledge and present interim findings	3. Weigh alternatives and make choices	4. Measure improvements and monitor progress
Flow diagrams	Key tool here	Revisit and update		Keep current
Cause-and-effect diagrams	Key tool here, especially after brainstorming	Stratify for detail		
Checksheets		Use to collect process data		Use to collect process data
Pareto diagrams or charts		Key tool here to stratify causes	Key to deciding on vital few	Use to show change
Frequency distributions (histograms)		Helpful in presentation		Helpful in monitoring
Run charts		Important to relate data temporally to changes		Key to knowing whether improvement has been associated with change
Regression analysis			Useful for testing hypotheses	
Control charts				Key to seeing whether the process is or remains under control

---

Demonstration

As an example, suppose a team selects the admission process for the area of inquiry. A flowchart graphically portrays the process of patient flow. Through a fishbone diagram, the group identifies delays in patients' departures from the admitting area as a possible cause of delays in the admission process. To proceed with their analysis, the team requires additional information on the delay time attributable to several steps of the process. For one week, staff in different parts of the organization record the time required by their step in the process for each patient. The greatest time delays are found to be related to transporter availability. The solution, achieved following some additional analysis by a team of transporters, is initiation of a silent beeper system for the transporters.

Source: Joann Genovich-Richards, "Selecting Topics and Methodologies," in *Improving Quality: A Guide to Effective Programs*, Claire G. Meisenheimer, ed., Aspen Publishers, Inc., © 1992.

Source: Susan Paul Johnson and Curtis P. McLaughlin, "Measurement and Statistical Analysis in CQI," in *Continuous Quality Improvement in Health Care*, Curtis P. McLaughlin and Arnold D. Kaluzny, eds., Aspen Publishers, Inc., © 1994.

Interinstitutional sharing will increase, making use of aggregate databases and standardized collection modes. Thresholds of evaluation established in the past on the basis of a single organization's experience will be enhanced or altered through the availability of the multi-organizational indicator database of peer group institutions. The database will be updated through the frequent and ongoing submission of institution-specific results of quality care monitoring. Therefore, evaluation will be continuous and,

---

Types of Review

Retrospective Review. Retrospective review is a critical examination of past or completed work with a view to improvement. Documentation in the patients' (medical) records is the source of data for the review.

Retrospective review has the advantages of use of data for the full continuum of care and evaluation of the results of care for a large series of comparable cases. Impressions gained by practitioners from single cases in which they are personally involved and without systematic study of quantifiable aspects are not always borne out by systematic review of a large number of cases.

Concurrent Review. Concurrent review is a critical examination of the patient's progress toward the desired alterations in health/wellness status (outcomes) and patient care management (activities) while patient care and treatment are in progress. Documentation of care in the patient's record and interview, observation, and inspection of the patient are the sources for data. Reviews required by the Social Security Amendments ask for certain preadmission, admission, and length of stay monitoring while the patient is receiving care. Concurrent review has the advantage of providing the opportunity to make corrective changes in ongoing care. It can also guide the work of the professionals.

although based on individual patient review, will address aggregate clusters of patients to focus more effectively on patterns and trends and to facilitate relevant conclusions regarding appropriateness of care, timeliness of services, efficient utilization of resources, and quality of patient outcomes.

Patient outcome standards will be the primary measure of quality and will determine the appropriateness of clinical practice. The expectation will be that the results of the ongoing monitoring of outcomes will have to be practitioner-specific in order to provide a database for the credentialing of the future. Evaluation methodology that links nursing and professional practice standards directly to patient outcome will anticipate the future in the continuing evolution of quality assurance.

Focus of Assessing Quality of Nursing Care*

To ensure quality, nursing care must be assessed in terms of outcome, content, processes, resources, and efficiency—in that order of priority.

1. Assessment of Outcome

Quality of nursing care received should principally be measured by the outcome of that care. The assessment of outcome focuses on the alteration in the health status of the consumer. Positive indices that can be used in assessing the alteration in the consumer's health status include the following:

- an increase in the consumer's health knowledge
- the degree of application of that knowledge
- the degree of the consumer's participation in his or her health decision making
- the degree of responsibility that the consumer assumes for his or her health behavior

---

*Source: Wisconsin Regional Medical Board, "Assessing Quality of Nursing Care," *Nursing Administration Quarterly*, Vol. 1, No. 3, Aspen Publishers, Inc., © 1977.

- the consumer's ability to maintain positive health behavior
- the degree to which the consumer's right to choices that affect his or her health are ensured
- the consumer's ability to use health services, both personal and community, with efficiency and economy
- the consumer's ability to function in work and personal roles
- longevity

Assessment of the outcome of nursing care also seeks to account for negative outcomes for the consumer of health services that may be attributed wholly or in part to nursing intervention or the lack thereof. Negative indices include the following: failure to maintain or improve patient's health status or patient's discomfort, dissatisfaction, complications, disability, unexpected prolongation of illness, or unwarranted death.

2. Assessment of Content

Second, the quality of nursing care should be assessed in terms of content. Content is the nursing care that is actually given in a specific instance. Content is assessed by the application of standards of nursing practice developed for specific nurse-consumer situations. For example, assessment of content involving a burn patient in an emergency department would differ from an assessment of content involving a coronary patient in the same setting. Similarly, assessment of content to improve the health status of a 2-year-old would differ from that for a 15-year-old.

3. Assessment of Process

Assessment of process in nursing care focuses on the nature and sequence of events in the delivery of that care. This assessment takes into consideration such aspects as the nature of the interactions among the consumer, nurse, other health care workers, and significant others; the extent to which nursing care objectives have been reached; the specific techniques or procedures used; the degree to which the consumer and significant others have been involved in the entire process; the degree of skill with which nurses have carried out the nursing care as compared with that established by clinical nurse specialists; the coordination among different components of the system and among members of the team; appropriate utilization of each of the available components of the system; and the continuity of care.

4. Assessment of Resources

Assessment of resources in nursing care focuses on the properties of the resources used to provide that care and the manner in which they are organized. Nursing care resources include staff, consultants, collaborating disciplines and services, physical structures, facilities, equipment, supplies, administrative structure, operating procedures and policies, and maintenance. A climate conducive to providing quality nursing care is a prime resource. Resources should be evaluated in terms of their accessibility, availability, appropriateness, and acceptability.

5. Assessment of Efficiency

Efficiency is the attainment of quality nursing care reviewed in relationship to the personnel, supply, equipment, space, and other resources of the provider and the appropriateness, acceptability, and cost to the consumer. Efficiency is frequently referred to as the cost benefit ratio. It is concerned with determining whether there is a less costly way to achieve the same quality nursing care.

Consumers must be ensured an equivalent standard of quality nursing practice in any care setting. It is the responsibility of practitioners to develop concordant standards of practice within the specific practice setting. (See Table 22–9.)

Assessment Monitors: The Clinical Indicator

Defining, understanding, and quantifying appropriate clinical indicators in nursing are critical to the comprehensive effectiveness of both

Table 22–9 Standard for Care: Dimensions of Performance

- *Appropriateness:* The degree to which the care/intervention provided is relevant to the patient's clinical needs, given the current state of knowledge
- *Availability:* The degree to which the appropriate care/intervention is available to meet the needs of the patient served
- *Continuity:* The degree to which the care/intervention for the patient is coordinated among practitioners, between organizations, and across time
- *Effectiveness:* The degree to which the care/intervention is provided in the correct manner, given the current state of knowledge, in order to achieve the desired/projected outcome(s) for the patient
- *Efficacy:* The degree to which the care/intervention used for the patient has been

shown to accomplish the desired/projected outcome(s)
- *Efficiency:* The ratio of the outcomes (results of care/intervention) for a patient to the resources used to deliver the care
- *Respect and caring:* The degree to which a patient, or designee, is involved in his or her own care decisions, and that those providing the services do so with sensitivity and respect for his or her needs and expectations and individual differences
- *Safety:* The degree to which the risk of an intervention and the risk in the care environment are reduced for the patient and others, including the health care provider
- *Timeliness:* The degree to which the care/intervention is provided to the patient at the time it is most beneficial or necessary

Source: © *The Measurement Mandate*. Oakbrook Terrace, IL.: Joint Commission on Accreditation of Healthcare Organizations, 1993, p. 69. Reprinted with permission.

---

unit-based and departmental quality assurance programs.

Clinical indicators are defined as a quantitative measure that can be used as a guide to monitor and evaluate the quality of important patient care and support service activities. Indicators should not be thought of as direct measures of quality, but rather as markers or barometers that can identify areas and issues that warrant closer evaluation.

Indicators should reflect and measure the structure, processes, and outcomes of nursing care. Structure indicators address the potential to deliver high-quality patient care. They evaluate structural aspects required for care, such as staffing requirements, necessary credentials, and equipment preparation or readiness. Process indicators focus on the actual manner in which care is delivered. Effectiveness, timeliness, and appropriateness of care rendered are examples of process issues. Outcome indicators assess exactly what the name implies: the end result (desirable or undesirable) of care delivered. It represents the composite of all other variables. While it is important to examine all three aspects of care

delivery, emphasis should be directed toward evaluating the outcomes of nursing care.*

*Basis for Measurements**

Indicators can be further refined and applied to nursing practice. According to the Joint Commission, there are two general types of indicators: sentinel event and rate based. A *sentinel-event indicator* identifies a grave, untoward process or outcome of care. Usually, and ideally, the incidence of this type of indicator will remain low (e.g., hospital-acquired decubitus ulcer). A *rate-based indicator* identifies patient care outcomes or processes of care that may require further assessment based on significant trending or variances from thresholds over time (e.g., percentage of patients prepared for discharge). Indicators may be expressed as either desirable or undesirable measures based on the aspect of care to be monitored.

---

*Source: Anne Dearth Williams, "Development and Application of Clinical Indicators for Nursing," *Journal of Nursing Care Quality*, Vol. 6, No. 1, Aspen Publishers, Inc., © 1991.

It is helpful to approach rate-based indicators as two more distinct types: occurrence indicators and compliance/performance indicators. *Occurrence indicators* are usually dedicated to identifying outcomes of care, while *compliance/performance indicators* are used to assess processes of care delivery. Occurrence indicators also can frequently measure the occurrence of patient complications. This is significant because a large majority of nursing activity focuses on the prevention of a wide variety of patient complications, thereby lending itself to measurement of the outcomes of the preventive nursing interventions.

*Designing Indicators**

Clinical indicators can be tailored to express almost any specialized patient process or outcome. Process and outcome indicators can be used simultaneously to evaluate any aspect of care more effectively. In fact, it is vital that indicators be as specific to the aspect of care as possible so that a thorough evaluation of nursing care can be implemented.

Quantifying indicators can be simplified when the aspect of care that is being measured is expressed in the form of a rate or ratio of events for a defined population and time frame. In other words, an indicator is measurable when a rate is used as follows:

$$\text{Outcome indicators} = \frac{\text{Number of patient care events}}{\begin{array}{c}\text{Total number of patients or total}\\ \text{number of times at risk for above}\\ \text{event (for a given period of time)}\end{array}}$$

$$\text{Process indicators} = \frac{\begin{array}{c}\text{Number of times "procedure}\\ \text{X" or "standard Y" is}\\ \text{successfully completed/}\\ \text{implemented by a nurse}\end{array}}{\begin{array}{c}\text{Total number of times}\\ \text{procedure or standards used}\\ \text{(for a given period of time)}\end{array}}$$

Indicators should also be flexible enough so that they can be revised periodically to reflect the most accurate and specific measure of the aspect of care being evaluated. Table 22–10 contains examples of specific clinical indicators.

To help ensure more valid indicator rates, several reliable data sources must be used. Consistent numerator and denominator definitions applied appropriately to credible data sources can strengthen the value of an evaluation. Specific, defined criteria must be used to assist in the measurement process of the indicator.

Data can be obtained from a combination of incident reports, direct observation and tracking on individual units, medical record reviews, unit event logs, and occurrence screening during utilization review activities.

*Triggering Evaluations: Established Control Limits?**

> Originally, a threshold was introduced as a mechanism that would trigger an intensive review of the cause(s) of variance in the monitoring and evaluation process. The threshold most often set a minimum standard as the point beyond which a tolerable allowance was acceptable.

The era of setting absolute threshold values and expecting staff members to hit the mark has passed. Currently, the trend is toward threshold parameters. Just as there is normal variance among patient parameters, there is normal variance among practitioners and systems.

Events that will always have a variance are termed *rate-based indicators* or comparative rate indicators. A control chart is an excellent way to record, track, and trend the variations of rate-based

Source: Anne Dearth Williams, "Development and Application of Clinical Indicators for Nursing," *Journal of Nursing Care Quality*, Vol. 6, No. 1, Aspen Publishers, Inc., © 1991.

Source: Eleanor Green, in "Quality Forum," *Journal of Nursing Care Quality*, Vol. 7, No. 2, Aspen Publishers, Inc., © January 1993.

Table 22–10 Examples of Clinical Indicators of Important Aspects of Care

Aspect of Care	Indicator	Indicator Type	Quantifiable Measure
Management of patients on ventilators related to (R/T) self-extubations	Occurrence of self-extubations	Outcome	No. of patients who self-extubate
			No. of patients intubated
	Compliance with standard of practice (R/T ventilator management)	Process	No. of times standard of practice (on ventilator management) is successfully followed/implemented
			No. of times standard of practice is used
Discharge education	Occurrence of well-prepared patients at discharge	Outcome	No. of patients who successfully completed discharge program
			No. of patients discharged
Discharge planning R/T continuity of care/support	Occurrence of discharged patients well prepared for community reintegration	Outcome	No. of patients referred to community support groups or resources
			No. of patients discharged
Medication administration R/T prevention of administration errors	Occurrence of medication errors	Outcome	No. of medication errors
			No. of doses dispensed
	Compliance with medication administration procedure	Process	No. of times procedure on medication administration is followed successfully
			No. of doses dispensed (no. of times procedure is used)
Patient safety R/T prevention of patient falls	Occurrence of patient falls	Outcome	No. of patient falls
			No. of patients at risk *or* no. of patient days
Management of premature infant with thermoregulatory problems R/T prevention of hypothermia	Occurrence of hypothermia events	Outcome	No. of hypothermia events
			No. of patients at risk *or* no. of patient days
	Appropriate implementation of management of thermoregulation protocol	Process	No. of times management of thermoregulation protocol is successfully followed or implemented
			No. of times protocol is used

indicators. A control chart is the tool most often used to record upper and lower control limits (parameters) and the data results. Each time data are collected and tabulated, the results are entered on the control chart at the appropriate spot with a dot. Then the dots can be connected to determine whether the trend is above or below the acceptable range set by the upper and lower parameter.

How are the upper and lower parameters established? This approach involves calculating the mean and the standard deviation of the mean for a data distribution and then setting the threshold at the mean, plus and minus one, two, or three times the standard deviation. Whether the con-trol limits are set at one, two, or three standard deviations from the mean depends on the seriousness of what is being monitored. The more critical the situation, the more narrowly the control limits should be set.

Parameters also permit a visual representation of common cause variations, which are the day-to-day ebb and flow of events in every organization. As long as data hover around the mean, the process is in statistical control.

Parameters established on a control chart also permit the immediate graphing of a special cause variation, in other words, one out of statistical control that should get immediate attention.

Chapter 23

Risk Management and Safety

NURSING'S ROLE IN RISK MANAGEMENT

The nurse manager should keep abreast of liability issues for nurses, be aware of state and federal legislation impacting nursing practice, monitor the quality of nursing care through regular reports, and keep informed of health care facility risk management issues. (See Table 23–1.) In an era of limited resources, risk management data can be extremely valuable in helping nurse administrators determine priorities and make decisions relative to resource utilization in their institutions.

The most important area of responsibility and potential liability for nurse managers is that of staff selection, orientation, and continuing education. Nurse managers are responsible for overseeing the quality of care provided by the nursing service and ensuring the competency of the nursing staff. The nursing service should have an established ongoing system for monitoring nursing licensure, nursing skills, and continuing education.

A participative approach to risk management should be fostered. This can be done by encouraging and involving nursing staff in risk management activities. Since the nursing staff are closest to the level of operations, they are most

Table 23–1 Functions of Risk Management

- Protection of financial assets of the health care facility
- Protection of human and intangible resources
- Prevention of injury to patients, visitors, employees, and property
- Loss reduction focusing on *individual* loss or on single incidents
- Loss prevention to prevent incidents by improving the quality of care through continuing and ongoing monitoring
- Review of each incident and the patterns of incidents through the application of the steps in the risk management process: risk identification, risk analysis, risk evaluation, and risk treatment

Source: Excerpted from *Hospitals,* Vol. 55, No. 11, by permission, June 1, 1981, Copyright 1981, American Hospital Publishing, Inc.

familiar with risks in the patient care delivery system. They serve as a valuable information source and can often suggest ways to prevent these risks. In addition, the chief nurse administrator should hold the administrative staff accountable for being familiar with risks in the environment through the use of risk management and quality assurance data collected by the facility. These data should be fed back to the staff nurses so that they also maintain an awareness of risks.

Programs to reduce patient risks should be developed in conjunction with the facility's risk management department. Generally, the highest risks are from slips and falls and medication errors.*

Components of a Nursing Risk Management Program**

Providing Proper Documentation

Adequate documentation can prevent malpractice claims from being initiated and is invaluable in a successful defense against them. The rules for appropriate documentation emphasize factual information presented as completely and as honestly as possible. A fraudulent record is difficult to defend in a malpractice case. Therefore, all health care providers are encouraged to alter records only if absolutely necessary for patient care purposes and only with the greatest of care to prevent even the appearance of misrepresentation. Accurately timing and dating nurses' notes and progress notes is especially important.

Using Reasonable Standards of Practice

A nurse's failure to document may lead to an erroneous judgment by a jury that the nurse failed to practice in a reasonable manner. Practicing in a reasonable professional manner and documenting that factor are the two best defenses against malpractice claims.

Risk management cannot prevent all malpractice claims. Those that cannot be prevented can be defended successfully by nurses' using rea-

sonable standards of practice. Nurses frequently ask what the standard of care is. This is a significant question, since the nurse's behavior in a specific malpractice case will be measured against reasonable standards of care.

These standards are formulated by the nursing profession. In fact, one of the characteristics of a profession is the ability to set its own standards. Nurses formulate their standards as they practice nursing on a day-to-day basis. Some standards are part of the custom of nursing practice and therefore are not necessarily in written form. Other standards are written, including job descriptions, policies, procedures, association guidelines, textbook material, and nurse practice acts. All of these may be admissible in a malpractice case to establish deviations from customary practice. An expert witness testifies in a malpractice case to assist the court in understanding the standard against which the nurse's actions should be measured.

Channeling Information Appropriately

To assist the health care facility board and administration in meeting their corporate responsibility, nurses frequently become the eyes and ears of the risk management program. Patient care information at the staff level must be channeled into the system appropriately so that action can be taken if necessary.

For example, if the nursing staff became aware of a physician who was impaired by alcohol (or drug) abuse and whose impairment was interfering with his or her ability to care for patients, such information must be communicated through appropriate departmental channels as well as to the risk management committee. This not only helps the institution meet its corporate responsibility, it also allows nurses to meet their own professional, legal, ethical, and personal accountability responsibilities for patient care. Once a staff nurse communicates the information, the situation then becomes a management or institutional issue to be resolved. If management or the administration fails to pursue appropriate action, the issue becomes one of institutional liability. The same principle applies when the nurse notifies the nurse manager that equipment is

---

*Source: Denise Pelle, "Risk Management," in *Current Strategies for Nurse Administrators,* Mary K. Stull and Sue Ellen Pinkerton, eds., Aspen Publishers, Inc., © 1988.

**Source: Janine Fiesta, "Nursing and Risk Management," in *Handbook of Health Care Risk Management,* Glenn T. Troyer and Steven L. Salman, eds., Aspen Publishers, Inc., © 1986.

deficient or unsafe for patient care or that staffing is inadequate. (See Table 23–2.)

Although it is well recognized that such events will occur on an isolated basis in even the best of institutions, the repetitiveness of such problems with no attempted intervention may signal the failure of reasonable standards of care for the institution.

Application of Standards of Care as a Preventive Strategy*

The best prevention/defense strategy against malpractice suits is thorough knowledge of the standard of care applicable in every clinical encounter. (See Table 23–3.) The legal standard of nursing care is to act as any other reasonable nurse would act under the circumstances. The client-nurse relationship, environmental factors (e.g., staff-client ratio), client acuity, and clini-

cal needs are factors to consider as part of the circumstances in determining what is reasonable. Reasonableness may be altered by the circumstances.

Reasonable can be defined by reviewing several sources, including nursing experience, education, state nursing practice acts and regulations, other legislation and regulations relevant to the practice area (e.g., home health agency, conditions for participation in Medicare/Medicaid, federal regulations), and previous case law (state or federal, depending on the practice setting and legal issues involved).

Evidence of the standard of care is usually developed by reviewing the facts of the case and applying the appropriate standard of care. Standards of nursing care can be found in organizational policy and procedure manuals, job descriptions, employment contracts and handbooks, accreditation criteria, American Medical Association certification requirements, statements of professional associations (e.g., the American Nurses' Association, etc.), and nursing journals and texts.

If there is inadequate documentation of what the nurse did and how the client responded, then

Source: Cynthia Northrop, "Malpractice and Standards of Care," *Nursing Outlook,* Vol. 34, No. 3, May–June 1986.

Table 23–2 Checklist of Risk Identifiers

Report If These Occur

____ Wrong dosage
____ Wrong medication
____ Medicine to wrong patient
____ IV infiltration
____ Wrong IV rate
____ Wrong IV solution/dosage
____ Other IV errors
____ Patient complaints
____ Left against medical advice
____ Suicide attempt
____ Self-inflicted injury
____ Other patient injury
____ Poor outcome/complications
____ Death/cardiac arrest

____ Infections
____ Fall from bed
____ Fall while ambulatory
____ Other falls
____ Untimely orders
____ Wrong treatment/test
____ Treatment/test to wrong patient
____ Delay in results
____ Lost orders/results
____ Delayed response/treatment
____ Orders unclear/contradictory
____ Improper criticism/jousting
____ Failure to follow policies/rules
____ Miscellaneous

Source: Tools for Quality Assurance Process, Colorado Hospital Association Trust, 1984.

Table 23–3 Guidelines for Nursing Activities in Risk Prevention

Minimizing Treatment-Related Injury	Monitoring/Observing/Supervising
• Adequately orient all personnel to a unit. • Test equipment regularly, provide routine maintenance for equipment, and keep records of equipment use. • Provide inservice education on treatment methods. • Organize a "buddy system" in which peers observe and evaluate each other's techniques and performance. • Provide close clinical supervision by peers and nurse managers. • Conduct clinical audits of nursing practice. • Conduct periodic performance evaluations by nurse managers, and conduct self-evaluations. • Develop and support employee assistance programs. • Urge prompt notification of the nursing administration of any problems with a physician or other health care team member.	• To facilitate monitoring, nurse managers should insist on prompt, complete, and accurate recording of data in patients' charts. Such a record makes it possible to recall the condition of the patient, the treatment given, the results of that treatment, and the follow up. • The nursing staff should have a thorough knowledge and understanding of the health care facility's protocols, rules, and policies and procedures. This could be encouraged by periodic review and/or testing. • Nurses should be expected to follow the current literature in their primary area of practice. • Workshops to enhance assessment skills and clinical judgment should be made available to all the nursing staff on a regular basis.

Source: Cynthia E. Northrop, "Nursing Actions in Litigation," © *Quality Review Bulletin.* Oakbrook Terrace, IL: Joint Commission on Accreditation of Healthcare Organizations, 1987, Vol. 13, No. 10. Reprinted with permission.

the issue becomes whether the standard of care was met. If the record is inadequate, the nurse may still convince the decision makers through testimony that the standard of care was met. One approach is to establish that the nurse knew the standard of care by using other evidence to show that the nurse regularly and routinely has met the appropriate standard of care. Adequate documentation, however, is part of a reasonable standard of care, and failure to meet a standard of care can be reflected simply by failure to record events properly.

An expert nurse witness is the most appropriate person to provide an opinion about whether a standard of care was met. In some situations in which a nurse's action is questioned, expert testimony may not be required. Figuring out when expert testimony is required usually rests on determining whether the decision maker needs information beyond what he or she possesses in order to make a decision.

INCIDENT REPORTS

Incident reports contain statements made by employees and physicians regarding a noteworthy deviation from what is considered acceptable patient care. Some state health codes provide that health care facilities must investigate incidents regarding patient care and require that certain incidents must be reported in a manner prescribed by regulation.

Although it may not always be clear as to when an incident report should be filed, appropriate procedures should be in place addressing how questionable events should be handled.

Source: George D. Pozgar, *Legal Aspects of Health Care Administration,* ed 5, Aspen Publishers, Inc., © 1993.

One component of a hospital's self-assessment is an evaluation of the types of data collected and analyzed in the effort to control risk exposures. The incident report is a central tool, used for both claims management and loss prevention activities. All occurrences resulting in actual or potential injury to the patient or that may lead to a claim or lawsuit should be reported to the risk management office. To ensure the completeness of reporting by health care providers, it is imperative to enhance reporting patterns through education of personnel and through efforts to streamline the reporting process for the convenience of practitioners. In addition to standard written reports, health care providers should be encouraged to call the office directly and/or to call a telephone answering service. Whether or not the incident reporting system is computerized, identification of trends and clusters of events is central to a loss prevention program (see Table 23–4).*

Responsibility for Completing Incident Reports**

Health care facilities should develop a clear policy with respect to who is responsible for completing the initial incident report and the more important incident investigation report. Generally, both the incident report and the incident investigation report forms should be completed by:

- the facility staff member involved in the occurrence (where more than one staff member is involved, it is preferable that the person with the most supervisory responsibility complete the report)
- the facility staff member who discovered the incident (where there is more than one employee involved, the person with the most seniority should complete the form)
- the facility staff member to whom the incident was reported

However, in those situations where the person who discovers the incident is involved in the incident or the person to whom the incident was reported is a registry nurse, temporary employee, or volunteer, that person's immediate supervisor should complete the form.

Incident reports should be completed as soon after the occurrence as possible, but in any event should be completed before the person responsible for completing the report form leaves the health care facility grounds.

MEDICATION ERRORS

There are inherent risks, both known and unknown, associated with the therapeutic use of drugs (prescription and nonprescription) and drug administration devices. The incidents or hazards that result from such risk have been defined as drug misadventuring, which includes both medication errors and adverse drug reactions (ADRs). Medication errors refer to episodes in drug misadventuring that should be preventable through effective systems controls involving pharmacists, physicians and other prescribers, nurses, risk management personnel, legal counsel, administrators, patients, and others in the organizational setting, as well as regulatory agencies and the pharmaceutical industry.

Medication errors compromise patient confidence in the health care system and increase health care costs. The problems and sources of medication errors are multidisciplinary and multifactorial. Errors occur from lack of knowledge, substandard performance and mental lapses, or defects or failures in systems (see Table 23–5). An understanding of the risk factors associated with medication errors should enable improved monitoring of patients and medications associated with increased risk for serious errors and should enable the development of organizational systems designed to minimize risk.*

Source: Barbara J. Youngberg, *Essentials of Hospital Risk Management*, Aspen Publishers, Inc., © 1990.

**Source:* Clemon W. Williams, "Guide to Hospital Incident Reports," *Health Care Management Review*, Vol. 10, No. 1, Aspen Publishers, Inc., © 1985.

Source: Originally published in *ASHP Guidelines on Preventing Medication Errors in Hospitals*, © 1993, American Society of Health System Pharmacists, Inc. All rights reserved. Reprinted with permission. (R9680)

Table 23–4 Sample Policy and Procedure for Incident Reporting

Policy

☐ Safety committee responsibilities:

- To assess how the internal reporting mechanism is working
- To code incidents according to their potential risk
- To review each incident report for completeness and quality
- To analyze the data obtained and prepare a bimonthly summary report to be sent to the assistant administrator for nursing, directors of division, clinical nurse specialists, the director of staff development and research, the nursing quality assurance/risk management director, and the nursing quality assurance/risk management committee

☐ Supervisory staff use information supplied by the safety committee to teach staff and correct problems.

Procedure

1. Complete an incident report for any unusual occurrence. If in doubt, it is always better to complete a report than not to file one.
2. Complete the report as soon after the incident as possible.
3. Have the staff person involved complete the report, and if more than one staff person is involved, all should participate and sign the report.
4. Make sure the report is accurate and complete.
5. *Never put the report into the patient's record or make a comment in the patient's record regarding the completion of a report.*
6. Identify only facts in the report.
7. Have the patient's physician sign the report.
8. Route the complete report as follows:
   - Initiator sends all copies to the clinical nurse specialist, who routes the report to the designated persons or committees.
   - Copy A is sent to the safety committee.
   - Copy B is sent to the director of the division and then to the assistant administrator for nursing.
   - Copy C is sent to the facility administrator, who will send copies to the facility's insurance carrier and attorney.

Source: Copyright © 1986, Anita Finkelman.

Detection and Classification of Medication Errors*

Though medication errors result from problematic processes, the outcomes of medication

*Source: Originally published in *ASHP Guidelines on Preventing Medication Errors in Hospitals*, © 1993, American Society of Health System Pharmacists, Inc. All rights reserved. Reprinted with permission. (R9680)

errors could range from minimal (or no) patient risk to life-threatening risk. Classification of the potential seriousness and clinical significance of detected medication errors should be based on predefined criteria established by the pharmacy and therapeutics committee (or its equivalent). The error classification should be based on the original order, standard medication dispensing and administration procedures, dosage forms available, acceptable deviation ranges, the potential for adverse consequences and patient harm, and other factors.

Classification of medication errors should allow for better management of follow-up activities on medication error detection. A simple classification of medication errors is the following: (1) clinically significant (includes potentially fatal or severe, potentially serious, and potentially significant errors) or (2) minor. Essentially, it is the effect on the patient (for a medication of any type) that really should determine what level of error is involved.

Medication errors should be identified and documented and their causes studied in order to develop systems that minimize recurrence. Several error-monitoring techniques exist: anonymous self-report, incident reports, critical-incident technique, disguised-observation technique. These may be applied as appropriate to determine the rates of errors. However, there are differences in the validity of data obtained by the various error-monitoring techniques or combined techniques. Managers should determine the best method for use in their organizations in consideration of utility, feasibility, and cost.

Improvement programs should provide guidance for patient support, staff counseling and education, and risk management processes when a medication error is detected. (See Table 23–6.) Incident-reporting policies and procedures and appropriate counseling, education, and intervention programs should be established in all health care facilities.

(*Note:* Other risk episodes have been identified in nursing care such as those connected with patient falls, improper use of equipment, lapses in infection, and employee substance abuse. Though these problems need to be addressed, space constraints do not allow further discussion of these issues here.)

Worker's Safety*

Health care workers are exposed to a variety of environmental risks from exposure to infec-

tion, chemicals, and physically onerous (e.g., lifting) or stress-related tasks.

Ideally, management should be committed to the concept of health and safety for all of its employees. But if it is not, legal demands may be placed on management to make such a commitment. Indeed, safety and health is a major issue for collective bargaining.

Ideally, a *collaborative team approach* should be taken to any potential or actual health and/or safety problems identified. The prevention, elimination, and control of these adverse conditions could involve input and action on the part of management (e.g., new hiring or shift work policies if psychological stress among the nursing staff is found to be a prevalent problem); labor (demanding safer and healthier working conditions, such as free hepatitis vaccine for all nurses who desire or require it); and workers (e.g., using the personal protective equipment provided at the worksite or no eating/smoking in the work area).

WORKPLACE ASSESSMENT*

Workplace assessment is defined as the process of observation and analysis of a workplace to identify conditions that may adversely affect the health and safety of workers. The benefits of worksite assessment include the following:

- *Detecting actual or potential hazards.* In the occupational health and safety field, the term *proactive approach,* which means identifying problems before they occur and doing something about them, is often used.
- *Pointing out problems unnoticed by employees themselves.* For example, the assessor, who knows that back problems are a major work-related problem for nurses, might walk onto a floor and observe that the newer members of the nursing staff are using improper lifting techniques.

Source: Denise C. Murphy, "An Introduction to Workplace Assessment," *Journal of the New York State Nurses' Association,* Vol. 18, No. 3, August 1987.

Source: Denise C. Murphy, "An Introduction to Workplace Assessment," *Journal of the New York State Nurses' Association,* Vol. 18, No. 3, August 1987.

Table 23–5 Checklist Review

Categories of Errors Related to Medication Administration Process	Risk Factors for Increased Medication Error
____ Omission error	____ Work shift (higher error rates typically occur during the day shift)
____ Unauthorized-drug error	____ Inexperienced and inadequately trained staff
____ Wrong-dose error	____ Medical service (e.g., special needs for certain patient populations, including geriatrics, pediatrics, and oncology)
____ Wrong-route error	
____ Wrong-rate error	
____ Wrong-dosage form error	____ Increased number or quantity of medications per patient
____ Wrong-time error	
____ Wrong preparation of a dose	____ Environmental factors (lighting, noise, frequent interruptions)
____ Incorrect administration technique	____ Staff workload and fatigue
	____ Poor communication among health care providers
	____ Dosage form (e.g., injectable drugs are associated with more serious errors)
	____ Type of distribution system (unit dose distribution is preferred; floor stock should be minimized)
	____ Improper drug storage
	____ Extent of measurements or calculations required
	____ Confusing drug product nomenclature, packaging, or labeling
	____ Drug category (e.g., antimicrobials)
	____ Poor handwriting
	____ Oral orders
	____ Lack of effective policies and procedures
	____ Poorly functioning oversight committees

- *Helping the assessor incorporate production needs* (i.e., facility/patient needs) *with the needs of the workers.* For example, a consumer need for an acquired immune deficiency syndrome (AIDS) unit should produce a corresponding need by workers for new or additional inservice education about the care of an AIDS patient.
- *Evaluating the effectiveness of existing controls.* Determining whether the ventilation system in the operating room is effectively removing anesthetic waste gases is an example.

The objectives of workplace assessment are to systematically identify high-risk personnel (such as a pregnant nurse lifting a heavy patient), high-risk areas (such as a dialysis unit for hepatitis), and high-risk materials and processes (such as the mixing of chemotherapeutic drugs). It should also determine the effectiveness of the existing health and safety program and engineering controls and suggest target areas for worksite modification and/or training and education for staff; for example, improper needle disposal may require education *and* the provision of the appropriate containers for needle disposal.

Table 23–6 Steps for Handling Medication Error Incidents

> Medication errors often result from problems in systems, rather than exclusively from staff performance or environmental factors; thus, error reports should not be used for punitive purposes but to achieve correction or change.

1. Provide any necessary corrective and supportive therapy to the patient.
2. Document and report the error immediately after discovery, in accordance with written procedures. For clinically significant errors, an immediate oral notice should be provided to physicians, nurses, and pharmacy managers. A written medication error report should follow promptly.
3. For clinically significant errors, fact gathering and investigation should be initiated immediately.
4. Reports of clinically significant errors and the associated corrective activities should be reviewed by the nurse manager and department head of the area(s) involved, the appropriate organizational administrator, the organizational safety committee (or its equivalent), and legal counsel (as appropriate).
5. When appropriate, the nurse manager and the staff members who were involved in the error should confer on how the error occurred and how its recurrence can be prevented.
6. Information gained from medication error reports and other means that demonstrates continued failure of individual professionals to avoid preventable medication errors should serve as an effective management and educational tool in staff development or, if necessary, modification of job functions or staff disciplinary action.
7. Nurse managers, department managers, and appropriate committees should periodically review error reports, determine causes of errors, and develop actions to prevent their recurrence (e.g., conduct organizational staff education, alter staff levels, revise policies and procedures, or change facilities, equipment, or supplies).

Source: ASHP Report, "Medication Errors," *American Journal of Hospital Pharmacy,* Vol. 50, February 1993, © 1993, American Society of Hospital Pharmacists, Inc.

Chapter 24

Space, Supplies, and Equipment

SPACE FOR HEALTH CARE

When considering facility space and design as part of the health care venue, what are the top considerations? There are four that benefit all concerned, and they are SAFE: strategy, assessment, flexibility, and efficiency. Exploring the interrelations will show how each element is required to protect another. For example, strategy includes the elements of organizational goals and project horizons, items that are critical to assessment. Likewise, flexibility is paired with efficiency because, if a facility is to meet the organizational goals, it will require design that can adapt to the needs of the organization on an ongoing basis.

Strategy encompasses architectural master planning and broader considerations of the facility's projected current and intermediate use as well as longer term flexibility.

Assessment suggests the programming phase of architectural design. As clients have learned, programming for facilities often allows organizations to reevaluate operations and just how things get done. As health care personnel are required to perform multiple tasks and greater attention is paid to a patient focus, programming is part of a health care organization's opportunity to implement total quality management and to measure outcomes.

Flexibility and efficiency can really be viewed as two sides of the same coin: architectural design. Flexibility allows qualitative enhancements to occur on an ongoing basis, whereas efficiency ensures a quantitative analysis. Both operate on a model of increasing productivity of the space designed, and both require highly creative solutions to be successful.

The SAFE elements will show how interrelated are master planning, programming, and architectural design. SAFE also orients a sensibility toward health care design in particular that is essential if the end result is to benefit the healing process.*

DESIGN OF FACILITIES**

Design of space for patient care involves both planning for new facilities and reorganizing extant facilities for new purposes. Whenever new facilities are planned for the health care institu-

---

*Source: Paul Westlake, Jr., "SAFE for Future Use? Stages in Master Planning, Programming, and Architectural Design," *Journal of Ambulatory Care Management,* Vol. 18, No. 4, Aspen Publishers, Inc., © October 1995.

**Source: Barbara Stevens Barnum and Karlene M. Kerfoot, *The Nurse as Executive,* ed. 4, Aspen Publishers, Inc., © 1995.

tion, be they patient care units or other structures, the nurse executive and the staff should be actively in on the planning. There are few aspects of a building that do not have an effect on nursing, even on non-nursing turf.

The nurse executive should be in on facilities planning *from the start*. If not consulted until late in the process, it may be too late to make revisions in plans without incurring great expense. Often, only late in the planning do others think to include the nurse executive; she should not wait for an invitation but should request to participate the moment any building plans are proposed.

Because facilities planning involves a special domain of knowledge, the nurse executive will want to become knowledgeable about this domain or else appoint a nurse specialist to work on renovation and construction projects. If a major building project is involved, someone in the nursing division should work permanently on the planning. There are nurses who have made a career specialization of design as it relates to patient care and architecture. Many firms specializing in health care architecture employ nurses to bring considerations of patients and staff to design.

All too often, plans have been made without the input of the users. Staff who will work in these areas every day can quickly critique what will and will not work and should be consulted at all phases of development. Significant costs can be saved by developing teams of these front-line people.

Now, we recognize the importance of patient input in the design of space. No longer do we design without considering the impact of the space on the patient. Everyone who will have to live within the space should be allowed to express his or her opinion.

Process of Building

There are several discrete stages in facilities building. The first is long-range planning. Here, the goals and needs of the community and the organization itself are considered, and future needs are projected. This part of the planning involves both long-range goal setting and the gathering of much demographic and other data to support the legitimacy of those goals.

Demographic data will describe the service area of the planned facility. It will also discuss subsidiary service areas expected to develop as the facility comes into being. Shifts in populations served may be due to changes in the community's population or due to an institution's plan to appeal to new groups within a community.

Changes in health manpower capabilities of the community (physician, nurse, technician, other) and growth or decline of other health service agencies in the community also need to be factored into the decision. Data concerning financing for the planned new facilities also must be gathered.

At the end of the planning phase, the institution is ready to make a knowledgeable decision as to whether the construction is feasible and logical. Typically, a certificate of need is required to build, and the data identified above provide the basis for this request.

The institution that hopes to put up new buildings also must deal with the community. Does the community want it? Are there groups that will contest it? Good relations with a community often make the difference between a building plan progressing smoothly or meeting insurmountable obstacles. Once an institution has determined to build, a good marketing plan usually is the next step: selling the notion to all potential interest groups.

In a resource-driven health care model, extensive financial analysis is necessary to ensure that the additional costs can be covered in an economically restrained environment. Revenue per square foot analysis is becoming as important to health care facilities as it is to retail stores. Overages can be reduced if the architecture can be turned into revenue generating space. This usually means that space is conserved; broad-scale plans are pared back. It makes no sense in this economy to bring more space onto the books if the space cannot generate the revenue to pay for itself over time.

While legal, political, and financial forces are being handled, the first phase of building involves development of a master site plan. This plan should take into account all foreseeable expansion, now and in the future. The site plan interrelates all lands owned by the institution, be they in geographic proximity or separated. Many institutions with tunnel vision have failed to acquire adequate land for expansion. In heavily built-up areas, it may be impossible to count on geographic expansion later, so that most planning will have to involve expensive vertical rather than horizontal extension.

An institution often walks a fine line with a community; although the community may want medical facilities to expand, it may balk at such a project if it involves the displacement of community residents or businesses. Now, many communities see new buildings as a symbol of escalating health care costs and actively oppose building programs.

The third phase begins the actual design of facilities. First, block schematics are drawn to show how major areas to be built will relate to each other, both horizontally and vertically. Figure 24–1 is a simplified block drawing. In an actual block drawing, the scale would be indicated. Computer-generated schematics allow planners to consider many different designs and design changes over a short period of time. In block schematics, the nurse executive must be careful to note the common pathways by which patients flow from one department to another.

An ideal structure would allow all departments immediate access to all other departments; unfortunately, the realities of space do not easily allow such construction. Any block design is a compromise, placing in close proximity those departments that most require it. For example, it makes sense if the recovery room is near the operating rooms, the nursery near postpartum, and so forth. On one set of block schematics, a nurse executive pointed out that the only way in which emergency department patients could be taken to the X-ray department was by moving them through the cafeteria or the front lobby (as in Figure 24–1).

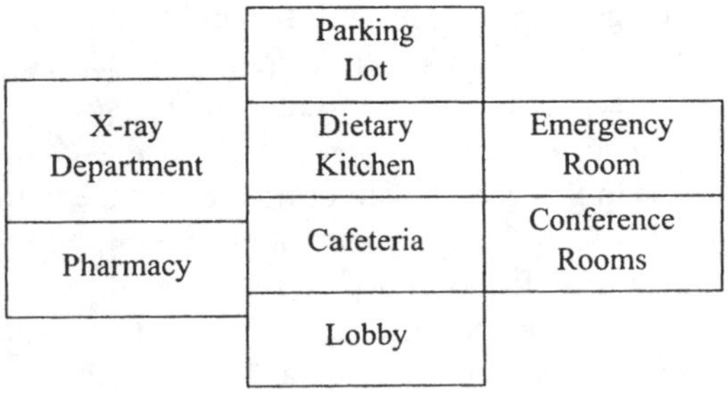

In the next phase of planning, single-line sketches are composed for all areas to be constructed. Actual space constraints such as internal columns, elevators, and corridors are drawn to scale, and rooms are designed with beds and room equipment also drawn to scale. Entrances and exits are indicated in the single-line drawings. The finished single-line drawings reveal the configuration of each unit, the size and shape of planned spaces, and the functional relationships (horizontal and vertical connections) between planned units.

Design development drawings are refinements of the single-line sketches. These drawings include such things as structural, mechanical, electrical systems, as well as built-in equipment. By the time the architects reach this stage of development, they are hesitant to make changes, and changes will cost significant amounts of money for the organization. The final planning stage is the development of blueprints—a refinement of the design development drawings.

Construction of facilities always is a compromise between what an institution wants and what it can afford. Few nurse executives have the privilege of having a building designed just as they desire. The nurse executive must beware of building savings that will cost money in the long run. For example, if the institution will have to pay extra nursing salaries over the next 20 or more years, a plan may end up costing far more than was saved by some architectural shortcut.

Suppose elevator service was limited because elevators are expensive to install: Thousands of nursing hours may be lost in waiting time. Similarly, if a work area is too small, nurses may have to wait until other nurses vacate an area. Nurse executives are successful in getting architectural

Figure 24–1 Block Schematic for the First Floor of a Hospital

plans changed by pointing out potential inefficiencies with cost benefit analysis data.

It is amazing how often the managerial needs of a nursing unit are overlooked by planners if nurses are not adequately represented on the planning committees. Head nurses' offices and conference rooms certainly should be included in any modern design, but even basics can be forgotten without nursing input.

One nursing vice president told of an institution that attempted to save money by hiring an architectural firm that had never worked on hospital designs previously. In the single-line sketch stage, she asked where the nurses' bathrooms were to be located, only to find that the architects had given thorough attention to patients' bathrooms but had totally forgotten that nurses might require such facilities. The architects argued in vain that the large nurses' bathroom in the basement locker facility would be adequate.

The nurse executive will need to be especially careful in the design of patient units. Many architectural horror stories are told by nurse executives. One moved into a new facility only to discover the door proportions somehow had been changed, making it impossible to roll a bed directly into a room; thousands of nursing hours would be spent in unnecessary stretcher-to-bed transfers.

Another new facility had bathrooms in which the patient had to be a healthy contortionist to use the bowl. Another had nurses' stations in a niche that could not be watched from the hall that led to patients' rooms. Worse, it was directly accessible to an elevator used by the public. Hundreds of dollars worth of equipment "walked off" before this nursing station was restructured.

Another, a critical care unit, had half partitions so that nurses could watch patients above the newest monitoring equipment installed in the lower portion. The only problem was that the heights were perfect for the average man, but many of the female nurses had to jump if they wanted to see over the partition. The area soon became cluttered with boxes, stools, and other contraptions for the shorter nurses.

Although common sense will prevent some errors of this sort, more refinement of judgment is required to do a good planning job. The nurse in charge of planning should know such things as the legal requirements for space usage, the norms of space footage for various facilities, state regulations and accreditation standards, and other tricks of facilities planning. If there is no one with such expertise in the nursing division, it may be wise to use a nurse consultant who is an expert in this area.

After blueprints receive final approval, the building phase is initiated. By then, it usually is too late for any changes unless a catastrophic error is discovered. If a major error is discovered at this late date, it means that the nurse executive did not give enough attention to the project at an earlier stage and costly revisions will be necessary.

Even with the best of planning, it is possible to become the victim of planning that fails to predict changes. For example, one facility was designed specially to keep the nurses at the bedside. One element in the building design illustrated this principle. A large 50-bed intensive care unit was designed around pods of three patients each. In each pod, the nursing station was centered among three highly visible patient rooms. The atmosphere was excellent; the latest of monitoring equipment was relayed to the mini-nursing stations. There was only one problem with the design; no pod had easy access to another pod. The stations were designed for separate staffing for each pod. The designer did not anticipate a time when costs would dictate reduced nursing staff. Now, this facility cannot safely afford to use this unit for intensive care, because it cannot afford to staff all these architecturally isolated pods.

Many buildings that applied the Friesen principle had similar problems. In this plan, all care equipment and records are kept adjoining the patient's room. The design was planned to allow the nurse to stay at the bedside. Many plans reinforced this method by eliminating the central nursing station. In most cases, however, nurses soon created their own nurses' station in halls, in treatment rooms, wherever a central meeting place could be created, however haphazardly. The designer simply failed to predict that nurses would not enjoy functioning in isolation. He failed to recognize the need for professional communication and consultation.

Many errors in design involve a failure to anticipate the security systems required today. One building, for example, was designed with large numbers of entry doors to facilitate traffic patterns. Now, because of security needs, most of these exits are locked. The resultant traffic patterns require great inconvenience on the part of many. And one can say without possibility of contradiction that no facility yet built has predicted how soon the planned number of elevators and parking spaces would be inadequate.

During the planning phases, the nurse executive will need to consider the architect's plan for (1) flow patterns for patients, staff, and visitors; (2) security needs of the facility; (3) facilities' proximity needs; (4) movement of equipment and supplies; (5) placement of nursing offices and managerial space as they relate to the space of other key managers; (6) educational and conference space needs; and (7) patients' convenience in use of the facilities.

Basic Plans for Patient Units

The design of patient care units needs special attention. The oldest and least satisfactory design is the single-corridor design, in which patient rooms as well as nurses' stations, treatment rooms, and other service areas all branch off the same long hall. Such a long-hall construction incurs many more man-hours spent in walking than is the case with the more compact designs. (Figure 24-2 is an illustration of this design. Here

and in subsequent illustrations, the dark areas indicate nurses' stations and other work areas.)

In the double-corridor design (Figure 24–3), patient rooms branch off halls located on both sides of a central core containing the work areas of the unit. Advocates of this design claim walking time is cut nearly by half compared with a long corridor with the same number of patient rooms. However, this design cuts down visibility of hall activities because only one-half of the unit can be seen at any one time.

Each variation in unit design has advantages and limitations. The triangle, circle, and square designs usually simplify walking but may devote more space to central work areas than is necessary (Figures 24–4 through 24–6). T-shaped units attempt to solve this problem while still shortening the length of any given corridor (Figure 24–7).

Figure 24–3 Double-Corridor Patient Unit (Dark areas indicate nurses' stations and other staff work areas.)

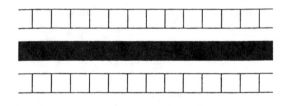

Figure 24–4 Triangular Patient Unit (Dark areas indicate nurses' stations and other staff work areas.)

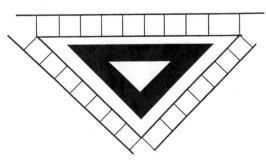

Figure 24–2 Single-Corridor Patient Unit (Dark areas indicate nurses' stations and other staff work areas.)

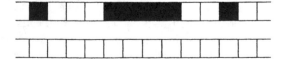

Figure 24–5 Circular Patient Unit (Dark areas indicate nurses' stations and other staff work areas.)

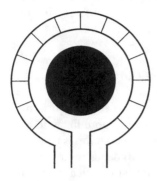

Figure 24–6 Square Patient Unit (Dark areas indicate nurses' stations and other staff work areas.)

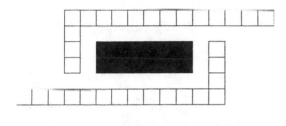

Figure 24–7 T-shaped Patient Unit (Dark areas indicate nurses' stations and other staff work areas.)

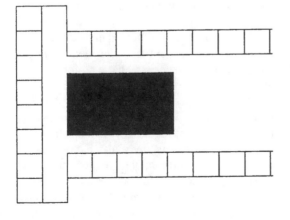

When deciding on the shape of nursing units, the nurse executive will want to consult people who have lived with the designs under consideration. Some of the newer designs may look attractive and efficient but contain subtle flaws. No one can anticipate how it is to inhabit a structure without visiting one and asking those who have worked there whether they like it and how it works.

Census is another issue. Builders generally prefer large-census patient units because they are less expensive to construct than small-census ones. The nurse executive will want a size compatible with the assignment system used. However, assignments systems change as other circumstances change.

Many nurse executives have managed to get smaller-census units or better designed facilities by quantifying the staffing costs incurred by the inferior design. A chief executive officer who favors a cheaper design because of cost factors is likely to be amenable to analyses that predict greater ultimate cost savings. If a building design causes the need for additional nursing staff, an institution will pay for a false economy many times over, every year that the building is in use.

A new initiative in many hospitals is to bring care to the patient instead of transporting the patient all over the health care facility for tests and procedures. In some settings, functions such as radiology and laboratory have been moved to the unit in an attempt to decrease transportation time and increase patient satisfaction. People on individual units have been cross-trained to do many functions that were once performed by people in centralized departments. In some cases this patient-focused redesign creates major renovation programs (e.g., when functions such as radiology are moved to the unit).

When architectural changes are *not* made but functions are moved to the unit, many hospitals must redesign. For example, centralized nursing stations have been replaced by bedside computers, and functions such as recording electrocardiographs have been moved to the bedside to be performed by cross-trained unit-based staff. In some facilities, this has meant overcrowding on the unit as more functions, people, and support equipment move there from formerly centralized departments.

In an attempt to move patients less often, some health care facilities are experimenting with rooms that can be upgraded to an intensive care unit or downgraded to a step-down or acute care unit, depending on the needs of the patient and the acuity. The concepts of patient-focused redesign force us to think in terms of designing care programs around the patient and not around the staff or personnel. As more functions are brought to the bedside, more creativity is demanded to create the support systems for these new patient care delivery models through innovation in architectural design.

Interior design also may present problems. Typically, the closet area in patients' rooms is inadequate. Another common fault is lack of counter space in bathrooms. Both of these problems arise out of attempts to save space, usually to increase the number of private over shared patient rooms. Another question in interior design is whether to go for built-in versus mobile equipment. Flexibility is maintained with mobile equipment, but such equipment typically needs more care and tending.

Carpeting is another issue that is usually debated in relation to patient rooms. Arguments *for* carpeting include aesthetic pleasure, noise reduction, fewer injuries in patient falls, and psychological satisfaction. Arguments against carpeting concern the difficulty of infection control, problems with moving stock such as stretchers and wheelchairs, and the difficulty of cleaning spills of various sorts. There is no single satisfactory answer, although the type of carpet used may make a radical difference in how satisfactory it is in patient rooms.

Interior design of the nurses' stations deserves attention; typically, these areas lack enough seating space. The need is greatest when physicians and nurses share the same space. As more professionals become unit-based, the need for writing, thinking, and conferencing space becomes critical.

Again, if the nurse executive or one of her staff has not had considerable experience in interior design, it is probably a good idea to hire a nurse consultant who specializes in this area. There are just too many possibilities of making mistakes that must be lived with for inordinately long times.

Redesign of Old Facilities

In an era when the nation is overbedded, a nurse executive is more likely to be involved in redesigning extant facilities than in the building of new ones. Indeed, with many institutions branching out into vertical integration of services, it is common that unused acute units be converted to other purposes. Adapting an old facility to a different purpose is probably even more challenging than designing a new facility.

One constructive way to begin such a challenge is to identify the requirements that one would have if a new facility were built. This forces one to identify the purposes of the proposed unit. Once these desirable traits have been identified, then one asks how or to what extent they can be realized in the redesign of the old facility.

Suppose, for example, that two old acute care hospital units are to be turned into a skilled nursing facility for long-term care patients. If one just rearranges without an overall plan, the results are likely to be bleak. With this haphazard method, one asks things such as, "Now where will I put the television room?" With the advised plan, instead, one starts with questions such as, "What are the requirements of persons who will make this facility their home for a sustained period? What are their abilities, their disabilities?"

Once one has identified the ideal arrangements, then one needs a realistic notion of what can and cannot be done with the old facility. This involves two aspects: what can be done from the point of view of cost, and what can be done given the architecture of the facility. Perhaps the most important questions involve what walls are weight-bearing and cannot be removed and what plumbing and service lines are permanent. When one has an idea of what cannot be changed, then it is easier to remember that all else becomes open to revision (at least within a feasible budget).

When deficits cannot be cured by revising space, then interior design becomes the challenge.

One should never underestimate the effect architecture and the arrangement of space on human activities and perceptions. For example, in one hospital renovated into a nursing home, residents were simply placed in rooms as the acute care patients before them had been. The nurses, not surprisingly, were treating the residents much as if they were acute care patients. The pull of the old facilities led to old behavior patterns, and the residents were treated as if they were ill.

Traffic patterns constitute another major consideration in redesigning facilities. In the nursing home example, the planners failed to recognize that permanent residents would be trafficking the halls far more than the previous inhabitants. Nor did the designers consider all aspects of mobility of the elderly well who would live there. Bright-colored handrails were put in, lining the halls for the walking elderly. Although these were useful, the planners failed to think about placement of communal rooms. These rooms were placed at the farthest ends of long corridors, making the walking distance formidable for many residents even with rails lining the corridors.

This mistake would not have been made if the planners had started with the needs of the residents. Instead, they asked, how can we use what is already here?

Esthetics are especially important in redesigning facilities. When the logistics may involve making do with less than ideal architectural designs, the environment can be made pleasant.

Using a Team Process for Planning*

Facility planning has traditionally been presided over by a small group from the health care facility senior staff that served as a coordinating group to oversee, review, and approve recommendations. The coordinating group typically may include the president and chief executive officer, the chief nurse executive, senior medical leadership, facilities administrator, and support services executive. However, most organizations now recognize that space planning requires a multidisciplinary approach, since each department is used by a variety of staff who have varying purposes and needs. Attention to these different perspectives will ensure a higher quality outcome in space design and functionality.

Consequently, a team process structure may be used, though the level or degree of participation may vary in different facilities. For example, a senior management group might serve as a supervisor of the planning process recommendations. It would first initiate the process for subteam development, outline the process parameters for planning, coordinate the multiple teams, and act as a communication link. Cross-level interdisciplinary teams are chosen from the actual users of the space being planned. Multiple levels of staff from all affected areas should be included. In general, it is advisable to identify not only the users of the space, but also those who provide a service to the space. Not all those identified may need to be full members of the team.

The base subteam should be limited to between 5 and 10 members to allow for maximizing the team process. A facilitator should be identified to ensure productive group functioning. The planners or architects sometimes serve in the facilitator role. It may be advisable to have a member of the senior management coordinating group as a member of each team. This is particularly important when there is more than one planning team and overlaps can easily occur. Senior managers can help to clarify issues and boundaries for the team, providing a broader perspective and an understanding of the integration of the larger building process.

When there are multiple department planning teams, it is necessary to develop special systems groups, with members from each department planning team. This may be necessary for systems like materials distribution, computers and communication, and transportation. These special teams are useful for major systems that affect more than one area or department. Without some coordination by an oversight group, individual teams could design their space based on different systems.

***Source:* Sheila Smith, "A Team Approach to Facilities Planning and Design," *Aspen's Advisor for Nurse Executives,* Vol. 9, No. 6, Aspen Publishers, Inc., © March 1994.

SUPPLIES

Analyzing Needs and Monitoring*

The first-line nurse manager may have significant responsibility for the ordering and monitoring of materials for the unit. The projected amount to request for supplies in the upcoming year will be based on the spending levels of the previous fiscal year. An effective manager won't wait until budget time to review material usage in the work area. Monthly expense reports, reports on supplies taken from central stores, and reports on supplies ordered directly from vendors provide baseline information for an analysis of material expenditures. The nurse manager should make a habit of reviewing all available reports for the essential data regarding supplies on the unit.

Advances in technology and the preference for disposable goods tend to increase the cost of supplies estimated per patient. In addition, new treatment modalities, the increased precautions taken with AIDS patients, physician preference for a particular, more expensive, brand of a given item—all have a direct impact on supply expenses. Not all of these influences can be predicted. The nurse manager should construct the budget with some leeway for these unplanned factors in mind. There is also a need to factor inflation into the cost of anticipated items for the next year. When limited resources are available, rather than increase expenditures the nurse manager may be expected to scale down the budget. Decisions will have to be made as to what will have priority. The purchase of a new kind of infusion pump may be postponed, while the plan to switch to digital thermometers remains in the budget.

Since accountability for supplies is at the unit level, the head nurse should review the ordering system and how usage is monitored in day-to-day practice. Staff members must be required to follow the correct procedure when ordering supplies and charging patients. Often staff consider these accounting procedures to be unnecessary paperwork that takes time away from patient care. What they fail to understand is that the hospital cannot be reimbursed when supplies are not charged to patients, and the money is then lost to the hospital and to the unit. If the processing of charge slips is in fact inefficient, the nurse manager must investigate new approaches to the problem. It would be interesting to find out how much money is lost because of an inconvenient system. It often proves worthwhile to spend time designing a more efficient means of charging patients for various care products that are used daily.

Supply Distribution Systems*

The majority of the hospital's inventory is kept in the main hospital storeroom. Items may be distributed via requisitions, par-level systems, or exchange carts. Using requisitions is a traditional system whereby individual departments or nursing units determine when and how much to order. In the par-level system, personnel from the approval of management or central supply section department go to each appropriate hospital department and nursing unit, count the supplies, write up orders, obtain the supplies, and bring them back to the unit. Supplies are brought up to the standard or par level. A variation of the par-level system is to distribute supplies on a movable cart. According to a predesignated schedule, depleted carts are exchanged with full carts. This is called an exchange cart system.

Evaluating Supply Delivery**

How does one measure the performance of the materiel management department? First and foremost, certain performance criteria should be

---

*Source: Barbara Stevens Barnum and Catherine O. Mallard, Essentials of Nursing Management: Concepts and Context of Practice, Aspen Publishers, Inc., © 1989.

*Source: I. Donald Snook, Jr., Hospitals: What They Are and How They Work, ed. 2, Aspen Publishers, Inc., © 1992.

**Source: C. Housely, "Let the Consumer Be the Judge," Dimensions in Health Service, Journal of the Canadian Hospital Association, September 1977. Reprinted with permission.

drawn up by the manager. This is commonly referred to as the statement of services for the department and should be distributed to all of the supply consumers. The following example represents such a statement.

Statement of Services to the Nursing Units

- A total supply cart exchange program for each nursing unit will furnish 95–99 percent of the supply requirements for each unit for a 24-hour period.
  - The supply quotas will be individualized according to the needs of each nursing unit.
  - These supply quotas will be reviewed and updated at least quarterly.
  - The carts will be exchanged daily at 6:00 AM.
- A 24-hour, seven-days-a-week delivery service will be provided for items that are not on the cart.
  - If you do not have a supply item for any reason, please use the supply hot line and you will receive an immediate response (within 15 minutes) around the clock.
  - Please do not send unit personnel to central stores to pick up supplies.
- Equipment rounds to each nursing unit will be made twice daily, seven days a week to check such items as suction machines, K-pads, and so forth.
- Monday morning of each week, a check of the miscellaneous equipment (flashlights, stethoscopes, scales, etc.) will be performed. You are to sign that this service was performed.
- Every attempt will be made to keep your units supplied with the proper items and equipment. To ensure this, the central stores supervisor will make daily supply rounds on each unit, Monday through Friday. If you should have any supply, process, or delivery problems, please bring them to his or her attention.
- A current supply reference catalog is filed on each nursing unit for your convenience and assistance.

After the evaluation criteria have been delineated, persons who use the service should judge the effectiveness. That means that nursing service will be a major contributor to the evaluation process. Periodically the nursing department should complete a questionnaire in reference to supply service. (See Table 24–1.) This information can be used by the materiel manager to improve services to the department and, ultimately, to the patient.

EQUIPMENT

One key area of supervisory involvement in the management of equipment is gathering and assembling the information required for justifying equipment needs and the potential allocation of capital funds for purchases. Depending on the scope of any undertaking and thus on the depth and extent of managerial involvement, the nurse manager may be called on to provide information on why a request is being made.

In most cases, regulation or accreditation requirements are sufficient justification for a purchase. If the equipment is requested to replace existing equipment, the justification for the request will proceed along the lines of demonstrating why and how the existing equipment is no longer adequate. The request for the addition of new equipment to perform a function not previously performed ordinarily involves the provision of a new service. The justification of the equipment purchase is, therefore, a part of the economic and clinical justification for adding the new service.

The manager should be able to explain why the equipment being asked for is the most efficient and effective way of performing the function or address the concern that triggered the request. A justification should attempt to deal with the potential usefulness or applicability of the proposed purchase under present circumstances, within the short run (up to one year in the future) and within the long run (looking perhaps four or five years into the future).

Table 24–1 Supply Survey

1. Are your supply and linen carts delivered on time (before 7:00 AM)?
   Yes ☐   No ☐

2. Generally, do the supply and linen carts contain all of your needs?
   Yes ☐   No ☐

3. Cart supply quotas are to be reviewed with you at least quarterly. How long has it been since someone in materiel management reviewed with you your supply needs?
   _____
   _____

4. Did you know that only "charge" items have charge tickets and need your attention to process them immediately?
   Yes ☐   No ☐

5. If the supply is not on the cart, can you use the telephone hot line and receive immediate (within 20 minutes) delivery?
   Yes ☐   No ☐

6. When you have a supply problem, do you feel free to call someone in central stores to get immediate action?
   Yes ☐   No ☐

7. When you call central stores, are the attendants courteous?
   Yes ☐   No ☐

8. Are they knowledgeable and helpful?
   Yes ☐   No ☐

9. When you phone central stores, what is the average delivery response time:
   10–20 Minutes ☐
   20–30 Minutes ☐   30–60 Minutes ☐

10. Do you ever have to send someone to central stores to pick up items?
    Yes ☐   No ☐

11. Does the linen cart meet your linen supply needs?
    Yes ☐   No ☐

12. If "No," what needs our attention?_____
    _____

13. Equipment rounds to check suction machines, K-pads, etc., are made on your unit seven days/week at 10:00 AM and 2:00 PM. Did you know this?
    Yes ☐   No ☐

14. In your opinion, are these equipment rounds effective?
    Yes ☐   No ☐

15. Also, we check and replace, if needed, items such as flashlights, blood pressure units, stethoscopes, etc., every Monday morning. Did you know this?
    Yes ☐   No ☐

16. Are these items being maintained well on your unit?
    Yes ☐   No ☐

17. In your opinion, what area of supply service needs our immediate attention to assist you most? _____
    _____

18. Generally, how would you rate our overall supply service?
    Poor ☐   Fair ☐   Good ☐   Excellent ☐

19. If you indicate "fair" or "poor," simply state why in 25 words or less. Please use the reverse side of this questionnaire.

20. Any other comments are welcomed:
    _____
    _____
    _____

Assessment of Clinical Implications*

It is often advisable to proceed beyond the general assessment of need to an additional clinically oriented assessment of the likely impact of the new equipment or service on both patients

*Source: Copyright © 1986, C.R. McConnell.

and staff. Any new personnel should be identified at least by skill level and pay grade and work status (full-time or-part time for some specific number of hours per week). This assessment should consider, in addition to the possibility of added personnel in the department, the use of existing personnel at present grade levels or the need to upgrade existing personnel.

Economic Analysis*

Economic analysis should take into account all costs of acquiring and using the equipment, including

- acquisition, which includes purchase price, cost of shipping, and total cost of installation
- estimated cost of all materials and supplies to be consumed in the operation of the equipment
- cost of additional personnel required or cost of essential upgrading of existing personnel
- cost, if any, of training personnel to operate the equipment
- estimated cost of maintenance, service, and repairs
- other applicable costs such as insurance premiums, license costs, various fees, additional power, and other utility requirements

Finally, a comparison of alternatives should be undertaken on the basis of equivalent annual costs, that is, the cost of owning and operating each alternative on a per year basis.

Collaboration with Materiel Management**

Nursing can be considered the materiel manager's biggest customer, as it is the highest volume end-user of health care facility products. There are two major contact points that emanate from this relationship. Nursing service is the object of supply deliveries, which may be late (or never arrive), may be sent to the wrong place, or may be a product that was ordered incorrectly. Nurses use the products and develop favorites or critical attitudes. They have learned, through

trial and error, what works clinically and have knowledge of new products from continuing education workshops and conferences. Nurses are highly qualified to participate in the purchase process. Nursing input can uncover serious deficiencies or advantages in competing products. Including nurses in product evaluation is now required by two major nursing organizations. In their published standards for patient care, both the American Association of Critical Care Nurses (AACN) and the Association of Operating Room Nurses (AORN) state that nurses must be involved in the evaluation process.

For each product evaluated, nursing can provide input and relay information to materiel management on a number of issues. In this process, even if a product looks good economically, if it will not work clinically, nursing has to stand its ground and make compelling arguments to reject it, thereby ensuring the best decisions for the patient and the institution.

Ideally, the purchasing decision should be a collaborative process with input solicited from all parties affected by the decision. The steps of such a process are shown in Table 24–2.

Conducting Equipment Trials*

Equipment trials are an option that should be strongly considered in any major departmental expenditure. Trials prior to selection of new equipment are a valuable means of evaluating both quality and costs in purchase decisions.

Establishing an equipment trial requires planning, staff education and cooperation, and evaluation procedures. The planning phase includes selecting the appropriate test population, establishing time limits, and coordinating sales representatives' activities to meet predetermined trial needs. The test population is determined by the use of the equipment; ideally it represents a sample of the nursing care units likely to use the equipment. A trial period should be long

Source: Copyright © 1986, C.R. McConnell.

**Source:* Adapted from Patricia Carroll, "Nursing Input into the Purchase Decision Reveals Cost Not Included in the Price Tag," *Hospital Materiel Management Quarterly,* Vol. 3, No. 4, Aspen Publishers, Inc., © May 1992.

Source: Phyllis Barone-Ameduri, "Equipment Trials Make Sense," *Nursing Management,* Vol. 17, No. 6, June 1986. Reprinted with permission.

Nursing's Role in Testing Products

Product comparison: Competitive products can be compared by nurses at the bedside, and benefits and problems with each product can be more easily determined.

Manufacturing claims: Nursing analysis can test the validity of manufacturer claims and whether they ring true at the bedside and in the clinical setting.

Evaluate ease of use: Products that require more time to use or are inconvenient to use will increase nursing time and increase the ultimate cost of the product. Nurses will be reluctant to use a product that makes their job more difficult and less efficient.

Safety features: What features are present to protect the nurse users as well as the patient? Nurses consider what can go wrong, how the device may be misused, and, most important, whether safety features can be defeated easily.

Manufacturer instructions: Nurses can test whether the manufacturer's instructions are clear and readily available.

Table 24-2 Product Evaluation Process

Step 1: New product is introduced by clinician, physician, or health care facility employee.

Step 2: Manager department head is informed.

Step 3: If there is sufficient interest, the product is introduced to materials management by the originator.

Step 4: Materials management contracts for vendor product information.

Step 5: Materials management presents the product to product standardization committee for approval of clinical trial and assignment of trial coordinator.

Step 6: Safety check is performed, if applicable to technology.

Step 7: Departments for trial are selected; clinical trial is conducted.

Step 8: Trial coordinator summarizes findings and reports to product standardization committee. Decision to adopt or not adopt is made.

Step 9: Trial coordinator informs originator, manager, and trial department of decision.

Source: Rhonda R. Stockard, Mary Murray, Martha McKee, Diane Stanfa, "A Practice Model for Evaluating New Products and Technology," *Aspen's Advisor for Nurse Executives,* Vol. 9, No. 5, Aspen Publishers, Inc., © February 1994.

enough to be fair to each product, but allowing an evaluation to drag on more than two weeks may decrease enthusiasm and input—especially when more than one company product is involved and the clinical trials will last for months.

A meeting should be held with each sales representative prior to the trial to review plans and discuss company responsibilities during the period. Based on the predetermined trial length and number of participating units, verify that the company is indeed willing and able to provide the equipment and supplies needed for a successful evaluation.

Clarify the inservice education that will be needed to acquaint staff with the product. Ascertain whether and when the sales representative will be able to meet staff education needs on all shifts. Will he or she be available as a resource person to field questions and solve problems that may arise during the trial?

An evaluation tool should be developed prior to the trial. This tool should measure staff opinion in areas that define gradations of performance from poor to excellent. Evaluation criteria include reliability, ease of learning, simplicity of operation, and/or features that are improvements over currently used equipment. These factors will later be balanced by considerations such as cost, service agreements, and the like.

Part V

Human Resources Management

Chapter 25

Personnel Policies, Salaries, and Benefits

THE LEGAL AND REGULATORY ENVIRONMENT

Nursing administration, in collaboration with the human resource department, must be careful to consult a wide range of documents before reaching any conclusions about the total legality of facility practices or policies for personnel.

Employment Laws*

The many laws relating to labor and personnel problems in the health care field include federal laws applicable uniformly to all institutions nationwide and state and local laws, which are applicable to their own particular geographic location. For the most part, when federal law and state law conflict, federal law will supersede, or preempt, the state or local law. Generally, when state or local law is more restrictive against the employer, the more stringent state law will be given effect.

It also should be noted that in addition to the statutes, many regulations, administrative inter-

pretations, administrative guidelines, and judicial interpretations exist and create a hugh document base on which a legal analysis must be grounded. Indeed, the actual laws and regulations provide only a small part of the legal system related to employment laws. The following list describes the types of federal and state employment laws that affect health care facilities.

Equal Employment. These laws deal with aspects of discrimination in employment because of race, color, religion, national origin, age, sex, sexual preference, handicap, or status as a disabled or Vietnam-era veteran.

Labor Standards. These laws establish minimum standards that employers must maintain with respect to working conditions. The principal laws in this field deal with minimum wages, maximum hours, child labor, and safety and health.

Fringe Benefit Administration. These laws regulate the standards for and taxability of fringe benefits such as health insurance, life insurance, pensions, profit sharing, vacations, holidays, disability insurance, and dental insurance. A detailed explanation of these laws is beyond the scope of this book.

Labor Relations. These laws establish the rights and duties of employers, unions, and em-

*Source: Skoler, Abbott & Presser, *Health Care Labor Manual*, Aspen Publishers, Inc., © January 1991.

ployees in relationship to each other; they are sometimes called "labor-management" or "collective-bargaining" laws. (See Chapter 27, "Labor Relations.")

Individual Employee Rights. Laws dealing with issues such as wrongful termination, unemployment compensation, workers' compensation, interference with contractual relations, negligence, libel, and slander constitute a large body of state contract and tort law relating to employment.

The Employee Handbook*

The employee handbook is a medium of communication. Its purpose is to define and explain the employees' relationship with the health care organization. The handbook presents the rules and procedures that all employees are expected to observe. It explains the organization's standards of appropriate conduct. It spells out the benefits and privileges offered in return for good work—along with the penalties for poor performance. It is an agreement that has many of the characteristics of a formal contract. That is why courts have found so often that a handbook *is* a contract.

As an instrument of communication, a well-written handbook can have many extremely valuable purposes. It can build a unified sense of purpose among the work force, since this is where the organization can express its mission in terms that make its employees want to "join the cause." A handbook can explain all the available procedures for claiming a benefit or the eligibility requirements. Those who find their answers in the handbook will not have to take the time to look elsewhere. It will be all there, in one reliable source.

An important preliminary to writing an employee handbook is to distinguish it from a policy manual.

- A policy manual is written for *managers and supervisors*. Its purpose is to tell them how to implement and enforce organizational policies.
- An employee handbook is written for *all employees*. Its purpose is to inform them about organizational policies and requirements and to explain benefits and procedures.

It has always been good practice to write two separate policy documents. An employee manual is designed to tell employees what the organization expects from them and, in return, what they can expect from the organization. This is the mutual exchange that has become so important, both in a legal sense and as a matter of good employee relations. A policy manual, on the other hand, is directed at the managers and supervisors who must implement the stated policies. It is intended for their guidance. The policy manual contains instructions. It does not represent an exchange of obligations and benefits.

One of the early decisions that must be made, then, is what subject matter to place in each type of manual (see Table 25–1), and how to treat each subject. The same subject will often appear in both manuals, presented typically as information to the employees and as policy guidance to managers and supervisors.

JOB EVALUATION AND WAGE DETERMINATION*

The need for scientific wage determination in health care facilities is no longer in question. Dissatisfaction about wages has three separate causes: inequities among wage rates paid within classifications and among classifications that employees consider similar to their own, individual or group pressure for higher earning power, and inappropriate market positioning. Health care facilities have come to accept that a

---

Source: The Employee Handbook, Panel Publishers, Inc., © 1993.

Source: Norman Metzger, "Human Resources Management," in *Health Care Administration: Principles, Practices, Structure, and Delivery*, ed 2, Lawrence F. Wolper, ed., Aspen Publishers, Inc., © 1995.

Table 25–1 Topics in an Employee Handbook

> To complete the planning process, the organization should identify the topics to cover. Here is a comprehensive list from which to choose. *Note:* The subjects marked (P) are best spelled out in the policy manual alone and should be treated lightly, or not at all, in the employee handbook.

Introduction to the Company
____ Welcome letter from senior official
____ History and philosophy
____ Organization, divisions, and departments
____ Products, services, and philosophy
____ General communication
____ Organization publications, bulletin boards, and other media for communication
____ Ethical standards of the business
____ Conflicts of interest
____ Information to be treated in confidence
____ Working hours
____ Employee rights
____ Health and safety requirements

Dispute Resolution System
____ Handling grievances
____ Counseling services

Hiring Policies
____ Equal opportunity
____ Probationary periods
____ When and how to distribute the employee handbook

The Disciplinary Program
____ Progressive discipline procedures
____ When exceptions are in order

Performance Appraisal
____ Frequency and method
____ How performance is measured
____ How the results affect retention, pay, and promotion

Progressive Discipline
____ Typical offenses and penalties
____ Normal steps in the process
____ Guidelines for exceptions

Discharge Procedures (P)
____ Guidelines for decisions
____ Procedural steps

____ Security and confidential information
____ Obtaining releases
____ Outplacement services

Work Rules and Standards
____ Hours, regular and overtime
____ Attendance standards and notification requirements
____ Vacations, sick leave, and personal time off
____ Time clock rules; breaks and lunches
____ Smoking
____ Solicitation and visitors
____ Telephone use
____ Alcohol and drug policies
____ Security requirements
____ Lunches, travel, and reporting expenses
____ Care of organization's property
____ Waste control and prevention
____ Safety procedures and equipment
____ Dress and appearance
____ Outside employment
____ Sexual harassment
____ Tools
____ Weapons

Pay Policies
____ Paydays and payroll periods
____ Salary administration
____ Payroll deductions
____ Overtime and shift premiums

Benefits
____ Available benefits
____ Eligibility standards

Other Personnel Policies
____ Jury duty
____ Leaves of absence
____ Sick leave
____ Employee classification
____ Assignments and transfers
____ Layoffs and recalls (P)

---

sound method of establishing wages is through job evaluation. Job evaluation has three purposes: to determine the relative worth of the various jobs in the institution, to establish a wage scale that incorporates fair differentials among jobs, and to correct pay inequities where necessary. When defensible job rates are established on a quasi-scientific and logical basis, the issue of compensation is removed from the world of conjecture, arbitrariness, and subjectivity, and personalized rates are abolished. By establishing a formal wage pattern that conforms to health care facility wage rates in the area and in general with community wage rates, job evaluation is a key tool for the administration in meeting competition.

Job Evaluation Principles

The primary objective of job evaluation is to determine the relative worth of each job in the institution according to the basic determinant of each job's requirements. Once the relationship among jobs has been established, fair pay differentials can be designed, and any existing pay inequities can be corrected.

Because the job evaluation plan is the cornerstone of the compensation program of the health care facility, it is essential that the following basic principles be agreed upon at the outset:

- Grant upward salary adjustments to currently underpaid employees to conform with the findings of the evaluation.
- Prohibit any downward salary adjustments to current employees as a result of the evaluation.
- Pay employees at rates equal to or better than the rates for positions requiring comparable skill, effort, and responsibility in the industry and the community.
- Establish and maintain fair wage differentials among jobs in all departments in terms of the value of each job to the institution.
- Pay all employees in accordance with all applicable federal and state legislation or regulations governing wages, hours, and other conditions of work.
- Follow the principle of equal pay for equal work assignments in the institution.
- Recognize and reward employees based on their individual ability, outstanding performance, and length of service within the rate range established for the job occupied.
- Develop a plan that is objective, simple, and acceptable to the personnel affected.

- Develop a plan that is flexible and adaptable to the unique needs of the institution.

The two most commonly used types of job evaluation programs are the point method and the factor comparison method or variations thereof. Both are quantitative systems, and both consider each job one element at a time.

Job Analysis

Job analysis is the scientific determination of the actual nature of a specific job. Each of the tasks that make up the job is studied, as well as the skills, knowledge, abilities, and responsibilities required of the worker. Job analysis examines the job *as it is*—its duties, responsibilities, working conditions, and relationship to other jobs. There are three steps in the analysis of any job: identifying the job completely and accurately, describing the tasks of the job, and indicating the requirements for a successful performance.

Through a job analysis, job facts are secured for the following purposes:

- *Job evaluation:* The facts assembled from a job analysis are used in the evaluation of jobs that will set the wages.
- *Selection and placement:* Job analysis results in job descriptions—specifications that are an orderly and effective guide for matching applicants to positions.
- *Performance evaluation:* Qualified job descriptions provide standards against which an employee may be rated.
- *Training:* Detailed information provided by job analysis can serve as a basis for a training department's curriculum.
- *Labor relations:* Job analysis provides specific breakdowns of duties, which can be used to answer grievances regarding the nature of the employees' responsibilities.
- *Wage and salary survey:* Job analysis provides a method of comparing rates of jobs in one institution with those in others.
- *Organizational analysis:* Job analysis can clarify lines of responsibility and authority

by a detailed breakdown of each job and can indicate functional organizational positioning of jobs.

Job Descriptions

Once all the requirements of a specific job are assembled, the job analyst reviews the questionnaire and notes from an interview or direct observation and organizes the information into a job description.

Job descriptions become indispensable to the process of classifying work into management components. These descriptions must be widely publicized, and the manager and incumbents in each position must be in complete agreement with their contents.

APPROACHES TO SALARY POLICIES*

Salary Range

The salary ranges and levels are key ingredients to a successful salary program. They must be substantial enough to attract and retain the most able employees yet modest enough not to waste the health care facility's resources.

Each salary range provides for a minimum, a midpoint, and a maximum. The minimum must be high enough for 80 to 90 percent of the candidates to accept it as a starting salary. It must be competitive. The midpoint must be enough to retain the employee once he or she has become thoroughly skilled and contributing to the job. The maximum must be sufficient to retain the employee, avoiding loss by piracy or disenchantment.

To achieve these objectives, the salary range will usually be narrower at entry-level positions, broadening out either on a dollar or percentage basis at higher grades. A common variance in salary ranges is from 20 percent (minimum to maximum) at entry-level positions to 35 to 40 percent at the senior positions (department head). This reflects a greater need at senior levels for

Source: Skoler, Abbott & Presser, *Health Care Labor Manual*, Aspen Publishers, Inc., © January 1991.

salary flexibility to reward a greater variety of skills and to minimize turnover, the impact of which increases dramatically at high levels. Such differences in the breadth of ranges and salary levels introduce a great emphasis on market requirements as opposed to equity requirements. (See Figure 25–1 for a sample set of salary and wage guidelines.)

Merit versus Longevity

What will be the basis for individual salary determinations and salary increments? There are two major alternatives for consideration: the merit system and the longevity system.

The Merit Approach

To many, the merit system has a very logical theoretical base: The hard-working employee should be rewarded for superior effort and ability, and the resources of the organization should be directed primarily to substantial contributors rather than to the indolent and mediocre.

The merit system is characterized by the ranges of salary increase that an employee may receive, based on relative achievement reflected by his or her manager's recommendation at predetermined review times.

Also common to this approach are the concepts of salary minimum, midpoint, and maximum. The salary minimum is the starting rate for employees not having exceptional experience. The employee then moves to the midpoint by two to three increases, occurring at, for example, six-month intervals. The midpoint of the range is also the competitive rate for similar work being done in the community. The spread between minimum and midpoint reflects the learning period necessary to become job competent. Once an employee arrives at the midpoint of the range, salary review periods are longer (at least 12 months), and the basis for any change is exceptional rather than competent performance. The maximum salary is the highest that can be received by a person in a particular salary grade.

Some administrators have taken exception to the merit system and its salary range concept based on problems they have experienced in its operation, for instance:

Figure 25–1 Sample Salary and Wage Guidelines Form

FROM:	Administrator
TO:	Distribution List
SUBJECT	SALARY AND WAGE GUIDELINES
PURPOSE	To provide for a sound, fair, and equitable system of compensating health care facility employees by paying the best possible wages based on job evaluation, area wages, effect on organizational costs, and employee performance.
PAY PERIOD AND WORKWEEK	*Pay Period*—will begin Sunday morning at one (1) minute after Saturday midnight and end fourteen (14) days later at midnight Saturday. *Workweek*—will begin at one (1) minute after Saturday midnight and end Saturday midnight seven (7) days later.
OVERTIME	Authorized overtime will be paid at 1½ times the employee's regular rate for all hours *worked* in excess of forty (40) hours per workweek. Exemptions to the time and one-half provision will be based on the revised Federal Wage and Hour Laws and facility policy. All overtime must be approved prior to the hours of actual overtime work by the department head and countersigned by administration.
LEAVE	Leave paid hours are hours not actually worked and *will not* be included in the computation of overtime.
GRADES AND STEPS	All non–department head positions have been assigned a grade of 1–20. Each grade has a minimum step and eight other steps. Employees may progress within their grade by receiving step increases.
WAITING PERIOD	A waiting period is the length of time an employee must wait before proceeding to the next step in grade. New waiting periods begin with promotions and/or step increases. Merit increases *do not* change the waiting period. The minimum time (waiting period) required to advance from the minimum step to step 1 is six (6) months; from step 1 to step 2, step 2 to step 3, step 3 to step 4, etc., is one (1) year.
EXCEPTION: MERIT INCREASE	The exception to the above waiting period is the employee who is recommended for and received a merit increase (1 step). A merit increase recommendation, however, must be based on at least six (6) months of observed performance.
PROMOTIONS	Promotions will normally result in an approximate 10 percent increase in salary.
MAXIMUM ADVANCEMENT	Employees will not normally be advanced more than two (2) steps in any twelve (12) continuous months.
WITHHOLDING INCREASES	Step increases may be withheld with proper justification for a period not to exceed forty-five (45) days. If not granted than, a *new* waiting period will begin.
HIRING RATES	New employees will normally be hired at the minimum step of the position they are filling. New employees may be hired at step 1 or step 2 of the appropriate grade provided the department head and the human resources director agree. Hiring at above minimum will be guided by the following:

1. Applicants with from two (2) to five (5) years of directly related recent experience or an additional education degree deemed appropriate without experience may be hired at step 1.

continues

Figure 25–1 continued

2. Applicants with over five (5) years of directly related recent experience may be hired at step 2.
3. Applicants with from two (2) to five (5) years' experience (as in guideline 1) and an additional education degree deemed appropriate may be hired at step 2.
4. The above guidelines apply to applicants who the department head feels will be outstanding employees.

TRAINEES

New employees hired as bona fide trainees will normally be paid at 90 percent of the minimum step established for the position. The trainee will receive an increase to the minimum step when satisfactorily completing the training period. A new waiting period will begin with that increase.

SHIFT DIFFERENTIAL

Additional compensation will be paid to the following nursing personnel who work in ICU, CCU, PCU, OR, RR, and ED:

	Evening	*Night*
1. RN, lab technologist, respiratory therapist (Reg.)	$.25 ph	$.30 ph
2. LPN, X-ray tech., lab technician, respiratory therapy technician	$.15 ph	$.10 ph
3. All others	$.15 ph	$.10 ph

SPECIALTY DIFFERENTIAL

Additional compensation will be paid to the following nursing personnel who work in ICU, CCU, PCU, OR, RR, and ED:

Staff nurse	$.15 ph
LPN	$.10 ph
Nursing assistant	$.10 ph
Unit secretary	$.10 ph

CALL PAY

Employees subject to call will be paid at a rate of $1.00 per hour of call. Employees on call who are called in to work will be paid at their normal base rate for no less than one (1) hour for the first hour and any time beyond for actual time worked. Call pay stops when the normal shift begins and/or the employee comes to the facility in response to being called in.

EFFECTIVE DATES

Salary changes will be effective *only* at the beginning of a pay period.

RESPONSIBILITY AND AUTHORITY

The administrator or his or her designee will approve any salary increases. The human resources director will be responsible for staff supervision of the salary and wage program.

Submitted by: Approved by:

_____   _____

Director of Human Resources   Administrator

Distribution List:
All Departments

- If the midpoint is the competitive salary in the community, and particularly if many employees in the area are on a single-rate (union) system, how can employees be recruited at less than that midpoint rate?

- If the range between minimum and midpoint is the learning period, does not the learning period differ from job to job and person to person? Can there be an arbitrary time between minimum and midpoint?

- Can the health care facility remain competitive and deny employees some annual increase after they arrive at midpoint? If not, the notion of exceptional performance is in jeopardy.

- Finally, the most common criticism of the merit system is management's imprecise ability to determine degrees of merit, and the resulting small differences in salary between employees. In practice, can management effectively measure the differences in contribution? Is it possible that the employee who is less of a rival to the manager and is more deferential receives the larger increase?

This latter criticism is particularly common at entry-level positions, where degrees of merit are more difficult to determine.

These challenges to the basic merit system have resulted in conversion by some health care facilities to other systems, such as longevity.

However, many who retain a belief in the efficacy of rewarding merit have developed modifications to meet the weaknesses in the merit program. These include the following:

- establishment of step increments rather than a range of possible increase and a "go/no-go" decision by the manager on whether a raise is merited or is to be delayed to another specified review date (often must be approved at the next level of supervision)

- establishment of quantitative bases for evaluation wherever possible (e.g., attendance, typing production speed, etc.)

- development of participating approaches to performance evaluation, including self-appraisal, objectives-related appraisal, or appraisal by several managers

- moving to a longevity approach for entry-level positions, where differences in performance are difficult to assess

Under this program, employees would receive modest longevity increases to midpoint, then be reviewed on the merit system. Other employees, in positions whose achievements are more measurable, would be eligible for merit increases from the minimum.

The Longevity Approach

Much of the structure described under the merit system also applies to any pay increase program based on longevity. There is still the minimum, midpoint, maximum concept, with a person eligible for salary reviews at stated intervals. The principal difference is that increases are based on length of service only, irrespective of achievement. The employee's manager has no significant say in determining the amount or appropriateness of the increase.

An interesting factor about longevity is the recent growth in its use and its application by various groups. Historically, there has been an emphasis on longevity for nonprofessional groups. Presently, there is a tendency toward a longevity base also among many professional groups.

The growth in the use of the longevity system suggests some important advantages that should be noted.

- It eliminates a source of real stress between employer and employee, to the extent that employees have been dissatisfied with their managers' salary recommendations.

- It effectively counteracts union-organizing claims of arbitrary management by adopting the salary increase approach espoused by unions.

- Finally, it demands that managers concentrate on other ways of motivating employees.

There are also disadvantages attributed to any longevity program, including the following:

- There is no tangible way to reward excellence within a particular job.
- There is no way to encourage the resignation of marginal employees by withholding increases.
- Longevity forgoes any leverage provided by the merit program for a continuous, formalized performance appraisal program. This could also lead to a breakdown in the informal day-to-day performance appraisal process. Without this, employees who have taken their jobs for granted may be terminated without what they feel is adequate warning.
- A manager has little opportunity to assume responsibility and authority in a highly judgmental area.
- Finally, longevity creates the tendency to have narrow salary ranges (minimum to maximum) to avoid overpaying the modest performer. The regrettable effect of this decision is that exceptional performers are also limited.

Job Changes

Changes in position also require salary administration policies. These can include promotions, lateral transfers, demotions, and reevaluation of positions.

Promotions, by implication, usually involve a higher salary. Frequently, however, due to salary range overlap, an employee already is within the salary range for the new position. Nevertheless, most programs will provide an increase unless the employee is higher than the midpoint of the new salary range, which is a rare situation.

Lateral transfers demand salary review and thorough communications. Usually the employee will transfer to the new position at the same salary, assuming that the same skills are used in the new position. If, however, he or she is using a new set of skills, the salary should be negotiable.

It may even be less than before, in fairness to the coworkers in the new department.

An employee may be *demoted* for cause or because of personal preference; the difference is important. Commonly, health care institutions may employ a senior employee who is no longer able to perform his or her old job, whether due to personal disability or a change in the demands of the position. Under these circumstances, many programs allow the employee to transfer, retaining his or her previous salary level, but exclude the employee from merit review raises until the new salary range catches up to the salary level carried over.

When an employee requests a change to a lower graded position (e.g., the registered nurse who wishes to treat patients rather than supervise), the salary should be adjusted to a level no higher than the maximum of the grade for the new position. This is a negotiated process and may result in a salary level lower than the maximum.

Finally, when a job is *reevaluated*, employees should be treated as though promoted. They should be brought at least to the new minimum. To provide a proper spread, increases should also be allowed within the new range up to midpoint.

EMPLOYEE BENEFITS*

Determining Employee Needs

An employer must consider the needs of different groups of employees in selecting desired benefits and in setting priorities. The health care facility work force consists of a mixture of full-time and part-time employees. Long-term workers may change their work schedules from time to time. The staff will include a wide variety of skill levels ranging from highly paid professionals to low-paid unskilled workers. Some of the workers will be planning a career in health care, and others will be temporary, with high rates of termination.

Source: Anna M. Rappaport, "Benefit Plan Design Issues Today and through the 1980s," *Topics in Health Care Financing*, Vol. 6, No. 3, Aspen Publishers, Inc., © 1980.

A benefit program should be able to accommodate workers in different circumstances and at different times in their life cycles.

The traditional approach to benefit design has been to develop a single pattern of benefits, with some completely paid for by the employer, some cost shared, and some paid for solely by the employee. The working husband, dependent wife, and minor children model served as the family prototype around which this pattern was built. The employee's only choice was whether to participate in contributory coverages. This benefit pattern was chosen to represent a compromise that would best meet the needs of a majority of the work force.

Flexible Benefits

A new approach to benefit plan design is currently developing in the United States. This approach provides for flexible benefits and permits individual employees to tailor a benefit package that best fits individual needs. This new approach is in the experimental stage.

Such programs involve a core of benefits provided by the employer for all employees, together with numerical credits that allow employees to select additional benefits beyond the core.

The factors that will determine the pattern of benefits that best fits a particular employee are

- family situation
- availability of other sources of benefits
- willingness to assume risks
- priorities of the individual
- general financial situation

Whether this method will work well over the long term remains to be seen.

Chapter 26

Interviewing Applicants and Orientation

OVERVIEW: THE EMPLOYMENT PROCESS*

Effective recruitment requires determination of future needs, the clear definition and description of the types of people needed, and an evaluation and determination of methods to be used in each particular case.

Most health care facilities have accepted the need for centralized screening and decentralized hiring based on departmental/unit in-depth interviews.

The selection process has as its hallmark the effective appraisal of applicants' qualities that are indicative of job success. The process necessitates the making of a value judgment, a forecast as to which applicant will turn into a productive employee. To aid the employment department in fulfilling such responsibility, five tools are widely used; the application blank, interview, personnel tests, reference checks, and preemployment physicals.

*Source: Norman Metzger, "Human Resources Management," in *Health Care Administration: Principles, Practices, Structure, and Delivery,* ed 2, Aspen Publishers, Inc., © 1995.

INTERVIEWING JOB APPLICANTS

The In-Depth Interview

Following the initial screening by the human resources department, nursing administration should interview all acceptable nurse applicants.

Interview Form

Sometimes the notes taken during an interview are more important than the application form information in determining a job applicant's qualifications. The written record of the interview could be a simple narrative report or a more defined check-off list or fill-in form. A combination of the two concepts may be preferable, namely, a form with check-off items as well as ample space for comments. Such a form provides consistency among interviews and reminds the interviewer of points to be observed, while the blank spaces allow room for qualifying or explanatory remarks.

Interview Plan

The interview often focuses on the "persona" of the applicant. Application forms supply the factual details but interviews supply the live impression of the applicant in action—thinking, organizing, and explaining. After the initial introductions, the following areas of inquiry should be pursued with the applicant.

Personal Past Experience. The applicant should be asked to discuss his or her experiences as a child, as a student, and as an employee in other work situations. Questions can be asked about the nature of the experiences—the benefits, obstacles, disadvantages, and assessments.

General Attitudes toward Nursing, the Position, and the Facility. The applicant should be asked to discuss his or her philosophy of nursing and special interest in the specific position and the health care facility in general. If there are criticisms or reservations, these should be explored.

Sense of Self. The applicant should be questioned on immediate and eventual goals and realistic plans to accomplish these objectives. Ask the applicant to evaluate his or her own strong and weak points in professional work and interpersonal relations. Discuss the applicant's responses to authority, responsibility, innovation, and participation.

Personal Current Experiences. The applicant may be asked about whether any conflict might occur between work and private life. Find out about the range of private interests and professional associations that occupy the applicant's leisure time.

Information Interchange. At this point, the applicant may have questions about the position, and the interviewer should respond with forthright answers. Additional information on areas not covered by the interviewer may also be offered by the applicant at this time.

Interview Flow

Careful reading of the interview plan will reveal a flow and ebb to the procedure, a movement from the general to the particular and back again to the general. The first part of the interview acts as a warm-up, but the open-ended quality of the questions should reveal a great deal about the applicant: his or her approach to problems, professional pride, sincerity, and so forth.

By introducing all major topics with a broad, neutral question, a spontaneous response can be elicited. The applicant is allowed to direct the conversation to areas that have relevance for him or her, thus offering the interviewer grounds for more specific questions. If the applicant persistently sticks to generalizations, he or she should be asked to provide illumination by describing a situation from his or her experience. The intent is to discover how the applicant handles situations in the working environment and whether these reflect potential personality conflicts, faulty reasoning, lack of understanding, or inability to cope.

In the last phase, when the applicant is more relaxed and is discussing his or her personal life outside of the health care setting, the interviewer should note those traits that may be of value in the health care facility unit. Is the applicant narrow in scope or curious, interested in learning? Are the applicant's interests diverse or focused? Will any interest contribute to his or her value as a worker? Observe also those questions asked and not asked by the applicant. The type of in-

---

Interview Questions

The questions developed for an interview should be determined by the goals for hiring and by the job description for the position. The interview questions should (1) address the job requirements, (2) solicit information about the skills and qualities management is seeking, (3) seek examples of the applicant's experience, and (4) help determine willingness or motivation to do the job.

Specific questions about the applicant's qualifications should be developed from a combined analysis of the job description and the information the applicant has presented on the résumé and application.

Source: Lillian R. Tibbles, "Structured Interview: An Effective Strategy for Hiring," *Journal of Nursing Administration,* Vol. 23, No. 19, October 1993. J.B. Lippincott Company.

formation actively sought by the applicant is indicative of his or her real concerns and of an attempt to assess the situation in terms of his or her needs.

Guidelines for Questioning*

Although common courtesy should prevail in interview behavior at all times, courtesy itself is not enough. One must be constantly aware of questions or comments that could be taken as discriminatory in some way although not intended as such. An applicant may *volunteer* information related to the following precautions, but you may not ask for this information.

Questions To Avoid

Questions that require the applicant to reveal *age, date of birth, race, religion,* or *national origin* must not be asked. The direct questions— "When were you born?"—should be easy to avoid. Watch out, however, for indirect questions through which a person can claim the interviewer was "fishing" for specific information. For instance, a question that is not allowed is one such as: "I'd say we've both been around about the same length of time—both early baby boomers, perhaps?"

The matter of *age* has become a particularly sensitive area in recent years, calling for heightened awareness on the part of the supervisor. Although the Age Discrimination in Employment Act (ADEA) has been in place since 1967, it was given added scope and influence by the Age Discrimination in Employment Amendments Act of 1986, effective January 1, 1987. Although mostly the concern of the personnel or human resources department, this law nevertheless has implications for the supervisor.

The 1986 act prohibits mandatory retirement for most employees and removes the age 70 limit on ADEA protection. Therefore, stay away from all questions related to an applicant's long-term

intentions, such as "How long would you plan on working before thinking about retirement?" because of the age-related inferences that one might draw.

There is no safe question that the supervisor can ask about age, except perhaps to inquire whether an apparently young person is of legal age to enter full-time employment under the circumstances required of the job in question (in most instances, at least 18 years of age). Avoid all questions that either directly or indirectly call for age-related responses. Also, the supervisor must be assured that all the qualifications sought are truly related to the job. Interviewers should evaluate individual applicants on their individual capabilities and qualifications, not on general beliefs or personal preferences ("An older person just couldn't keep up," or "Someone her age would resist new technology," or "I want someone who's more likely to stay 10 or 20 years").

Similar to concerns about age, there are few if any safe questions the supervisor can ask about *disability,* whether a job candidate's disability is evident or not. The Americans with Disabilities Act (ADA) (1990) provides a national mandate barring bias against persons with disabilities This act calls for supportive and accommodating behavior by employers in maintaining disabled persons in the work force. Concerning the employment selection interview and the disabled person, the supervisor should ask questions about the applicant's qualifications and experience that focus strictly on the *essential functions of the job.* The job's peripheral activities that have no bearing on its essential functions—for example, occasional filing or report delivery related to the position of a billing clerk—are subject to "reasonable accommodation" by the organization and have no bearing on the person's capabilities as a billing clerk.

The supervisor may not ask if the applicant has a *recommendation* from a present employer. This may be taken as discriminatory, since it may be difficult for the applicant to secure such a recommendation because of reasons other than job performance (e.g., race, religion, political affiliation).

Interviewers can no longer ask the identity of the person's *nearest relative* or *"next of kin,"* even

---

*Source: Charles R. McConnell, *The Effective Health Care Supervisor,* ed 3, Aspen Publishers, Inc., © 1993.

for the simple purpose of having someone to contact in case of illness or accident. This can be taken as probing into the existence of spouse or family, which you cannot do. Even asking about "the person to be notified in case of illness or accident" is risky until the applicant is actually employed.

It is generally permissible to ask if an applicant is a *U.S. citizen* or is *legally eligible for employment.* However, this should not be an active concern of the supervisor if the personnel department is fulfilling its proper role in complying with the Immigration Reform and Control Act of 1986 (IRCA). This law requires employers to hire only U.S. citizens and lawfully authorized alien workers, and provides penalties and sanctions for employers who knowingly hire or continue to employ illegal aliens or who fail to verify legal eligibility for employment.

In compliance with IRCA, the personnel department must require an applicant to produce certain proofs of identity and employment eligibility within three working days *after* an offer of employment is made. For a supervisor's part in helping the organization comply with IRCA, one should resist the temptation to prevail on the personnel department to allow a much-needed new employee to begin work before the necessary proofs are produced.

Immigration reform has provided the work organization with a set of risks and pitfalls of a kind never previously experienced, and these risks and pitfalls cannot be avoided by backing away from the problem. The supervisor who might seek to avoid IRCA problems by not considering an applicant because of foreign appearance or language can face discrimination charges as defined by other laws.

In asking about the applicant's *military service,* the interviewer may inquire only into the general training and experience involved. One may not ask the character of the person's discharge or separation. Whether the discharge was honorable, dishonorable, general, or otherwise remains privileged information, which the applicant may reveal voluntarily but which the interviewer may not request.

The *marital status* of the applicant at the time of the interview may not be asked. Particular

sensitivity has developed along these lines in recent years. Many women have been able to claim, with considerable success, that they were denied employment because of marital status. Employers often proceeded on the assumptions, sometimes statistically substantiated, that:

- young women recently engaged often quit shortly after they got married
- young, recently married women may leave after a year or two to begin families
- ummarried women with small children tend on the average to have poorer attendance records than other workers

Even if an applicant, male or female, has willingly revealed marriage on a résumé, it is not permitted to ask what the spouse does for a living. In the case of a married female applicant, it is also forbidden to ask her maiden name because this question can be interpreted as probing for clues to national origin.

The interviewer may not ask if the applicant *owns a home or a car.* This may be interpreted as seeking to test affluence, which may in turn be taken as discriminatory against certain minorities. One may, however, ask if the applicant has a driver's license—*if* driving is a *bona fide occupational qualification* (BFOQ), that is, a requirement of the job. (Generally, one is on the soundest footing when all questions of a personal nature relate to BFOQs.)

Interviewers may not ask if the applicant's *wages were ever attached or garnished.* Credit information is privileged information; it may be volunteered by the applicant but not requested by the prospective employer.

Interviewers may not directly ask any applicant's *height* or *weight.* Neither of these factors should have a bearing on the applicant's suitability for the job unless there is a specific job-related requirement (BFOQ) that is uniformly applied to all applicants.

Beware of requesting an applicant to take *qualification* tests. Preemployment tests have been under fire as discriminatory in matters of age, race, and economic background. Preemployment testing is best left to professionals who design tests that are specifically related to the requirements of the job, statistically validated as nondiscriminatory, administered consistently and in good faith, and evaluated impartially.

There are also pitfalls to be encountered in asking an applicant's *educational level,* such as completion of high school or possession of a college degree. An employer may require specific educational levels when these are directly related to job performance (again, BFOQs). Otherwise, it may be possible to show a pattern of employment discrimination. One can require, for instance, a nurse to possess a diploma or degree and a state license since these are essential to the performance of the job as it is structured. However, one cannot require a housekeeping maid or kitchen helper to have a high school diploma since it is possible to demonstrate that people in these job categories may perform equally well with or without the diploma. Effective personnel department procedures should take most of the burden off the interviewer in this matter.

Interviewers can no longer ask if an applicant has ever been *arrested.* An arrest is simply a charge, not a conviction. It has even become risky to ask if a person has ever been convicted of a crime. Most courts have ruled that after a few years have passed following conviction and correction, the individual need not be called on to reveal this information. Unless the job is clearly related to safeguarding money or security (a BFOQ), it is best to refrain from this line of questioning.

Interviewers may not ask whether an applicant is or has been a member of a *union* or has been involved in organizing or other union activities.

Interviewers may not ask any obviously older applicants if they are receiving *Social Security* benefits. It has been demonstrated concerning older persons applying for part-time work that some employers have discriminated in favor of applicants receiving Social Security payments, since a person receiving a combined income may be more likely to remain on the job longer than one to whom the part-time job is the sole means of support.

Questions To Ask

The questions one is permitted to ask are broad and in many instances open ended. This is as it should be; remember, one is interested in learning as much as possible about the applicant in a limited amount of time and the way to do this is to listen to the person talk. Try these in conversation with the applicant:

- What are your career goals? What would you like to be doing five or ten years from now? How would you like to spend the rest of your career?
- Who have been your prior employers, and why did you leave your previous positions?
- What did you like or dislike about the work in your previous positions?
- Who recommended you to our institution? How did you hear about this job opening?
- What is your educational background? What lines of study did you pursue? (Be careful, however, of attempting to delve into specifics as cautioned in the list of questions to avoid.)
- What do you believe are your strong points? What do you see as your weaknesses?
- Have you granted permission for us to check references with former employers (see following section)?

If the personnel department has not already done so, ask the applicant to explain any gaps of more than a few weeks duration that appear in the résumé or application. Some applicants will omit mention of unsuccessful job experiences or other involvements that they believe might reflect negatively on their chances of being hired. The hiring supervisor should be in a position to make a fully informed decision based on more than just selected pieces of a candidate's background. Also, the supervisor shares a responsibility for ensuring that the organization is protected from possible negligent hiring charges should an employee who was hired without reasonable background verification cause harm.

Psychological Barriers at Interviews*

Unequal Power

The emotional state of each party in an interview is likely to be entirely different. The interviewer can afford to be relaxed and comfortable—perhaps even blasé. The interviewee cannot enter into this relationship in such a relaxed manner, however; it is far too important. Given this situation, it is perhaps even naive to expect that the typical applicant can be at ease during the interview. On the contrary, managers should expect in many cases to see an applicant who is ill at ease, uncomfortable, and nervous. This is certainly a very natural way to react to a stressful situation. If managers convince themselves that the seemingly comfortable, self-assured applicant is somehow "better" than the uncomfortable and nervous applicant, they run the risk not only of basing their decision on largely superficial personality traits but also of potentially succumbing to the second psychological barrier: "phoney" behavior.

"Phoney" Behavior

Related to the power imbalance inherent in job interviews is what can best be termed "phoney" behavior. Phoney behavior is familiar to anyone who has done extensive job interviewing—the feeling that the applicant is attempting to project an "image," to convey an impression of being a certain type of person. To get a job, many applicants seem to feel, one must be perceived as sociable, highly intelligent, considerate, and so on. They love to "work with people," never have problems with superiors, and are universally liked; they are seeking a job with challenge, responsibility, and an opportunity to prove themselves. The clichés runneth over.

*Source: Richard G. Nehrbass, "Psychological Barriers to Effective Employment Interviewing," Personnel Journal, February 1977. Reprinted with the permission of Personnel Journal, Costa Mesa, California; all rights reserved.

Questions without Answers

The third psychological barrier to effective employment interviewing is the tendency of some interviewers to ask questions that do not really have answers. Some examples include "Tell me something about yourself," "How would you describe yourself?" and "Where would you like to be 10 years from now?"

Given the power imbalance in the situation and the emphasis on phoney behavior, there is little reason to believe that answers to these questions are completely honest anyway. This puts the interviewer in the position of providing a probably incorrect analysis of a dishonest answer from a tense and uncomfortable applicant.

Overcoming the Barriers

Awareness of these three barriers can aid an interviewer. Awareness, by itself, will not solve the problem, but it can emphasize to the interviewer the need to create (to the extent possible) a psychologically safe and supportive atmosphere for the interview. The interviewer can show by behavior and active attention to the applicant that he or she considers the interview to be as important as the applicant does.

A short introductory statement to the effect that the organization is looking for the best person to fit the position, rather than any particular personality type, can also partially alleviate the applicant's felt need to project a certain image.

Perhaps, most importantly, the interviewer can ensure that the interview stresses facts and not opinions or feelings. Through an emphasis on questions that require the applicant to relate factual events from the past, the interviewer can steer the conversation away from projecting an image and toward reality.

A number of these factually oriented questions exist and have been used by some interviewers for years. It is usually a good idea to pair a "positive" with a "negative" question to further reduce the uneasiness of the applicant. An example would be "There are always some things about our jobs we like and some we dislike. Tell me a couple of things about your last job that you particularly liked and a couple of things you particularly disliked." This question can also be asked about the applicant's previous superiors. Another such question is "What were some of the things about your last job that you felt were particularly difficult to do? What were some of the things you did best?"

OVERVIEW: INDUCTION AND ORIENTATION

A new employee forms permanent and, too often, irreversible attitudes toward the job, the manager, and the health care facility much earlier than management believes. The preliminary task of induction and orientation has been assigned to human resources departments, with special emphasis on the social adjustment to a new milieu. If an induction and orientation program is to succeed, it must have clearly stated and publicized objectives, must be thoroughly understood, and must be carefully planned.

In general, objectives are to reinforce the employee's confidence in his or her ability to cope with the new work assignment, to communicate complete and detailed conditions of the person's employment, to inform the person of rules and regulations governing his or her employment, and to instill in the employee a feeling of pride in the organization. A formal induction program is held on the institutional level to fulfill the second and third objectives. The nursing department and unit conduct their own program to meet the objectives related to work assignments and "local" team pride.

The premise one builds upon in an orientation program is that an employee who is informed—who knows the what, why, how, and when of his or her role in the large organizational structure—is likely to be more efficient, motivated, and sympathetic to the total goals of the health care facility than one who does not possess this knowledge. Essentially, the expense of a sound and effective formal induction and orientation program is infinitesimal when com-

pared to the cost of employee turnover and inefficiency.*

Program Scope**

The number of nursing instructors and clerical staff required depends on the number and type of training programs needed, which may be as various as on-the-job skill training for nursing assistants or inservice education for inexperienced nurses requiring special preparation in clinical specialties.

All newly employed personnel are entitled to be oriented to the health care facility as a total institution and specifically to the nursing service. (See Table 26–1.) The orientation program usually includes a tour of the physical setting, as well as information on the philosophy, goals, and structure of the overall facility, and is conducted by the human resources department.

The nursing department conducts its own tour. Functions of the various members of the nursing team and nursing care standards are usually emphasized. Under normal circumstances, it takes only a few days to orient new employees to the work situation and setting. However, since many new graduates lack sufficient clinical practice in the generic nursing programs, many health care facilities have had to combine orientation and inservice education during the initial period of employment to prepare the nurse to function as a beginning-level practitioner.

Individualized Training**

The inservice education program to help the new nurse become proficient in clinical nursing skills must be individualized, since nurses differ in their educational background and work expe-

---

Source: Norman Metzger, "Human Resources Management," in *Health Care Administration: Principles, Practices, Structure, and Delivery,* ed 2, Aspen Publishers, Inc., © 1995.

**Source:* Reprinted with permission from G. Matsunaga, *Concerns in the Acquisition and Allocation of Nursing Personnel,* © 1978, National League for Nursing.

Table 26–1 Outline: Self-Learning Manual for Nursing Department RN Orientation

Section A—General Information
RN/GN Competencies
Organizational Chart
Department of Nursing—Purpose and
   Objectives
Department of Nursing Statement of
   Philosophy
Facility Map
Policy and Procedure Review Worksheet
Patient's Bill of Rights
Code of Nurses

Section B—Documentation
Charting Guidelines
Guidelines for the Use of Nursing Diagnosis
Flowsheets
Patient Teaching Records

Section C—Transcription of Orders
Transcription Process
Transcription of Medication Orders
Use of the Medication Sheet
Medication Administration Times

Section D—Pharmacy Information
Medicated Large Volume IVs
Ordering Intermittent IVs
Pharmacy Forms
Pharmacokinetics
Aseptic Technique
Unit Dose System
Medication Calculations

**Section E—Admitting, Transferring, and
Discharging Patients**
Routine Scheduled Admissions
Transfers: in house, to a hospital or home
   health care agency, to a long-term care
   facility
Discharges: routine, against medical advice,
   deceased

Section F—General Communication
Shift-to-Shift Report
Patient Classification
Communication with Nutritional Services
Communication with Family Practice
   Center—Residents
Laboratory Reports
Incident Reports
Central Distribution System

Section G—Emergency Plans/Safety
Fire Fighting Plan
Procedure for Evacuation of Patients,
   Visitors, and Staff
Tornado Alert
Bomb Threat Plan
Disaster Plan
Hazard Communication

Section H—Suicide Policy
Identifying Suicidal Patients
Suicide Precautions
Case Study

Evaluations

---

rience. The observed and felt learning needs can best be identified through the use of a checklist that involves the active participation of both the trainee and instructor. This type of basic preparation may extend from two weeks to over a month, depending on the learning needs of the nurse. However, if the new nurse is to be assigned to an intensive care unit, he or she will probably require much more time in the training program. The preparation of the new graduate, however, is not the sole responsibility of the inservice education staff. Nurse managers, clinicians, and head nurses on the services on which the nurse is assigned are also responsible for closely working with the nurse to further develop his or her com-

petencies in nursing practice and to reinforce knowledge acquired in the formal teaching situation. The supportive help and guidance given to the new nurse in this early phase of employment is crucial for further development of the potentials of the nurse and for a healthy adaptation to the work situation.

If unskilled workers employed as nursing assistants will be involved in direct patient care services, they must be provided with on-the-job skill training. They must be taught the knowledge and skills required to perform their defined functions, with measures taken to safeguard the quality of nursing care. To continue their employment, nursing assistants should successfully pass paper-and-pencil tests and a practical examination on skill performance.

Supervised Practice*

The appropriate allocation or assignment of newly recruited nurses cannot be based solely on the staffing requirements of the various clinical services if the goal is to retain qualified and competent nursing personnel. A number of health care facilities place new graduates on selected general medical-surgical units to gain basic nursing care experience under close supervision and guidance prior to assignment to other clinical specialties. Also, it is often found essential to rotate new nurses to evenings and nights during the initial phase of employment. Nursing administration is responsible for ensuring that these new graduates receive sufficient orientation, supervision, and support in rendering patient care and in carrying out their other assigned functions. The new graduate is vulnerable and will be greatly influenced by the attitudes, expectations, and behavior of the head nurse. The relationship that is established between the new graduate and the head nurse is a key factor in determining the adaptation, productivity, and satisfaction of the staff nurse. Nursing administrators must give thought to assigning the impressionable new staff nurse to head nurses who can serve as healthy role models and who have the interest and patience to work with newly employed nursing personnel.

Department Orientation Activities

- Support the new employee during the transition period to the assigned area.
- Assist the new employee in identifying individual strengths and weaknesses.
- Provide an ongoing appraisal of the new employee's performance during orientation via regularly scheduled meetings.
- Provide an introduction, review of basic skills, and selected learning experiences based on individual needs.
- Act as a liaison between the employee and the staff, assisting and encouraging the staff to participate in teaching the new employee.

Source: Copyright © 1987, Ellen Lewis.

---

*Source: Grace Matsunaga, *Concerns in the Acquisition and Allocation of Nursing Personnel,* National League for Nursing, Pub. No. 20-1709, 1978. Reprinted with permission.

Chapter 27

Labor Relations

UNIONIZATION IN HEALTH CARE FACILITIES

Status of Union Organizing in Health Care*

Since health care employees were given the right to organize and bargain collectively for wages and benefits under the National Labor Relations Act (NLRA), about 20 percent of health care workers have joined unions. About the same percentage of U.S. hospitals have one or more bargaining units. Most of the union organizing activity occurred in the late 1970s and early 1980s, and organizing activity has been on the decline ever since. The rate of union victories has remained fairly constant, however, with around 55 percent of elections being won by unions.

There are indications that union activity may increase, however. The recent National Labor Relations Board (NLRB) rule that established eight categories of hospital workers as separate bargaining units is perceived as an opportunity for significant gains for unions. (*Note:* Registered nurses are one of the separate bargaining units.) The economic climate and the uncertainty of health care financing may also motivate employees to seek the protections promised by organized labor. These conditions will serve to exacerbate an organization's vulnerability to unionization. However, unions are still most likely to target organizations that have weak, insensitive supervision and arbitrary, inconsistent practices concerning pay, promotions, and grievance resolution.

Labor Relations Responsibilities

Where unions have successfully organized a segment of workers, there is a need for specialists in collective bargaining and contract administration. Understanding the applicable laws, advising managers on appropriate actions relative to unionized employees, and maintaining effective union and employee relations are part of the labor specialist's role.

In the *unionized organization,* a key labor relations responsibility is negotiating the contract on behalf of the employer. Other key responsibilities include preparing the organization to handle work stoppages or strikes, administering the contract on a day-to-day basis, and dealing with grievances and arbitration.

Source: Laura Avakian, "Human Resource Management," in *Manual of Health Services Management,* Robert J. Taylor, ed., Aspen Publishers, Inc., © 1994.

In a *nonunionized setting,* staff must also be familiar with labor law and know legal, effective ways to respond to union organizing attempts. When organizing efforts are under way, those responsible for employee relations need to educate managers regarding their responsibilities according to the NLRA. In nonunionized organizations, key employee relations tasks include developing supervisory policies and writing employee handbooks that define fair treatment and the rules of the organization. Many of the policies are similar to those found in union contracts. The handbooks delineate conditions under which employees may be laid off, disciplined, or discharged and include policies on such subjects as overtime, uniforms, and lunch and break periods.

Management and Union Campaigns*

> The percentage of wins for unions depends on the amount of institutional communication. The institution's win rate goes up appreciably if it has an extensive communication program.

Management failures are the root cause of the majority of successful union campaigns. Management failures include the lack of understanding of employees; the lack of salary and fringe

---

Source: Norman Metzger, "Addressing Employee Needs in the 1990s," *Hospital Materiel Management Quarterly,* Vol. 11, No. 4, Aspen Publishers, Inc., © May 1990.

Unions in the 1990s

Unions are discovering that old approaches to union organization, particularly in health care facilities, are not working. New forces emerging in the work environment will affect union organization. To start with, there is a changing configuration of employer-employee relationships. Management structures are experiencing a major redevelopment; more attempts are being made to address commitment, to provide fulfilling and meaningful work, and to increase motivational opportunities. Quality-of-life programs are more prevalent today than in the past. Empowering workers, which means giving them more ability for independent judgments regarding discipline, promotions, job assignments, and so forth, blurs the line between the manager and workers. Shared governance and self-directed work teams, which appear to be an anathema to unions, are increasing and may well be a factor in the decline of the union movement.

Confrontational approaches to solving work problems, at which unions were so adept, have little or no appeal to old or young workers. The name of the game is not adversarial labor relations. Many workers are now turned off by the constant threats and rhetoric surrounding employer-union confrontations at negotiating time. The strike as a useful process for settling disputes is now in question more than ever before. Workers' needs are rarely addressed through the strike mechanism. Profit sharing, gain sharing, employee stock option plans, and bonus incentive and performance-based pay systems have much more interest to workers than is obvious from the negative reaction of unions to such plans.

Under new work conditions, the traditional package of union services has little appeal and is often irrelevant. It is clear that unions must reassess their approaches to organizing due to the most serious challenge to their power and influence they have faced for many decades.

Source: Norman Metzger, "Addressing Employee Needs in the 1990s," *Hospital Materiel Management Quarterly,* Vol. 11:4, Aspen Publishers, Inc., © May 1990.

benefit competitiveness; the lack of clear and usable communication lines; the lack of sound personnel policies; the lack of a formal and understandable grievance mechanism; the lack of appropriate and acceptable working conditions; the presence of arrogant, insensitive, overworked, and harried managers; and the presence of management that is not employee centered. When groups of employees are faced with a choice of voting for or against the union, they often think in terms of the relationships with their managers. If health care institutions are to meet the challenge of the 1990s, not only in maintaining a nonunion status, but also, more importantly, in dealing with falling productivity, they must provide an environment that gives employees

- more individual job freedom
- greater input into matters that affect their jobs
- greater control over their work schedules
- more enlightened supervision
- opportunities for advancement and educational experience

CONTEMPORARY ISSUES AND UNIONS

Participative Structures in a Labor Context*

Participative management via employee teams and shared governance structures have been practiced in an increasing number of work organizations. Total quality management (TQM) programs are spurring even greater emphasis on participative management, tending to bring more and more employees further into self-determination on the job. More and more is being done with the involvement of employees by way of employee teams.

---

*Source: Charles R. McConnell, "Getting Maximum Value from Employee Teams—and Keeping Them Legal," *The Health Care Supervisor,* Vol. 13, No. 1, Aspen Publishers, Inc., © September 1994.

There are, however, areas of employee involvement in which teams are seen as intruding on the territory of labor unions. There is a constant risk that a given employee team could be adjudged an illegal labor organization under the National Labor Relations Act.

Some ideas for employee involvement could readily lead to group structures that might be considered as infringing on the rights of collective bargaining organizations.

What the NLRB Apparently Looks For

The reason for this stance by the NLRB is the interpretation that in establishing the National Labor Relations Act years ago, Congress prohibited employer interference with labor organizations to ensure that such groups were free to act independently of employers in representing the interests of employees.

An employee team or committee might be considered an employer-dominated, illegal labor organization for any of a number of reasons. These reasons include the following:

- whether the group is perceived to be dealing with wages, hours, benefits, grievances, or other terms and conditions of employment (the issues most frequently subject to collective bargaining)
- if committee suggestions or recommendations result in management decisions but the group itself does not have the power to actually make the decisions
- if employees are elected to the group as representatives of larger bodies of employees
- if employees see the group as a means of resolving their concerns with management
- if meetings appear to involve "negotiation" between employees and members of management

The NLRB decisions should not be allowed to deter the use of employee teams in health care organizations. The active use of employee participation and input via teams or committees is near the heart of every total quality and empowerment initiative.

Steps To Take

Short of actually establishing teams or committees to wrestle with certain issues, there are a number of steps that can be taken to encourage employee participation and avoid union-related conflict.

When establishing a team or committee, identify it up front as *not* intended as an employees' channel to management. Have a clear mission or charge in place before soliciting team membership, and have the team's functions and limits identified before any team activity begins.

Keep the team focused on process improvement topics only. This requires plenty of continuing vigilance. It can be difficult to talk about quality, efficiency, productivity, and similar issues without conditions of employment becoming involved, so be constantly aware of the potential need to periodically redefine the team's boundaries.

Staff teams with volunteers, or use rotating membership selected by some means that is not management dominated. If a team is empowered to make a final management decision, that is, the team decides in place of management, not just recommends to management, it can be seen as *acting as management*. This is acceptable. In fact, it has been suggested that the ultimate protection against being ruled an illegal labor organization exists when the team can make final decisions in its own right.

If an issue is sufficiently narrowly defined that all persons affected by it can be included in a single group, a "committee of the whole" including everyone is usually legally safe. In such an instance, nobody can be seen as "representing" anyone else.

For standing committees or long-lived teams, maintain a majority membership of managers. A committee or team composed of a majority of managers stands less chance of being adjudged illegal under the National Labor Relations Act, but it is also far less likely to be seen as a legitimate vehicle for employee participation.

Consider establishing specific problem-solving or work improvement ad hoc groups, each with a specific, well-defined charge and a specific problem to solve, and disband each group after its goals have been attained. Management representatives can serve as observers or facilitators, without the power to vote on proposals or dominate or control the group.

Union Issues in Work Design*

Within the past few years, significant numbers of health care facilities have been forced to realign human resource utilization with shifts in patient volumes from inpatient to outpatient services. Such realignment has typically included restructuring of operations, elimination of management positions and/or layers, and decreased numbers of employees at the point of care or business encounter within the organization. These activities have frequently coincided with elements of work redesign: specifically, the identification of new roles within resized or restructured organizations to deliver patient care effectively and efficiently. For all health care workers, fear associated with job change or insecurity has heightened union awareness. For nursing professionals, labor organizations have stimulated interest in unions by suggesting potentially adverse effects of work redesign on the quality and safety of patient care.

Because of the extent of work redesign currently occurring in health care organizations and the corresponding perceptions about job security and potential representations about quality of patient care, unions are being provided with fertile ground for employee consideration of union representation in health care organizations. In preparation for project initiation, leadership teams should conduct an analysis of the features typically found in a work reengineering initiative that contribute to union awareness in health care organizations.

Source: Carol Boston, "Reengineering in Health Care: Labor Relations Issues," in *Reengineering Nursing and Health Care: The Handbook for Organizational Transformation,* Suzanne Smith Blancett and Dominick L. Flarey, eds., Aspen Publishers, Inc., © 1995.

Downsizing. Nationwide health care reform endeavors, driven by political agendas and the private sector, have resulted in a tremendous shift in inpatient versus outpatient utilization of health care services within health care organizations and systems. Efforts to redesign clinical services that focus on health instead of illness and the need to deliver more cost-effective services in the wake of increased managed care/capitated payer arrangements have spearheaded substantial reductions in hospital inpatient utilization and the simultaneous need to adjust human resource utilization according to service needs.

Union experts agree that loss of position, pay, or job is ample incentive for health care workers to rebel and seek union representation for protection of their overall welfare.

Skill-Mix Changes. Human resources (wages and benefits) typically exceed 50 percent of a hospital's operating budget. Nurses are the largest group of employees; hence, nursing costs are the largest expenditure in the human resource budget. As a health care organization seeks opportunities for improving its overall cost structure to ensure financial viability in an increasingly competitive, managed care market, utilization of all resources comes under scrutiny, including the largest resource—human resources. In particular, how nursing professionals, specifically registered nurses, are being used in the care delivery setting has become a prime consideration as part of the major work reengineering projects. Customarily, an organization undergoing work redesign seeks to create jobs that call for all professionals, including registered nurses, to function at the upper limits of licensure. Such redesigning requires the simultaneous commitment to assign an unlicensed worker to patient care activities that could be performed by someone other than a registered nurse.

Organizations that conduct work reengineering, depending on various internal factors, are demonstrating substantial changes in skill mix that comply with relevant state nurse practice acts and simultaneously yield substantive, annualized savings in labor costs.

Skill-mix changes within a health care organization as part of a work redesign initiative will undoubtedly result in decreased numbers of jobs for licensed professionals, including registered nurses. Two areas in which heightened sensitivity to the need for a union can be anticipated are (1) the loss of job availability for incumbents because of skill-mix changes and (2) the delegation to unlicensed caregivers of tasks that have been historically assumed by licensed professionals.

The Process of Redesign. The process or methodology a health care organization selects to guide its work reengineering design initiative can be a major determinant of union-organizing activity. Employees in contemporary health care organizations desire an active role in organizational decision making. Hence, the more participative the process is for employees, the more likely it is that union sensitivity will be appropriately controlled during a work reengineering initiative.

Labor Relations Strategy in a Changing Work Environment

The manner in which employees are treated is significant on an ongoing basis, but when change initiatives are undertaken—facility mergers or structural/work redesign—a union "hot spot" is created. Developing an effective labor relations strategy as part of work reengineering should be a mandatory component of the overall plan in order to achieve organizational outcomes, mitigate union sensitivity, manage union relations, and avoid charges of unfair labor practice.

Whether a health care organization is unionized or not is irrelevant. Nonunion organizations will want to remain union free. Unionized organizations will desire union cooperation and the avoidance of any adversarial union-management relationships. The following labor relations strategies are applicable to all health care organizations—unionized or union free:

- *Communication:* Communicate openly, honestly, and frequently about the organization's commitment to work transformation.
- *Involvement:* Use a work reengineering process that provides for relevant and compre-

hensive involvement of employees and managers.

- *Recruitment and staff selection:* Design a solid human resources strategy for the recruitment and selection of staff into newly designed jobs.
- *Employee opportunity:* Provide relevant and sufficient opportunities for employee education and training.
- *Management education:* Provide management education for all managers and department heads regarding union prevention strategies and tips for detecting potential union activity.

LABOR RELATIONS AND THE NURSE MANAGER*

The nurse executive must understand laws relating to the organizing of workers into unions, the negotiation of a labor contract between employees and management, and the administration of a contract by the nurse executive.

This is only part of the task. He or she must also consider the intermix of personnel relations and labor relations, with the former based on constitutional law and the latter originating in contract law. Although good personnel relations do not necessarily protect an institution from contract disputes, poor personnel relations leave an institution open to unionization, many grievances, and costly suits.

Errors in Personnel Relations

Three personnel systems affect staff attitudes toward unionization and grievances: the wage and salary administration system, the performance appraisal and disciplinary system, and the supervisory system.

Inequitable salary distribution is a major factor. A worker may be drawing a high salary, but

Source: Barbara Stevens Barnum and Karlene M. Kerfoot, *The Nurse as Executive,* ed 4, Aspen Publishers, Inc., © 1995.

if a coworker with less seniority and less responsibility draws a higher one, he or she will be discontent. In a nursing division, inequities may lead to unionization or, when a house is already unionized, in attempts to dictate salary by labor contract. When unions enter into salary distribution, the principle of seniority is inevitably advanced.

Although seniority sounds like a principle a nurse executive could live with, it is not that easy. First, salaries fixed by seniority tie the executive's hands as to merit pay, and that removes one of the performance incentives. Worse, once a principle of seniority takes precedence in job retention—a logical extension of pay by seniority—the successful operation of the institution may be jeopardized.

An example is an acquired immune deficiency syndrome (AIDS) unit where an intelligent, committed head nurse had worked diligently to build a well-working team. The staff gave excellent care and each member was devoted to working with AIDS patients. Then, the institution experienced downsizing. Because of a labor contract based on seniority, nurses on closed units were allowed to "bump" nurses with less time in the system.

Nurses on this unit were vulnerable—they were among the more recently hired, the unit being only three years old. In an era when nursing jobs were scarce, the bumping privileges were exercised. More than half the staff of the unit were replaced with nurses from other specialties as distant as obstetrics and orthopedics.

For the most part, the replacement nurses resented having to work with AIDS patients and could not wait for other opportunities to open up in the system. The spirited working team of the unit was destroyed. Then, bit by bit, the nurses who had bumped them returned to their regular units as vacancies opened up by attrition. This left the unit in flux for more than year. At about the time the unit stabilized, another downsizing occurred, initiating the process all over again. The difficulties experienced by the AIDS unit were played out on many other units as well—all in the name of seniority.

The goal of equity (as intended by a seniority system) may be easier to apply in the employee disciplinary system. If some employees constantly ignore policies (e.g., those relating to tardiness and absenteeism) without any penalty while others are penalized according to the rules, then morale sinks. Because inequity of treatment is a major factor inciting unionization and grievances, nurse managers simply cannot implement policies discriminately.

An institution needs a good grievance procedure available to the employee who believes he or she has been unfairly judged or disciplined. The grievance procedure should be clear and simple to follow; it should not have too many steps until final resolution is achieved. If a licensed practical nurse has a dispute at the unit level that is not settled to his or her (or the union's) satisfaction, it should not be necessary that it be heard at every intervening level—head nurse, supervisor, department director, vice president for nursing, and president. Most grievance procedures sidestep the usual chain of command, shortening this procedure. Often, the final hearing officer is appointed from the personnel department, although this is not invariable. The nurse managers of an institution must not deviate from the established pattern for grievance hearings.

The executive must see that the grievance procedures are applied precisely. Most grievance procedures have time limits for how soon after an incident a grievance must be filed and for how soon after a hearing the hearing officer must respond. The procedure must be applied without exceptions.

Because the hearing officers in grievance cases are managers of the institution, hearings must not be loaded in favor of management. If the grievance is merely a *pro forma* event, with the outcome easily forecast, then the procedure will cause more discontent than would exist without it. Where there is such bad faith, *pro forma* hearings result in a large number of expensive arbitration cases. When there is not a union contract, unfair grievance hearings may result in moves to unionize. Unfortunately, some hearing officers are so threatened by employee action that they are prejudiced in favor of the grieving employee. In this case, the institution makes a travesty of management by undercutting their power.

The aim of any grievance hearing should be that of fair resolution.

Managerial Principles for Labor Relations

When labor contracts already exist or when the potential for contractual relations exists, the nurse executive must know what laws are applicable. All private hospitals, both profit and nonprofit, fall under the provisions of the Labor Management Relations Act (LMRA). The act incorporates the National Labor Relations Act (NLRA), the Wagner Act of 1936, the Taft-Hartley Amendment of 1947, and the Health Care Amendment Act of 1974.

If the nurse executive is in a federal institution, then labor relations are covered by Executive Order 11491 as amended and the Federal Personnel Manual. This order functions in the federal public sector much as the LMRA does in the private. However, the provisions of the two documents are not identical, so the nurse executive will need copies of the legislation that affects her institution. If the nurse executive is in an agency in the public sector but under a state or political subdivision rather than in a federal institution, then he or she must check on the laws of the state to find out the status of collective bargaining. Both the LMRA and the aforementioned executive order make collective bargaining mandatory. When collective bargaining is *not* mandatory, the agency still may elect to enter into bargaining on a voluntary basis.

The nurse executive must know whether he or she must bargain with an elected union and what enabling rules he or she must follow. He or she should have access to an expert labor relations consultant if new to the collective bargaining process. Consultation is needed long before negotiation begins and consultation should be sought at the start of any unionizing activity. Some institutions handle unionizing within the personnel department, but if part of the nursing staff are involved in unionizing, there will be impacts on the nursing division that go beyond the interests and attention of the typical personnel department.

Often, the nurse executive seeks expert help only after a contract has been negotiated that is virtually impossible to execute. One director who had relied on others to negotiate a contract discovered the agreement allowed all vacation time to be taken at the employees' discretion. This seriously affected the budget, incurring unanticipated replacement salaries.

Finally, the nurse executive must realize that labor relations are bilateral; they divide people into two camps—managers and employees. Labor relations work on the principle of balance created by the push and pull of the vested interests of the two sides. Many nurses and even nursing organizations are hesitant to admit to this division between worker and manager. It fights against the sense of unity created among professional colleagues. It can also be difficult to determine who is in management and who is in staff. Indeed, a recent case raises new issues by calling a bedside nurse a manager.

The nurse executive recognizes that his or her role as manager necessarily gives a unilateral position at the negotiating table on management's side. If he or she is ambiguous in an attempt to show unity with the nursing staff, all sides will suffer from an imbalance in the bilateral relationship. Labor relations are based on the principles of conflict and negotiation, not on principles of synergism and cooperation, and this is difficult for some nurse executives.

PHASES IN LABOR RELATIONS

The process of establishing a labor contract will be reviewed in four steps: the organizing phase, the recognition phase, the contract negotiation phase, and the contract administration phase.

Organizing Phase

The organizing phase takes place when a union builds a base of support among workers. Managerial responses to this activity depend on whether the institution legally must bargain with a duly elected union, whether the management favors unionization (or *this* union), and whether unionization is perceived as inevitable or preventable.

The typical management response to incipient union organizing is to try to defeat the movement. Counteractions may involve correction of wrongs—if any—that led to the union activity and attempts to propagandize against the idea of unionizing. If an organization waits until the threat of unionization to correct blatantly unfair policies, the action may come too late.

When a nurse executive is involved in an anti-union propaganda campaign, he or she must be careful not to overstep legal boundaries. Under the LMRA, one cannot institute employee surveillance (e.g., identifying employees entering a meeting on unionizing), interrupt employees promoting unionization on their free time and on property where the work of the organization is not being disrupted, nor allow biased disciplinary action against leaders of the unionizing movement. Under the law, one can stop unionizing activities when they impinge on the work of the institution and when they use the work hours of employees.

The organizing phase of unionizing includes solicitation (oral encouragement to form a union) and distribution (written encouragement to form a union). Groups organizing under the LMRA are able to demand an election if they can produce signed cards showing that 30 percent of the employees of the given class are interested in holding an election. Although such an election cannot be held more than once a year, any group with a constituency can constitute a union. Where more than one union is interested in representing a group, the winner of the election will get sole representation rights (providing that unionizing is not voted down).

The Recognition Phase

A union is recognized as the sole representative of an employee group if it wins the majority of votes in an election, no matter how many or how few qualified voters actually vote. Often, employees think that not voting speaks against unionizing. Given the way that votes are counted, failure to vote works in the union's favor and staff should be made aware of this fact.

In the recognition phase, one may ask who is to be recognized? A union group is considered to be formed by a community of common interest. In the health field, it is typical that groups divide between professional and nonprofessional roles.

Ideally each small group would like to have its own union because each group thinks that its issues and needs are unique. However, if each and every group were granted the right to bargain separately, management would be forced to spend unreasonable time and resources in bargaining. The National Labor Relations Board decides who must be in the same union to limit the number of bargaining agents in any one institution. In nursing, it may be difficult to identify where management responsibility starts and employee functions leave off. Is the primary nurse a manager? What about the case manager? Further, employees may fill a managerial function (team leading) one day and a staff position (bedside care) the next.

Under the LMRA, a supervisor/manager is anyone with the authority to make personnel decisions such as assignment, hiring, suspending, promoting, and firing, or even anyone who has the right *to recommend such action*.

In the recognition phase, the institution must recognize as the bargaining agent any legitimate union that wins election under the appropriate procedures and laws. When an agent is recognized, under the LMRA, the institution cannot legally refuse to enter into the next stage: collective bargaining.

The Contract Negotiation Phase

Major issues in negotiation, from the manager's perspective, include managerial rights and employee salaries. Because nurses have been very successful in winning increased salaries in recent years, often "increases" are asked for in benefits.

Workers often try to win concessions in nonsalary issues such as every other weekend off, greater medical benefits, or more paid education days. These are not really divorced from cost; they have major cost implications. Many proposals hope to limit managerial flexibility. If the nurse executive must allow one-half of the staff off every weekend, for example, weekend quality of care may be jeopardized. Unions also try to limit management's right to reassign staff. If the nurse executive agrees to a contract that does not allow staff to move according to patient acuity, larger staff will need to be hired. The nurse executive must look at the real cost when she gives up such managerial prerogatives as flexibility in scheduling and assigning of staff.

Obviously, as nursing moves into an age of specialization, flexibility declines naturally. For example, one cannot assign a regular medical-surgical nurse to a specialized intensive care unit and expect him or her to assume responsibility for the specialized care that goes on there. One can, however, assign such a nurse to such a unit if he or she is to work there under the supervision of a nurse who knows that specialty and if the transferred nurse is accountable only for performance of familiar routine nursing acts.

The nurse executive or the agent should sit at the bargaining table to ensure that others do not give away nursing managerial prerogatives without recognizing that they are doing so. For example, a non-nurse negotiator may not recognize the potential impact on care of an every-other-weekend-off policy. Certainly, no contract should be signed without the approval of the nurse executive if it deals with nursing personnel. The nurse executive will want to watch developments as contracts are negotiated outside of the nursing division as well. If another group of workers bargains out of a given duty, the assumption may be that the nursing division will pick up the task. Nursing is the hub of the organization's services; it is usually affected by changes made in any other section of the institution.

Dynamics of Collective Bargaining

The nurse executive who sits on a negotiating team for the first time needs to be prepared for the negotiating process itself. He or she must recognize the process as an adversarial one in which the other side may use unpleasant tactics. Unfortunately, personal attacks are used at times. The nurse executive should be prepared to cope with such tactics, although this is easier to say than to do, and many nurse executives refuse to sit at the negotiating table because these tactics tend to alienate them from their nursing staff. It is a difficult problem, and the director who cannot deal with such tactics with a cool head probably does not belong at the table. Nevertheless, it is important that nursing top management be represented and that the nurse executive follow the happenings in the negotiations in detail.

Negotiations take place with each side giving up some lesser goals to achieve its major goals, negotiating in good faith. Give and take does not mean, however, that management must give in to unreasonable demands. Management must consider labor's demands; it need not cave in to them. And certainly, management should get something for every item it gives to the other side.

A word about unions: Union leaders are elected on the basis of the benefits they obtain for their membership. Although the professional union claims it is bargaining for patients' rights as well as staff members' benefits, it is typical that when those rights and benefits clash, the union opts to support staff benefits, claiming that it is management's job to find a way to achieve high-quality care.

The Contract Itself

The nurse executive must be careful concerning what is included in the contract. For example, if the contract inadvertently mentions certain personnel documents, a director may subsequently be unable to change even a job position description without agreement by the union (because those outside documents are legally included in the contract by reference). Conversely, one might fail to include some critical clause, such as a managerial rights statement, a scope clause, or an exclusionary clause.

The contract itself primarily covers such items as salaries, fringe benefits, and working conditions. Some nursing contracts also refer to con-

trols on patient care quality that may be exerted by the employee. There are different levels of employee participation in setting standards for care. Recently, some contracts have included clauses limiting an employee's assignment. For the executive, this is a double-edged sword, beneficial in demanding a better staffing ratio, disastrous in emergencies when additional staff simply cannot be found.

Clear language is essential in a contract. It prevents disagreements between management and labor concerning the issues included. If the contract's language is ambiguous, it will present as many problems as it solves. The contract must be carefully checked for contradictory clauses, another potential source of future problems.

One important clause in almost every contract is the arbitration clause. In exchange for a guarantee of no strike during the life of the contract, management agrees to arbitration of disputes that are not satisfactorily resolved in the grievance procedure. In an arbitration, an outside party makes the judgment in a dispute, and both parties—labor and management—agree to abide by the arbitrator's decision. Two methods are used in seeking an arbitrator: Either an arbitrator is sought for each separate case, or the two sides agree on a permanent arbitrator to hear all cases within the institution. The second method allows the arbitrator to become more familiar with the institution and thus more likely to be able to resolve disputes to everyone's satisfaction.

The Contract Administration Phase

Once a contract has been negotiated, the administrator is responsible for seeing that its provisions are upheld. The nurse executive will need to know intimately any contract that she administers as well as to educate new managers to the necessity of preserving the contractual agreements. The nurse executive cannot afford a manager who fails to implement the contract carefully, for consequent grievances and arbitrations could be costly.

The nurse executive does not derive rights to make managerial decisions from the contract. Relations with union representatives only concern those matters legitimately within the contract. Two major responsibilities fall to the nurse executive: to see that the contract provisions are upheld and to provide the appropriate grievance channels when there are disagreements as to whether the contract was enacted. When grievances are not satisfactorily resolved through the usual channels, most contracts provide for arbitration. Only matters contained within the contract are subject to this route. Any items not contained within the contract remains a managerial prerogative. There are at least two major sources of arbitrators: the American Arbitration Association and the Federal Mediation and Conciliation Service. Both will provide lists of possible arbitrators and their qualifications. Ideally, an arbitrator with previous experience in the health field would be selected.

Table 27–1 Limits on Management's Right To Oppose Unions

Under the Taft-Hartley Act, there are four management unfair labor practices that pertain to the organizing stage.

- **Interference, restraint, and coercion.** Seven major types of management conduct are proscribed: (1) violence, (2) espionage, (3) surveillance, (4) threats, (5) promises of benefit, (6) coercive interrogation, and (7) interference with the right of employees to communicate with each other.
- **Assistance to or domination of a labor organization.** This prohibition is intended to protect the integrity of unions. For example, management may not assist a union's organizing efforts by giving it money, free office space, free legal counsel, information about employees, or the like. Moreover, management may not apply its rules in a disparate fashion among unions. It may not, for example, permit professional organizers of one union to enjoy ready access to the institution's premises while barring a second union's organizers.
- **Discrimination to discourage or encourage union membership.** The classic example of discrimination to discourage union membership is the discharge of a leading union adherent shortly after management becomes aware of his or her role in an organizing campaign. Less obvious but equally illegal types of discrimination to dis-

courage union activity are closing a facility to avoid union activity, blacklisting union adherents, demoting union adherents, reducing wages or fringe benefits, withdrawing traditional overtime opportunities, supervising employees more strictly than has been customary, increasing the severity of penalties for minor employment offenses, and withholding wage increases promised before the organizing campaign began. It is equally illegal to discriminate against employees *to encourage* union membership by taking hostile action against employees who decline to support a union favored by the employer or granting benefits to employees who agree to support the union favored by management.
- **Discrimination against an employee because he or she filed charges or gave testimony under the NLRA.** This is a rarely used prohibition, intended to protect employees' *access* to the NLRB. An employer may not retaliate against an employee who has either filed unfair labor practice charges or given testimony that the employer does not like by engaging in any form of discrimination in the terms or conditions of employment.

Source: Skoler, Abbott & Presser, *Health Care Labor Manual,* Aspen Publishers, Inc., © November 1988.

ORGANIZING CAMPAIGNS AND THE HEALTH CARE PROFESSIONAL*

An organizing campaign among health care professionals differs in several ways from one involving nonprofessionals. A professional campaign, for example, typically involves the circulation of a huge number of letters and memoranda, far more than in a campaign involving nonprofessionals. Both sides emphasize the potential impact of unionization on patients, whereas in a campaign among nonprofessional health care facility employees, the parties emphasize the impact of unionization on employees virtually to the exclusion of patients. And throughout the campaign, issues of professionalism are raised over and over again. Management typically questions whether high professional standards can be maintained in a unionized health care setting, whereas the union (or association) maintains that unionization is consistent with high professional standards.

The typical campaign involving nonprofessionals is fundamentally a contest between management and the union. They alone circulate letters and other written materials. Only they call meetings to explain their views. But, in an organizing campaign involving professional employees, individual professionals—usually on their own initiative—write long, argumentative letters to their colleagues for or against unionization. Committees of employees spring to life to advocate and oppose collective bargaining. In short, a campaign involving professionals is far more lively and unpredictable.

The professional association that undertakes to organize nurses for collective bargaining purposes has a supreme advantage that traditional labor unions do not enjoy: It is not a complete stranger either to the employing organization or to professional employees. The crux of the professionals' campaign, therefore, usually involves the association's claim that it is still the custodian of the traditional values of the nursing or medical profession, contrasted with management's claim that the association should be seen by professional employees for what it has become and seeks to be (namely, a labor union that, like the Teamsters, calls strikes and disciplines members).

POSITION OF THE NURSE ADMINISTRATOR IN LABOR ORGANIZING DRIVES

Caught in Between*

Staff nurses ordinarily look to their nurse managers and director for the support, problem solving, and decision making needed to keep any organization, large or small, functioning smoothly. They expect nurse leaders to serve as an open communication channel to administration, passing on information regarding both their personal needs—such as salary and benefits—and their professional interests—such as education, career development, and relations with the medical staff and other health care facility personnel and departments. These ex-pectations are quite realistic. Indeed, the role of intermediary comes with the managerial territory. And, provided nurse leaders can maintain the confidence of both the staff below and the hierarchy above, it can be a rewarding role to play.

But the picture changes when a union organizing campaign begins. Supervisory and staff nurses suddenly become adversaries and find themselves on different sides of the fence. This "we" against "them" atmosphere is created because under labor law, supervisory personnel are defined as "management," while those being supervised are considered "labor."

Source: Skoler, Abbott & Presser, *Health Care Labor Manual,* Aspen Publishers, Inc., © November 1988.

Source: Anthony Lee, "How To Rise above the Cross-Fire of a Union/Hospital Battle," *RN.* Reprinted with permission of Medical Economics Company, Inc., Oradell, N.J.

A Manager's Active Role

The guidelines pertinent to supervisory behavior during a union organizing campaign make up a sizable collection of dos and don'ts. Refer to Table 27–2, "What the Supervisor *Can* Do," and Table 27–3, "What the Supervisor *Cannot* Do." It is to a manager's advantage to be sensitive to the limitations these requirements place on actions and comments in dealings with employees. Ideally, the supervisors in an institution undergoing organizing pressure should receive classroom training in these guidelines from a labor attorney or a labor relations expert.

It is also to one's advantage—at all times, but especially during a union organizing campaign—to know employees as individuals, and know them well. Although people cannot be stereotyped and there are few reliable generalizations concerning employees' receptiveness to a union, it is nevertheless possible for you to make some reasonable judgments as to how certain employees might react under organizing pressure. Often the employee sympathetic to the union's cause may:

- feel unfairly treated by the organization and believe that reasonable work opportunities have been denied
- feel that the organization has been unsympathetic regarding personal problems and pressures
- express a lack of confidence in supervision or administration and be unwilling to talk openly with members of management
- feel unequally treated in terms of pay and other economic benefits
- take no apparent pride in affiliation with the institution
- exhibit career-path problems, having either changed jobs frequently or having reached the top in pay and classification while still

---

Table 27–2 What the Supervisor *Can* Do When a Union Beckons

- Campaign against a union seeking to represent employees, and reply to union attacks on the institution's practices or policies.
- Give employees opinions about unions, union policies, and union leaders.
- Advise employees of their legal rights during and after the organizing campaign, and supply them with the institution's legal position in matters that may arise.
- Keep outside organizers off institution premises.
- Tell employees of the disadvantages of belonging to a union, such as strikes and picket-line duty; dues, fines, and assessments; rule by a single person or small group; and possible domination of a local by its international union.
- Remind employees of the benefits they enjoy without a union, and tell them how their wages and benefits compare with those at other institutions (both union and nonunion).
- Let employees know that signing a union authorization card is not a commitment to vote for the union if there is an election.
- Tell employees that you would rather deal directly with them than attempt to settle differences through a union or any other outsiders.
- Give employees factual information concerning the union and its officials, even if such information is uncomplimentary.
- Remind employees that no union can obtain more for them than the institution is able to give.
- Correct any untrue or misleading claims or statements made by the union organizers.
- Inform employees that the institution may legally hire a new employee to replace any employee who strikes for economic reasons.
- Declare a fixed position against compulsory union membership contracts.
- Insist that all organizing be conducted outside of working time.
- Question open and active union supporters about their union sentiments, as long as you do so without direct or implied threats or promises.
- State that you do not like to deal with unions.

Table 27–3 What the Supervisor *Cannot* Do When a Union Beckons

- Ask employees about their union sentiments in a manner that includes or implies threats, promises, or intimidation in any form. Employees may *volunteer* any such information and you may listen, but you may *ask* only with caution.
- Attend union meetings or participate in any undercover activities to find out who is or is not participating in union activities.
- Attempt to prevent internal organizers from soliciting memberships during nonworking time.
- Grant pay raises or make special concessions or promises to keep the union out.
- Discriminate against prounion employees in granting pay increases, apportioning overtime, making work assignments, promotions, layoffs, or demotions, or in the application of disciplinary action.
- Intimidate, threaten, or punish employees who engage in union activity.
- Suggest in any way that unionization will force the institution to close up, move, lay off employees, or reduce benefits.

- Deviate from known institution policies for the primary purpose of eliminating a prounion employee.
- Provide financial support or other assistance to employees who oppose the union, or be a party to a petition or such action encouraging employees to organize to reject the union.
- Visit employees at home to urge them to oppose the union.
- Question prospective employees about past union affiliation.
- Make statements to the effect that the institution "will not deal with a union."
- Use a third party to threaten, coerce, or attempt to influence employees in exercising their right to vote concerning union representation.
- Question employees on whether they have or have not signed a union authorization card.
- Use the word *never* in any statements or predictions about dealings with the union.

having a significant number of working years remaining

- be a source of complaints or grievances more often than most other employees
- exhibit a poor overall attitude

As a supervisor it is extremely important for you to know your employees' attitudes toward the institution so you may develop a sense for how well you are communicating. Ultimately, a labor union has little to offer if employees already feel that the organization is responding to their needs.

How To Prepare for Negotiations*

Preparations should commence several months before negotiation time. There should be a discussion with the facility administrator about

the role of the nurse administrator in contract negotiations. The nurse administrator is in a position to do all of the following:

- Predict the impact of the contract on patient care.
- Predict the impact on personnel and financial resources.
- Be aware of personnel issues that will arise to be dealt with at contract time.
- Be familiar with the goals, personalities, and idiosyncrasies of the personnel involved in negotiations.
- Implement the contract legally and fairly.
- Deal with issues that are a focus of conflict during negotiations throughout the upcoming year.

After establishing your involvement in the process, prepare for the time of negotiating.

Know your own contract thoroughly. List the difficulties it has created, both from an admin-

Source: Donna K. DeGraw, "Role of the Nurse Administrator in Labor Negotiations," *Nursing Administration Quarterly,* Vol. 6, No. 2, Aspen Publishers, Inc., © 1982.

istrator's perspective and from the staff view-point. Define changes that would make staffing the facility easier, be beneficial to patient care, and not take too large a proportion of resources. Read the minutes and notes taken during past negotiating sessions. This may be very helpful in giving a perspective on previous negotiations and a sense of the probable direction of future negotiations. List the changes that you anticipate the negotiating team will propose. Assess the importance of each area to the team. Communicate this information to the management negotiating team.

Be familiar with any other contracts that exist within your facility. Obtain copies of contracts from other facilities within the community, especially those that are in competition with yours for personnel and those that were negotiated by the same labor organization. If your facility is a corporation, be familiar with other contracts within the corporation, especially those negotiated by the same union. Extract from all these contracts their positions on all major issues, especially wages and major problem areas, and prepare a simple data sheet that compares and contrasts these items.

Be familiar with labor laws, especially the Taft-Hartley Act and the Fair Labor Standards Act. Contact both state and federal offices and obtain all pamphlets on wage and hour laws, employment, discrimination, employment of minors if this is applicable, and safety.

Be knowledgeable about the management team and who will be the primary spokesperson. It is definitely preferable that the spokesperson be experienced through previous contract negotiations. (You can be certain that the union representative will be an experienced person.) Discuss the plan for negotiating and determine what areas are negotiable. Most administrators seem to have their "pet peeves" on which they are inflexible. Identify these in advance and estimate the impact on the contract, the employees, and the nurse administrator's task.

Assess the community's attitude about unions and collective bargaining. Know whether there is a climate for settlement or strike.

Identify the staff who will be part of the union collective bargaining team. Find out whether the primary motivation is patient care, working conditions, wages, unresolved feelings of conflict and anger, or peer pressure. Predict what areas are essential to them individually and collectively to settle. Predict which areas are negotiable and which are extras.

Identify the needs of nursing administration. What will help to provide good care to patients, to attract and keep well-qualified staff, and to facilitate the goals and objectives of the nursing department of the facility? Identify areas that are essential and those that are advantageous. Ideally, vital areas of common concern should be discussed months before contract negotiations time. For example, if a contract change is needed to make it possible to implement 10-hour shifts, discuss the advantages, implications, and problems of the 10-hour shift with appropriate groups from the staff long before it is a part of negotiations.

Communicate with other departments that will not have direct representatives to determine any needs and problems they have identified that might be different from those identified by nursing.

When you have gathered sufficient data, prepared data sheets, and considered the implications for your facility, define for the management team areas important to nursing administration to negotiate. This will be very general at this point but will give your team a purposeful direction. You can negotiate more effectively regarding nursing administration needs on the basis of accurate facts, statistics, and analysis.

As you meet with the management team, listen carefully to what others are saying and strive to understand their viewpoint. It is important to negotiate from a common position.

Prior to moving to the negotiating table, know your team's strategy. Which member will assume the position of spokesperson? How will you communicate concerns to the spokesperson? What is the system for having conferences?

During Contract Negotiations*

During negotiations, the first step will be a proposal submitted by the union. While first proposals tend to be gross exaggerations of expectations, they do serve as an indicator of the direction of the group. Management will normally use this first time together just to seek clarification on all the issues, take good minutes, and then set dates and times for further negotiations. Management will then withdraw to prepare the first counterproposal.

Compare each proposal to the data sheet previously prepared and calculate the cost of all proposals for the immediate and distant future. Realize that some expenses (e.g., a significant increase for employees with longevity or step increases for education and/or experience) may result in a greater cost in several years than in the immediate future.

Determine if there are significant needs that have not been addressed. This is likely to occur because the union committee is rarely representative of all employee groups and can never speak for all employees. Determine if management's strategy is to introduce these areas into the contract. There may be a real advantage to including some of these in the counterproposals or saving these as trade-offs. Areas such as holiday pay, shift differential, or on-call differential may be much more significant to the nurse administrator than to others. Clarify this to the management team and supply facts to support your position.

Totally avoid negotiating management rights that are essential to the management of the facility. These issues usually represent a current concern within the facility and are often related to a single incident or several incidents. It is important to hear those concerns and address them away from the table. Contracts rarely, if ever, settle conflicts about staffing, safety, determination of quality of work, or job descriptions.

Source: Donna K. DeGraw, "Role of the Nurse Administrator in Labor Negotiations," *Nursing Administration Quarterly,* Vol. 6, No. 2, Aspen Publishers, Inc., © 1982.

Union Contract Negotiation Issues

- Discharge
- Suspension
- Layoff
- Recall
- Seniority
- Discipline
- Promotion, demotion, and transfer
- Assignment within bargaining unit
- Safety
- Health practices
- Hours of work and overtime
- Vacations
- Holidays
- Leaves of absence
- Sick time and other benefits

Avoid building these matters into the contract as they may return to haunt you in situations neither side ever anticipated.

As negotiations progress or deteriorate, remember the following guidelines:

- Deal with issues, not personalities.
- Keep all notes and minutes under lock and key.
- Do not talk about negotiations, especially in a negative manner, except with the other members of your team in a closed room.
- Be completely fair with the members of the union team in other situations. Do not expect more or less from them than you normally would.
- Recognize your role as a valuable one and do not accept responsibility for the feelings of others.
- Accept the fact that you are experiencing extra stress during this time, and have a tangible plan for dealing with this.

Always deal with the issues completely and be very certain not to be libelous, derogatory, or careless. Many grievances are lost on both sides because procedure was not followed exactly, or lost by management for publicly saying or writing something critical of the staff member.

Dealing with grievances and conflicts will normally take only a small portion of the administrator's total time if the communication systems are open. Most time will be spent creating a good environment in which to work. The most effective way to obviate the need for a strong labor union organization is to apply good management techniques, stressing that employees are valuable people. This is especially effective in a small health care organization where the nurse administrator knows all the staff and is able to have a direct impact on the staff members' perceptions of their roles, their jobs, and management.

ADMINISTRATION OF A COLLECTIVE AGREEMENT

In the eyes of the law, a collective agreement is legally enforceable, just like any other commercial contract. In fact, if a collective bargaining agreement contains no grievance arbitration procedure, the contract is enforceable *only* in the courts or through strike action by the union. The vast majority of collective bargaining agreements, however, provide for enforcement through a multistep grievance procedure that terminates in final and binding arbitration.*

Training the Management Team*

Management should act promptly after a contract becomes effective to ensure that its own representatives—especially first- and second-line managers—understand its significant aspects. If managers are ignorant of the institution's contractual rights and obligations, management's rights may be eroded and the union's rights may be violated, both at high cost to the employer.

A practical way to communicate the terms of a newly negotiated labor agreement to the managerial-supervisory staff is through a formal training and orientation program.

Training should include instructions about how to respond to grievances. Under the typical collective bargaining agreement, all grievances by the union are first filed with the manager. Managers must be careful to note whether the union has observed the contract's time limits and must respond to the union within the contract's time limitations. Training should also prepare managers to reply to a grievance with such clarity that there can be no doubt about the institution's position. Any defect in the union's handling of the grievance should be expressly noted because, if the grievance is carried to arbitration, the institution's defenses may be limited to those set forth by the first-level manager in the initial response to the grievance.

To ensure that discipline is administered for the right reasons and by the right procedures, managers should be trained in the uses of progressive (corrective) discipline under the contract.

Every manager should be encouraged to keep a copy of the collective bargaining contract handy. When questions arise, they should consult the contract and not rely on memory. Moreover, managers should be encouraged to consult with the institution's labor relations or human resource director when novel or difficult questions arise. Further, first-line managers should consult with the institution's labor relations or human resource director whenever possible before imposing discipline, such as discharge, since under collective bargaining, acts of discipline are usually subject to review by outsiders, labor arbitrators, whose sole interest is to decide whether discipline was just or unjust.

Reviewing the Contract*

As the manager in the nursing unit and as the person responsible for contract enforcement and interpretation, you should use the following principles when you review and interpret provisions of the contract:

---

*Source: Health Law Center, *Health Care Labor Manual,* Aspen Publishers, Inc., © November 1995.

Source: Virginia K. Baillie, Louise Trygstad, Tatiana Isaeff Cordoni, *Effective Nursing Leadership: A Practical Guide,* Aspen Publishers, Inc., © 1989.

- Read and reread those sections that affect the employees under your supervision.
- Note limitations, restrictions, or qualifying language.
- Never assume that the language as presented is superfluous or unimportant.
- If you are unclear about an interpretation, *ask for help.*
- Verify your understanding of a contract provision with someone in authority (e.g., your superior or the human resource/labor relations director).

There are several principles used to guide interpretation of the contract, particularly if a disagreement appears before an arbitrator.

Residual Rights Theory. What management has not given away, it retains. The contract cannot cover all policies, rules, and procedures concerning the day-to-day activities of employers and employees. Because the contract does not cover all issues, the concept of "residual rights" exists to aid in contract interpretation. This concept may not be agreed upon by the union.

Clear Contract Language versus Past Practice. Clear and unequivocal contract language cannot be ignored nor given a new interpretation by the arbitrator. In situations where contract language is unclear, ambiguous, or incomplete, arbitrators can go beyond the literal wording in the contract.

Past Practice. This relates to a consistent and long history of handling similar questions in one particular way. For example, the way in which management and the union have settled similar grievances is investigated as a potential precedent.

Steps in the Grievance Procedure*

The grievance procedure itself is negotiated and clearly described in the labor-management

---

Source: Copyright 1977, The American Journal of Nursing Company. Reprinted from *American Journal of Nursing*, February, 1977, Vol. 77, No. 2. Used with permission. All rights reserved.

contract. Ideally, it provides for a series of progressive steps and time limits for submission and resolution of unresolved grievances to higher and more authoritative management levels. The grievance procedure also will define what a grievance is and the manner of its presentation. This is to guard against emotional excesses on the part of either party.

In one institution, a grievance is first initiated through an informal discussion. This is just a talking stage during which the employee informally presents his or her complaint to the nurse manager, usually as soon as possible after the violation has occurred. The collective bargaining agent has the right to be present. The following sequence of steps is then used.

Step 1. If the grievance is not adjusted by informal discussion, written notice of the grievance is given within 5 to 10 workdays to the nurse manager. A written response from this level of authority should be received within 3 to 5 workdays. Many institutions have forms on which formal grievances are submitted. The employee, delegate, and nurse manager are present for any discussions at this time.

Step 2. If the response to step 1 is not satisfactory, a written appeal may be submitted within 10 workdays to the director of nursing or his or her designee. Parties to discussions at this stage are the employee, the (SNA) representative, the grievance chairperson and/or delegate, and the director of nursing or designee. Again, written response will be provided in 5 workdays subsequent to these meetings. In many bargaining units, the positions of delegate and grievance chairperson are separated. Generally, the grievance chairperson is an officer in the bargaining unit, and though apprised of the grievance at the early stages, he or she may become more actively involved at the later stages. Whether the person is a delegate or grievance chairperson will depend on how the bargaining unit is structured.

Step 3. The employee, SNA representative, grievance chairperson, and/or delegate, director of nursing, and director of human resources meet for discussions. The 10- and 5-day time limits for appeal and answer are again observed.

Step 4. This final step is arbitration. It is invoked when no solution suggested is acceptable at all. Present at these meetings are an arbitrator who is a neutral third party selected by both parties involved, the SNA representatives, employee and facility representatives, and any others who may be called as witnesses. The submission of a grievance to this step may be required in 15 days of step 3. In some contracts, there is a step between 3 and 4 that provides that the grievance be taken to someone in the health care facility's management before going to arbitration; however, this is not usual.

Often a statement included in each of the steps states that if the time limits are not observed by one party, the grievance may be considered resolved and further action barred. The contract also usually specifies how an arbitrator is selected. One should remember that, in some cases, the employer also has the right to state a grievance and use the procedure to resolve it.

PROACTIVE STRUCTURES FOR HARMONIOUS UNION RELATIONSHIPS*

Standing Grievance Committee

One of the best ways to avoid grievances is for management and the union to meet often and share interpretations of contract clauses. This can be accomplished through a special grievance committee in which management and union officials share their interpretations and work together to establish mutual agreements of language interpretations. Problems that rise can often be discussed at this level and agreements

Source: Adapted from Dominick Flarey, Susan K. Yoder, and Mark C. Barabas, "Collaboration in Labor Relations: A Model for Success," *Journal of Nursing Administration,* Vol. 22:9, September 1992. J.B. Lippincott.

can be reached regarding ways to avoid contract violations. This will help the union to "weed out" inappropriate grievances from members and assist management to develop policies and procedures that prevent contract violations.

Open-Door Policy

Nurse executives should establish an open-door policy with union officials. This will go a long way in building support by the union for management. An "open door" communicates to the union that nurse management accepts and acknowledges the union's position of representing nurses and that they need to establish effective communications and foster teamwork. Most union officials request to see the nurse executive when there is a significant problem to be solved or a particular nurse has a real need. An open-door policy to union officials shows that union and employee problems are shared, are important, and deserve attention.

Advisory Council

An advisory council of management and union officials and members should be established. Such a council mirrors the concept of shared governance but at a higher level. When negotiating a union contract, administration should propose specific contract language regarding the council. This shows support of the concept and cooperation between the union and the organization.

Care must be taken to ensure that issues focus on patient care. Any semblance of bargaining issues as defined in the NLRA must be avoided. Quality-of-care issues should focus on problem identification and mutual support to seek resolutions. Input from staff nurses is imperative.

Communication and Interpersonal Relations

COMMUNICATION

Experts say we only hear one-quarter of what people say to us.

One researcher who studied 100 American industries discovered that the president of the average company got only 90 percent of the information the board of directors wanted the president to give company employees. The department heads (listen well, nurse managers) got only 50 percent of the information. The foremen (are you listening, head nurses?) got 30 percent. And the nonmanagement employees—for whom the information was intended—got only 20 percent of the information.

Misunderstandings are usually caused by the fact that whenever communication is attempted between two people, there are at least six messages—each somewhat different—involved in the communication.

- what you mean to communicate
- what you actually communicate
- what communication the other person *receives*
- what communication the other person *thinks* he or she receives
- what the other person *says*
- what you *think* the other person says

Improving the Communication Climate*

Communication climate is the degree to which an organization permits—and preferably promotes—a free and open exchange of ideas and information among its members.

There are three key components of communication climate: the amount or *quantity* of information exchanged among people, its *quality*, and the number and nature of *channels* available for relaying the information.

Quantity. Essentially the communication climate in an organization is favorable when the quantity of information exchanged among people is sufficient to allow them to carry out their assigned jobs knowledgeably and confidently. When too little information is exchanged, whether among superiors and subordinates or among peers in the same or different departments, confusion and uncertainty could well result. People may not know what is expected of them in their jobs and so will not be able to meet expectations, and further, they might not understand how their jobs relate to others' work.

---

*Source: Corwin P. King, "Keep Your Communication Climate Healthy," *Personnel Journal*, April 1978. Reprinted with the permission of *Personnel Journal*, Costa Mesa, California; all rights reserved.

Among peers, this may lead to a failure to cooperate in solving common problems.

Though it is usually less of a problem, exchanging too much information can also be harmful, for it can easily create a state of information overload for people. Faced with more information than they can conveniently handle, they may simply ignore most of it, and in the process ignore essential information that is needed for their jobs. Additionally, when it comes from superiors, too much information may have negative motivational effects, implying that people are too dull and irresponsible to do anything on their own. In time, this may cause them to "live down to the label," refusing to take initiative and passively waiting for instructions on even the simplest of tasks.

Quality. Essentially, the quality of information is good when it is clear, relevant, accurate, and consistent from the standpoint of those who receive it. The value of clarity and relevance should be obvious, for information that fails to meet the needs of people's jobs, at least in terms that they can understand, is worthless. The value of accuracy and consistency should also be obvious, since staff cannot rely on inaccurate and inconsistent information.

Channels. Information is exchanged through two kinds of channels in an organization, vertical (including downward from superiors to subordinates as well as upward) and horizontal (including internal, among peers in the same department, and external, among peers in different departments). Regardless of classification, however, good channels for information have the following characteristics.

First and foremost is the fact that channels exist where they are necessary, and second is the fact that people who need to use them have access to them—preferably easy access. When channels do not exist, or when people are not aware that they do, employees may not know where to turn for important information about their jobs and so may be denied that information. When channels do exist but people do not have access to them, the situation may be even worse, for it is highly aggravating to know where to find information but not be able to get it. If people must spend too much effort to get information, they may just do without it and trust to their own resources, however good or bad they may be.

Another characteristic of good channels is that they are direct and official. Direct channels are desirable because they are simpler, faster, and usually more reliable. When information is conveyed indirectly through third parties, there is little guarantee that those who need the information will receive it accurately and on time.

As a rule, the more channels people have access to in an organization, the more they are likely to communicate. When people are asked to suggest ways of improving an organization's communication climate, they often suggest ways of improving the frequency of communication by developing more and better channels or by better using the channels that exist.

How To Communicate*

How an individual responds to others in the communication process has a great deal to do with their reactions. There are three ways of responding to people and problems. First is the repressive level, where the response is very unsatisfactory. The second is to minimize what the other person feels to be a legitimate problem. In the third way, the individual tries to understand what is being said. Try to identify with the person and his or her view of the situation.

Climate and communication work hand in hand. Be open and interested. Try to de-emphasize the hierarchical differences, play down the power differentials. Level more with people in an open way characterized by frankness, integrity, and openness. If you lay out the problem and get the people themselves involved in solving it, they are better able to pass judgment on themselves than you are. There is nothing you need to tell a person about his or her shortcomings and deficiencies that you cannot convey indirectly and without demeaning the person. If you demean people, they will only become defensive and fight back.

Source: Robert K. Burns, "Techniques for Strengthening Intra and Interdepartmental Operations and Coordination," *Hospital Topics*, March-April 1975. Reprinted with permission.

If you ask two or three pertinent questions, the individual can come up with the problem him- or herself. It is psychologically much easier for the person to find and state the problem and take corrective action on his or her own than for you to tell the person, for that is self-imposed control.

The Art of Asking Questions. When you ask an employee a question, you are indicating that you think it would be valuable to hear the employee's ideas and suggestions, and that should make him or her feel valuable as a person. It is better to ask than to tell.

When asking people questions, use the kind of methods that give you the kind of information you desire. If you need the facts about something, ask a factual question. To get the facts, do two things: First identify and isolate what you need to ask, and then differentiate and separate it in terms of the desired answer. Ask the questions what, when, which, where, why, who, how, and how many until you get all the information you need.

Involving Subordinates. One test of leadership is getting the other person to do the work that needs to be done the way it should be done because that is the way he or she wants to do it. That exemplifies authority based on cooperation instead of authority imposed from above.

Try to clarify the work by taking a look at the job, decide what the mission is, then break down the job into key areas. Talk things over with the people you work with—boss and subordinates. Get agreement and commitment from everyone and work together as a team. Many people say that to do that is giving up one's prerogatives. Hogwash! You are not giving up anything, you are getting something: ideas, suggestions, and motivated people.

Manager-Employee Communication*

The relationship between nurse manager and employees should be congenial, show mutual caring without undue familiarity, be personal but not show favoritism, and be relaxed but purposeful. From this relationship the nurse manager can be as directive as the situation requires while allowing employees all the freedom and flexibility in the performance of duties as their competence allows. Good communication builds a relationship that strengthens the nurse manager's ability to motivate the best efforts of the team because the members are satisfied with the relationship.

Supervisory relationships can be considered in four phases: meeting, knowing, enabling, and directing. These are somewhat sequential but are also intertwined.

The tasks of the *meeting* phase are for the manager to learn about the employees' experience, aptitudes, and skills; to help them become oriented to the job; to create expectations for instruction and feedback processes that the manager will use; and to establish expectations about work attitudes and quality of performance. This usually is a short phase occurring at the beginning of the relationship.

Skills include the ability to give information clearly, to model appropriate action, to listen, and to communicate empathy, respect, and warmth. Basic friendship skills are used. Generally, the human resource department helps with some of these tasks.

The effect of the meeting phases is that both levels obtain information about each other, size each other up, and lay the basis for the relationship. The employees are introduced to the job and become part of a work group.

The task of the *knowing* phase is to know the person. This means going beyond biographical and vocational facts to such intangibles as attitudes and motivation.

The manager learns the employees' capacity for doing assigned work and gains an understanding of how to improve that capacity. The manager finds out who the employees are; their attitudes and opinions; preferences for work, for fun, and for people; and their motivators—what makes them tick. It also is important for managers to learn to accept characteristics that were disliked at first but that do not hurt the employees' work performance.

Source: George M. Gazda, William C. Childers, and Richard P. Walters, *Interpersonal Communication: A Handbook for Health Professionals*, Aspen Publishers, Inc., © 1982.

In the *enabling* phase, the manager uses the skills of giving encouragement and praise, pointing out performance problems or missed goals, giving advice and instruction frequently, and in other ways using the transition dimensions. The primary task here is informal. Later formal performance reviews will show what the employees need to change in order to be more successful on the job. These efforts all are directed toward helping the employees see how personal success comes by helping the organization advance by providing opportunities for staff members to grow professionally through work, which results in their working hard because personal needs are met through the job. This has benefits for productivity and effectiveness, especially over the long term.

In the *directing* phase, the manager enforces rules, sets deadlines, gives ultimatums, and takes disciplinary measures as appropriate. Here the action dimensions, especially confrontation, may be used. This includes dealing with inappropriate talk and responding to an angry person.

The use of the directing phase dimensions usually results in some resistance, which is in proportion to how meaningful the relationship has been. This may strain the relationship, either temporarily or longer.

The manager's behavior, for the most part, is nondirective in the knowing phase and becomes increasingly directive in moving through the enabling phase to the highly directive behaviors of the directing phase. Nondirective, gentle supervisory behaviors of persuasion, encouragement, asking, listening, and cooperating are in sharp contrast to the directive, tough, supervisory behaviors such as forcing, demanding, telling, and coercing. These, however, also are legitimate under certain conditions.

Using only gentle behaviors or only tough behaviors works for a while, but good supervision requires the full range of actions. Optimal performance comes when the manager can concentrate on enabling employees to do their best but can shift to the gentler approach of the knowing phase or the tougher approach of the directing phase when either of those are indicated.

Confrontation

Probably the most difficult task in supervision is talking with an employee about problems such as deficiencies in performance of duties, infractions of rules, or undesirable interpersonal relationships.

The acceptance of any confrontation depends on (1) a good base relationship and (2) skillful use of the confrontation itself.

The confrontation occasion does not need to be extremely uncomfortable for either manager or subordinate. It can, in fact, be a time of constructive advance in skills and understanding for both parties. These suggestions can maximize the benefits of these occasions. The manager should do the following:

- Be careful not to get overly caught up in the crisis of the moment but keep the long-range relationship in mind.

- Take care not to accuse prematurely, listen to the employee's story, and be alert for new data that are relevant to the situation.

- Give employees an opportunity to take the initiative in explaining and correcting the situation, follow the principle of allowing them to do as much for themselves as they are capable of doing.

- Put the criticism and the problem area in perspective by discussing employees' areas of strength. To let employees mistakenly feel that they are doing nothing right is tragic, but it happens frequently. Again, stay alert for the effect of the interaction on the employees.

- Provide the best protection against remedial supervisory work by prevention of problems through clear task assignment and other preparation of employees to carry out their duties.

- Avoid "hit and run" confrontation. Things rarely are as simple as they appear on the surface, so allow for explanation of the problem and ample time for interaction.

Nurse Administrator's Guidelines for Communication

Identification of Weaknesses

The effective use of information depends on effective communication links. Every administrator plays a vital role in this system, both as a transmitter and as a recipient of information. To help you assess and identify communication weakspots, review the questions below.

Do you receive information from *your staff* that is excessive, minimal, inaccurate, or basically routine? Do you hear requests for supplementary information or further explanations? Do you hear complaints about information arriving too late?

Do you receive information from *facility management* that is untimely, insufficient, overabundant, garbled, or imprecise? Do you hear (or do you recognize) that your communications are late, unnecessarily time consuming, or in need of revision?

Do you receive reports from *other department heads* or send reports to them that are purposeless, inconsistently informative, or inappropriate? Are your conferences overlong, excessive in number, vague in objectives, or indecisively concluded?

Effective Leadership Communication

Behind the exchange of information in the communication process are larger concepts that the nurse administrator hopes to convey to his or her staff: standards of performance, motivation toward effective functioning, and acceptance of innovations. Communication is a force for influencing staff direction. Indirect and direct means can be used. Indirectly, the nurse administrator sends out signals by his or her own behavior. Lectures about standards and attitudes will be ineffective if subordinates observe contradictions and lapses in the nurse administrator's own actions. Most people learn to communicate through example.

For direct communication, it is important that messages are not only given but heard as well. The first step is to promote a responsive communication climate in the department where staff members feel comfortable in expressing their underlying reactions, attitudes, and problems. The following steps may help you communicate clearly with your subordinates:

- Consider your objectives in advance, forming a plan for communication: why, when, how.
- Express yourself with unmistakable clarity. Be concise and tick off main points by emphasizing them.
- Formulate messages in a manner that is attuned to the subordinate's self-interest, creating greater acceptance.
- Be sensitive to differences in needs, experiences, and frames of reference among various subordinate levels; adjust messages accordingly.
- Avoid didactic language. Use conversational language, but be aware that words have different shades of meaning, assuming coloration from the type of situation or the background of the listener.
- Be a listener as well as a talker. Encourage openness and observe accurate criticisms and fresh approaches. Strive for feedback from subordinates to confirm whether the message has been comprehended.
- Follow up conversations and meetings with memos or reports to the staff. Let them know that action has resulted from communication or, in the case of individual criticisms, that progress has been noted.
- Use a variety of communication methods to reinforce an important message or select a single most appropriate method according to the nature of the message: conversations, notes, official memos, meetings, conferences, and reports.

The Skill of Listening

Many nurse administrators are trained to communicate effectively, but few are prepared properly to receive the wealth of information found in the attitudes, opinions, and suggestions of others. By learning to listen well to the words of staff members in conversations and meetings, by learning to read the manner of expression with which these words are conveyed, the administrator is able to keep in contact and to direct activities more successfully. (For a self-assessment of your listening habits, see Table 28–1.)

The groundwork of effective listening is built on the practice of the three As.

Availability. Be accessible to your staff, willing to listen to statements in meetings, impromptu conversations in the hall, or discussions from drop-in visitors.

Attentiveness. Be receptive in your manner of listening, maintain eye contact and bodily attention. During the conversation, listen nonevaluatively, encouraging the speaker to express him- or herself freely and nondefensively. Avoid the raised eyebrow or other comments of skepticism of the moment. Reserve judgmental assessment until after the speaker has delivered his or her piece in full. Practice courtesy and request clarification if anything is unclear.

Acceptance. Understand the speaker's frame of reference. Sense how background and experience influence a point of view. Perceive and accept the emotional content as well as the verbal message. Suspend any prior prejudice to a particular mode of expression or the delivery of contrary ideas. Last, guarantee the right of others to speak out, focusing disagreement or criticism on the message content and not on the speaker's "outspokenness."

Using Feedback Constructively

An incident occurs, an attitude is expressed, and you are sufficiently annoyed with the behavior of a worker to set on a course to change that behavior. How do you communicate that message?

Step 1. Suggest a private talk at an appropriate time in a place where the discussion will not be interrupted or overheard.

Step 2. Present the facts, not an evaluation, of the behavior observed. Shore up the facts with accurate details.

Step 3. Give the worker time to draw his or her own inferences, such as "I guess I didn't control my temper." If none are forthcoming or there is disagreement with the worker's inference, then express your own.

Step 4. Double-check the validity of your inference and the communication of your message. Ask the worker to comment on the accuracy and meaning of what you said. Is his or her response in line with what you were trying to convey?

Step 5. Describe the impact of the worker's behavior on coworkers and let him or her judge whether this is a desirable reaction.

Step 6. Ask the worker for plans or actions that will be taken to correct the behavior. Guide the discussion with discreet suggestions of your own. Check if these messages are accurately perceived.

How To Prepare a Speech*

One of the most important elements of successful speaking is the speaker's preparation. Most speech experts agree that preparation for speaking is a simple step-by-step process. The first task that any speaker faces in preparing a speech is to determine and limit the purpose of the speech. The speaker then assembles relevant support materials, plans the organizational pattern, and decides how to begin, develop, and conclude the speech.

Purpose

Every successful speech has a clear and definite purpose designed to achieve a particular audience reaction. This purpose is the goal or objective for the speech. Like other goals, the purpose serves to guide the speaker in all phases of speech preparation and final delivery.

Within such limitations as the occasion, place, time, speaker's ability, and audience background, all speeches have been traditionally classified

---

*Source: Principles and Techniques of Instruction, U.S. Air Force (AF 50-62), 1974.

Table 28–1 Quiz on Listening Habits

Assess your own listening abilities by answering whether you find yourself acting in the following ways.

Do you . . .
- Act impatient, fidget, or seem poised in midflight while others are speaking? Yes___ No___
- Pretend attentiveness, barely tracking the conversation while your mind is on other thoughts? Yes___ No___
- Selectively listen, picking out partial facts, ideas, or underlying feelings but ignoring the whole content? Yes___ No___
- Fail to ask questions when a statement is unclear? Yes___ No___
- Frequently have to check back and verify details because you misunderstood the information? Yes___ No___
- Become easily distracted from the conversation by nearby noises and activity? Yes___ No___
- Judge a message as unworthy because of the speaker's appearance or delivery? Yes___ No___
- Pride yourself on predicting what the speaker will say before it is said? Yes___ No___
- Dismiss statements or arguments of others without a hearing because you are certain you are right? Yes___ No___
- Stifle conversation by making constant corrections or asserting your own viewpoint? Yes___ No___
- Spend more time in forming your answers than in concentrating on what is being said? Yes___ No___
- Prefer talking, speaking, telling, lecturing, or sounding off to the state of listening? Yes___ No___

If your honest response to all the questions is an unqualified no, then you have attained perfection as a listener. Most people cannot make claim to that ideal; they admit to several of these bad habits. However, if you answer yes to half the questions or more, you are losing contact with your subordinates. Start listening to yourself and start changing your listening habits.

---

according to one of three general purposes: to inform, to persuade, or to entertain.

The speaker's purpose is *to inform* when he or she helps an audience to understand an idea, a concept, or a process or broadens the range of the audience's present knowledge. All informative speeches have a clear organization, supporting facts, and illustrative examples and comparisons.

In the speech *to persuade*, the speaker wishes to change or reinforce existing beliefs, stimulate activity, or increase emotional involvement. A distinguishing feature of the persuasive speech is its appeal to an audience's emotions in addition to its appeal to their intellectual reasoning.

The speech *to entertain* has as its objective the enjoyment of the audience. This type of speech, then, is characterized by information that is interesting, unusual, or humorous.

Once the general purpose has been selected, the speaker is ready to form the specific purpose by stating the precise response desired from the audience. When writing the specific purpose, the speaker must conform to the needs of the audience, the limitations of time, and any limitations inherent in the situation.

Research

With the purpose of the speech in mind, the speaker now proceeds to the second step—gathering material on the subject. The source of this material is the speaker's own experience or the experience of others gained through conversation, interviews, and written or observed material. The person concerned with giving a good speech will probably draw from all of these sources.

The next step is to evaluate the material gathered. The speaker will probably find that there is enough material for several speeches. The speaker must now combine some ideas, eliminate others, and perhaps bolster some ideas that appear in the research materials. At this time, the speaker will probably see that the ideas are beginning to form into some type of pattern.

Determining the Pattern

The *time* or *chronological pattern* is used when the material is arranged according to the order in which a number of events took place.

The *spatial* or *geographical pattern* is very effective in describing things. When the spatial pattern is used, the speech material is developed in some directional sequence.

The *topical pattern* is used when the subject has within itself divisions well known to the speaker and the audience.

The *cause-and-effect pattern* is also used in speaking but does not lend itself to all topics. When using the cause-and-effect pattern, the speaker may first enumerate specific forces, then point out the results that follow; or the speaker may first describe conditions, then discuss the forces that caused them.

The *problem-solution pattern* organizes material in terms of problems (needs) and solutions (plans). The problem-solution pattern is particularly effective with a persuasive speech.

The Outline

An effective outline helps to make a good speech. By establishing the structural form of the speech, the outline facilitates evaluation. Is the thinking clear? Is each point treated according to importance? Does the speech need more support material? Are ideas in the proper sequence? Such evaluation questions will ensure that the speech has unity, is coherent, and has a smooth progression from beginning to end.

The first step in the rough draft is listing the main points and arranging them in a systematic sequence. Once this is accomplished, the speaker inserts subpoints and decides which support material will best verify and/or illustrate each point. Then comes the crucial question: Does the draft cover the subject and fit the purpose? If not, the speaker revises the draft.

Delivery

One object of speech delivery is to achieve a sense of direct communication with the audience. Both the speaker and the listeners must feel that they are in touch with each other. The speaker must believe in both the content and the need to communicate the same. This may not be a permanent conviction, but it must be the conviction of the moment.

Variety in voice is one secret to effective delivery. The speaker may vary the loudness, pitch, and rate of utterance, but the variations must be in harmony with the meaning, emotional content, and emphasis. One effect of movement is that the audience tends to follow the speaker's body as he or she moves across the platform. This effect can be used to gain attention or to aid in the transition from one point to the next. Too much movement becomes distracting, while too little movement becomes boring for lack of change.

Gestures should appear natural, definite, and well timed. They should never draw attention from the point they are emphasizing. Any gesture should be harmonious with the speaker's attitude, conviction, and topic.

Use of Notes

Through the use of notes in delivery, the speaker can remain flexible and responsive to the needs and attitude of the audience.

The use of notes allows the language and phrasing of the speech to remain flexible. The speaker is not restricted to reading a set speech. He or she can vary the support material collected during the preparation to meet the needs of the audience. Notes used wisely have certain advantages, namely, to stimulate memory, to help with the reporting of complicated information, to help vary the support material to meet the needs of the audience, and to ensure organizational accuracy during delivery.

CONFLICT

One of the main characteristics of any organization is that it is made up of human beings in interaction with each other. In such circumstances it is well known that conflicts will arise, and will sometimes result in detrimental side effects to the parties involved or to the organization as a whole.

In fact, conflict in organizations is probably inevitable due to the nature and design of the structure itself. The modern progressive organization recognizes the fact, however, that conflict, both internal and external, exists in any healthy organization and attempts both to benefit by desirable types of conflict and to resolve or eliminate detrimental conflict. A certain degree of conflict among individuals and groups may increase creativity, satisfaction, performance, and effectiveness (see box).

Conflict is a dynamic process, a type of behavior, involving two or more parties in opposition to each other. It can be overt or covert. Of the two, the covert is the more dangerous, because the harbored feelings of individuals can drain an untold amount of energy, both physical and psychological. Once conflict is acknowledged, then energies and resources can be channeled to dealing with and resolving it.

To be able to deal effectively and constructively with conflict, the manager must understand and must be able to analyze the various sources of conflict that may be found in people, things, or conditions. It is important to diagnose as correctly as possible the underlying causes of conflicts, because they are not always what they appear to be on the surface.*

Sources of Conflict*

A typical source of conflict is when two people or two units have mutually exclusive goals—goals that cannot be reached simultaneously. An example would be when two or more managers of equivalent ranking are competing to replace their superior who is about to retire. Another example would be a person justifying failure by pointing to the errors of a colleague.

Groups or individuals that are committed to reach their goals will want to ensure that they have all the resources required. In any organization, resources are limited and all demands cannot be satisfied to the same degree. This is a frequent area of conflict.

---

*Source: Ross Smyth, "The Sources and Resolution of Conflict in Management," *Personnel Journal,* May 1977. Reprinted with the permission of *Personnel Journal,* Costa Mesa, California; all rights reserved.

Is Conflict Good or Bad? It Depends.

- Conflict can be good if it is recognized and not ignored. Conflict is usually the manifestation of some fundamental problem that needs addressing. Effective managers face conflicts rather than avoiding them. Conflicts that are avoided seldom go away; in fact, they get worse.

- Some types of conflict are detrimental. These divert energy away from goal attainment, deplete resources (time or money), damage individuals, and make cooperation difficult.

- Some types of conflict are beneficial. Conflict, for example, can lead to constructive problem solving, a search by people for ways of changing how they do things, and a greater acceptance of change in general.

- Too little expressed conflict leads to stagnation, but uncontrolled conflict invites chaos.

- Conflict can sometimes be handled by a conflict resolution process, and use of such a process can have benefits other than mere resolution of the conflict.

Source: David P. Starkweather and Donald G. Shropshire, "Management Effectiveness," in *Manual of Health Services Management,* Robert J. Taylor, ed., Aspen Publishers, Inc., © 1994.

Competition for status often leads to conflict. The concern of people with their position relative to others has much influence on their behavior and performance. An example of frequent conflict is when a young, highly educated person is called on to supervise the work of older persons who have gained their status through their years of experience with the organization.

In a large organization, people will have different backgrounds and different value systems and will perceive things from different viewpoints—a possible cause of conflict, especially when not understood. Those in different functional departments will have varying beliefs and opinions on what is best and how it should be done. Perceptual differences between people in different areas can be accentuated because they interact with a different public. Difference of position in the hierarchy can also give rise to significant differences in perception of events.

Conflict also occurs frequently between first-line managers and managers at higher levels. The nurse manager will seek short-term solutions to immediate problems, whereas the nurse administrator will consider longer term solutions.

Table 28–2 summarizes the basic types of organizational conflict. Knowing the type of conflict and the level at which it is operating is crucial to conflict resolution.

Dealing with Conflict*

How conflict is managed often determines whether it has beneficial or destructive effects on the organization and the people involved. Effective conflict management starts with diagnosis, since conflict that is manifest may not be real. For conflict that is real, there is an array of techniques that can be brought to bear, each appropriate to different types and levels of conflict. The effective manager tries to find the resolution that lets all parties win.

---

*Source: David P. Starkweather and Donald G. Shropshire, "Management Effectiveness," in *Manual of Health Services Management*, Robert J. Taylor, ed., Aspen Publishers, Inc., © 1994.

Table 28–2 Basic Types of Organizational Conflict

Organizational conflict occurs when there is discord caused by the way jobs are designed or allocated. In the following list, the first three, seemingly interpersonal, conflicts become organizational because the conflictive individuals represent organizational units and levels that are in contest over resources, how best to render care, or who has authority and power.

- *Goal conflict* occurs when desired end states or preferred outcomes are incompatible. For instance, gains on one side are seen as losses on the other.
- *Cognitive conflict* occurs when ideas or opinions are perceived as incompatible. This kind of conflict is due to a misunderstanding or misperception. Once the cognitive dissonance is cleared up, the conflict can be resolved.
- *Affective conflict* occurs when feelings or emotions are incompatible (i.e., people or groups become angry with one another).
- *Vertical conflict* occurs between levels. It often arises when subordinates resist attempts by superiors to restrict their autonomy. But it also arises from misunderstandings, lack of consensus on goals, and so on.
- *Horizontal conflict* occurs within the same hierarchic level (e.g., when each team, unit, or department strives for its own goals regardless of the effect on other departments).
- *Line-staff conflict* sometimes results when line managers feel that staff managers are using their technical knowledge to intrude on the line managers' areas of legitimate authority. Open conflict is particularly likely when staff managers control resources used by line managers.
- *Role conflict* occurs when there is inconsistency or misunderstanding about the job a person is supposed to be doing. Such a misunderstanding can take place between a subordinate and a superior, between different groups that depend on each other, or between an individual's notions of acceptable behavior and his or her job.

Source: David P. Starkweather and Donald G. Shropshire, "Management Effectiveness," in *Manual of Health Services Management*, Robert J. Taylor, ed., Aspen Publishers, Inc., © 1994.

Five styles (for methods) are identified by their location in two dimensions: *concern for self* and *concern for others*. A person's desire to satisfy his or her own concerns depends on the extent to which the person is *assertive* in pursuing personal or unit goals. The person's desire to satisfy the concerns of others depends on the extent to which he or she is *cooperative*. The five styles thus represent different combinations of assertiveness and cooperativeness.

Avoiding involves behavior that is unassertive and uncooperative. People use this style to stay out of conflicts, ignore disagreements, or remain neutral. Sometimes conflict is avoided out of a calculation that "it will work itself out."

Forcing is an assertive and uncooperative method of dealing with conflict. It reflects a win-lose attitude: The forcing person feels that one side must win and the other must lose. This method usually helps a person achieve his or her goals, but its regular use by a manager develops fear, lack of respect, and hatred by those affected.

Accommodating is a cooperative but unassertive method. Accommodating is often called the lose-win strategy. It may reflect unselfishness or simple submission. Accommodators are usually viewed favorably by others, although also being seen as weak and submissive.

Most interpersonal relationships in organizations are enduring (i.e., they have a past and a future). Therefore, accommodation in one conflict may have the purpose of buying reciprocal accommodation in the future, in which case accommodating would be part of a long-term strategy of cooperation.

Collaborating is a highly cooperative and assertive method. It is a win-win method. It represents a desire to maximize joint outcomes. For it to work, both parties to a conflict have to be committed to the joint outcome.

Compromising is an intermediately cooperative and assertive method. It is based on give and take and typically involves a series of negotiations and concessions.

Negotiation is based on the concept of interdependence: Both sides recognize that they mutually have needs and that they must work together after the conflict. The two parties are aware that each is trying to influence the other and that

---

Characteristics of Managers Who Use Collaboration Methods

- See conflict as natural and leading to a more creative solution if handled properly.
- Trust others and exhibit candor.
- Believe that the parties at conflict have an equal role in resolving the issues, and view the opinions of all parties as legitimate.
- Recognize that when conflict is resolved to the satisfaction of all parties, there results a greater commitment to the solution.
- Do not sacrifice any one person simply for the good of the group.

---

agreement is a function of the power they bring to the situation and their skill at bargaining.

Compromise is commonly used and widely accepted; indeed, many managers feel it is the only method available. Reasons for this include the following:

- It can be seen primarily as a cooperative gesture even though it is also a holding back.
- It is a practical approach and appeals to those who regard themselves as practical.
- It usually results in a legacy of good relations for the future.

On the other hand, compromise can yield subsequent doubts about the fairness of the outcome and the equality of each party's concessions. Compared to collaboration, compromise does not maximize joint satisfaction; rather, it results in moderate but partial satisfaction for each party.

STAFF DIVERSITY IN A MULTICULTURAL CONTEXT

The nation's work force is becoming increasingly diverse. This diversity may be based on gender, culture, or age. Differences among workers in an organization may result in conflict and tension among the labor force. In light of these factors, managers and leaders must learn to respect and manage their employees' differences in order to be successful. The health care environment is especially vulnerable to the issue of work force diversity.*

Managing Diversity*

Many reasons have been provided to support diversity management as a success strategy. A particularly interesting reason is that, by valuing and using employees' diversity, an organization will be able to interact more successfully with its diverse public. Health care facilities serve all types of individuals and, therefore, should see this factor as an important reason to put effort into managing the diversity of their employees.

Problems Associated with Work Force Diversity

A work force diverse in gender, culture, and age has the potential to create conflict in an organization. Communication difficulties, including language and literacy issues, may arise. Communication is a particular problem for foreign-born workers due to the dependence of performance ratings and promotions on the ability to communicate both orally and in writing. Along literacy lines, communication between individuals of differing educational and professional levels is a challenge. This concept is especially true for health care facilities, in which a range or spectrum of individuals from physicians to cleaning staff is working.

Orientation and integration into the culture of the organization can be problematic issues. Groups other than the predominant group may encounter barriers when attempting to adapt to the interpersonal environment. Organizations may have preconceived negative expectations of nontraditional workers. This situation may be particularly true for older or foreign-born nurses.

---

*Source: Laurie Ashmore Epting, Saundra H. Glover, and Suzan D. Boyd, "Managing Diversity," *The Health Care Supervisor*, Vol. 12, No. 4, Aspen Publishers, Inc., © June 1994.

A lack of faith on the part of the organization may result in unchallenging assignments that lead to low credibility and visibility, which, in turn, lead to poor ratings and poor advancement opportunities. This negative spiral can continue indefinitely.

Stereotypes represent an additional problem resulting from work force diversity. Traditional managers, in many cases, trust those workers most like themselves more than they trust other groups. Stereotypes related to an employee's age or gender may also be encountered.

Respecting Diversity and Valuing Differences

Diversity is far from a passing fad. It is a significant issue in the health care labor force. Managing diversity entails the use of a comprehensive managerial process for developing an environment that works for all employees. While legal requirements demand that organizations offer equal employment opportunities and follow affirmative action guidelines, managing diversity goes a step further toward valuing the differences among workers. Traditionally, many organizations have done just enough to meet their legal obligations. Diverse employees were assimilated, or required to "fit in," to the culture of the organization. Management of diversity requires emphasis on the importance of integrating workers into the organization instead of assimilating them. *Assimilation of employees is not effective* for three reasons:

- People are now celebrating their differences and are not as willing to assimilate into one homogeneous group.
- Diversity among workers offers a "richness" not found in a uniform work force.
- There is growing recognition that some factors are beyond assimilation.

Managing diversity successfully requires placing a value on diversity in order to enhance interpersonal relationships among individuals and to minimize blatant expressions of racism and sexism. Managers should be encouraged to tap the fullest potential of the diversity of their subordinates and to recognize that treating all employees the same is not the best policy. Diversity requires managers to develop a greater understanding of employee differences. This understanding will enable them to interpret gender-associated and culture-associated traits correctly as individual characteristics, and not as signs of incompetence. Valuing differences is the best way to obtain optimum performance from a mixed work force.

Managers should develop a strategy for handling front-line diversity issues. General guidelines for managing diversity have included suggestions meant to do the following:

- Improve communication between employees.
- Reduce bias toward nontraditional workers.
- Orient all employees to an organizational culture that values diversity.
- Meet the needs of all groups of workers.

Other guidelines are listed in Table 28–3.

Figure 28–1 shows the three major stages that are necessary to achieve a fully multicultural organization. Achievement of the first stage requires widespread, continuous training and orientation throughout the organization to increase awareness of differences and to teach employees to value the differences that will benefit the organization and its employees. The leaders of the organization need to be highly visible participants at this stage.

Stage 2 is a period of change. The development of this stage parallels that of the other stages, as change is continuous. Basic changes should be observed in employee attitudes, behaviors, and values. Unplanned social interaction begins to accelerate as employees begin to feel comfortable with each other and with each other's skills and abilities. The organization needs to institute a strong effort to reward and reinforce employee changes during this phase.

At Stage 3, the organization fully incorporates diversity into its public and private language and its policies, and the mobility of employees from all walks of life is evident in the organization. Management is managing diversity fairly, and it is well known that diversity is highly valued.

When an organization reaches Stage 4, it no longer needs to make an effort to make diversity explicit; it has become a part of doing business. The organization has become a multicultural organization.*

UNDERSTANDING PEOPLE'S VALUES**

Based on 16 years of observation and research, Professor Graves of Union College found that people seem to evolve through consecutive levels of "psychological existence" that are descriptive of personal values and lifestyles.[1] Relatively independent of intelligence, a person's level of

---

Table 28–3 Staff Diversity Tips for Managers

- Do not avoid the diversity issue—discuss it openly.
- Recognize and understand the importance of each employee's uniqueness and combination of background influences.
- Be "intercultural ambassadors," using respect as the organizational rule.
- Meet Equal Employment Opportunity Commission (EEOC) requirements.
- Mediate between personal and professional needs of employees.
- Explain the unwritten rules of the organization to nontraditional workers.
- Ensure a well-rounded perspective by having employees from the "diverse" group talk with coworkers who have resolved a similar problem.

Source: Adapted from J. Goldstein and M. Leopold, "Corporate Culture versus Ethnic Culture," *Personnel Journal* 69, November 1991.

Source: "Creating an Organizational Climate for Multiculturalism," John G. Bruhn, *Health Care Supervisor*, Vol. 14, No. 4, pp. 11–18, Aspen Publishers, Inc., © 1996.

**Source:* M. Scott Myers and Susan S. Meyers, "Adapting to the New Work Ethic," *Business Quarterly*, Winter 1973. Reprinted with permission.

[1]Clare W. Graves, "Levels of Existence: An Open System Theory of Values," *Journal of Humanistic Psychology*, Fall 1970.

Figure 28–1 Indicators of Progress Toward a Multicultural Organization

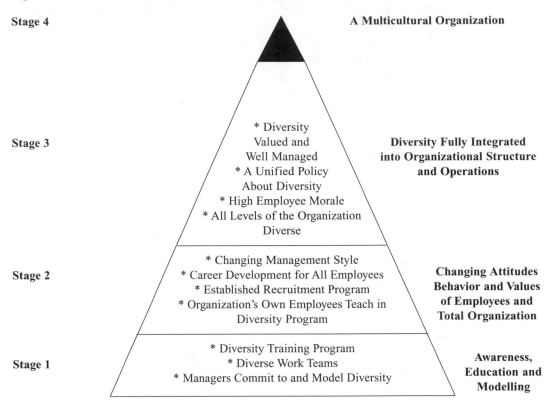

Stage 4   A Multicultural Organization

Stage 3
* Diversity Valued and Well Managed
* A Unified Policy About Diversity
* High Employee Morale
* All Levels of the Organization Diverse
Diversity Fully Integrated into Organizational Structure and Operations

Stage 2
* Changing Management Style
* Career Development for All Employees
* Established Recruitment Program
* Organization's Own Employees Teach in Diversity Program
Changing Attitudes Behavior and Values of Employees and Total Organization

Stage 1
* Diversity Training Program
* Diverse Work Teams
* Managers Commit to and Model Diversity
Awareness, Education and Modelling

Source: "Creating an Organizational Climate for Multiculturalism," John G. Bruhn, *Health Care Supervisor*, Vol. 14, No. 4, pp. 11–18, Aspen Publishers, Inc., © 1996.

psychological existence can become arrested at a given level or it can move upward or downward depending on that person's cultural conditioning and perception of the opportunities and constraints in the environment. A diagrammatic version of Graves's framework is presented in Figure 28–2.

Level 1. The *reactive* level of existence is most commonly observed in newborn babies or in people psychologically arrested in, or regressed to, infancy. They are unaware of themselves or others as human begins, and simply react to hunger, thirst, urination, defecation, sex, and other periodic physiological stimuli. Few people remain at this stage as they move toward adulthood; however, those at the threshold of subsistence may be little beyond this stage of existence. People at this level are generally not found on payrolls of organizations.

Level 2. Most people, as a matter of course, move out of the reactive existence to a *tribalistic* stage. Tribalism is characterized by concern with feelings of pain, temperature control, and safety and by tacit submission to an authority figure, whether a supervisor, police officer, government official, teacher, priest, parent, big brother, or gang leader. Tribalism is commonly observed in primitive cultures where magic, witchcraft, ritual, and superstition prevail. For example, the Bantu, who work in the coal, gold, and diamond mines of South Africa, are largely tribalistic. People at this level are locked into the rigid traditions of their tribe and are dominated by the tribal chieftain or his or her substitute.

Figure 28–2 Levels of Psychological Existence

EXISTENTIAL

High tolerance for ambiguity and people with differing values. Likes to do jobs in his or her own way without constraints of authority or bureaucracy. Goal-oriented but toward a broader arena and longer time perspective.

MANIPULATIVE

Ambitious to achieve higher status and recognition. Strives to manipulate people and things. May achieve goals through gamesmanship, persuasion, bribery, or official authority.

EGOCENTRIC

Individualistic, selfish, thoughtless, unscrupulous, dishonest. Has not learned to function within the constraints imposed by society. Responds primarily to power.

REACTIVE

Not aware of self or others as individuals or human beings. Reacts to basic physiological needs. Mostly restricted to infants.

SOCIOCENTRIC

High affiliation needs. Dislikes violence, conformity, materialism, and manipulative management. Concerned with social issues and the dignity of human beings.

CONFORMIST

Low tolerance for ambiguity and for people whose values differ from his or her own. Attracted to rigidly defined roles in accounting, engineering, and the military and tends to perpetuate the status quo. Motivated by a cause, philosophy, or religion.

TRIBALISTIC

Found mostly in primitive societies and ghettos. Lives in a world of magic, witchcraft, and superstition. Strongly influenced by tradition and the power exerted by the boss, tribal chieftain, police officer, schoolteacher, politician, and other authority figures.

Level 3. Egocentrism is an overly assertive form of rugged individualism. This person's behavior reflects a philosophy that seems to say, "To hell with the rest of the world. I'm for myself." He or she is typically premoral—thus unscrupulous, selfish, aggressive, restless, impulsive, and, in general, not psychologically inclined to live within the constraints imposed by society's moral precepts. To this person, might is right, and authoritarian management, preferably benevolent, seems necessary to keep him or her in line. Typical group techniques are not usually successful for this type of person, but structured participative management, properly administered, promises to be an effective strategy for getting the person out of this egocentric mode.

Egocentrism and tribalism are not a function of ethnic determinants but a result of cultural disadvantage or individual background. Egocentric and tribalistic behavior has become more prevalent in organizations.

Level 4. Persons at the *conformity* level of existence have low tolerance for ambiguity, have difficulty in accepting people whose values differ from their own, and have a need to get others to accept their values. They usually subordinate themselves to a philosophy, cause, or religion and tend to be attracted to vocations circumscribed by dogma or clearly defined rules. Though often perceived as docile, the conformist will assert or sacrifice him- or herself in violence if his or her values are threatened. Conformists prefer authoritarianism to autonomy, but will respond to participation if it is prescribed by an acceptable authority and does not violate deep-seated values. They like specific job descriptions and procedures and have little tolerance for supervisory indecision or weakness.

Level 5. The fifth level of psychological existence is characterized by *manipulative* or materialistic behavior. Persons at this level are typically products of the Horatio Alger, rags-to-riches philosophy—striving to achieve their goals through the manipulation of things and people within their environment. They thrive on gamesmanship, politics, competition, and entrepreneurial effort; measure their success in terms of materialistic gain and power; and are inclined to flaunt self-earned (as against hereditary) status symbols. Typical of level 5 persons are business managers, who define their goals and strategies in terms such as cash flow, return on investment, profits, share of the market, and net sales billed and generally focus on short-term targets such as the quarterly review or annual plan. They tend to perceive people as expense items rather than assets.

Level 6. People at the sixth, or *sociocentric*, level of existence have high affiliation needs. Getting along is more important than getting ahead, and the approval of people they respect is valued over individual fame. At this level, people may return to religiousness, not for its ritual or dogma, but rather for its spiritual attitude and concern with social issues. On the job, the sociocentric person responds well to participative management, but only on the condition that he or she and valued others believe in the product or service. The sociocentric person tends to articulate protests openly, but characteristically dislikes violence and would counter authoritarianism with passive resistance. Sociocentrics are frequently perceived as cop-outs by persons at levels 4 and 5, and their behavior is not generally rewarded in business organizations. As a result, persons at this level who do not ultimately capitulate by regressing to the organizationally accepted modes of manipulation and conformity or adapt by evolving to the seventh level of psychological existence may become organizational problems because of alcoholism, drug abuse, or other self-punitive behavior.

Level 7. Individuals at the *existential* level of existence have high tolerance for ambiguity and

for persons whose values differ from their own. On the job, their behavior might say, "OK, I understand the job to be done—now leave me alone and let me do it my way." In some respects they are a blend of levels 5 and 6 in that they are goal-oriented toward organizational success (level 5) and concerned with the dignity of fellow human beings (level 6). Like individuals at level 5, they are concerned with organizational profits, the quarterly review, and the annual plan, but they are also concerned with the 10-year or 50-year plan and the impact of the organization on its members, the community, and the environment. Like those at level 6, they are repelled by the use of violence. However, their outspoken intolerance of inflexible systems, restrictive policy, status symbols, and the arbitrary use of authority is threatening to most level 4 and 5 managers, and they may be expelled from the organization for reasons of nonconformity or insubordination.

RELATIONS WITH STAFF

Personnel Cliques*

Satisfying the individual's need for belonging, prestige, recognition, and so forth, is the primary function of the informal group. The informal group is a natural unit in which work decisions and judgments are reached. It provides an atmosphere for testing new procedures and creates standards of conduct for its members.

Group standards of behavior pervade the informal social organization. Management may either benefit or suffer from the group's standards and group pressure to conform. It depends on how close the goals of the group are to the goals of management.

Members

The group member experiences certain pressures to conform to group standards and norms.

---

*Source: Richard S. Muti, "The Informal Group—What It Is and How It Can Be Controlled," *Personnel Journal*, August 1968. Reprinted with the permission of *Personnel Journal*, Costa Mesa, California; all rights reserved.

The individual point of view becomes aligned with the group's point of view, and since the group satisfies the member's social needs, he or she accepts the group's goals. The member wants to be "well regarded" by the other members. A member who exceeds the group's accepted level of output may find him- or herself ostracized. Any deviation from group standards may cause the member to be isolated and be given the "silent treatment." The member may be left out of group activities. More direct methods of pressuring the individual to conform include letting management know of the deviant's "mistakes," flooding his or her desk with work, or even sabotaging his or her equipment.

Leaders

It is sometimes hard to identify the group leader. The group spokesperson is not necessarily the leader. There may be different leaders for different group functions.

The group's leader tends to be the member who most closely conforms to the group's standards and norms, or the one who has the most information and skill related to the group's activities. The leader must enable the members to achieve their private goals as well as the group's goals.

The informal leader can sometimes mold and change the group's goals and norms. When the leader speaks, the group listens and is influenced. But if the leader tries to change things too fast, he or she can lose the role of leader.

Managing Cliques

Management must recognize that informal groups exist. Once this is acknowledged, management should gather as much information as possible about the existing groups. Who belongs to which informal groups? What are the goals of the different groups? Are they opposed to the organization's goals? What are the operating techniques of the groups? How cohesive are they?

The nurse manager can gain cooperation only by respecting the group's standards and norms. Managers have been characterized as the "people in the middle." They are formal leaders, but must rely on more than the authority of the formal

organization to get successful results. They must build acceptance of themselves by the informal group and, in effect, attain some portion of the role of informal leader.

A good manager knows what the group expects and adjusts his or her behavior accordingly. The manager must make *fair* demands of the group and emphasize getting the job done rather than use authority for its own sake. Rules imposed on the group should be reasonable. Time-honored customs should be respected whenever possible. The manager must weigh the implications carefully before taking a position at odds with the accepted practices of the group.

Informal leaders should be given a chance to gain recognition by working with rather than against management. It is important to build good relations with informal leaders—pass information to them, ask their advice, have them train others. However, it is necessary to be aware of the danger of cooperating so far that it becomes favoritism.

Social Dynamics of Teams

Team structures are a persistent part of delivering care in the contemporary health care facility, from bedside care items to improvement teams to multidisciplinary teams. Socialization and communication within teams and between teams are important parts of interpersonal relations today. (*Note:* The goals and mechanics of teamwork are discussed in Chapter 8.) The social interactions of teams require the development of communication skills, whether for the evolution of the team itself or to facilitate work.

Development of Team Relations*

The socialization process in team development involves forging and unifying a group of people into an effective and efficiently functioning work unit so that specified goals are accomplished. It is a continuous process that goes through sev-

---

*Source: Mary J. Farley and Martha H. Stoner, "The Nurse Executive and Interdisciplinary Team Building," *Nursing Administration Quarterly*, Vol. 13, No. 3, Aspen Publishers, Inc., © Winter 1989.

Table 28–4 Questionnaire: Manager's Interpersonal Relations

1. Do you have a thorough understanding of the institution's goals and your part in meeting the objectives of the institution?	Yes	No
2. Do you avoid confusion and have a clear understanding of what is expected and how to do it?	Yes	No
3. Do you offer suggestions or constructive criticism to your immediate supervisor and ask for additional information when necessary?	Yes	No
4. Do you build team spirit and group pride by getting everyone into the act of setting goals and pulling together?	Yes	No
5. Do you schedule time for meetings with your subordinates and with your superiors?	Yes	No
6. Do you encourage each of your employees to come up with suggestions about ways to improve things?	Yes	No
7. Do you make it easy for your employees to approach you with job or personal problems?	Yes	No
8. Do you keep your employees informed on how they are doing?	Yes	No
9. Are you too busy with operational problems to be concerned with your employees' personal difficulties?	Yes	No
10. Do you give your employees a feeling of accomplishment by telling them how well they are doing in comparison with yesterday, last week, or a month or a year ago?	Yes	No
11. Do you build individual employee confidence and praise good performance?	Yes	No
12. Do you use personnel records and close observation to learn exactly which skills each employee has so that his or her best abilities may be used?	Yes	No
13. Do you let your employees know how jobs are analyzed and evaluated and what the job rates and progressions are?	Yes	No
14. Do you attempt to rotate employees on different jobs to build up skills for individual flexibility within the group?		
15. Do you train your employees for better jobs?	Yes	No
16. Are you developing an understudy for your job?	Yes	No
17. Do you hold a good person down in one position because he or she may be indispensable there?	Yes	No
18. Are you doing things to discourage your subordinates?	Yes	No
19. Are you aware of sources of discontentment or discouragement or frustration affecting your employees?	Yes	No
20. Do you listen to the ideas and reactions of subordinates with courtesy?	Yes	No
21. If an idea is adopted or not adopted, do you explain why?	Yes	No
22. Do you usually praise in public, but criticize or reprove in private?	Yes	No
23. Is your criticism constructive?	Yes	No
24. Are you aware that a feeling of belonging builds self-confidence and makes people want to work harder than ever?	Yes	No
25. Do you ever say or do anything that detracts from the sense of personal dignity that each of your employees has?	Yes	No

Source: Copyright © 1988, Norman Metzger.

eral stages and takes time, energy, and effort to accomplish.

Nurse executives who are familiar with individual member tasks as well as group tasks are in a better position to help the team to achieve the ideal outcomes of each stage. Table 28–5 presents a compilation of the stages of team growth, the identifying characteristics of each stage, and the member tasks.

Nurse executives need to be aware of the negative forces and actively work to alleviate them so that teamwork may be effective and successful. The forces that may tear a team apart include such things as different needs, values, and world views of team members; professional rivalries; contradictory institutional priorities; misunderstandings between team members; and lack of commitment to team goals. Therefore, the nurse executive must be sensitive to individual needs and must use diplomacy in managing conflict.

NEGOTIATION AS A COMMUNICATION STRATEGY*

Due to the increased use of cross-functional activities, health care professionals now deal less with their superiors and subordinates and more with colleagues. In other words *horizontal* negotiations are now of paramount importance. Negotiation has become part of the nurse administrator's life, whether participating on an executive team or trying to impart skill to nurses participating in a team structure of care.

The ability to negotiate is a vital part of interpersonal skill. The paradigm of negotiation strategy is undergoing a profound shift from power pressure to an egalitarian form of problem solv-

ing or a value-added approach that is much more likely to result in win-win outcomes.

Preparations for a Negotiation

At its worst, negotiation is battling with opponents; at its best, it is an interaction that enables both parties to gain what they want—a win-win outcome.

As with any worthwhile activity, planning is essential to successful negotiations. Too often people walk into a negotiation unprepared. Each person has different interests, and being prepared increases understanding of these different interests.

The Wish List. You must know what you want and what you are willing to concede. Try to find out what the other side wants, how badly they want it, what they are likely to propose, and what cards they hold.

Data. Effective negotiators have the necessary data. These may be copies of laws, policies, protocols, or written and unwritten guidelines. Negotiators must have up-to-date information gleaned from formal and informal communication channels. Nothing will shoot down a proposal quicker than a valid document that proves that what has been proposed violates a law or the organization's mission statement.

Information must be organized and presented in a concise understandable fashion. This often requires handouts, graphs, charts, and other visual displays.

Complete a Plan of Action. Several steps should be taken before negotiating. You should sketch out the possible options you can offer, prepare your opening remarks, and prepare the arguments you can make to maximize the positive aspects and to counter the other person's arguments. Before meeting, review your approach with an associate or mentor. Then try to pick the best time and place for you for the meeting.

Source: William Umiker, "Negotiating Skill for Health Care Professionals," *The Health Care Supervisor*, Vol. 14, No. 3, Aspen Publishers, Inc., © March 1996.

Table 28–5 Stages of Social Working Relations in Teams

Stage	Characteristics	Member Tasks
1. Orientation	Opinions expressed cautiously Artificial politeness Ambiguous relationships Efforts unfocused	Learning what is expected and relating this to self Making social comparisons (including needs) Asking, "How do I belong to this group?"
2. Adaptation	Social mechanisms developing that serve to differentiate members Team identity beginning	Finding appropriate role for self, both personally and professionally
3. Emergence	Bargaining Alliances forming Power struggles Dispute, disagreements, and defending of opinions	Finding identity as a team member with ability to communicate, differ, confront, and collaborate
4. Working	Achievement of complementarity and gestalt	Making honest disclosure Reaching individual decisions and negotiating solutions

Major Steps in a Negotiation

Step 1: Clarify Interests. Interests may be objective (special service, sharing of equipment, turnaround time) or subjective (goodwill, long-term relationships). Ask the person with whom you are negotiating how the situation is viewed and what is important. Paraphrase the message you get and ask if you have interpreted the view correctly. Then, state your view. Do not proceed until these viewpoints and desired outcomes are crystal clear.

Step 2: Focus on Perceived Points of Agreement. Center on points of agreement and work from there. Only after covering each of these should you get into the problem areas.

Step 3: Formulate Possible Options—The More the Better. Verify that each deal offers a different way to balance interests through a different arrangement of the value elements.

Articulate the benefits of each option to the other person.

Do not get stuck believing that your solution is the only good one. Be gracious; if the person has a valid argument, say so.

Step 4: Agree on the Best Option. If you cannot reach complete agreement, be willing to compromise, *but not until you have explored all win-win solutions.*

In some situations, it is best not to make a definite commitment. Each of you may need more information or to consult with other individuals. View the initial meeting as an exploratory session.

Step 5: Perfect the Deal. It is important to refine the selected deal, to make sure it is balanced in terms of total value, and to ensure that each of you is comfortable with it.

Step 6: Wrap It Up. Close the negotiation by reviewing what has been agreed upon and documenting it.

- Agree on exactly who is going to do what—and when.
- Get commitments for deadlines for completing specific responsibilities.
- Get it in writing. A carefully typed statement demonstrates commitment and provides a reference for the future when memories get hazy.
- Decide how long results will be monitored, what will be measured, how, by whom, and for how long. What will constitute a successful outcome?
- Discuss a series of "what if" situations.
- Help the other person sell the agreement to associates and superiors.

The box lists several things one should and should not do when involved in negotiation.

General Tips for More Effective Negotiation

Do

- State objectives or interests, not positions. Make certain that you understand the other party's interests.
- Regard the other person not as an enemy but as a partner in problem solving. Attack the problem, not the other person.
- Remember that the other person is usually willing to accept a solution if you can make it sufficiently attractive. Phrase requests in terms of the other person's best interest.
- Listen carefully for what is said and what is not said. Watch the body language.
- Keep things simple. Distill your ideas into a few sentences.
- Anticipate objections.
- Know what you can give.
- Present several options.
- Model openness and compliance and act as if you expect the other party to do the same.
- Remain assertive but not aggressive.
- Remember your veto power. You can always say no or walk away.
- Use your body language. A simple shudder when the other person makes an offer may change the offer in your favor.
- Persist when you know you are right.

Avoid

- Putdowns, sarcasm, gloating, cynicism.
- Manipulation and dirty tricks.
- Distortions, exaggerations, or falsehoods.
- Revealing that you have been taken by surprise.
- Rushing the negotiation process.
- Jumping at the first offer; you can almost always do better.
- Making just one offer.
- Giving away the store. Do not be a pushover.
- Trying to score all the points. Your position is strengthened and cooperation is much more likely if you accede to some of their ideas.
- Allowing the other party to pick the best parts from all the deals in order to make a new one ("cherry picking.")

Chapter 29

Job Satisfaction and Motivation

JOB SATISFACTION AND JOB PERFORMANCE

Job performance is the result of the interaction of two variables: (1) ability to perform the task and (2) amount of motivation. Ability to perform the task is an obvious variable. To the extent that people are put in jobs that demand skills and abilities that they do not possess, or possess to a degree below that required, lower-than-desired levels of job performance should be expected. Increasingly, this requires a complete understanding of job requirements and a thoroughness in screening applicants to ensure that they have the necessary skills and abilities.

Motivational Factors*

The second determinant of job performance is the amount of motivation. This in turn is a function of the following motivational factors:

- need for achievement
- belief that one is being well paid

Source: Burt K. Scanlon, "Determinants of Job Satisfaction and Productivity," *Personnel Journal*, January 1976. Reprinted with the permission of *Personnel Journal*, Costa Mesa, California; all rights reserved.

- job requiring skills and abilities valued and believed possessed
- feedback
- opportunity to participate
- performance instrumental to promotion, wage increases, coworker acceptability, and so forth

Several factors deserve special comment. The individual's need for achievement is one. Unfortunately, no way has been determined to precisely pinpoint this. Once the person is employed, the need can change as a result of many factors: the kind of training programs, how the job is designed, the style of supervision received, changes in motivational patterns, and so forth.

Also, individuals enter jobs with certain preconceived ideas about "how good" they are—their skills and abilities. Right or wrong, if a person thinks his or her skills and abilities are not being used and developed, a motivation problem occurs. It is perhaps worth noting that most people overestimate themselves and therefore tend to perceive themselves as being underutilized. Truth or falsity is not the issue; an individual's perception of the situation is the important factor.

The importance of feedback and having an opportunity to participate has been widely publicized. Motivation requires more than just physical involvement in a job. It demands mental and emotional involvement also.

Environmental Factors*

Environmental factors also play a key part in motivation. Among these factors are

- communication
  - appreciation of one's efforts; praise when it is due
  - knowledge of the organization's activities and intentions; inclusion in the employer's goals and plans
  - knowledge of where one stands with the organization at any given time; appraisal
  - confidentiality in personal dealings with management; tactful disciplining and reasonable privacy
- growth potential
  - the opportunity for advancement; career ladders and promotional paths
  - encouragement in growth and advancement; skill training, tuition assistance for formal education, and management training for potential managers
- personnel policies
  - reasonable accommodation of personal needs, as in work scheduling, vacation scheduling, sick time benefits
  - reasonable feeling of job security
  - organizational loyalty to employees
  - respect for an individual's origins, background, and beliefs
  - fair and consistent treatment relative to other employees
- salary administration
  - fair salary and benefits relative to others in the organization, in the community, and in one's specific occupation
- working conditions
  - the physical working conditions relative to what is expected or desired

The Manager's Role*

The department manager can have an influence on both motivating factors and environmental factors. However, the extent of possible influence depends partly on the job—specifically what the manager has to work with—and partly on the organization—how much latitude the individual manager is allowed.

For all employees, the manager has at least some ability to arouse motivation and to prevent dissatisfaction from taking over.

The true motivating factors—those listed previously—represent that capacity for the fulfillment of needs that are largely, if not entirely, psychological. As compared with the nonprofessional, the professional employee is more likely to be operating on a level of psychological need fulfillment. This should suggest to the manager that the professional employee would be more effectively managed through an open, participative management style that allows the employee the maximum possible opportunity for self-determination.

The manager is likely to have an impact on the five environmental factors surrounding the professional's work.

1. Communication. The immediate manager is always the key to communication with employees at all levels. Whether professional or non-professional, an employee's overall level of satisfaction often hinges completely or at least in large part on communication that is controlled by the manager. Communication serves many important needs in answering for the employee many questions, such as "How am I doing?" "Am I appreciated?" "Am I trusted and regarded with respect?" "Am I kept advised of what is happening in the organization?" "Am I treated as truly a part of the organization?" These questions and more are answered both directly and indirectly by the manager in the all-important one-to-one relationship with the employee.

2. Growth Potential. The manager has somewhat limited influence in the area of growth potential. Quite simply, the manager cannot create opportunities that may not be there because there are few openings for promotions or because short, restrictive career ladders are involved. The manager can, however, adopt a positive attitude that encourages employees to fix their sights on the existing opportunities.

3. Personnel Policies. As a member of the larger management group, the individual manager may have input into the formulation of personnel policies. Regardless of the extent of the manager's involvement in setting policy, however, he or she always has a key role in ensuring the consistent application of personnel policies in all employees. Inconsistency of treatment tends to be a major dissatisfier for many employees.

4. Salary Administration. Ordinarily the manager has little or no role in determining the salary structure of the organization. However, in hiring and promoting people and in granting pay raises, the manager may well have a key role in the consistent and equitable application of the salary structure. Often the principal determinant of an employee's level of satisfaction with the job's pay is that person's perception of how well he or she is paid relative to others, especially others of comparable skill who do the same kind of work.

5. Working Conditions. The manager has an active role in watching out for the well-being of the employees. Something as seemingly simple as inadequate lighting in the office or insufficient space in the parking lot can lead to dissatisfaction if not addressed. The manager, in many ways the advocate of the employee, partly ensures that the work gets done by ensuring that working conditions are reasonable or tolerable. The manager should serve as a channel through which complaints about working conditions are aired and problems are reported and corrected.

MOTIVATION

Motivation Theories*

Motivation comes from within the individual. Motivation is described as the effort with which an individual applies his or her abilities to the job. One of the beginning professional nurse's roles in organizational management is to create an environment and implement strategies that facilitate the development of the human potential of the patient care work group. Each person has needs and wants. Creating a work environment and implementing motivational strategies that support both organizational outcomes for effective, efficient patient care and individual outcomes for job satisfaction as well as personal and job growth can be facilitated by the behaviors of the beginning professional nurse.

Organizations must be designed to make individuals feel like winners. Motivation comes from within, but managers can influence motivation by providing effective feedback that supports growth and productivity. Managers and peers can give effective feedback using positive reinforcement by:

- giving specific and relevant examples of a positive performance (e.g., "I appreciate your helping care for Mr. Y today. Your assistance with his physical care really added to his comfort.")
- providing immediate and timely feedback and reinforcement
- setting achievable goals and celebrating small wins privately and publicly
- providing intermittent and unpredictable (spontaneous) reinforcement in recognition of the power of small rewards

Motivational theories may be characterized as content theories, based on human needs and motives, and process theories, based on how and why behaviors occur. Content theories include

*Source: C.E. Loveridge and Barbara Cummings, *Nursing Management in the New Paradigm,* Aspen Publishers, Inc., © 1995.

Maslow's hierarchy of needs and theory of motivation, which many nurses have utilized as a framework for planning patient care. Maslow's hierarchy of needs includes:

- physical needs (hunger, thirst, and physiological drives)
- safety needs (freedom from harm or danger; security)
- love and belonging needs (nurturing, acceptance, and respect)
- esteem needs (perceived self-worth)
- self-actualization needs (realization of one's potential)

Within Maslow's hierarchy, lower-level needs must be met before higher-level needs can influence human behavior. If the lower-level needs are not met continually, they will again become priority needs. For example, meeting physiological needs for food and rest will be more important to an individual than self-actualization needs if the individual has not eaten or slept for a prolonged period of time. Self-actualization can become a motivator if the environment is such that opportunities for individual development occur. These hypotheses are equally applicable to patients and health care team members. Maslow's theory, although not empirical, has been widely used as a motivational theory.

Alderfer's ERG needs-based motivational theory focuses on three categories of need: existence, relatedness, and growth. Alderfer's theory is simpler than Maslow's in its taxonomy of needs, and it rejects Maslow's concepts by stating that multiple needs may be activated over a short period of time.

Probably the most controversial content theory of motivation is Herzberg's two-factor theory. This theory, also known as the motivational hygiene theory, is based on research involving engineers and accountants. Herzberg's premise is that hygiene factors keep employees from being dissatisfied but have little or no positive impact on motivation. These hygiene factors, also called extrinsic factors, include working conditions, salary, security, and interpersonal relations with workforce peers. Motivating factors that are in-

herent in the individual include job challenges, achievement, recognitions for accomplishments, opportunity for career growth, and responsibility. When these factors are not present, an individual may not be dissatisfied but on the other hand is not experiencing satisfaction. When motivator factors are present, Herzberg believes, individuals can be satisfied. Herzberg's implications are that motivation can be enhanced via job enrichment. In reality, hygiene factors must also be met before intrinsic motivator factors are operant.

Process theories of motivation include Vroom's expectancy model, which considers an individual's preferences or valences based on social values, which can be defined as positive, negative, or neutral; expectancy, or beliefs about actions and work outcomes; and instrumentality, the belief that personal consequences result from work performance. Stated differently, expectancy theory focuses on an individual's belief that performance affects results, consequences are linked to individual performance, and consequences are valued by the individual.

Adams focused on equity as a process theory of motivation with two dimensions. One is the perceived ratio of personal outcomes to work effort (input), and the second is the outcome-input ratio compared with that of individuals in the work group, that of similar groups, or industry standards. This theory influences motivation by causing individuals to seek to maintain equity and reduce actual or perceived gaps. Beginning professional nurses should not underestimate the power of comparison as a motivational factor for health care team members as well as themselves.

Motivation in Health Care Settings

It has been suggested that individuals are an organization's most valuable asset. Key to successful motivation of health care team members in empowered organizations is the identification of the overlap of both organizational needs and necessary outcomes and individual needs and goals. Agreements can then be created with team members that clearly define expectations related to outcomes, guidelines or boundaries, resources, accountabilities, and consequences. Beginning professional nurses can facilitate individual and group success by determining key success factors and using work group impact to modify processes and the environment to support positive outcomes. Clarifying objectives, outcomes, expected actions, and the coaching necessary to attain them, and providing both individuals and groups positive reinforcement or constructive feedback as appropriate, can improve motivation and performance. In health care settings, employees value recognition but often do not receive recognition or rewards for what they accomplish.

Supporting, Recognizing, and Rewarding Individuals and Groups

Rewards should motivate employees toward higher levels of performance. Intrinsic rewards are associated with the job itself and include:

- a feeling of personal responsibility
- work outcomes that utilize skills and abilities
- perception of work as meaningful
- credible feedback regarding the amount and quality of work

Extrinsic rewards are supplied by the organization and include:

- monetary rewards
- professional or peer recognition
- career development and promotion
- compliments and recognition from supervisors

Recent studies of staff nurse perceptions of reward and recognition practices indicate that, although money is clearly motivating, if salary is commensurate with responsibilities nurses value and desire personal feedback. Registered nurses in a recent study preferred to be rewarded for performance, including private verbal feedback, written recognition of performance, assistance toward professional goals, and participation in unit planning and management activities.

(See Table 29–1 for other factors in job satisfaction.)

Role Activities, Recognition, and Reward Strategies

The beginning professional nurse with responsibilities for organizational management functions with the patient care unit manager and advanced practice nurses, who have the responsibility to create an environment that maximizes human potential. By the nature of their roles, the beginning professional nurse, patient care unit manager, and advanced practice nurse act as role models and coaches, supporting staff in attaining individual and organizational outcomes and recognizing and rewarding successes.

How *Not* To Motivate*

Incompetent workers are often made, not born. With a little effort, you can squelch enthusiastic workers' initiative and cut their efficiency in half.

You can actually demolish their common sense so that they will apply your instructions to obviously inappropriate situations. The quality of their work will decline while their errors increase. Then, when their confidence plummets, you can let them go.

You can even get their replacements to follow the same path. If any of your workers retain their capabilities, you can make sure that they find better jobs elsewhere or are promoted out of your department.

As a result, you will become busier and busier, buried under a burden of work, completing tasks that your subordinates should have completed and reinstructing them in procedures that they should have learned long ago.

How can you accomplish this unfortunate situation? How can you destroy your subordinates' confidence and watch it crumble? The answer lies in your attitude toward them and the way you treat them.

---

*Source: "Sure-Fire Ways To Wreck Employee Competence," *Hospital Topics*, November-December, 1975. Reprinted with permission.

Table 29–1 Key Factors in Job Satisfaction

Twelve key factors emerged from two major research projects that examined the attitudes of health care workers and the factors that made them satisfied with their jobs.

- *Input.* Workers want the opportunity to speak up about their jobs. They want the chance to suggest change and to perceive that they are heard by management and supervision. In the studies, this was a particularly strong concern of registered nurses.
- *Worker-manager relations.* The manager is the key to organizational harmony and the success of motivational programs. Managers must know how to accomplish their jobs and how to be fair, understanding, mature, and helpful. In the studies, this factor was a particularly strong concern of registered nurses and allied health professionals.
- *Discipline/grievance.* Workers desire policies and procedures that are fair and unbiased. Policies and procedures can act as powerful motivators.
- *Work environment.* The environment has to be perceived as clean, comfortable, and safe. These items often emerge as particular concerns of allied health professionals.
- *Breaks and meals.* Workers feel the need for time off during working hours. Breaking away appears essential to registered nurses, who often get little or no time to rest because of staffing situations.
- *Discrimination.* Workers of all job classifications display a general aversion to racial, sexual, and professional discrimination. Fairness in this dimension is highly critical and is more of an issue for female workers than for male workers.
- *Work satisfaction.* Workers will be motivated if they have jobs that make them feel good

about themselves. Individuals need to feel they have a future in the organization, and their workload must be perceived as reasonable. This dimension presents a particular challenge for the manager in areas where workers have limited upward mobility because of training or educational constraints.
- *Performance appraisals.* Appraisal and feedback must occur on a regular and timely basis and must be equitable. Managers must be thoroughly trained in appraisal methods.
- *Clarity of policies, procedures, and benefits.* Workers must understand and possess *working* knowledge of policies and procedures and particularly of their benefits. It is the manager's responsibility to serve as a teacher and a resource person in this area.
- *Pay and development opportunities.* Workers want pay that is fair in comparison with the pay of competing health care institutions and with the community in general. Nurses are particularly concerned about development opportunities, including both continuing education and the opportunity to grow within the organization.
- *Decision making.* Workers want something to say about how the institution or agency is managed; they want to experience a true vested interest.
- *Style of management.* The attitude projected by top management through the individual managers is an important factor. Health care workers want to be associated with an organization that cares about workers and patients alike.

Source: Paul E. Fitzgerald, Jr., "Worker Perceptions: The Key to Motivation," *The Health Care Supervisor*, Vol. 3, No. 1, Aspen Publishers, Inc., © 1984.

Sure-Fire Techniques

Be so vague about what you want your subordinates to do that they cannot pinpoint precisely what you want. In other words, do not mention any specific cases or show any examples to which they can refer. Give your instructions matter-of-

factly, as if you had no doubt that anyone of minimum intelligence would understand them. Give criticism in the same way so that they will not know what they can do to correct their performance.

Give an audible sigh of resignation if they ask you to clarify something you have explained.

Imply that no one has ever asked you to clarify such simple instructions. Remember to avoid giving them any examples that would clear up the problem.

If they ask the same questions more than once, point out that you have already answered those questions. Sometimes you can do this even when a subordinate asks the question the first time—especially if his or her confidence has already been shaken. You may be able to convince the subordinate that his or her memory is failing—which should make him or her feel guilty for having unnecessarily taken up so much of your valuable time.

Make an obvious effort to contain your impatience if the subordinate still does not understand what you mean. This time, instruct him or her so slowly—in minute detail, with very simple words—that you underscore your low opinion of his or her intelligence. Continue to give the subordinate this kind of explanation and impression on other occasions—even when the subordinate insists that he or she understands.

Be sure to criticize specific acts—even where the error is minor and would have been corrected in the normal course of events with no harm done. You can, in fact, make a game out of trying to catch subordinates in "errors" of procedure. Monitor their work closely and point out minor details that they could have accomplished "better" some other way.

Always give them step-by-step instructions, but leave out an explanation of the purpose or expected results. This makes it impossible for them to claim that another procedure would better serve the purpose. Be specific enough to prevent them from exercising their initiative.

Change your instructions from time to time as subordinates proceed with a project. It may help sometimes to deny having given the earlier instructions—particularly if the results do not seem to be turning out too well.

If unforeseen problems arise from following your instructions, insist that the subordinates always return to you for the solution. Do not let them solve the problem themselves, even if they claim they know how to do so. If they challenge this restriction, tell them that there are many details you cannot give them because of lack of time.

Give subordinates deadlines that you know they cannot meet. When they fail to meet them, as expected, you can blame it on their lack of efficiency.

Improve on everything subordinates do. Tell them that you do this only to make their work acceptable. Then if they start taking two or three times as long to complete tasks in a futile attempt to meet your "rigorous" standards, point again to their lack of efficiency. Or, if they give up and do each task carelessly, point out how slovenly they are.

Following these guidelines will ensure two things: (1) Your subordinates will be totally demoralized, and (2) you need not worry about being promoted to a position that you cannot fill.

JOB ENRICHMENT

Job Design: A Strategy for Improving Satisfaction*

After nurse managers have determined that their nursing program or organizational climate is less than desirable, they must devise strategies to promote its potential well-being. Numerous strategies are available. Many concentrate on motivation and reward strategies. One strategy that has been recommended for improving the nursing program or organizational climate is job design. The premise underlying job design is that job variety and flexibility in assignments decrease boredom and increase staff satisfaction. (See Figure 29–1.) Job design consists of three ingredients.

Source: Judith F. Garner, Howard L. Smith, and Neill F. Piland, *Strategic Nursing Management: Power and Responsibility in a New Era,* Aspen Publishers, Inc., © 1990.

Figure 29–1 Variables Contributing to Satisfaction and Affecting Retention

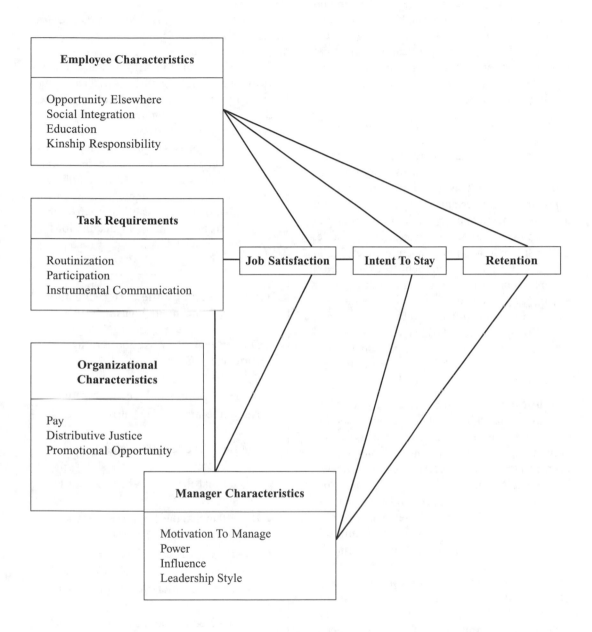

Source: Reprinted from "Manager Impact on Retention of Hospital Staff: Part 1" by R.L. Taunton, S.D. Krampetz, and C.Q. Woods, *Journal of Nursing Administration*, Vol. 19, No. 3, p. 15, with permission of J.B. Lippincott Company, © March 1989.

Job Enlargement. Nurses are assigned more tasks to improve the challenge of their job and to reduce boredom. For example, instead of just performing triage, a nurse may be delegated the responsibility of defining a treatment plan and schedule for patient follow up. This instills variety in the task and relieves the boredom of repeating a single task.

Job Enrichment. Nurses are incorporated into decision-making processes of the nursing department and are assigned more meaningful tasks. By sharing decisions about the service delivery process, their work tasks acquire more meaning. They are no longer simply repeating tasks but are active in and appreciative of the complexity surrounding health care services. For example, a licensed practical nurse at a clinic may log in patients and then assign them to examination rooms. Under a job enrichment strategy, he or she might participate in determining which patients will be scheduled for return visits during the following week and which will be scheduled for another week because of an excessively busy schedule. The job includes more tasks that require decision-making discretion.

Job Rotation. Nurses periodically rotate in assignment in completing the various tasks that are included in a service. In this strategy, nurses come to know, appreciate, and complete all the tasks in a specific service. Variety prevents boredom. In addition, there is greater flexibility because more nurses are capable of filling in at any specific point if illness or absenteeism occurs. Bottlenecks can be prevented. For example, a nurse executive in a consulting firm may be required to write proposals, to present the proposals to clients, to undertake the proposed analysis, to write up the analysis, to present the results to clients, and to undertake the follow up. After rotating through each of these tasks, spending perhaps four months on each task or a combination of tasks, the nurse executive can fill in at any point in the process as necessary. Further, by purposefully scheduling rotation it is unlikely that the nurse executive will be bored with any assignment.

Job Redesign Measures*

An effective job design meets both the requirements of the tasks and the social and psychological needs of the workers.

The actual introduction of job redesign measures to enhance staff members' satisfaction may be formal or informal, planned well in advance or on the spur of the moment. Certain times, however, are more opportune than others. These include the latter phases of probationary employment, at the time of performance reviews, when salary discussions are initiated by employees, when new services are contemplated, when employee cutbacks are necessary, and when organizational expansions, mergers, acquisitions, or other restructurings take place.

Guidelines and Cautions To Using Job Enhancement Measures

- Do not attempt to use job redesign or enrichment as a cure-all.
- Tailor the changes to the needs and wants of the employees and the organization.
- Know the motivational drives of each person.
- Consider the effect of the change on others.
- Ensure that the employee endorses the measures.
- Be certain that the employee has a good chance to succeed.
- Make the goals and plans flexible and reversible.
- Update the position descriptions as appropriate.
- Provide feedback and support.
- Do not promise what you cannot deliver.

Source: William Umiker, *Management Skills for the New Health Care Supervisor*, ed 2, Aspen Publishers, Inc., © 1994.

Table 29–2 Methods for Transfer of Power to Front-Line Service Providers

There are many ways that an organization can shift power downward.

- transferring authority from central headquarters to branches or satellites
- eliminating layers of management (flattening the pyramid), which forces individuals in the lower echelons to assume more responsibility and authority (Organizations that have carried this restructuring to the fullest extent have organized semiautonomous, self-managing teams that perform not only the technical tasks but also the administrative ones. These work groups answer only to the top administration.)
- using selection and training procedures that ensure requisite technical, linguistic, and social influence skills
- having open communication systems that create extensive network-forming devices

- instituting policies and culture that emphasize self-determination and collaboration more than competition, high performance standards, and nondiscrimination
- letting employees evaluate the performance of their superiors, or getting employee input via frequent anonymous morale surveys
- discouraging bureaucratic factors such as manipulation, managed information, or penalizing people for telling the truth
- redesigning jobs to provide variety, autonomy, low levels of established routines and rules, and high advancement prospects
- rewarding the performance desired with salary and promotional strategies that are valued by the recipients, for when organizations do not provide rewards that are valued by employees and when rewards are not offered for competence, initiative, and innovativeness, employees' sense of powerlessness increases

Source: William Umiker, "Empowerment: The Latest Motivational Strategy," *The Health Care Supervisor*, Vol. 11, No. 2, Aspen Publishers, Inc., © 1992.

Job redesign measures include

- cross-training
- rotation of work stations, departments, or shifts
- job transfer
- changed work hours (flextime)
- switches from full time to part time, or vice versa
- deletion or addition of specific duties
- new locations of work stations
- improved instrumentation, flow patterns, communication, and methodology
- changed team membership or roles
- support of creativity and entrepreneurship
- delegation or more challenging assignments
- appointments to committees, quality circles, or other work groups
- involvement in research or development
- assignments to teaching or training roles

EMPOWERMENT AND MOTIVATION

Empowerment as a Motivational Strategy*

Supervisory Component of Empowerment

Underlying a motivational strategy is the manager's goal to enhance people's belief in their self-efficacy. To achieve this, managers must satisfy needs for self-determination, competency, power, and self-actualization.

Employees must have reason to believe that they are competent and capable of more. Their self-esteem and feelings regarding their personal efficacy are strengthened when they know that they are technically or professionally competent, they note that their performance is as good as or better than that of their colleagues, and they receive positive feedback from superiors and as-

---

*Source: William Umiker, "Empowerment: The Latest Motivational Strategy," *The Health Care Supervisor*, Vol. 11, No. 2, Aspen Publishers, Inc., © 1992.

sociates. To help upgrade your empowering process, ask yourself these questions: May any of my employees call for a meeting or send out a memo? At performance reviews after I say what I want from the employees, do I ask what they want from me? Are my subordinates committed or only complying? Do they have job "ownership"? Do they say "I" or "we," or is it "they"? Do they have any input into work hours, assignments, priorities, vacation schedules, and the selection of new instruments, procedures, policies, and new employees? Do I encourage self-expression and assertiveness? Do I model what I want from others? Do I avoid manipulation, favoritism, and saying yes when I mean no? Do I eschew bureaucratic or autocratic leadership? Do I devote time at each staff meeting to issues dealing with attitude, morale, and motivation, that is, identifying things that have made them proud?

Risks of Empowerment

Empowerment does involve risks. Whenever there is a transfer of authority, there is risk. Only managers who are not afraid to take risks will empower their subordinates. Some managers feel threatened by an empowered person or an empowered group of people because there is some loss of control.

Some empowered subordinates are going to come up with worthless ideas and are going to do silly things. Empowering managers must accept this and chalk them up to learning experiences.

Because empowered employees take new risks when they use their new powers, not everyone wants to be empowered. It is difficult to empower nonassertive people or people who cannot accept guilt ("It's not my fault"). Blame avoidance is also characteristic of the bureaucratic mindset, while innovative individuals have no difficulty accepting responsibility without being immobilized by fear or guilt.

On the other hand, empowerment may lead to overconfidence and misjudgments. Some empowered individuals abuse their prerogatives or have difficulty defining the limits of their authority.

Chapter 30

Absenteeism and Turnover

THE IMPACT OF ABSENTEEISM

To the nurse manager, absenteeism is an immediate problem of sometimes significant dimensions. Even a modest percentage of absenteeism in the department is likely to upset schedules and cause much supervisory time and effort to be devoted to juggling personnel and assignments to cover necessary tasks.

When someone fails to show up for work, usually one of three things happen: (1) the employee's work goes undone that day, (2) someone else must be assigned to cover for the absent employee, or (3) someone extra is hired to replace the absent worker. In any case, significant cost can be involved.

It has been estimated that absenteeism costs the country in excess of $10 billion per year in lost output and other costs. For example, sick leave benefits are paid, replacement employees are hired, or revenue is lost because employees are not there to perform. Numerous rippling inefficiencies occur that ultimately have a dollar impact on the organization.*

---

*Source: Charles R. McConnell, *The Effective Health Care Supervisor*, ed 3, Aspen Publishers, Inc., © 1993.

Management Response

How do administrators go about the job of combating the drain on staff caused by excessive turnover and absenteeism? The administrators who have been most successful in meeting these problems preplan their work and allow for absences. They keep accurate and complete records of attendance. They provide for exit interviews and analyze separations to find the real reasons for discharges, voluntary quits, and absences from the job. They carefully select new workers; make use of training, safety, and health programs; and cooperate with community agencies to provide child care, shopping, banking, transportation, and recreational facilities. They make careful analyses and evaluations of the facts and take steps to identify and relieve or eliminate the causes of employee dissatisfaction because they are aware that management cannot afford to ignore either excessive rates of turnover or unrealistic reasons for absenteeism or lateness.

Excessive turnover and absenteeism are expensive to both employers and workers in terms of money, morale, and wasted human resources. Some turnover and absenteeism must be expected, but excessive rates can be reduced by sound human resource policies in which management and labor work closely together.

RELATIONSHIP BETWEEN ABSENTEEISM AND TURNOVER*

Absenteeism and turnover are generally seen as forms of employee alienation or withdrawal from an organization. The nature of the relationship between absenteeism and turnover consists of three parts. In the first case, absenteeism is a form of withdrawal behavior that represents an alternative to turnover. Here employees do not desire termination nor do they believe the employer will terminate them for their behavior. Some condition related either to the job or to an employee personally seems to justify the absence and restores the individual or the employment relationship to equilibrium. The second position identifies a continuum of withdrawal, with absenteeism preceding turnover. The individual's decision to be absent from the job is just a miniature version of the more important decision made when the employee quits the job. In the third case, there is no consistent relationship between absenteeism and turnover. An individual's decision to terminate will depend on (1) the relative importance of a particular job to other factors in the person's life or (2) the person's perception of alternative employment opportunities that are superior to his or her current job.

Factors in Absenteeism

Personal Life. Traumatic experiences or abnormal pressure levels in employees' personal lives can result in higher absenteeism rates as they take the time required to restore some semblance of psychological equilibrium.

Need State. If individuals obtain most or all of their need satisfaction off the job, they will subordinate both the job and the time spent on it to their outside projects.

Source: Donald L. Hawk, "Absenteeism and Turnover," *Personnel Journal*, June 1976. Reprinted with the permission of *Personnel Journal*, Costa Mesa, California; all rights reserved.

Organizational Policy. Salary continuance or sick pay plans may contribute to absenteeism in two ways. First, if employees feel that they are contributing more to the organization than others are, the existence of a liberal sick pay program may help encourage them to stay home. Although a sick leave policy does not necessarily encourage absenteeism, it does seem to authorize it. Second, in a case where the sick pay program provides no payment for the first two or three days of absence, employees are enticed to remain off the job until they become eligible for sick pay for their total absence.

Work Planning and Scheduling. The natural work cycle, which creates substantial differences in an employee's workload, may result in absenteeism immediately following the peak level. Employees feel that this absenteeism is justified because it represents a return to equilibrium; that is, the job requires intensive work during a period of time and thus the employee rests to return to normal prior to the next peak.

Factors in Turnover

General Economic Conditions. Historically, studies have shown that turnover follows directly (with practically no lag time) the peaks and troughs of the general economy.

Local Labor Market Conditions. The concept of a local labor market applies not only to a limited geographic area but also to the supply-demand ratio for a particular occupation or profession.

Personal Mobility. In addition, individuals' skills or background will greatly influence their mobility and thus be a potential cause of attrition.

Job Security. The number of involuntary transfers and terminations in a department directly affects individuals' perceptions of job security and affects their feelings about the fairness or equity of policy. If employees perceive the work environment to be volatile, that is, unstable or unpredictable, then their tenure may well be affected.

Factors in Absenteeism Leading to Turnover

The level of job dissatisfaction will directly influence the rate of both absenteeism and turnover.

Supervisory Style. Supervisory style can affect job satisfaction in several ways. First, when work planning and scheduling is perceived as arbitrary and/or inefficient, employees react to the "punishing" supervisory incompetence by withdrawing. Second, role ambiguity created by unclear performance expectations can cause high levels of psychological stress. Third, the lack of feedback on performance and the perceived inequity of performance appraisal can often reduce job satisfaction.

Interpersonal Relationships. An organizational structure that creates and/or reinforces destructive competition will reduce team spirit, group pride, or group cohesiveness and cause job dissatisfaction.

Working Conditions. A working environment that is unsafe or that interferes with efficient, productive work contributes to job dissatisfaction.

Salary. Two elements related to salary can affect the individual's satisfaction level. The first of these, and perhaps the most obvious, is wage rate. If an individual's wage rate is substantially below that of the area average, he or she will be dissatisfied. The second case, and perhaps the more important, is the intraorganizational dimension of salaries, that of wage level. If there are substantial differentials in wage levels, employees may perceive the wage structure to be arbitrary and inequitable when compared to the work required.

Job Expectations. From interviews, orientation training, and perhaps job descriptions, individuals develop preconceptions of what a job will be like. If individuals' job expectations are a great deal different from what they find the job is really like, they are apt to be dissatisfied with their decision to join the organization.

Job Fit. When through selection, placement, and/or promotional practice, individuals' capabilities are systematically underutilized and/or there is no career path available to them, they become dissatisfied. The contrary is also true. Should the job require more ability than an individual has, the individual will feel incompetent and be dissatisfied.

Job Design. Jobs with low motivating potential (i.e., low skill variety, low task identity, low task significance, little autonomy, and little or no feedback from the job itself) produce employee dissatisfaction.

Developing an Absenteeism/Turnover Reduction Strategy

After discovery of an absenteeism or turnover problem, most organizations react in one of the following three ways:

- They develop an elaborate "control" program.
- They adopt a current fad.
- They implement a program that worked well for some other organization.

Since the causes or the circumstances surrounding absenteeism or turnover problems are not necessarily the same, these programs inevitably have less than the desired effect or fail outright.

For this reason, careful diagnosis of management's absenteeism/turnover position must precede the formulation of any plans to deal with the problem. The first step in this diagnosis should be a detailed analysis of both absenteeism and turnover data.

Next, the costs of the problem should be identified. If the cost is significant enough to merit an investment in change, the next step is to iden-

tify which of the major variables listed are contributing most to the absenteeism/turnover problem.

In determining which are the most significant
causal variables, valuable information can be
obtained from the following:

- a review of exit interview data, especially
  where similar reasons for termination occur frequently
- an analysis of current performance problems
  (e.g., substandard work output)
- the administration and analysis of an appropriate attitude survey

Implementation of the most appropriate and
direct solution will then provide the best return (i.e., maximum results for minimum investment).

ABSENTEEISM

Rate and Cause

The rate of unscheduled absenteeism reported
for hospitals in one extensive survey was an average of 2.8 days per year per employee for small
hospitals and 3.9 days per year per employee for
large hospitals. The average for all hospitals was
3.2. Almost 40 percent of hospitals indicated their
rate as less than 1 day per employee. On the other
end of the scale, 2 percent of hospitals reported
a rate of 12 or more days of unscheduled absences per year per employee. Illness was clearly
the most frequent cause of absence listed by all
hospitals, regardless of size or geographic region.
Other causes, in order of importance, were family health, other problems, and injuries.*

Note: The Family and Medical Leave Act
(FMLA), enacted in 1994, provides legitimacy
to the number of absences caused by personal or
familial health conditions, including the birth or
adoption of a child. A total leave time of 12 weeks
in a year is allowable. It may be taken on an intermittent basis instead of one continuous period of time. For example, the leave may be for
an hour or more over an extended period of time
(ideal for medical treatment appointments for the
employee or a sick relative).

This aspect of permissible intermittent absenteeism may cause as much havoc as traditional
absenteeism and is a much criticized aspect of
the federal leave legislation. It is an area that
could be vulnerable to employee abuse.

Most health care employers will adopt special
controls as they reformulate absence, sick leave,
and maternity leave policies to comply with the
FMLA. Utilization reports, trends in abuse, and
management training in the new system will
probably be made available by a centralized
FMLA division within the human resource department.

Documenting the Absenteeism Problem*

A four-step tool can be used by the nurse manager to examine whether a problem of absenteeism exists at any level—institutional, departmental, or individual employee.

The first step is to calculate the average number of full-time employees assigned to the
department. Counting the employees at the beginning and end of any month and averaging provides a mid-month number of employees. Or
even simpler, the number of full-time equivalents
(FTEs) of a department can be used.

In *the second step*, this work force (either FTEs
or mid-month number of employees) is multiplied by a constant number of days scheduled
per employee per month. This number can be
computed by subtracting the number of vacation,
holiday, and other days off allowed by the institution from the number of theoretical days an
employee can work annually (see box).

---

*Source: NIOSH *Hospital Occupational Health Services
Study*, U.S. [Survey of 5,298 Hospitals] Pub. No. (NIOSH
75-154).

*Source: Kip DeWeese, "Absenteeism: A Nurse
Manager's Concern," *The Health Care Supervisor*, Vol. 5,
No. 3, Aspen Publishers, Inc., © April 1987.

Example

Assuming an employee is scheduled to work 5 days per week for 52 weeks, the maximum number of days the employee could work annually would be 260. By subtracting 10 vacation days, 8 holidays, and 2 other benefit days, the employee will work 240 days per year, or 20 days per month. This constant, 20 days per month, is then multiplied by the average number of employees assigned, thus equaling the total number of days scheduled per month for a department.

The third step is to figure the number of unplanned absences during the month by simply keeping track of who is absent and when.

The fourth step is to compute the absence rate. The method most frequently used and recommended by the Bureau of Employment Security of the U.S. Department of Labor is:

$$Absentee\ rate = \frac{Total\ days\ lost\ due\ to\ absence \times 100}{Total\ days\ scheduled}$$

Control Methods

Nurse managers must assume the bulk of responsibility for reducing absenteeism. Often nurse managers are aware that certain employees are chronic absentees, but the human resource department must make sure that nurse managers have adequate training in handling problems of this kind. (See Figure 30–1.) The human resource department also should provide the manager with statistical information reflecting absenteeism patterns in the department.

Many health care facility administrators handle short-term absences in a systematic fashion, using selected rewards, penalties, and surveillance devices. The following control methods are used.

Bonus for Health. Employees receive full pay for any of the allotted sick days they do not take.

Another method gives one day's pay for accruing a given amount of sick days.

Checkup and Surveillance. This method takes the one-day sickness excuse at face value and sends the returned absentee down to the employee health clinic to explain the causes (symptoms) to the physician. A more concerned attitude is seemingly displayed in a variation of this method where a nurse hired for this purpose actually visits the absentee worker's home to find out how the worker feels or if medical help is needed.

Penalties. Many health care facilities deduct the first day of illness but some use a system of makeup work. For example, absences unaccompanied by a physician's note on scheduled weekends must be made up by work on the employee's next off weekend.*

Practical Unit-Level Supervisory Actions **

The key to control of absenteeism lies in maintaining records, paying ongoing attention to attendance, and making sure that the unit staff know that attendance is monitored. A second principle is consistency, particularly in applying attendance policies consistently across the work group regardless of personal knowledge of individual circumstances. New employees should be informed of the attendance policy and other staff should be reminded periodically.

- Telephone absentee who is approaching need for counseling.
- Require absentees to report directly to nurse manager upon return.
- Maintain absentee report in department.
- Develop list of chronic offenders and remain aware of their status.
- When possible, institute practice of requiring makeup of missed work.

---

*Source: NIOSH *Hospital Occupational Health Services Study*, U.S. [Survey of 5,298 Hospitals] Pub. No. (NIOSH 75-154).

**Source: "A Supervisor's Checklist: Absenteeism," *The Health Care Supervisor*, Vol. 12, No. 3, Aspen Publishers, Inc., © March 1994.

Figure 30–1 An Absenteeism Control Program for Chronic Abusers

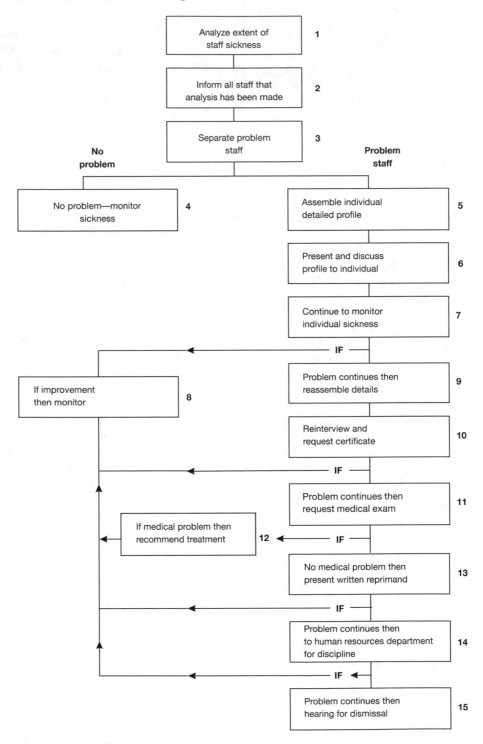

Source: Romeo Circone, "Controlling Sick Leave Abuse," *Dimensions in Health Service*, Journal of the Canadian Hospital Association, April 1978. Reprinted with permission.

- If rotating scheduling is involved, reschedule weekend sick call to work the following weekend (so fair share of weekends is not avoided through sick call).
- Following multiday absences, have employees cleared through employee health service.
- Require use of employee assistance program (EAP), if available, at the stage of written "attendance-problem" warning or suspension.
- Establish a clear policy for calling in sick (time limits in which to call, to whom to report, etc.).

TURNOVER

A certain degree of attrition is healthy, especially when it leads to refinement of practices. If there were no terminations, there would be no room for new and fresh ideas. However, nursing service leaders must be aware of the costs of turnover to the health care facility, the department, and clinical units. In addition, although nonquantifiable, the resulting effect on patient care should also be taken into consideration.

In metropolitan areas, where job change is easier due to proximity and number of choices, the turnover rate sometimes reaches 150 to 200 percent. It would seem that many nurses change jobs, hoping to find a difference, but generally find the new position quite like the previous one—and quite as frustrating.

One neutral study found that the mean number of workdays a new, inexperienced registered nurse spent on the job before assuming full responsibilities was 39.1, or about eight workweeks. Therefore, if a health care facility's turnover rate is, for example, 70 percent, the average position is filled each 68 weeks and the new, inexperienced employee is not fully productive 12 percent of his or her average tenure.

Another factor to note in reckoning with turnover issues is that turnover is considered voluntary when the nurse has control over leaving a position, involuntary when departure is for reasons beyond his or her control.

Factors in Nurse Turnover*

The *health care environment* consists of all factors outside the health care facility that affect and are affected by the organization. There are four primary means by which this external environment affects the health care facility: regulatory factors, such as those for accreditation; political factors, such as the prevailing climate regarding care reimbursement (Medicare, Medicaid); economic factors, such as the current availability of nurses or cost containment; and social factors, such as competitiveness between health care organizations.

The *health care facility environment* consists of factors within the facility that are unique to its internal interaction. The internal environment continuously responds to external environmental changes. Factors that make up the health care facility environment and influence the nursing department environment include political factors, such as internal resource allocation; economic factors, such as the facility's profit margin; policy; and organizational dynamics, such as departmental structures, interaction, and competition.

The *nursing department environment* is the aspect of the internal health care facility environment composed of nursing personnel working toward common nursing service goals. More specifically, the nursing department encompasses those elements that influence nursing turnover behavior, including goals and philosophy, such as formalized departmental objectives; departmental resources, such as financial and personnel components available within the department; departmental structure, such as the articulation of nursing divisions and units within the nursing department; and working conditions, such as scheduling, employee job satisfaction, and leaders' management style.

A conceptual framework of the turnover cycle is illustrated in Figure 30–2.

Note: According to studies, in a stable era with high nursing shortages, nurses list personal and

---

Source: Cheryl Bland Jones, "Staff Nurse Turnover Costs: Part 1. A Conceptual Model," *Journal of Nursing Administration*, Vol. 20, No. 4, April 1990.

Figure 30–2 Conceptual Framework for Nursing Turnover

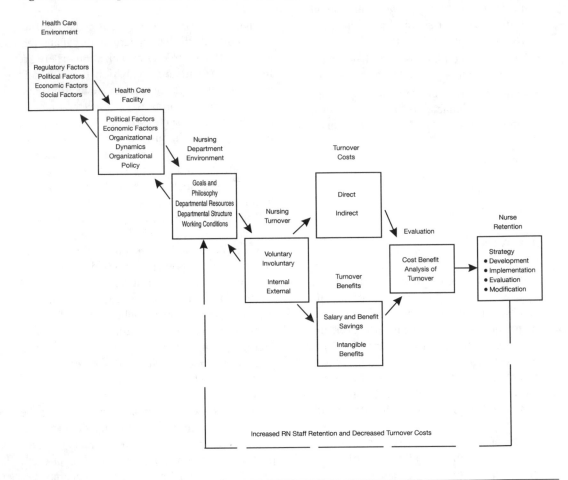

professional reasons for resignation and turnover more frequently (see data in Figures 30–3 and 30–4). In an era of organizational restructuring, new arrangements might lead to a new and complex set of reasons based on three levels of environmental influences. How these factors are played out will determine the priority order given to standard turnover reasons.

Factors in Management Turnover*

Professional employees generally know or believe that they can change employment more easily than others, so they are less likely to tolerate what they see as unsatisfactory conditions and less likely to balk at stepping out into the unknown territory represented by a job change.

The manager must recognize that the same kinds of needs that first brought the worker into the profession—the need to achieve, to do interesting work, to be challenged, to do something of value, and so forth—are often the same kinds of needs that stimulate the professional to change organizations. This claim of the impact of professionals' psychological needs on turnover can be supported by a simple examination of the reasons why higher level employees quit their jobs for new employment.

Figure 30–3 Reasons for Nurse Resignations

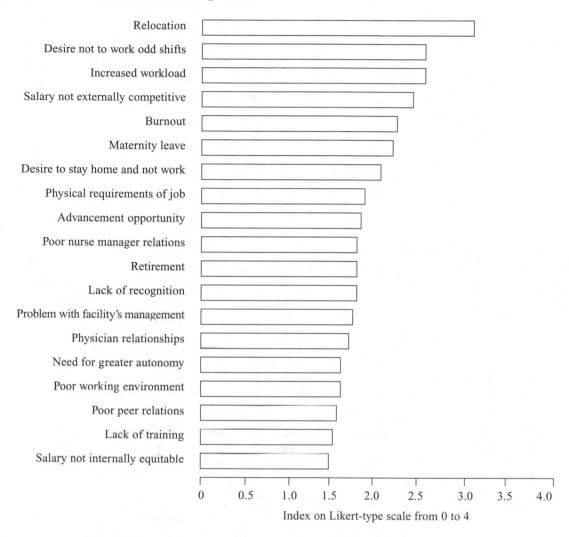

Index on Likert-type scale from 0 to 4

Note: These reasons were offered in more than 14,000 exit interviews over a four-year period in seven southeastern states. In analyzing the exit interviews with registered nurses, this study noted how often each reason for resigning was given and scored them all on a scale of 0 ("never") to 4 ("always").

Source: Reprinted from "Hay Study Ties Shortage to Ancillary Cutbacks; Finds Quality of Care 'Directly Threatened,'" *American Journal of Nursing*, Vol. 88, No. 9, September 1988. Copyright © by the American Journal of Nursing Company. Used with permission. All rights reserved.

Why Valued Employees Quit

A brief report appearing in the monthly news publication of the American Society for Personnel Administration (ASPA) discussed turnover under the title of "Eight Reasons Why Good Employees Leave Jobs." According to the report, the reasons why top-level people leave jobs are, in order of importance, the following:

1. Lack of Job Satisfaction. This was given as the most common reason for people leaving

Figure 30–4 Factors Contributing to Nursing Turnover

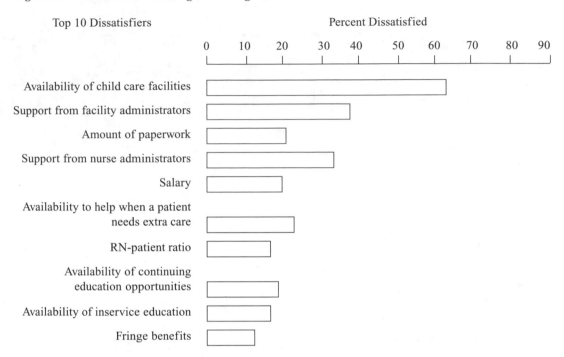

Top 10 Dissatisfiers   Percent Dissatisfied

Note: Nurses who will leave and those who will stay agree that lack of child care facilities is the worst part of the job. On nearly every item, more leavers are dissatisfied, but high percentages of stayers also are dissatisfied. Are the dissatisfied stayers the nurses who skip from one job to another in search of better conditions? Or are they trapped and disgruntled? Will they one day join the leavers?

Source: Reprinted from Florence L. Huey and Susan Hartley, "What Keeps Nurses in Nursing: 3,500 Nurses Tell Their Stories," *American Journal of Nursing*, February 1988. Copyright © by the American Journal of Nursing Company. Used with permission. All rights reserved.

supposedly good jobs. Indeed it has been established time and again that employees who are unhappy because they do not feel useful or valued, who are generally dissatisfied with what they are doing, are likely to seek employment changes that appear to offer greater job satisfaction.

2. Lack of Challenge. An organization's best potential producers are usually those people who need to have the limits of their knowledge and skill tested regularly. An organization that does not use the full talents of its employees, and does not listen to these employees and take their suggestions seriously, tends to lose precisely those employees whom it should be most interested in retaining.

3. Dissatisfaction with Supervision. Uncommunicative or authoritarian supervision—or bossism—makes employees feel that they are not allowed to think for themselves. A style of management that demands blind obedience and prohibits active participation eventually drives away quality employees, precisely those employees whom the organization should most wish to keep.

4. Dissatisfaction with Organizational Image. An organization that develops an image as a loser, perhaps through shrinkage of its volume of business or its share of the market or the loss of vital or prestigious services, experiences continual difficulty retaining employees who are strongly growth oriented. The professional who sees him-

or herself as going places or making a name eventually seeks an organization that also appears to be on the rise (if not already there).

5. Incompatibility within the Work Group. This reason for leaving can surface at any time within any organization and at any level. It essentially involves personality clashes between and among persons who must work together on a regular basis. Although no worker is immune to possible incompatibility, the professional, with more interorganizational mobility, is more likely to seek active relief by changing jobs.

6. Inadequate Pay. An organization that does not remain competitive in regard to salaries and benefits stands to lose a number of its valued employees. The notion of equity in compensation is particularly important; what is important is not so much what a person may be paid in absolute amounts but rather what the person is paid relative to others. Money sometimes holds persons longer in the face of other dissatisfactions. However, if the pay is the only satisfactory condition of a person's employment, it never ensures contentment with employment.

7. Lack of Confidence about Eventual Success in the Job. Employees who may feel that they are in over their heads often tend to escape that feeling by quitting. The organization that fails to take active steps to develop its employees and demonstrate that it wants them to succeed eventually loses many potential long-term employees.

8. Location of the Organization. Some organizations—health care organizations among them—inevitably find it necessary to move the primary business to a new location. Though much more pertinent to nonhealth businesses in general, this can be a factor in employee resignations in any organization. Depending on the distance of the move—whether a few blocks, across town, or across the country—some employees may choose not to move with the organization.

Costs of Turnover*

Turnover is expensive to an institution because the costs of turnover include recruiting and selecting a replacement, socializing the replacement with regard to organizational norms, overpayment of the replacement during the period of learning when he or she cannot produce at full capacity, overtime work performed by others during the period between the turnover and the replacement's achievement of full capacity, and achieving social adjustment between the nursing unit and its new member.

For these reasons, nursing administrators require up-to-date records of the turnover rate so they can more accurately estimate their total budget. It also allows them to identify areas of weakness as well as opportunities for cost reduction.

Three distinct cost components are usually examined: recruitment, on-the-job training, and termination. By estimating the appropriate wage rate for the amount of time spent by health care facility personnel in each of these phases of employment, nurse managers can determine organizational costs for nurse turnover.

Recruitment Costs

Interviewing. Time is spent by human resource department staff in handling applications, holding preliminary interviews, and processing initial forms.

Physical Examination. Time is spent by medical personnel in conducting routine health examinations.

Clerical Staff. Time is spent completing records and payroll forms.

Orientation. Time is spent off regular job duties (nonoperational) by one or more staff members and the new employee, based proportionately on the wage rate for each person involved.

---

*Source: Suggestions for Control of Turnover and Absenteeism, U.S. Department of Labor.

On-the-Job Training Costs

Time To Reach Proficiency. The complexity of duties and the difference in worker backgrounds affect the amount of time needed to reach proficiency. However, the nurse manager should be able to provide an average time estimate.

Excess Wages Paid for Duties Performed. Until the new staff member learns the job requirements, he or she cannot be working at full capacity.

Estimated Costs of Supervision during Training. Wages of supervisory staff during instruction periods are based on the amount of time spent in direct contact and the number of trainees involved during the training period.

Termination Costs

Payment of Wages. A departing employee is paid for nonproductive time, that is, salary is received through checkout and exit interview periods.

Exit Interview Expenses. Depending on how elaborate the health care facility's system is, costs vary but are essentially based on salary time for the interviewee.

Clerical Staff. Again, time is spent for completion of records and payroll forms.

The High Cost of Turnover. When all these factors are calculated to arrive at a turnover cost, expenses can be quite high, particularly for personnel in the nursing department.

Based on these cost components, a nursing department may have an average turnover cost of thousands of dollars—which, when multiplied by the total number of terminated personnel, can add up to a substantial sum. Considering the high rates of turnover frequently reported by nursing departments, it would appear necessary for reasons of cost as well as efficiency to investigate methods of reducing staff turnover.

Formulas for Determining the Turnover Rate*

Health care facilities may use the following formulas for compiling, computing, and recording turnover.

Separation Rate. The number of separations (includes all persons who left for any reason—resignation, dismissal, layoff) during the month is divided by the total number of workers on the payroll in the pay period ending nearest the 15th of the same month; the result is then multiplied by 100.

$$\frac{S\ (separations)}{E\ (employment)} \times 100 = T\ (separation\ rate)$$

Example:

$$\frac{20\ separations}{100\ employees} \times 100 = 20\%\ separation\ rate$$

Quit Rate. The number of quits or resignations during the month is divided by the total number of workers on the payroll in the pay period ending nearest the 15th of the same month; the result is then multiplied by 100.

$$\frac{Q\ (number\ of\ quits)}{E\ (employment)} \times 100 = R\ \begin{matrix}(resignation \\ rate)\end{matrix}$$

Example:

$$\frac{10\ resignations}{100\ employees} \times 100 = 10\% \begin{matrix}resignation \\ rate\end{matrix}$$

In addition, the American Hospital Association encourages hospitals to consider calculating the stability factor, which reflects the number of positions with no changes in staffing related to total authorized positions for a given month. This figure counteracts distortion caused by the turnover of one position several times. When one position turns over three times, this is

---

*Source: Suggestions for Control of Turnover and Absenteeism, U.S. Department of Labor.

reflected in the turnover rate, tending to make the staff appear unstable. (See Table 30–1 for a summary of different methods of calculating turnover rates.)

Reducing Turnover

Computerized accounting systems can develop turnover data into useful management tools by correlating them with personnel and job characteristics. Detailed data collection can result in recommendations for hiring and allocation of personnel.

A number of techniques have been adapted to reduce turnover. The exit interview can provide significant assistance in determining which approach might be best for the specific department.

1. The Exit Interview*

The exit interview can be a valuable source of information concerning reasons for labor turnover. A few factors contributing to turnover, for example, death or retirement, are not controllable. However, numerous factors that give workers cause for leaving an organization are controllable, and a carefully conducted exit interview will help bring these to light. The exit interview is not intended to absolve the nurse manager of the responsibility to maintain conditions that keep turnover low. It is intended to provide additional assistance after the nurse manager has done his or her utmost toward retaining a desirable worker.

_____

*Source: Suggestions for Control of Turnover and Absenteeism, U.S. Department of Labor.

Table 30–1 Summary of Different Methods of Calculating Turnover Rates

Profile of a Nursing Department

At the beginning of the year, 290 nurses were employed. During the year, 100 nurses left and 120 nurses were hired. By the end of the year, 96 of the new nurses were still employed.

	Definition, by Method	Calculation	Rate
Accession rate	$\dfrac{\text{Number of new employees}}{\text{Average number of employees}}$	$120 \div \dfrac{290 + 310}{2}$	40.0%
Separation rate	$\dfrac{\text{Number of employees leaving}}{\text{Average number of employees}}$	$100 \div \dfrac{290 + 310}{2}$	33.3%
Stability rate	$\dfrac{\text{Number of beginning employees remaining}}{\text{Number of employees at beginning}}$	$\dfrac{190}{290}$	65.5%
Instability rate	$\dfrac{\text{Number of beginning employees leaving}}{\text{Number of employees at beginning}}$	$\dfrac{100}{290}$	34.5%
Survival rate	$\dfrac{\text{Number of new employees remaining}}{\text{Number of new employees}}$	$\dfrac{96}{120}$	80.0%
Wastage rate	$\dfrac{\text{Number of new employees leaving}}{\text{Number of new employees}}$	$\dfrac{24}{120}$	20.0%

Source: Paul B. Hoffman, "Accurate Measurement of Nursing Turnover: The First Step in Its Reduction," _Journal of Nursing Administration_, November-December 1981. Reprinted with permission.

Exit interviews offer opportunities to do the following:

- Determine the real reasons employees wish to resign.
- Retain competent employees by exploring the causes of the dissatisfaction and trying to find a solution for their grievances or problems.
- Clarify complaints against employees who are separated involuntarily.
- Promote good relations with employees who separate voluntarily or involuntarily.
- Obtain reliable data on problem areas that will enable management to set up corrective measures.

A person with a mature and sympathetic outlook should be selected to conduct the interview. A friendly atmosphere is important. The interviewer's purpose is to get information, not to argue with the employee over his or her reasons for leaving. With understanding and tact, valuable information concerning causes of separation may be obtained. Even though the employee leaves, he or she may leave with friendly feelings and a better understanding of the health care facility and with the assurance that the exit interview will not be detrimental to getting a good reference.

To offset the reluctance of an employee who has not given frank and candid statements during the exit interview, a questionnaire may be sent to the employee 30 to 60 days after termination. (It should be accompanied by an explanatory letter and a self-addressed, stamped envelope.) This form should contain questions concerning the employee's feelings about the organization and his or her job and manager.

If the employee has become established in a new job, he or she may feel freer to give candid, objective answers. These answers can be checked against information given in the exit interview and discrepancies noted. These additional comments can supplement the information gathered in the exit interview. Analysis of information gathered in this manner over a period of time will pinpoint areas in which corrective action may be taken.

Exit interviews should be held in a private office where the employee will feel at ease and may speak without fear of being overheard. Where this situation is impossible, conditions of maximum privacy should be arranged.

Since so many eventualities are considered in an outline for an exit interview, the process may appear rather complicated and time consuming. An experienced interviewer can usually conduct a satisfactory interview in from 15 to 30 minutes. Interviews with employees, for the most part, follow a general pattern by progressing through the following stages.

Informal Conversation of General Interest. Every effort should be made to establish rapport with the worker. An atmosphere of "quizzing" will elicit little useful information. A chat about something of general interest can be steered around to the principal reason for the interview in a pleasant and informal manner.

The Employee's Own Statement. The employee should be given every opportunity to tell why he or she wishes to resign, if that is the reason for the interview. Interrupting the employee to influence his or her statements should be avoided. Attention to all remarks is important for subsequently directing the interview to an effective conclusion.

Questioning by the Interviewer. When the employee finishes his or her statement, the interviewer should ask appropriate questions in an attempt to determine, in the case of an employee who plans to resign, the true reasons for the dissatisfaction—the employee's attitudes, feelings, and motivations. The interviewer should do the following:

- Ask for specific information about the situation described and evaluate it in view of statements made by the nurse manager.
- Ask the employee if he or she has (1) explored the possibility of taking training to

obtain greater satisfaction in his or her present position or to prepare him- or herself for promotion or (2) explored the possibility of transfer to another unit in the nursing department.

- Suggest ways in which the present situation might be improved to the worker's satisfaction, or state what arrangements might be made to transfer him or her to another job, paying careful attention to the employee's reaction to all suggestions.
- Attempt to restate in specific terms the problems the employee may encounter in leaving the organization and encourage him or her to try to adjust to the present situation with whatever changes or improvements are suggested. Sometimes, stimulating interest in the importance of the employee's job to the completed product or services of the organization or pointing out the loss in seniority that will result from his or her separation will be effective in retaining the worker.

Final Stage of Informal Conversation. Closing stages of the interview are important to ensure a mutual understanding of any arrangements agreed upon and to plan for any follow up required. The interview should close on a friendly basis, even if the employee persists in the decision to leave. The employee should be made to feel that he or she will be given every consideration if he or she cares to return.

2. Rewards*

In one investigation, the influence of specific safety, social, and psychological rewards and incentives on the rate of nursing staff turnover was studied. Results indicated that 59 percent of the registered nurses who left their staff positions could have been influenced to stay on the job by rewards and incentives—of which 34 per-

cent could have been easily held on the job. The remaining 41 percent could not have been influenced to stay on the job. The categories of rewards were specified as follows:

- *Safety rewards and incentives:* salary, vacation time, sick leave, weekends off, opportunity for part-time work, hours per day, insurance, and retirement programs
- *Social rewards and incentives:* maternity leave; child care facilities; a different nurse manager; a different head nurse; social contact with coworkers, nursing superiors, and physicians; and opportunities to share opinions and feelings with other registered nurses and physicians
- *Psychological rewards and incentives:* educational opportunities, job responsibility, recognition of work, help from peers and superiors, career advancement, and participation in research

The data revealed that psychological rewards were perceived as more important than safety or social rewards. The unanimous choice of psychological rewards over safety and social rewards strongly indicates that nurses left jobs for lack of internal rewards. In other words, while external rewards may draw a person to a job, internal rewards keep the person there.

Higher pay did not retain nurses, and they were not influenced by a specialty area. Most nurses wanted opportunities to attend educational programs, to continue course work for credit, to seek career advancement, and to have their work recognized by peers and managers.

3. An Ombudsman*

Before creating an innovative new program, the yearly attrition rate at Beth Israel Hospital in New York was 37 percent or more. A few years later it had dropped to 14.5 percent.

A position was created for a nurse recruitment and retention coordinator who really func-

---

Source: Methods 2, 4, and 5 are excerpted from Joanne McCloskey, "Influence of Rewards and Incentives on Staff Nurse Turnover," *Nursing Research*, May-June 1974, © American Journal of Nursing Company. Reprinted with permission.

Source: Regina Bloch, "The Nurse Ombudsman," *American Journal of Nursing*, October 1976, © American Journal of Nursing Company. Adapted with permission.

tions as an ombudsman for the professional staff.

The coordinator is expected to emphasize helpfulness and empathy and encourage staff members to seek solutions to problems rather than to seek other employment.

Interviews are scheduled at three months, six months, one year after employment, and yearly thereafter. They provide nurses with an opportunity to express themselves freely and offer them a release from problems that might otherwise be suppressed.

A great deal of counseling takes place during the interview. Personal problems may involve baby sitting, housing, or finances; occupational problems may relate to a change of assignment, interpersonal relations, or simply a clarification of policy.

Reports in writing are sent to the director of nursing. Urgent problems are reported orally. Frequently, a problem brought to the ombudsman can be resolved then and there merely by bringing it into the open and talking it out. At other times the director of nursing may feel that intervention is necessary and ask an associate director to investigate or to resolve a complaint. But all complaints are studied to identify any pattern of repetitive problems. All complaints are categorized under major headings, such as orientation, administration, policies, staffing, promotions, and the like. Under these major headings, statements by staff are listed anonymously. When a problem has been resolved, the manner of resolution also is entered into the record.

Twice a year the problem list is reviewed, and changes are made accordingly.

4. A More Intellectual Atmosphere

To hold staff nurses on the job, nursing service administrators might try to provide a more intellectual atmosphere by providing inservice education programs that allow nurses to participate actively, providing time off and tuition waivers to nurses who wish to continue their education, and hiring a nurse research coordinator to plan and participate with staff nurses for nursing research on their units.

5. Career Advancement

Changes might be made from the traditional career advancement pattern—staff nurse to team leader to head nurse to nurse manager—to a pattern related more to levels of practice, such as staff nurse to clinician to clinical specialist. Nursing administrators might provide a more positive working atmosphere to help maintain staff nurses' self-esteem by emphasizing team nursing or instituting primary nursing care; allowing nurses to have more decision-making power, especially in primary care; insisting on problem-oriented charting for nurses; and training nurse managers and head nurses in leadership skills.

6. Using the Nurse Recruiter*

One emerging response to the need to understand and control nursing turnover is the expanding role of the nurse recruiter. Nurse recruiters are in an ideal position to monitor the flow of nursing personnel into and out of the system, to compute turnover and vacancy rates, and to map resignations by location within the health care facility. Further, nurse recruiters frequently conduct employment interviews with newly hired nurses and exit interviews or follow-up interviews with resigning nurses. These activities provide important information about nurses' expectations for their jobs and their assessments of their work experiences within the health care facility.

Other Strategies for Reducing Turnover**

A number of hospitals in the United States has no difficulty recruiting and retaining RNs. In 1981 and 1982 the American Academy of Nursing Task Force on Nursing Practice in Hospitals identified what attracts RNS to these hospitals.

---

*Source: Carol Weisman, "Recruit from Within," Journal of Nursing Administration, May 1982. Reprinted with permission.

**Source: F. Theodore Helmer and Patricia McKnight, "Management Strategies To Minimize Nursing Turnover," Health Care Management Review, Vol. 14, No. 1, Aspen Publishers, Inc., © 1989.

The ANA published the results of that study in 1983. What these hospitals offer RNS, making these nurses eager to join the staff and content to remain in their employ include:

- A nurse–patient ratio that assures quality patient care.
- Flexible staffing to support patient care needs.
- Flexible scheduling and elimination of rotating shifts.
- A strong supportive nursing administration—and hospital administration—at all levels.

- Primary nursing.
- Clinical advancement opportunities (so that RNs can stay at the bedside, but still advance professionally).
- Participative management.
- Open communication in all directions.
- Inservice and continuing education opportunities on all shifts.
- Good nurse–physician professional relationships.
- Longevity benefits for staff RNs.
- Tuition reimbursement.

Chapter 31

Recruitment and Retention

OVERVIEW*

Recruitment and retention are parts of a continuous process. Recruitment is supported by a satisfied and stable nursing staff who "sell" their institution to the students and experienced nurses with whom they interact. Retention is fostered by the recruitment of nurses who see themselves "fitting" the culture of the health care facility and who find that their career aspirations may be met by the opportunities for professional growth and advancement provided by the organization.

To successfully obtain and maintain its share of the dwindling nursing resource, a health care facility must match the incentives provided by its competitors while differentiating itself in one or more areas as a progressive leader that visibly supports its nursing staff. The special niches created by the facility must be marketed aggressively to both its existing staff and potential recruits. The organization not only must focus its efforts in the immediate geographic area but also must compete regionally and nationally.

To track its efforts, the health care facility must decide in advance what are acceptable attrition rates and maintain records on the costs of registered nurse replacements and programs aimed at retention. While a 0 percent turnover is not only unrealistic but also undesirable, the institution should decide what its target rates are for turnover so that allocation of resources for recruitment can be planned. The comparison of costs of recruitment and retention can assist the organization to ensure that a disproportionate amount is not directed toward recruitment. The facility must focus continually on the fact that retention is the most cost-effective way to maintain an adequate nursing resource.

Health care facilities cannot be satisfied with currently successful recruitment and retention activities but must work with other health care organizations and agencies on long-term ways to address the shortage of nurses. One method may be to cooperate with community efforts to introduce high school students to nursing as an attractive profession. Another approach may be to work with businesses and schools of nursing in efforts to retrain a displaced work force from another industry.

The institution must address administrative, organizational, professional practice, and professional development characteristics to compete successfully with others for the limited nursing

---

*Source: Catherine DeVet, "Nurse Recruitment and Retention in an Urban Hospital," in *Managing the Nursing Shortage: A Guide to Recruitment and Retention*, Terence F. Moore and Earl A. Simendinger, eds., Aspen Publishers, Inc., © 1989.

resources available. The organization that involves its own staff in the planning of the retention program will be the one that selects those characteristics that are most meaningful to its particular nursing population and creates a program that meets the widest variety of individual preferences. As the nursing work force becomes more diverse in types of personalities and career stages yet more specialized in practice, the retention factors will need to become more individualized. Refinements of the program should be planned to meet the changing expectations of nurses.

The philosophy of the health care facility must be articulated clearly so that a nurse may select an environment that is congruent with his or her own values. The organization must establish an identifiable "corporate culture" and consistently act in congruence with the norms of the culture. A nurse employed in an institution that shares his or her value system is less vulnerable to the recruitment efforts of another organization since the work environment is part of the nurse's own identity.

Nurses must also see that their jobs are recognized and valued by nursing and health care facility administrators and physicians as well as by their colleagues and patients. Therefore, facilities must plan and implement recognition and reward programs for their nursing staff as part of a comprehensive approach to retention. Adequate compensation alone will not retain nurses. The environment in which the nurse works must convey a sense of esteem and worth for the nursing care provided to patients.

Early career nurses need an opportunity to perform well on the job through the support of nurse managers and peers and to receive adequate feedback on the contributions they are making to the organization. Midcareer nurses need autonomy to make decisions and to work more independently. Advanced career groups need incentives that maintain or rekindle their excitement in their jobs.

Any program must be based on the needs as expressed by nurses in assessments conducted by the institution and by the needs expressed by individual nurses to their managers. (See Table 31–1.)

RECRUITMENT FROM THE NURSE'S POINT OF VIEW

Nurse Expectations*

The most qualified nurses graduating from baccalaureate and master's programs are seeking positions in institutions that offer salaries and work responsibilities commensurate with their educational preparation, work experiences, and clinical interests. What new graduates are seeking in a position is perhaps best reflected in the advertisements published in the nursing journals. Some cater to the nurse's desire for self-development or to the nurse's wish to function as a nursing practitioner. Some stress the opportunity for advancement.

It is interesting to note that comments regarding the fringe benefits and salaries are usually at the end of the advertisement. While these items may be minimized, experience has shown that they are extremely important in attracting nurses, but not necessarily in retaining them.

Increasingly, nurses are interested in greater specialization in the various clinical fields—intensive care, medicine, pediatrics, psychiatry, and others—and are less willing to function as generalists who rotate to any service in the facility.

How Nurses Select a Health Care Facility**

In studies conducted at one hospital, nurses were asked to assign a weight to the criteria used in selecting an organization for employment. In order of importance, they were listed as follows:

1. spouse working/studying in the area
2. assigned to the service of my choice
3. pay

Source: Reprinted with permission from G. Matsunaga, "The Nurse Executive and Nursing Manpower," *Concerns in the Acquisition and Allocation of Nursing Personnel,* © 1979, National League for Nursing.

**Source:* C. David Hughes, "Can Marketing Help Recruit and Retain Nurses?" *Health Care Management Review,* Vol. 4, No. 3, Aspen Publishers, Inc., © 1979.

Table 31–1 Variables Influencing Employee Retention and Turnover

Job Dimension	Factors Encouraging Retention	Factors Encouraging Turnover
Career or job attitudes (employee motivation)	Organization provides a sense of respect for the work completed Pay equity exists with external labor markets Pay equity exists within the organization Jobs are structured to be challenging Employees perceive that their work units are allocated a fair share of total budgets, resources, and rewards	High salary expectations by employees Low utilization of employee skills relative to education and training Failure to integrate employee work goals with organizational goals
Environmental favorability (job situation)	Management gives employee relations a high priority Personnel receive periodic training and development Flexibility exists for defining work hours Task variety is high Performance is linked to objectives and periodic assessment Efforts are made to develop work teams Technology supporting tasks is periodically updated or replaced	Failure to acknowledge accomplishments, which pertains to personal attainments as well as organizational achievements Limited employee knowledge of organizational benefits Limited opportunities for employees to express dissatisfaction regarding their jobs Lack of a formal system for disseminating important information
Employee selection (employee capabilities)	Past performance is analyzed before employees join organization	Inability to judge job candidates' motivation and goal sets Failure to involve peers of the candidates in the selection process

Source: Howard L. Smith and Richard Discenza, "Developing a Framework for Retaining Health Care Employees: A Challenge to Traditional Thinking," *The Health Care Supervisor*, Vol. 7, No. 1, Aspen Publishers, Inc., © 1988.

4. responsibility consistent with my training
5. workload
6. fringe benefits
7. teaching facility
8. social life
9. opportunity for university courses
10. reputation of the organization
11. modern equipment
12. research facility

The most important criterion was the fact that the spouse was in the area. This finding suggests that nurse recruiters will want to work with the human resource offices of local companies and graduate school admission officers to identify nurses whose spouses will be moving into the area.

The second most important dimension, and more important than pay, was the desire to be assigned to the service of one's choice. Closely related to this dimension, and only slightly less important than pay, was the desire to have responsibility that is consistent with training. The career dimensions of the job are clearly important to the nurse during the *selection* of a health care facility. They are also important considerations for *staying* with the facility.

THE RECRUITMENT PROGRAM

Scope*

Before establishing a sound recruitment program, sources of personnel must be identified and developed. Modern employment departments carefully research the market. Sources of recruitment include present employees, employee referrals, walk-in applicants, applicants who send in written résumés, public employment agencies, private employment agencies, retired military personnel, other retired individuals, schools and colleges, and unions.

Often, health care facilities have a written policy that requires the posting of all available positions. Posting provides present employees the opportunity to apply or to recommend others for the positions. An institution's present employees are an excellent source of referral of qualified applicants. Many health care facilities offer bonuses to present employees for recommending successful applicants for difficult-to-recruit vacancies. The largest single group of candidates are those who apply to the institution's human resource department without any formal solicitation by the institution. Private employment agencies are widely used, once again for difficult-to-recruit classifications. Successful recruitment of professional positions can be achieved by visits to college campuses. The most widely used recruitment technique is that of placing classified ads. This method brings in applicants, but the "sell" is up to the interviewer and the "fit" is between the applicant and the department.

Recruitment Strategy*

Recruitment is an ongoing process, not something done only during staff shortages. Recruitment strategies may change during shortages, but the successful organization continually works on recruitment.

The first step in developing a recruitment strategy is to identify the current level of recruitment. Next, the external environment should be assessed. What changes are occurring that will affect the necessary level of recruiting? Are enrollments increasing in nursing and allied health schools? What specific factors in the environment may affect the health care facility's ability to recruit? Have competing organizations offered salary increases? After assessing the external environment and internal needs, an organization can establish a recruitment goal and develop a specific recruitment plan. (See Table 31–2 for some tips.)

It is important to identify the existing strengths of the health care facility so that the information can be conveyed to a target group. Communicating the facility's strengths, whether by advertising or other means, will often result in inquiries from potential employees. The package of material the organization develops to respond to those inquiries is a critical element of the overall marketing strategy. (See Table 31–3 for a list of some recruitment benefits).

Another important point to emphasize is that only a part of current advertising should be aimed at current recruitment. Another, equally substantial part should be aimed at long-term image building. People often associate with an organization because it is well known; such reputations are built over a period of years, through

---

*Source: Norman Metzger, "Human Resources Management," in *Health Care Administration: Principles, Practices, Structure, and Delivery*, ed 2, Lawrence F. Wolper, ed., Aspen Publishers, Inc., © 1995.

*Source: Steven A. Finkler et al., "Minimizing the Costs of Employee Turnover," *Hospital Cost Management and Accounting*, Vol. 4, No. 5, Aspen Publishers, Inc., © August 1992.

Table 31–2 ABC's of Nurse Recruitment

A — Acquire an effective nurse recruiter.

B — Budget to allow adequate funds for competitive recruitment programs carefully conceived and based on a realistic projection.

C — Convey a positive image in your ads and literature.

D — Develop strong internal recruitment resources.

E — Encourage promotion from within to fill leadership positions. Appoint the best-qualified candidate regardless of source.

F — Foster a climate of openness so that problems surface and are solved before they result in turnover statistics.

G — Generate effective advertising that reflects not only high professional standards but an administrative philosophy that bespeaks concern for the individual.

H — Heed the advice of advertising experts concerning the selection of media, copy developing, timing, and general strategy for placing advertisements.

I — Immediately respond to employment inquiries with a personal letter; a well-prepared, informative, and persuasive brochure; details about specific opportunities available, salaries, benefits, housing, and so forth; and a clear statement of qualifications expected. Send follow-up correspondence at regular intervals.

J — Judge the effectiveness of your nurse recruitment efforts in terms of the "average cost per hire." Use this index as a basis of comparison with previous results and with other employers' results.

K — Keep records of inquiries by origin (journal, newspaper, in-house, etc.) and by summary of their disposition (interviews, hires).

L — Learn which recruitment resources provide the greatest yield in quality as well as numbers of candidates.

M — Maximize the use of these resources.

N — Negotiate with other health care facilities to recommend qualified applicants for whom current vacancies do not exist.

O — Offer assistance to out-of-state applicants in finding convenient, reasonably priced housing. This is often essential in metropolitan areas.

P — Promote positive public relations by participating in and sponsoring events that involve potential candidates and present staff members.

Q — Query terminating staff members concerning reasons for resignation, and consider their recommendations for improvement.

R — Reward exceptional performance by added responsibility and commensurate authority, compensation, and recognition.

S — Schedule regular performance reviews to assess individual progress, to identify problems, and to agree on appropriate job objectives.

T — Tell your nurse recruitment representatives and advertising agency about any changes or problems affecting your staffing situation so that suitable adjustments can be made in your recruitment campaign.

U — Understand the hidden costs of inadequate or inappropriate staffing.

V — Vitalize your orientation, inservice, and continuing education programs to provide the latest information.

W — Work with school and college guidance counselors and conduct "career day" programs.

X — X-ray your staffing and scheduling patterns to deploy your present nursing group most effectively.

Y — Yield to constructive criticism in the development of solutions to your recruitment and staffing patterns.

Z — Zero in on a unifying theme that distinguishes your facility as a place to learn and to practice nursing. Promote this theme in all aspects of your recruitment program.

Source: Adapted from Edin Hoffman, "ABC's of Nurse Recruitment," *American Journal of Nursing*, April 1974, © 1974 American Journal of Nursing Company.

Table 31–3 Features and Benefits for Nurse Recruitment

Permanent shifts
Shift bonuses
Cafeteria-style benefits packages
Attractive wage range
Salary bonuses
Profit-sharing
Tuition reimbursement
Clinical ladders
Retirement programs
Child care
Adult care
Recognition programs
Shared governance

Source: Data from Moore and Simendinger, *Managing the Nursing Shortage,* Aspen Publishers, Inc., © 1989 and Rebecca Jones and Sharon Beck, *Decision Making in Nursing,* Delmar Publishers, © 1996.

---

an effort of getting the message out year after year.

Employment Agencies and Headhunters*

Although they operate differently, search organizations and employment agencies offer several common advantages. They provide a measure of confidentiality and enable the employer to limit advertising expense and exposure. With good fortune and competence, the pool of applicants ultimately interviewed by the employer is restricted to those likely to be offered work.

Search organizations normally operate on a fixed fee to the employer or offer an estimate of cost based on a daily charge plus out-of-pocket expenses. Often, an hourly charge is made in

*Source: Skoler, Abbott & Presser, *Health Care Labor Manual*, Aspen Publishers, Inc.

addition to expenses and a placement fee. They will also provide some idea of how long the search might last. In most cases, you can terminate the arrangement if you decide not to fill the position or you locate a suitable candidate from some other source. As is true with search firms, private employment agencies normally charge only the employer.

Agencies customarily operate on a contingency basis—no placement, no fee. As a rule, they screen a larger volume of candidates and tend to refer more applicants for employer consideration.

Search firms bear the undignified sobriquet of "headhunters" because they do only minimal advertising and use their contacts to reach into competing organizations—including yours—for likely candidates. The ritual requires, among other things, that the candidate react first with surprise and then reluctance to change jobs. This is calculated to sweeten the compensation package, and if played with adroitness, does. Search firms have reached a level in recent years that has made them increasingly useful adjuncts in the difficult task of locating and recruiting scarce professional talent. Their charges have more than kept pace, however, and tend to run upward of 25 percent of the successful candidate's first-year gross salary. Employment agency fees have also increased rapidly. They usually run 10 to 25 percent of the initial annual rate of pay and are contingent upon a successful placement. Some guarantee of satisfaction on the employer's part is customary.

Questions to be asked in dealing with search firms and employment agencies include the following: What are the obligations of each party? How long has the firm been in business? Can the owners give you the names of client firms they now serve? Are the people you will be dealing with sensitive to the needs of the health field as well as the specialized jobs for which they will be asked to recruit? Do you and your people understand that by using an outside source for recruiting purposes you cannot abdicate your responsibility to critically examine the credentials and representations of all job candidates, however referred?

ORGANIZING FOR RECRUITMENT*

Nurse Recruiter

Selection of a nurse recruiter should be based on qualifications such as

- the ability to sell and persuade
- the ability to relate well to applicants
- an affinity for administrative detail
- a knowledge of labor laws and general hiring and employment practices
- a ready knowledge of nursing or the ability to grasp job qualifications and licensure requirements
- complete honesty in presenting the facts to interested applicants
- freedom and willingness to travel

The basic job description in Table 31–4 should be helpful to a health care facility in establishing the new position or reevaluating the position as it currently exists.

Recruitment Budget

Useful guideposts in budget planning are the surveys by the National Association of Nurse Recruiters (NANR). These surveys provide information on budgets allocated for recruitment by health care facilities grouped according to size and geographic location.

Basic expense categories to consider when planning your recruitment budget and/or determining your average cost per hire at the end of the recruitment year are the following:

- salaries and fringe benefits for the recruiter and clerical support staff
- cost of office space and utilities
- telephone charges (including the flat rate as well as long distance and collect calls)
- postage for first class letters and recruitment packets
- printing costs for all recruitment materials
- exhibit costs
- travel costs to conventions and career programs for the recruiter and assistants
- booth fees at conventions and job fairs (including rental of furniture for the booth)
- advertising fees (local and national)
- advertising/public relations agency fees for brochures, advertisements, and other materials (if you hire an agency)
- staff time of your facility's public relations department
- staff time for those involved in the interviewing process
- expenses incurred in interviewing
- entertainment of prospects, both in-house and on the road
- cost of preemployment physicals
- cost of orientation
- relocation expenses (if your institution offers them)

NURSE RETENTION

Overview

Health care facilities must redirect their energies and resources from short-term, stopgap recruitment efforts to long-term retention efforts. Another way of putting this is that organizations will have to learn to recruit from within—that is, to retain those productive nurses in whom the facility has already invested time and money.

*Source: Tina Filoromo and Dolores Ziff, *Nurse Recruitment: Strategies for Success*, Aspen Publishers, Inc., © 1980.

Table 31–4 Basic Job Description for Nurse Recruiter

JOB SUMMARY

Meets, screens, interviews, and refers registered nurse (RN) applicants. Collects and keeps current listing of RN vacancies. Reviews RN applications and follows up on initial inquiries, interviews, and job offers. Works directly with department heads, nurse managers, and others in establishing rapport and cooperation with, offering jobs to, screening, and employing RN applicants. Periodically assists various members of the department and the director of the department in completing projects and research studies.

DUTIES AND RESPONSIBILITIES

- Keeps in constant contact with department heads to maintain current records of their needs.
- Responds to written inquiries about RN positions available; corresponds with RN applicants regarding interviews, openings, and any other questions applicants may have.
- Greets and initially interviews RN applicants who come to the nurse recruitment office, fully explains the facility's benefits, and sees that applicants have a chance to interview with a member of the department of their interest; provides information for callers in regard to RN vacancies; schedules appointments.

- Acts as the coordinator between department heads and RN applicants for job openings and job offers.
- Informs department heads when an RN applicant is acceptable or not acceptable by checking references and evaluating results; makes available the references to the department heads.
- Informs the proper departments when an RN applicant does not accept a position.
- Notifies RN applicants if they are unacceptable for employment.
- Keeps a tally of the source of inquiries about RN vacancies and the number of job offers that can be traced back to each source.
- Maintains other files and records as required.
- Works directly with an advertising agency or the facility's public relations department to coordinate recruitment materials; maintains the materials in up-to-date form.
- Travels to annual RN and student nursing conventions, career days, and other career-related activities to recruit registered nurses; makes arrangements for, assembles materials for, attends, and is in charge of recruitment at these conventions.
- Keeps the director of the department informed of any consistent problems and new developments in RN recruitment.
- Performs additional tasks as assigned and requested by the director of the department.
- Adheres to all organizational and personnel policies of the facility.

It is highly unlikely that a health care facility can get a "quick fix" by adopting a single innovation, such as salary bonuses or primary nursing, to attract and keep nurses. Changes that merely throw money at the problem are particularly unlikely to work as retention devices. Many health care facilities are now using such recruitment gimmicks as salary increments for baccalaureate nurses, bonuses for nurses who work weekends or nights on a regular basis, or bounties for recruited nurses. These methods may help a facility compete with others in its locale or with temporary agencies to recruit more nurses in the short run, but they are unlikely to help retain nurses in the long run unless other job factors are also addressed. This is not to argue that competitive nursing salaries are not desirable and deserved, only that salary improvements must be combined with other strategies in a serious effort to retain nurses.*

Manager's Role in Staff Retention**

Management control and management style heavily influence areas from which staff job satisfaction is derived: autonomy, effective communication, and attainment of an identified standard of patient care. Managers must also take into account the areas that contribute to nurses' discontent and stress (see Figure 31–1).

Therefore, an appropriate retention plan should first address the management style used in a particular area, and the person managing the area should be evaluated regarding appropriateness of style. For example, determining which managers are unable to promote autonomy can be accomplished by listening to the staff in the managers' departments. These staff members usually develop frustration about their practice and refer to "the system" as the problem. Once it can be determined how the style of management affects the department, a targeted retention plan can be developed to correct deficits and strengthen positive attributes.

Development of a plan should include a review of present policies and management practices and a survey of staff opinions. A retention plan is an integral part of the day-to-day functioning of the unit. The management style should be synchronized with the retention plan, and particular attention should be focused on increasing staff autonomy and increasing effective communication. A retention plan developed with input by the staff is the most effective plan for staff retention.

Implementation of such a plan is not easy. It is a restructuring of present policies, attitudes, and behaviors. The manager must be willing to change the method of managing. Rigid policies need to be adjusted so that staff growth and development can be fostered. Important areas to evaluate include patient care assignments, scheduling policies, the work environment, and how problem solving occurs in the area.

Improving Retention Factors*

A nursing environment that satisfies and retains staff members should stress certain elements.

Excellence in Nursing Practice. Knowledge, skills, and attitudes of the nursing staff should build the image of excellence. These elements should be the building blocks in a retention program. The drive toward excellence in practice can be enhanced with a complete and thorough orientation to organizational mission and purpose and by ensuring that staff are sufficiently versed in requirements and basic skills. Staff nurses should be given opportunities to grow, to learn, and to change directions if that is the stimulus needed. For example, the organization could provide clinical, educational, and management tracks.

Autonomy. A structure for autonomy also implies responsible decision making and self-governance. Professional nurses with responsibility for clinical decision making must also have the authority to make those decisions within a supportive framework.

Supportive Management. Those who are responsible for resources, whether human or material, should create and support an atmosphere that allows for optimal patient care. Management should promote mutual support interdepartmentally and use appraisal systems to promote lateral and vertical growth.

Benefits. There should be a just, competitive, and variable reward system that recognizes the value of service provided. The system should speak to the needs of the employee, be flexible, and allow for consistent and frequent reviews.

(Suggested activities are listed in Table 31–5.)

---

*Source: Carol Weisman, "Recruit from Within: Hospital Nurse Retention in the 1980s," *The Journal of Nursing Administration*, May 1982. Reprinted with permission.

**Source: Joan H. Goodroe, "The Manager's Influence in Retention," *The Health Care Supervisor*, Vol. 11, No. 2, Aspen Publishers, Inc., © December 1992.

---

*Source: Adapted from Mary Ann Sorensen, "New Strategies in Nurse Recruitment," *Aspen's Advisor for Nurse Executives*, Vol. 7, No. 9, Aspen Publishers, Inc., © June 1992.

Figure 31–1 Factors Contributing to Nurse Retention

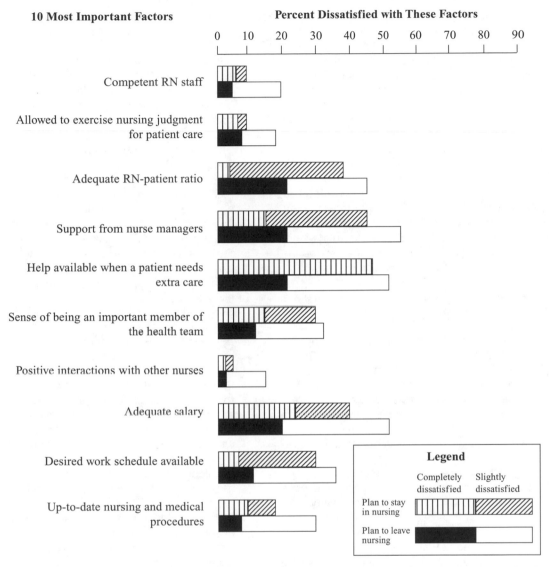

Note: Nurses who said they are not likely to stay in nursing three more years clearly do not have what they want—though they agree with those who will stay on what is most important. Over 90 percent of all nurses rated the top four items as very important. Where leavers and stayers part company is on satisfaction with what they say is important: For each item, a higher percentage of leavers than stayers are dissatisfied.

Source: Reprinted from Florence L. Huey and Susan Hartley, "What Keeps Nurses in Nursing: 3,500 Nurses Tell Their Stories," *American Journal of Nursing*, February 1988. Copyright © by the American Journal of Nursing Company. Used with permission. All rights reserved.

Table 31–5 Suggestions for Nurse Retention Activities

The following suggested procedures would remedy job factors that research has shown to be dissatisfying to nurses:

- Provide realistic job previews during the hiring process, emphasizing both the positive and the negative aspects of the job. Assessment center–type selection, especially for supervisory positions, is a good approach.
- Offer summer positions to nursing students to expose them to the variety of jobs in your facility.
- Provide career planning for registered nurses. Develop a career ladder so that those who want to remain at the bedside can do so and yet progress. (An educational advisor in the staff of the education department can be a valuable adjunct in setting career goals.)
- Make certain that wages and benefits are comparable to other health care facilities in the area.
- Establish a "retention position" and appoint a staff member to help personnel with things such as counseling, transfers, promotion, and relocation within the institution. This appointee should be a staff person, preferably not reporting directly to the director of nursing.
- Develop a nursing advisory committee as part of nursing administration and include staff nurses among its members.
- Consider centralized scheduling and post the results prominently and well in advance of work dates. As part of this process, institute a program to train those responsible for making these decisions.
- Introduce an incentive system with rewards for exceptionally good work. Consider, for example, a quality circle program or a financial reward system.
- Assess your orientation program to make certain it focuses on realistic expectations, and encourage its presentation by your education services department. This step should be necessarily preceded by the recruitment of a departmental staff with full professional and educational credentials.
- Maintain communication with nurses, both upward and downward, through the use of conferences, quality circles, newsletters, and so forth.
- Enhance the status of head nurses and respect the influence you allow them.
- Institute sound behavior-based management skills training for *all* supervisory personnel, which should include coaching, counseling, delegating, discipline, handling employee complaints, taking a problem to the boss, performance appraisal, on-the-job training, and so forth. These problems will be resolved best through the behavior-modeling process.
- Redesign nursing jobs so that nurses can use all of their skills adequately. This should be done to increase autonomy, feedback, skill variety, task significance, and task identity.
- Provide adequate staffing. Staffing needs to reflect a realistic pattern of nursing coverage. Allow for meeting time, downtime, sick time, vacation time, and so forth.
- Offer substantial opportunities for continuing education on the premises, and provide the highest tuition reimbursement possible, especially for those aspiring to a baccalaureate degree.
- Eliminate rotating shifts, if possible, and/or use a flextime schedule.
- Approve RN hires at the unit level.
- Consider the establishment of quality day care and early childhood learning centers.
- Assess the possibility of using a part-time float pool or temporary agency nurses as an alternative to understaffing.
- Design a sabbatical/leave policy.
- Pay full-time hourly wages and benefits to nurses willing to work weekends only.
- Educate the medical staff to cooperate and communicate better with the nursing staff.

Source: Used with permission from *Hospital and Human Services Administration*, Vol. 27, No. 6: pp. 18–20 (Chicago: Health Administration Press, 1982).

Chapter 32

Criticizing, Correcting, and Disciplining

CRITICIZING*

Criticism in its highest sense means trying to learn the best that is known and thought and measuring things by that standard.

Criticism can be used and met constructively or destructively. It can be the means by which people receiving it climb, or it can be used to bolster the critic's vanity. Captious criticism takes note of trivial faults; its author is usually unduly exacting or perversely hard to please. Carping criticism is a perverse picking of flaws. Caviling criticism is the habit of raising petty objections. Censorious criticism means a tendency to be severely condemnatory of that which one does not like.

Ordinary faultfinding seems to indicate less background and experience than the art of criticism requires. It is wholly concerned with tearing down and scolding, whereas criticism is the art of analyzing and judging the quality of something.

Silence is sometimes the severest criticism.

What Is Fair Criticism?

Fair criticism does not judge without factual information. It considers the event on which it is

---
Source: John R. Heron, "On Criticism," *Monthly Letter*, November 1977, Royal Bank of Canada. Reprinted with permission.

to pass judgment in the light of these factors: What was said or done? What did the person mean to say or do? What was his or her reason for saying or doing it? What is the effect of what he or she said or did? Why do I object to it?

Fair criticism does not exaggerate. All but a few careful and considerate persons seem to be urged either to overstate things by 100 percent or to understate them by 50 percent in order to criticize with greater enjoyment.

Fair criticism does not include common gossip. Gossip may be merely friendly talking or useless chatter, but it too often degenerates into mischievous comment on neighbors or business associates.

The Ideal Critic

The ideal critic would know the topic, would be dispassionate in weighing the evidence, would have ability to see clearly what follows from the facts, would be willing to reconsider the facts if that seemed advisable, and would have courage to follow his or her thoughts through to the bitter end. The ideal critic would not, in all this process, brush aside the help of advisors. He or she would retain a keen and lively consciousness of truth.

In making his or her criticism known, the ideal critic would have regard for the feelings of the other person. Courtesy is easily the best single quality to raise one—even a critic—above the crowd.

Charming ways are quick winners. When an end is sought, why browbeat and shout and storm if one can persuade?

The good critic will not force the person being criticized too far. It is always good strategy to let the other person save face.

CORRECTING ERRORS*

The *purpose* of correcting errors is to help employees improve their work performance.

Correction must be focused on helping employees identify and understand their errors and learn how to avoid repeating them. They must know what the manager expects and feel confident that they can live up to these expectations.

There are three steps in correcting errors: (1) review the standards by which the job was to be done, (2) point out the error, and (3) indicate what must be done to correct it. These steps should be followed in sequence. Unfortunately, most managers start by pointing out the error. This usually results in defensiveness, excuses, or an attempt to focus on the things that the employee does do right. The employee tries to justify his or her poor performance rather than to correct it.

Reviewing Standards

The importance of reviewing standards as the first step in correcting errors cannot be overemphasized, even though it is seldom done.

When an employee ignores step-by-step procedures for accomplishing a particular task, the manager should review the procedures with the employee and ensure that the worker understands the standards. But what about standards that govern certain behavior or practices but are not in writing? Health care facilities often have no written policies, procedures, or rules about gossip-

ing, passing along rumors, arguing with other employees, improper personal appearance, and so on.

Here the manager must fall back on broad policies of the organization, some of which may only be implied, not available in writing. The manager may even point out that management does not tolerate gossip and rumor because they waste time, affect morale, and reduce the quality and quantity of work.

Step-by-Step Guidelines

Effective guidelines have been developed for carrying out the three steps of correcting errors. Managers who follow these guidelines can make corrections far more objectively and are less likely to become involved in personalities and personal problems.

1. Correct the first error. No employee should be allowed to get by with a work error, even once. If he or she does, other employees will be encouraged to put forth less than their best effort.

2. Choose the proper time and place. Corrections should be made as soon after the error as feasible. Waiting a few days lessens the effectiveness of the correction. Correction interviews should be in private, never before fellow employees.

3. Be objective. To be objective, the manager must correct errors when not angry or irritated. Being objective means correcting the *situation*, not a personality. It is important not to criticize the employee as a person. Correction should be made for the sake of improvement.

4. Be specific. The manager should never make general statements. General statements make employees defensive. They respond by pointing out the things they do correctly and believe they can defend. The manager should focus on specific errors.

5. Stick to the facts. The manager should never base a correction on hearsay. It is essential to get all sides of a story before acting.

6. Do not react to excuses. Employees often try to justify their errors, to explain that errors were not their fault. The manager should never let the listener divert attention from the specific

---

*Source: Winborn E. Davis, "Correcting Errors in Work Performance," *Hospital Topics*, August 1973. Reprinted with permission.

work error under discussion, but should stick to the three steps, saying, "These are the standards you agreed to follow, this is what you did wrong, and this is what must be done."

7. Be serious. Joking or teasing should be avoided. If a work error is serious enough to call to an employee's attention, it is worthy of a serious approach.

8. Spell out the remedy. The manager should be as specific about the remedy as about the error and should not leave the employee uncertain of what is expected.

9. Allow employee questions. Letting the employee ask questions gives immediate feedback on whether he or she understands the standards, the error, and the remedy.

10. Do not make excuses yourself. Managers often lessen the value of correction by being apologetic. Managers are paid to deal openly with errors in work performance. It is part of the job.

11. Individualize the employee. Sensitivities vary: the manager should approach employees differently, yet follow the same steps and guidelines.

12. Tie up loose ends. The manager should get immediate feedback on whether the employee truly understands what went wrong and what is expected.

DISCIPLINING

The Goal of Disciplining*

Disciplining is not punishing, at least not at first. Disciplining is an educational effort to nudge unsatisfactory performance up to an acceptable level while preserving employee perceptions of self-worth. The initial goal is not to grease the slide to separation. It is to provide traction for employees to climb back—to correct behavior and to salvage the employee.

Punishment breeds resistance, encourages subterfuge, and undermines employees' willingness to make future contributions to the organization.

The nonpunitive or *positive disciplinary* approach has been successful in overcoming many of these adverse effects.

The theme of the nonpunitive approach is building commitment instead of enforcing compliance. It is congruent with the principle of participative management in that it, too, is treating employees as adults, not children.

Encouragement replaces threats. Rules are referred to as employee responsibilities; oral and written warnings are expressed as suggestions. Discussions are low key with emphasis on problem solving.

When these discussions fail, the suggestion is made that there may be a poor employee-job fit and that a change in employment may be beneficial for all parties.

The Meaning of Discipline*

Discipline first meant complete and total obedience to rules and regulations and to the directives and orders of superiors. Failure to comply resulted in punitive actions. Closer examination of discipline reveals that the most constructive and effective forms of discipline involve something more than mere obedience to authority. The second and higher discipline, then, involves self-control and a sense of personal responsibility for behavior and performance.

Traditional discipline is achieved through the authority of the individual in a supervisory capacity. The self-control form is achieved through the influence of a systematic frame of reference that is held in common by all individuals in the organization and that guides their actions.

Factors Influencing Discipline

Several factors influence the learning of self-discipline. They can be considered to be conditions that must be satisfied if discipline is to be developed and maintained within an organization.

Understanding of Requirements. Good discipline rests on the security of understanding. Each individual in an organization must know and understand the ground rules, the limits, and the actions and behavior that are approved and disapproved. And those requirements must remain relatively consistent if subordinates are to learn them.

Atmosphere of Confidence. Good discipline rests on a foundation of mutual trust and confidence. That confidence includes the confidence of managers in their subordinates, of subordinates in the decisions and actions of their managers, and of everyone in the organization in his or her own ability to perform effectively.

Informal Sanctions. Good discipline is the result of the operation of informal sanctions—social pressures generated within a group or organization to enforce informal norms of performance and conduct. The extent to which norms allow a group to accept or resist organizational rules and principles plays an important part in the development and maintenance of discipline. The concept of group norm is comparable with such concepts as codes, customs, and traditions.

Formal Sanctions. When authority is used to enforce discipline, formal sanctions must play an important part in the process. But it is not just the sanctions themselves that exert an influence on the development and maintenance of discipline. The way in which they are used to enforce compliance with decisions, rules, and principles is even more important. Two principles apply: First, justice and fairness to all concerned must be ensured; second, the sanctions must be applied consistently. Subordinates must be confident that they will be treated fairly, and they must know that punishments come to them because of what they *do* and not because of how someone in authority *feels*.

Goals, Cohesion, and Morale. When individuals develop a strong commitment to the objectives of an organization, they are more likely to be highly motivated. Such motivation leads to acceptance of organizationally approved standards of conduct. Cohesion is related to

---

Analyzing Discipline Problems

Seriousness of Problem. How severe is the problem or infraction?

Time Span. Have there been other discipline problems in the past, and over how long a time span?

Frequency and Nature of Problems. Is the current problem part of an emerging or continuing pattern of discipline infractions?

Employee's Work History. How long has the employee worked for the organization, and what was the quality of performance?

Extenuating Factors. Are there extenuating circumstances related to the problem? For example, if there was a fight, was the employee provoked?

Degree of Orientation. To what extent has management made an earlier effort to educate the person causing the problem about the existing discipline rules and procedures and the consequences of violations?

History of Organization's Discipline Practices. How have similar infractions been dealt with in the past within the department and within the entire organization? Has there been consistency in the application of discipline procedures?

Implications for Other Employees. What impact will your decision have on other workers in the unit?

Management Backing. If employees decide to take their case to higher management, do you have reasonable evidence to justify your decision?

---

identification with the organization and to the capacity of the unit to exert influence without the use of punitive measures. In general, cohesion results in greater conformity with the norms of conduct of the organization. Morale influences discipline because attitudes affect behavior. Poor morale and poor discipline are often partners in the disintegration of an organization.

Discipline Approaches*

The two most widespread problems in the administration of discipline are a broad managerial failure to act promptly in dealing with discipline problems as they occur and overreaction when a long-overdue action is finally taken. The basic foundation of any sound disciplinary program must be a set of procedures that are tailored to achieve the particular objectives of a given organization.

However, a well-written discipline policy is only as effective as its enforcement. And this is where most organizational efforts at effective discipline administration break down or are less than fully successful. Implementation is only successful when discipline is characterized by (1) promptness, (2) impartiality, (3) consistency, (4) nonpunitiveness, (5) fairness, (6) advance warning, and (7) follow-through.

The single efforts of a manager acting alone are quite insufficient to make an organizational discipline program effective. Any successful program must include the following elements: (1) an organizational set of discipline policies and procedures, (2) a uniform application of discipline rules, (3) managers who are trained in the knowledge and skills related to implementing a discipline policy, (4) an orientation program that informs all new employees about management's expectations of appropriate performance and behavior, and (5) a continuous management effort that communicates to employees all changes and revisions in personnel and discipline policies *before* changes are actually put into effect.

Problem Solving

A basic idea in contemporary management practice is that discipline should not be used as a substitute for effective supervision. The first approach to most employee-caused problems should be characterized by problem solving.

Managers are expected to aid their employees in analyzing work problems, obtaining information not readily available to the employees, and in some cases serving as a counselor on personal problems affecting an employee's work problems.

In other words, the manager has an obligation to attempt to deal with the root cause of an employee's discipline problem. This approach does not preclude expressing management's concern over the employee's infraction; therefore, a problem-solving effort by the manager should be part of an oral warning discussion. In other cases, depending on the judgment of the manager, he or she may want to try a counseling problem-solving interview without resorting to a disciplinary action.

Disciplinary Action

While problem-solving efforts can eliminate or significantly minimize future employee discipline infractions, problem solving will not always work. At this point, a disciplinary action should be taken. The typical sequence of steps under "progressive" or "corrective" discipline is as follows:

1. oral warning
2. written warning
3. suspension

Dismissal, the final stage of disciplinary action, will be discussed later in this chapter.

1. Oral Warning. As a rule, the oral warning should be conducted in an informal atmosphere. The purpose of this informality is to encourage the employee to relate his or her view of the problem with an opportunity for a reasonably complete statement of the facts as the employee sees them. The manager may expect to question the employee during the discussion but normally should avoid interrupting the employee. It is important to obtain all relevant facts.

After the manager knows the relevant facts, and after these facts have been analyzed and evaluated against the employee's past record, the employee should be informed of the manager's determination. This includes any expected improvement in future behavior; assistance, if ap-

556   NURSING ADMINISTRATION HANDBOOK

propriate, that the manager plans to give to the employee in correcting the problem; the disciplinary penalty being imposed (assuming there is one); and any follow-up action that will be taken.

2. Written Warning. The written warning is the second step. It is preceded by an interview similar to the oral warning–type discussion. Employees are told at the conclusion of the interview that a written warning will be issued. The key points that should be included in a written warning are a statement of the problem, identification of the rule that was violated, consequences of continued deviant behavior, the employee's commitment to make correction (if any), and any follow-up action to be taken.

3. Suspension. Suspensions can only occur for minor discipline violations after there has been a record of oral and written warnings established. Suspension, of course, can be applied without such a record if a major discipline infraction has occurred. Suspension rather than dismissal is used when management believes that there is still some hope for "rehabilitating" the employee. Or, because of a union presence, management may feel that it could not sustain a discharge if that discharge was taken to arbitration.

Suspension may be for a period of one day to several weeks. Disciplinary layoffs in excess of 30 days are rare.

Other Kinds of Steps and Systems*

Although the sequence of oral and written warnings, suspension, and dismissal is considered to be the standard in the discipline process, some organizations have developed embellishments of the process by adding other elements to that sequence. For example, there is the "corrective" interview. This step is designed to precede any formal disciplining act. The corrective interview is used to instigate an improvement in behavior without having the interview necessarily go on the employee's personnel record.

*Source: Wallace Wohlking, "Effective Discipline in Employee Relations," *Personnel Journal*, September 1975. Reprinted with permission of *Personnel Journal*, Costa Mesa, California; all rights reserved.

Another device that is occasionally used in a progressive discipline policy is the "final warning." The final warning is a step inserted between the written warning and suspension. The effect of this extra step is to allow the employee additional and more gradual notification that he or she is approaching a point where severe punishment (suspension and/or dismissal) is about to be imposed.

Some employers use a two-step approach: immediate discharge for a listed "serious" offense and a progressive disciplinary process for less serious infractions.

Other organizations attempt to eliminate judgments that a manager is required to exercise in disciplinary cases by developing a "slide rule" set of dischargeable offenses. For example, discipline policy based on this concept might state, "The second time an employee is found smoking in the work area, he or she will be suspended for three days."

Slide rule policies remove much of the traditional considerations that must go into analyzing and assessing a determination in discipline cases. Factors normally considered in evaluating most discipline cases are ignored for a mechanistic, formularized approach.

Wrongful Discharges and Cautions in Disciplining*

An ill-advised decision to discipline an employee can invite serious legal complications and potentially costly back pay awards.

The discharge of an employee is sometimes necessary, and the corrective disciplining of an employee is often useful. However, given the growing number of antidiscrimination laws and collective bargaining agreements, the increasing number of cases brought by employees, and the substantial burden of proof placed on employers in such cases, it is prudent to review and revise disciplinary procedures to minimize the risks involved. Most employers who lose disciplinary cases before a government agency or before an

*Source: Health Law Center, *Health Care Labor Manual*, Aspen Publishers, Inc., © March 1993.

arbitrator can usually trace their lack of success to one of three areas: inadequate or procedurally defective investigation, the existence of disparate treatment, or the lack of documented evidence. (See Table 32–1.)

In most states, wrongful discharge theories must be considered in every termination of employment situation. It must be emphasized that wrongful discharge is a function of state law and varies from state to state. While there are some universally applied legal theories, to be certain that your conduct comports with the law in your jurisdiction, you should contact competent legal counsel.

Table 32–1 Avoiding Litigation: Review of Appropriateness of Disciplinary Actions

The manager who takes hasty or improper action against an employee is usually involved in a grievance charging him or her with "unfair, discriminatory, and unjust" action. The burden of proof falls on the manager and the institution to justify the discharge. A "No" answer to any of the following questions could mean that just cause for an action does not exist—or, at best, that there is a questionable case.

Rules or Orders	Yes	No
• Is the rule or order violated published in writing?		
• Is it posted on institution bulletin boards easily visible to this and other employees?		
• Did this employee ever receive a personal copy of this rule or order?		
• Is the rule or order stated in clear, concise, easy-to-understand wording?		
• Is the violated rule or order reasonably related to the orderly, efficient, and safe operation of the institution?		

Enforcement

	Yes	No
• If other employees have violated this rule or order, did they receive the same disciplinary action as this employee?		
• Does this employee have the worst record of all employees on violation of this rule or order?		

Warnings

	Yes	No
• Has this employee been warned previously for violation of this rule or order?		
• Has this employee ever received a final warning for the violation of this or any other published rule or order?		

Investigation	Yes	No
• Was the incident that triggered the final warning or discharge carefully investigated prior to taking serious or final disciplinary action?		
• Was the institution's investigation conducted fairly and objectively?		
• During the investigation did the "judge" obtain substantial evidence or proof that the employee was guilty as charged?		

Facts and Documentation

	Yes	No
• Is there a factual, written record showing the steps taken by the institution to correct this employee's improper actions prior to serious disciplinary action?		
• Have similar written records been kept and similar steps taken by the institution to correct the improper actions of all employees?		
• Does the institution's evidence include names of witnesses, dates, times, places, and other pertinent facts on all past violations, including the last one?		

Reasonableness of Penalty

	Yes	No
• Was the degree of discipline imposed on this employee related to (1) seriousness of the proven offense, (2) the employee's past record, and (3) his or her length of service?		
• Is the institution's disciplinary action in this case consistent with its past practice for violations of the same rule?		

Source: Health Law Center, *Health Care Labor Manual*, Aspen Publishers, Inc., © March 1993.

Chapter 33

Troubled and Troublesome Employees

TROUBLED EMPLOYEES

Alcoholism, drug abuse, emotional illness, and family crisis are employees' personal problems that spill over into the environment of the health care organization and ultimately affect job performance. A personal crisis situation involving marital, family, financial, or legal troubles is considered the most prevalent problem among all employee groups.

Adopting the Proper Manner*

Employees with personal problems—those that people cannot help but bring to work with them—are rarely able to do their best work. As an administrator, you should be interested in the employee as a whole person, but the employee's private life and personal problems are none of your business; they represent an area you cannot enter without specific invitation.

In dealing with the apparently troubled employee, do not prod and do not push. Make yourself available to the employee, and make known your willingness to listen. You may have to go as

---

*Source: Charles R. McConnell, *The Effective Health Care Supervisor*, ed 3, Aspen Publishers, Inc., © 1993.

far as to provide the time, the place, and the op portunity for the employee to talk with you, without specifically asking the employee to "open up." Quite often, if your openness is evident, the troubled employee will turn to you.

In relating to the troubled employee, the following attitudes should be adopted.

Listen, but be aware at all times of the temptation to give advice. Some of the most useless statements you can make begin with "If I were you. . . ." Also, although many troubled employees could use advice, it is usually advice that you are unqualified to deliver. The best you can do under most circumstances is to suggest gently that the employee seek help from qualified professionals.

Be patient and show your concern for the employee as an individual. Although you should naturally be concerned with an individual's impairment as a productive employee, do not parade this before the troubled person. Rather, be patient and understanding. Perhaps, when possible, you can even be patient to the extent of easing off on tight deadlines and extra work requirements until the person is able to work through a problem.

Do not argue and do not criticize an employee for holding certain feelings or reflecting certain attitudes. Avoid passing judgment on the employee based on what you are seeing and hearing.

Be discreet and let nothing a troubled employee tells you go beyond you. Be extra cautious if an employee tends toward opening up to the extent of revealing much that is extremely personal and private. While it often is good for a person to be able to simply talk to someone else about a problem, the individual often runs the risk of saying too much and afterward perhaps feeling extremely uncomfortable about having done so. If you can, try to demonstrate that you sympathize and understand without allowing the employee to go too far. Always provide assurance that what you have heard in such an exchange is safe with you.

Reassure when you are honestly able to do so. Provide the employee with reasonable assurance of things of importance, such as the security of the employee's job, the absence of undue pressure while problems get worked out, and the presence of a friendly and sympathetic ear when needed. You need not even know the nature of the employee's outside problem to supply very real assistance by reducing the job-related pressures on the individual.

In dealing with the troubled employee in general, listen honestly and sympathetically and do what can be done to reduce pressure on the employee, but leave the giving of specific advice related to the problem to persons qualified to deal with such matters.

Troubled Employees and Employee Assistance Programs*

Even if you are trained as a licensed psychologist or psychiatric nurse, your job as a manager is not to give therapy to employees under your supervision. However, you can, and should, refer troubled employees to an employee assistance program (EAP) if one is available. Some health care facilities have their own internal EAPs; oth-

ers use independent EAPs. The point is, the health care organization has a vested interest in salvaging, not terminating, valued employees; in reducing, not increasing, employee stresses; and in being informed, in advance, when employees' personal problems place them and others in the health care organization at risk should a personal problem develop into workplace violence.

If an EAP is not available, for whatever reason, refer the employee elsewhere for appropriate counseling and intervention. These types of referrals are easier to accomplish in urban or metropolitan areas, and more difficult to accomplish in small, rural areas, where resources may be limited. You may have to refer the troubled employee to the closest geographic area where appropriate resources are available. In any case, appropriate referrals should be made, regardless of the geographic area. Referral is in the best interests of all concerned: the troubled employee, coworkers, the health care manager, the health care organization, and the patients and the community served by the health care institution.

Stress*

The classic definition of stress, attributed to Dr. Hans Selye, probably the world's leading authority on the subject, is *the nonspecific response of the body to any demand made on it.* In 1914, years before Selye's work, Dr. Walter B. Cannon defined stress as *the body's ability to prepare itself instantaneously to respond to physical threat.* The latter definition describes the oft-cited "fight-or-flight" response.

We now know, of course, that the "threat" Cannon referred to can be emotional as well as physical. Indeed, the demand that triggers stress in the body can be purely physical, purely emotional, or a combination of the two. And we should all be more than passingly familiar with the fight-or-flight response—increased heart rate, faster breathing, tensed muscles, flowing adrenaline, and other signs that the body is ready for action.

*Source: Carol A. Distasio, "Employee Violence in Health Care: Guidelines for Health Care Organizations," *The Health Care Supervisor*, Vol. 13, No. 3, Aspen Publishers, Inc., © March 1995.

*Source: Charles R. McConnell, *The Effective Health Care Supervisor*, ed 3, Aspen Publishers, Inc., © 1993.

We cannot avoid experiencing a certain amount of stress. It is inextricably related to change. Stress is largely the way we respond to change, not through our conscious actions but involuntarily, both physically and emotionally.

Perhaps one of the most useful ways to describe stress is as a feeling of loss of control. When some outside influence—some change—disturbs our equilibrium, we react involuntarily in ways that suggest we no longer have the measure of control we need over events and circumstances.

Stress can be both positive and negative. It is positive when you are "up" for something, prepared and alert and determined to regain control. People who seem to perform at their best when under pressure usually do so out of response to positive stress. Consider, for example, a key presentation you are required to make to top management. The future of your department, as well as your own future in the organization, may depend on how well you do. You feel "up" for the occasion—tense, perhaps anxious, maybe experiencing butterflies in the stomach. In your knowledge of how much is riding on your presentation, you are thoroughly prepared (or one would hope you are) and determined to do a good job. You are taking control, reacting positively to positive stress.

Much stress, however, can be negative. And no one can say with any certainty which events constitute positive stress and which constitute negative stress. People vary greatly in their ability to cope with stress in general and to perform well under pressure in a job situation. Whether stress is positive or negative depends largely on how you react *after* the stressful event has passed. Positive stress, or "good" stress, is invariably followed by relaxation. Negative, or harmful, stress is not followed by relaxation, and you continue to experience tension, anxiety, and the like.

Sources of Stress

Stress emanates from three general sources: your personal life (life outside work), the total job environment, and yourself—your personality, inherent capabilities, and approach to daily living whether at work or away from work.

Stress arising in our personal lives is highly likely to influence our job performance in some way. We have all known people who seem incapable of leaving the problems of the job at work, instead carrying their frustrations home and allowing them to affect their personal lives. And we have certainly known employees who regularly bring their personal problems to work and allow them to affect their performance. Some of the most frequently encountered employee problems a supervisor faces arise with employees whose performance and interpersonal relations are adversely affected by personal difficulties.

We need to recognize that it is not possible to separate the person on the job completely from the person off the job. People vary greatly in their ability to keep the work side of life from influencing the nonwork side and vice versa. To some people home is a welcome respite from the problems of the job; they can literally leave their worries on the doorstep. To others, work is a refuge, an escape from a chaotic personal life. To a great many people, however, trouble at work usually means trouble at home, and trouble at home usually spills over into their employment in some way.

The total job environment can induce stress in a number of ways. Factors that seem as simple as physical working conditions—heating, lighting, furnishings, space, noise, and the like—can create stress. So also can organizational policies and practices that are inconsistent or unpredictable. These are common sources of stress in supervisors.

A supervisor's feeling of having less than total control over the work situation can induce stress, especially when the supervisor has total responsibility for a given situation without having full authority over all the elements that must be brought to bear to address the situation. It is common among supervisors to find that they have responsibility—at least *implied* responsibility—but that they have not been given authority consistent with that responsibility.

Much supervisory stress comes from negative practices of higher management. "Bossism"; management that pushes rather than leads; and management that is authoritarian, unreasonably demanding, or fault finding all create supervisory stress. And although not necessarily negative itself, a change in management that leaves a supervisor reporting to a new superior can be a stress producer. Virtually guaranteed to produce considerable supervisory stress is frequent change in the chain of command or organizational structure that leaves the supervisor reporting to a new manager every few months.

Finally, a major potential stress producer for supervisors is work overload—the fact or at least the perception of having too much to do, not enough time to do it, and not enough resources for its accomplishment. Many supervisors have learned the hard way that they cannot be all things to all people in a finite amount of time.

As functions of personality, capabilities, and approach, the stress producers that can be at work within ourselves include:

- self-doubts; a lack of confidence in our own abilities
- lack of personal organization
- inability to plan out our work and to establish priorities and address them appropriately
- perfectionism; placing excessive and unrealistic demands on ourselves
- the inability to say no to any request or demand
- the tendency to take all problems as indications of our own shortcomings; the tendency to take all criticism personally

If you are never stressed on the job, you may have too little to do and little or no true responsibility. Also, if you are never stressed by the demands of the job, you are probably falling short of doing your best work. Positive stress, in urging you to perform under pressure, produces learning and growth.

To a considerable extent, stress goes with the supervisory territory. But if you are always stressed, if you are chronically on the verge of anxiety, depression, or panic, this stress can lead to personal ineffectiveness and ultimately to physical or emotional illness.

Burnout

Vulnerability to Burnout*

Personnel who deliver direct medical or nursing care are vulnerable to the burnout syndrome, in which their personal resources for coping with and managing stress are exhausted. Supervisory and administrative employees also become susceptible to burnout because of pressures to maintain an adequate support system for those who deliver direct health care services.

Some health care professionals attain burnout early in their careers because they experience physical and emotional exhaustion and no longer are able to experience empathy, respect, or positive feelings for patients. They become extremely critical of patients and of the professional and deal with individuals in a demeaning and derogatory manner. They view their patients as being worthy of their illness since the burnout changes some of their perceptions and makes it extremely difficult for them to practice their role in a humanistic, helping, positive manner.

One way in which health care personnel maintain their psychological equilibrium and at the same time attempt to keep stress at a minimum is to maintain a psychological distance from patients. They often behave in ways that justify patients' complaints about the care being received, since they are too impersonal and fail to give adequate explanations concerning the nature of the patients' problems and other pertinent factors.

Signs of Burnout**

Some of the signs of burnout are the following:

- when nurses' capacity to solve problems and satisfy cognitive requirements of the work are impaired by burnout and they consider job termination
- when nurses begin to perceive patients, families, and clients from a negative, judg-

---

*Source: Steven H. Appelbaum, Stress Management for Health Care Professionals, Aspen Publishers, Inc., © 1980.

**Source: Excerpted from Hospitals, Vol. 53, No. 22, by permission, November 15, 1979, Copyright 1979, American Hospital Publishing, Inc.

mental perspective and label them as problems or troublemakers

- when nurses feel the administration is not supporting them or understanding their job performance and these feelings are directed through anger toward the work environment, peers, and administrators

- when interpersonal contact between the emotionally exhausted nurse and patient is affected adversely and the nurse experiences lower job satisfaction and self-esteem

- when perceptions of self-image begin to change drastically (negatively), accompanied by swings in emotional disposition

- when rigidity increases and nurses' personal and social life changes via withdrawal and isolation

- when nurses have been trained to be aware of and sensitive to the needs of patients and then do not apply these skills

- when nurses increase self-imposed restrictions and experience stresses in their own lives, such as marital and financial problems, parenting difficulties, social pressures, and other disruptive influences

Preventive Mechanisms*

Preventive mechanisms include rap sessions, lectures on stress, management development, job restructuring, supervisory training, job discussion, variable work schedules, and health education and promotion. See Figure 33–1 for a model for assessing burnout.

PROBLEM EMPLOYEES

Guidelines for Dealing with Problem Employees**

1. Listen. Make it clear that you are always available to hear what is bothering your employees. Display an open attitude, conscientiously avoiding the tendency to shut out possible unpleasantries because you "don't want to hear them." Many employees' doubts, fears, and complaints are created or magnified by a closed attitude on the part of the manager, so your obvious willingness to listen will go a long way toward putting some troubles to rest.

2. Always be patient, fair, and consistent. However, retain sufficient latitude in your behavior to allow for individual differences among people. Use the rules of the organization as they were intended, stressing corrective aspects rather than punishment. Apply disciplinary action when truly deserved, but do not use the threat of such action to attempt to force change by employees.

3. Recognize and respect individual feelings. Further, recognize that a feeling as such is neither right nor wrong—it is simply there. What a person *does* with a feeling may be right or wrong, but the feeling itself cannot be helped. Do not ever say, "You shouldn't feel that way." Respect people's feelings, and restrict your supervisory interest to what each employee does with those feelings.

4. Avoid arguments. Problem employees are frequently ready and willing to argue in defense of their feelings or beliefs. However, by arguing with an employee you simply solidify that person in a defensive positive and reduce the chances of effective communication of any kind.

5. Let resistant employees try something their own way, if possible. As a manager you are interested first in results and only secondarily in how those results are achieved (as long as they are achieved by reasonable methods). There is no better way to clear the air with the employee who "knows better" than to provide the flexibility for that person to try it that way and either succeed or fail. In other words, the employee who appears stubborn or resistant may not be so by nature but may rather be reacting to authoritarian leadership. More participative leadership might be the answer.

6. Pay special attention to the chronic complainers. These are the employees who seem to grouch and grumble all through the day and spread their gloom and doom to anyone who will listen. Chronic complaining is, of course, a sign

---

*Alice D. Seuntjens, "Burnout in Nursing," *Nursing Administration Quarterly*, Vol. 7:1, Aspen Publishers, Inc., © 1982.

**Source: Charles R. McConnell, *The Effective Health Care Supervisor*, ed 3, Aspen Publishers, Inc., © 1993.

Figure 33–1 A Model for Assessing Burnout

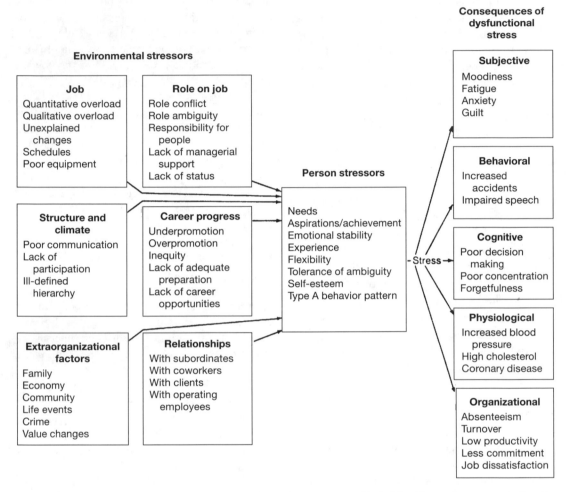

Source: Reprinted with permission from J. Ivancevich and M. Matteson, "Optimizing Human Resources: A Case for Preventive Health and Stress Management," *Organizational Dynamics,* Autumn 1980.

---

of several potential problems and also breeds new problems of its own. The chronic complainer can affect departmental morale and drag down the entire work group. You should make every effort to find out what is behind the complaining and perhaps even consider altering assignments so that the complainer is semi-isolated or at least has limited opportunity to spread complaints.

7. *Give each employee some special attention.* The manager-employee relationship remains at the heart of the manager's job, and each employee

deserves to be recognized as an individual as well as a producer of output. Honest recognition as individuals is all that some so-called problem employees really need to enable them to stop being problems.

The Whole Person

In the long run you will find it practically impossible to separate the person off the job from the person on the job. To a greater or lesser extent, people bring their outside problems onto the job and carry their job-related problems off the job. With some employees this crossover is minimal. With others, however, a small crisis in either facet of their existence can affect attitudes and behavior in the other. Thus the employee who becomes sullen and withdrawn may have done so either because of some job-related experience or because of something that happened off the job. If someone has become "moody" or "stubborn" or invited the application of some similar label, that alone should give you cause to wonder what is behind the behavior.

The behavior projected by an employee can be an emotional defense against treatment received on the job. Because people are different, some distinctly so, the same approach will not work with everyone. As a supervisor, do you make it a practice to remain on friendly terms with everyone—friendly, but impersonal and businesslike—conscientiously trying to play no favorites while you avoid getting "too close" to your employees? To some of your employees this will be appropriate behavior; you will be seen as a good supervisor. However, some employees will see this same behavior as artificial and perhaps label you as "cold" or "phony." (It is not just the supervisors who do the labeling.)

Do you make an effort to get to know all your employees, openly expressing interest in them as individuals and inquiring into their personal interests? Again, to part of your employee group this behavior will make you a good supervisor. To others, however, you will seem nosy, inquiring into things that are "none of your business." Is it your practice to circulate about the group during the workday to simply show people you are there, available, and interested? If so, this behavior will be accepted by some employees as appropriate supervisory behavior while some others may see you as distrustful because you are constantly "checking up" on them.

Whatever you do in your efforts to be a good supervisor, a few employees are likely to react negatively. These negative reactors are likely to be your "problem employees."

Dead-End Employees

The dead-end employee is that employee who can go no further in the organization. Promotion to supervision may not be possible because basic qualifications are lacking; promotion to a higher level is not possible because the employee is already at the top of grade; pay raises are infrequent because the employee has reached the top of the scale and can move only when the scale itself is moved. In short, the dead-end employee is blocked from growth and advancement in all channels. Motivating this employee is a special problem because there are no more material rewards left with which to prevent creeping dissatisfaction from setting in and other rewards, the true motivators that should be inherent in the job, are limited.

It is unfortunate that many dead-end employees become problems because these employees very often have the most to offer to the organization. It falls to the nurse manager to deal with the problem by appealing to the individual through true motivating forces that stress job factors rather than environmental factors.

In dealing with the dead-end employee, use the following strategies:

- *Consult* the employee on various problems and aspects of the department's work. Ask for advice. It is possible that an employee with years of experience in the same capacity has a great deal to offer and will react favorably to the opportunity to offer it.
- Give the employee a bit of additional *responsibility* when possible, and let the person earn the opportunity to be more responsible. Some freedom and flexibility may be seen as recognition of a sort for the employee's past experience and contributions.
- *Delegate* special one-time assignments. Again, years of experience may have prepared the employee to handle special jobs above and beyond ordinary assignments.
- Use the dead-end employee as a *teacher*. The experienced employee may be quite valuable in one-on-one situations, helping to

orient new employees or teaching present employees new and different tasks.

- Point the dead-end employee toward certain *prestige* assignments, such as committee assignments, attendance at an occasional seminar or educational program, or the co-ordination of a social activity such as a re-tirement party or other gathering.

- Conditions permitting, cross-train the dead-end employee on several other jobs within the department. The employee is thus given a chance to do a variety of work and be-come more valuable to the department.

Note that all of the foregoing suggestions deal with ways of putting interest, challenge, variety, and responsibility into the work itself. In deal-ing with the dead-end employee, special atten-tion must be given to true motivating forces because the potential dissatisfiers, that is, the en-vironmental factors such as wages and fringe benefits and working conditions, are present in force. If the employee has come to regard an oc-casional pay increase as deserved reward for putting up with the same old nonsense, when the top of the scale has been reached and pay raises stop, then dissatisfaction will begin. All the sug-gestions made relative to the dead-end employee are intended to help the person find sufficient motivation in the work itself and avoid the weight of the dissatisfiers.

There are other potential solutions to the prob-lem of the dead-end employee, conditions per-mitting. Maybe it is possible to transfer the per-son to a completely different assignment or perhaps set up a rotational scheme in which sev-eral employees trade assignments on a regular basis. Also, the dead-end employee may be cross-trained on several other jobs within the depart-ment and thus be given a chance to do a variety of work and become more valuable to the de-partment.

Perhaps it is unfair to discuss the dead-end employee in a chapter on "troubled employees," since many such employees may present no trouble at all. However, it is to the supervisor's advantage to recognize the dead-end employee as at least a slightly special case that a bit of con-

scientious supervisory attention can keep from becoming a real problem.

The Impaired Nurse*

The Situation

Nurse managers must consistently and law-fully confront the problem of an alcohol- or drug-impaired nurse practicing in the health care fa-cility. The nurse must be identified and disci-plined according to the facility policy and state law. The appropriate action taken discreetly and promptly will protect patients from being injured by a drug-impaired nurse and lessen the facility's risk of liability for corporate negligence in con-tinuing to employ a nurse it knew or should have known was impaired. In addition, it will elimi-nate the nurse's drug source and remove him or her from practice. It may also encourage the nurse to admit the problem and seek medical assistance.

The Drugs Most Often Diverted by Nurses

- Meperidine (Demerol), 25.7 percent
- Diazepam (Valium), 18.9 percent
- Codeine products, 9.6 percent
- Flurazepam, 6.6 percent
- Morphine, 6.5 percent
- Propoxyphene products, 5 percent
- Pentazocine, 4 percent
- Barbiturates, 3 percent
- Cocaine, 1 percent

Note: Most state nurse practice acts list a variety of drugs that may be involved in a disciplinary proceeding. Some states in-clude the use or abuse of any drug as grounds for discipline.

---

*Source: Carmelle Pellerin Cournoyer, *The Nurse Man-ager & The Law*, Aspen Publishers, Inc., © 1989.

Identification of the Problem

The proximity of drugs in a health care facility makes the leap between temptation and addiction a very short step. Those health care professionals who take that step are people who are initially burdened with problems. The addiction—whether alcoholism or other substance abuse—then becomes the final feather.

Nurse administrators should be in a position to recognize the problem (see Table 33–1), prevent access to the temptation, provide assistance where possible, and institute legal action when necessary. The recommended stance is to be alert, firm, and helpful. Nurses often seek treatment voluntarily, and there is an incentive in having a profession that they may return to after they have been rehabilitated.

Legal Approach

The most frequent legal proceeding involving alcohol- and drug-impaired nurses is an administrative hearing conducted by the state board of nursing for the purpose of determining whether there are grounds to suspend the nurse's license to practice nursing. The nurse has a right to due process and a fair hearing and in most states can obtain a judicial review of the board's final decision.

The board of nursing must prove the specific offense with which the nurse is charged. In most jurisdictions, the board's order to suspend a nurse's license must include a statement of law, a specific reference to the section of the nurse practice act or regulations that the nurse has violated, and a statement of fact, which is a citing of the evidence on which it based its decision.

The Dysfunctional Manager*

Nothing can sabotage the efforts to create a healthy workplace more than dysfunctional behavior at the top of the organization. The culture of the workplace is shaped from the top, and

---

*Source: Francine S. Hall, "Managing the Dysfunctional Manager in Times of Change," *Aspen's Advisor for Nurse Executives*, Vol. 10, No. 2, Aspen Publishers, Inc., © November 1994.

it is at this level that healthy, reality-centered modes of dealing with people and change are needed.

For nursing executives, the ability to identify dysfunctional managers and intervene to help them begin a course of "recovery" is crucial. Nursing executives not only can curtail managerial styles that foster unhealthy behavior, but can also develop a workplace culture that is consistent with accepting reality and confronting change.

Several characteristics of a manager's style may be symptomatic of dysfunctional patterns (see box). Alone, any one of these characteristics does not suggest a problem. However, when a manager manifests a cluster of these behaviors, attention must be focused on whether the behaviors are affecting the culture of the workplace and its subunits.

Behaviors of a Dysfunctional Manager

- Willingness to tolerate rather than resolve problems
- Avoidance of conflict and conflict resolution
- Overdeveloped sense of responsibility
- Tendency to take on the role of "martyr"
- Workaholic lifestyle and pace
- Inability to express feelings and emotions
- Inability to delegate effectively
- Tendency to establish and retain control of situations
- Difficulty with intimate relationships
- Denial of reality

Intervention Strategies

Although it is not the role of the nursing executive to change individual dysfunctional behaviors, the organizational culture can be modified by leaders to create an environment in which recovery is accepted and facilitated. But first, the nurse executive must deal with the immediate issue.

Table 33–1 Chart for Identification of Chemical Dependency Behavior

Note: There is increasing documentation that individuals are addicted to more than one chemical substance. The following list is not all-inclusive.

	Alcoholic Nurses	*Drug-Addicted Nurses*

Personality/ Behavior Changes	• More irritable with patients and colleagues; withdrawn; mood swings
	• Social isolation: wants to work nights, lunches alone, avoids informal staff get-togethers
	• Elaborate excuses for behavior, such as being late for work; unkempt appearance
	• Blackouts: complete memory loss for events, conversations, phone calls to colleagues; euphoric or "glossed over" recall of events on floor (e.g., arguments or unpleasant events)
	• Frequent use of breath purifiers; drinks high volume of "sodas"
	• Flushed face, red or bleary eyes, unsteady gait, slurred speech
	• Signs of withdrawal; tremors, restlessness, diaphoresis
	• As disease progresses: jaundice, ascites, spider veins, cigarette burns and bruises caused by carelessness and clumsiness during intoxication, and gastritis from gastrointestinal effects of alcohol
		• Extreme and rapid mood swings: irritable with patients, then calm after taking drugs
		• Wears long sleeves all the time
		• Suspicious behavior concerning controlled drugs:
		  – consistently signs out more controlled drugs than anyone else
		  – frequently breaks and spills drugs
		  – purposely waits until alone to open narcotics cabinet
		  – constantly volunteers to be med nurse
		  – disappears into bathroom directly after being in narcotic cabinet
		  – vials/medications appear altered
		  – incorrect narcotic count
		  – discrepancies between his or her patient reports and others' patient reports on effect of medications, and so forth
		  – patient complaints that pain medications dispensed by him or her are ineffective
		  – defensive when questioned about medical errors
		  – abnormal number of syringes used, missing, or found in bathroom

Job Performance Changes	• Job shrinkage: does minimum work necessary • Difficulty meeting schedules and deadlines • Illogical or sloppy charting	• Too many medication errors • Too many controlled drugs broken or spilled • Illogical or sloppy charting
Time and Attendance Changes	• Increasingly absent from duty with inadequate explanation: long lunch hours, sick leave after days off • Calls in to request compensatory time at beginning of shift	• Frequently absent from unit • Comes to work early and stays late for no reason—hangs around • Uses sick leave lavishly

Source: Commission on Nursing Administration Ad Hoc Committee on Chemical Dependency, *WSNA Position on the Need for Employee Assistance Programs for Chemical Dependency*, Washington State Nurses Association, 1983.

- *Confront the individual* with the dysfunctional behavior and its consequences in the workplace.
- *Avoid giving professional counseling*; instead, get the individual in touch with the variety of support structures available in your community. This may be an EAP, a support group, or a group specializing in dysfunctional issues.
- *Help the individual recognize underlying problems*, for the behavioral pattern is symptomatic of a deeper problem or issue. Real

behavior change depends on dealing with the root cause.
- *Set realistic goals and expectations* with managers regarding plans for working on recovery. Follow through with support, interest, and reinforcement.
- *Establish a compassionate culture* in which it is acceptable for people to talk about and deal with recovery issues. These issues may include dysfunctional family syndrome, alcoholism, addictions, or any disability.

Chapter 34

Learning:
Staff Development

OVERVIEW

In today's environment in which consumers are greatly concerned about the cost and quality of health services, health care organizations must be innovative, learn, or languish.

To meet the challenge, health care executives will be compelled to create a learning environment that encourages continuous learning and motivates personnel to develop new skills, adapt to change, increase job competency, and deliver customer-driven service. Continuous learning must occur simultaneously at the individual, work group, and organizational levels.*

Management Principles To Support a Learning Environment*

The continuous development of the work force is a major challenge for nurse executives. There are several management principles that will help guide the development and nurturing of the learning organization.

Management should support an environment that facilitates individual, work team, and orga-

nizational vitality. A high-performance environment is characterized by the following:

- a clear vision and a strategic direction that focuses on meeting customer needs
- delegation of responsibility and authority to self-managed work teams
- quick resolution of conflict to the satisfaction of all parties
- honest and open communication up, down, and across organizational chains of command
- individual and work team skill in using information for problem solving, decision making, and goal attainment
- a culture and process that supports continuous quality improvement
- rapid and creative adaptation to change

Guidelines for adult learning are used in the design and implementation of all training programs. These guidelines stress the following:

- Adults have varying levels of knowledge and expertise because of different levels of experience. Each person should have an individualized assessment of his or her experience to determine the type and content of training.

---

*Source: Barbara P. McCool, "Organizational Learning," in *Manual of Health Services Management*, Robert J. Taylor, ed., Aspen Publishers, Inc., © 1994.

- Adults tend to be oriented to the concrete and useful. Therefore, instruction should include active participation of the learner and a focus on demonstrating skill in the workplace.
- Adults learn best in environments that are physically comfortable and support trust, respect, freedom of expression, and diversity. Learning is also enhanced when nurse managers find ways to reinforce newly learned behaviors of workers so that these behaviors will start to be used immediately on the job.
- Adults are usually motivated to learn quickly when they recognize they suffer from a work skill deficiency that can be corrected through job training.

Training should be a means of improving the quality of services offered to patients and solving organizational problems. The content of training programs should flow from the needs of the organization and its clients and should stress competency development for meeting clearly stated standards of performance.

The human resource development function should be supported by management, adequately staffed and financed, and continually evaluated for effectiveness.

Using a Decentralized Staff Development Program*

In many nursing divisions, the task of staff development has been primarily delegated to a specific education/staff development department. The functional components of such a department include

- periodic needs assessment activities
- an orientation program (centralized and decentralized)
- an inservice and continuing education program
- a patient and community education program

However, as nursing units become more specialized, it is increasingly difficult for the staff development department to provide specific educational programs for individual staff members. Therefore, it is recommended that staff development activities be shared between the nurse manager and the staff development department.

Under such an arrangement, the staff development department retains primary responsibility for centralized orientation and community education, while the nurse manager is responsible for decentralized orientation and patient education. Although assessment of educational needs is conducted jointly by the nurse manager and the staff development department, the nurse manager has primary responsibility for targeting which inservice and continuing education programs are needed by his or her staff. The nurse manager continues to rely on the staff development department staff for material and human resources to help with planning, conducting, and evaluating the programs he or she designs for the unit staff. As staff developer, the nurse manager performs the following key role functions:

- sets staff development goals
- enhances and encourages decision making
- provides education and training opportunities
- monitors staff growth and development through the evaluation process
- serves as a mentor to staff by facilitating career advancement and development

INSERVICE EDUCATION

Steps in Planning an Inservice Education Program*

Planning really takes place on *two levels*— the overall inservice education plan for a 6- or 12-month period, perhaps, usually developed by, or with the help of, a program planning commit-

---

Source: Virginia K. Baillie, Louise Trygstad, and Tatiana Isaeff Cordoni, *Effective Nursing Leadership: A Practical Guide*, Aspen Publishers, Inc., © 1989.

Source: Reprinted with permission from E.S. Popiel, "Education Program Planning," *Problem Oriented Systems of Patient Care,* © 1974, National League for Nursing.

Table 34–1 Demonstration of Education Compliance

To comply with the strong proeducation stance taken by the Joint Commission on Accreditation of Healthcare Organizations, health care facilities should have evidence of periodic departmental review of staff training needs and of planned provisions to address those needs.

___ Departmental education plan
___ Orientation checklists
  _ Patient rights
  _ Safety
  _ Department quality improvement
    activities/individual responsibilities
___ Continued competency
  _ Job descriptions
  _ Skills validation
___ Annual required inservices
  _ Table of projected dates
  _ Departmental education calendar
  _ Trending summary of required
    inservices/status of department
___ Individual education profiles
  _ Appraisal period

_ Annual required inservices
_ Unit meetings
_ Continuing education
_ Destination of profile: What is date of
  implementation of new profiles format?
  What will happen to the profile at the
  end of the employee's appraisal period?
___ Agency personnel
  Are agency staff used?
  _ If yes, show policy/procedure for use of
    agency staff.
  _ If yes, show documentation for licen-
    sure, orientation records, and other
    training/skills validation, and so forth.
  _ If no, is it possible that agency staff
    could be used in the future?

Source: Theresa Korycan, "Hospital Redesigns Staff Education Process," © *Joint Commission Perspectives.* Oakbrook Terrace, IL: Joint Commission on Accreditation of Healthcare Organizations, January/February 1994, p. 15. Reprinted with permission.

---

tee and involving as many people as possible, and, on another level, the specific steps that the inservice education director needs to take to carry out the plan, to put together interesting and effective education programs. Following are the steps to be taken from the inservice education director's point of view. (A flowchart to demonstrate the process is presented in Figure 34–1.)

Assess Needs

Inservice education directors need to realize the importance of early recognition of changes in nursing service, technology, legislation, research, economics, public demands, and the changing patient load within the institution, all of which affect what nursing personnel need to know to give effective and comprehensive nursing care.

Observations of the nursing care given on the units will assist in assessing needs. But a word of warning—if an inservice program is planned only in response to expressed interests, desires,

and needs of nursing personnel, educational activities may prove to be limited in scope and remedial in nature, dealing with problems that are already deeply entrenched in the established system and are difficult to solve. Such educational offerings may be too little and too late, both to meet present needs and to forestall future problems. The director of inservice education is in a unique position and can view the total nursing situation in a manner detached from the immediate problems and pressures of the job of the nurse practitioner and with a degree of objectivity not available to most others. An education program planning committee and the nursing service administration may provide a great deal of assistance in outlining future, as well as present, needs for educational courses.

Set Goals and Define Specific Objectives

The program planning committee can also assist in setting the goals of a staff development or inservice education program. These objectives

Figure 34–1 Flowchart: Education and Training Planning Process

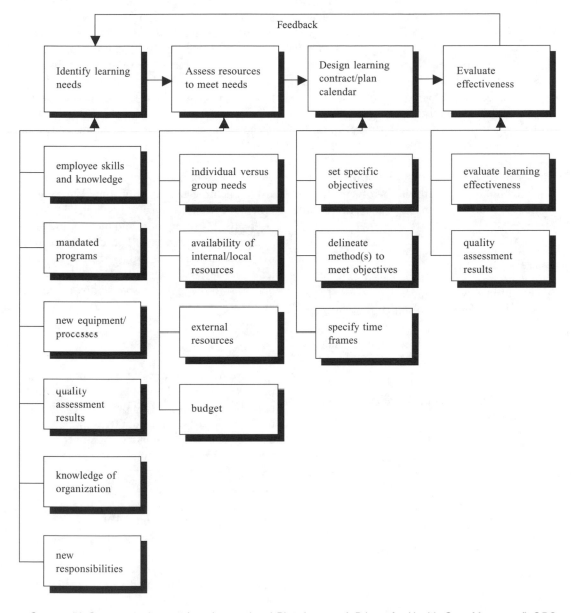

Source: "A Systematic Approach to Instructional Planning . . . A Primer for Health Care Managers," *QRC Advisor*, Vol. 9, No. 1, Aspen Publishers, Inc., © November 1992.

should express expected outcomes, because evaluation of the effectiveness of the overall program will be easier if the objectives are stated so they can be evaluated. Once the goals and objectives are formulated, they should be subjected to periodic scrutiny to keep them relevant.

Plan Courses and Design Learning Experiences

It is important to leave plans and schedules flexible enough that changes and additions can be made as short-range needs arise during the year. The planning and designing of learning experiences challenge the inservice coordinator to draw on the rich methodologies of adult education. Since the primary goal of inservice education is more than merely imparting information and is geared to changing the way a person performs, thinks, or feels, the plan calls for helping personnel to integrate the new knowledge or skill into their immediate experience and stimulating them to set future learning goals for themselves. Role-playing, simulated games, small group work, "alone-time," lectures, independent study, pilot projects, and other methods facilitate the involvement and response of the total person to the learning situation.

Select Resource People

Several attributes should be kept in mind when selecting individuals as resource persons.

- expertise and clinical competence in the area to be covered
- ability to serve as a model for learners
- knowledgeable about the concepts of adult learning
- relates well with adult learners
- knows how to communicate knowledge without a belittling or pompous manner
- starts where the learners are and lets them progress at their own pace
- willing to assist in the evaluation process
- an accepting, listening person who is willing to change the course in midstream if necessary to meet learner needs

Implement Plans

This phase centers around designing the curriculum. Content requirements, learning experiences, and expectations of the participants provide input for the program outline and schedule.

Once the year-long program has been projected, it is then time to decide how to implement the activities. Again, the planning committee can be very useful here. Some of the planned activities would be done best on the nurse manager, head nurse, or team leader level, that is, decentralized rather than institutionwide. When this is true, the task is to train, support, and assist the head nurses or team leaders in planning the decentralized activity. Everyone in the institution needs to be aware of the courses and educational activities scheduled so they can plan ahead to meet their own continuing education goals.

This is the time to ask the nursing personnel what courses or activities they would like to assist in planning and implementing. The committees for each educational activity can be selected at this time, getting more and more of the nursing personnel involved. The more personnel involved, the easier it will be to get good attendance at the activities. Involvement also enhances staff feelings of responsibility to the program.

Evaluate Program

There are many ways of performing evaluation, and everyone should be involved—the director of the program, the planning committee, resource persons, the committees for each educational activity, the nursing personnel who attend the courses, their nurse managers, and their peers. The most important questions to be answered are: Did this educational activity make a difference in the knowledge, skills, and attitudes of the participants? Was there a change in behavior so that better nursing care was given?

Having specific objectives for each activity that clearly delineate the desired outcomes will assist evaluation immensely.

Some evaluative methods include diaries; process recordings; tapes; reaction sheets; participant satisfaction ratings; personnel relations surveys; pre- and posttests of knowledge, skills, and attitudes; and specific rating of achievement of course objectives by the participants. Six-month or one-year postevaluations are helpful, as are interviews of peers and nurse managers and observations of the nursing personnel at work.

Identification of Training Needs*

The process of identifying training needs is accomplished through the collection of evidence or data. Numerous methods are used, but the sources of information can be divided into two categories: staff input and focused observations.

Staff Input Methods. Staff are canvassed, as individuals or as a group, to determine their own awareness of inadequacies. They may identify shortages of particular skills in their own background or on the unit in general. Among the methods used are

- individual interviews by inservice director
- self-evaluation checklists of required performance skills
- survey polls on specific functional areas
- establishment of a suggestion box system

Focused Observations. The talents of a perceptive inservice educator are used to match nursing care functions and standards to the priorities expressed by the health care facility and nursing administration. Observations may be geared to uncovering problem areas on the unit, for example, in charting or in distribution of drugs or in determining trouble spots in a staff member's performance. Among the methods used are

- direct observation of unit/individual in performance
- inspection of incident reports
- review of previous performance evaluations of staff members
- checklist observations of specific functions

As the problem spots are revealed, the inservice educator should start to correlate needs with educational answers and be prepared to marshal available resources for effecting solutions to the problems presented.

Questions for Evaluating Impact of Training on Job Performance

- Did training making a difference?
- Are individuals able to perform the tasks that formed the basis of training?
- Did training solve the problem or fill the need identified during the needs analysis process?
- Do nurse managers, head nurses, and those receiving training feel that completion of the program by the employees made a difference?
- Did training affect the product produced by those completing training?

Note: If job performance has not improved, each phase of the training process must be examined through an internal evaluation. The internal evaluation process examines the instructional design, delivery, and evaluation phases of training. Even when job performance has improved, the evaluator may decide to monitor the training process to identify the strengths and address any concerns within the program.

Source: Richard L. Sullivan, Jerry L. Wircenski, Susan S. Arnold, and Michelle D. Sarkees, *The Trainer's Guide: A Practical Manual for the Design, Delivery, and Evaluation of Training*, Aspen Publishers, Inc., © 1990.

General Guidelines for Inservice Programs*

- Provision should be made for nurses to participate in the identification of their continuing education needs and in plans for meeting the needs.
- Programs of continuing and inservice education should be relevant to both the educa-

Source: Reprinted with permission from E.S. Popiel, "Education Program Planning," *Problem Oriented Systems of Patient Care,* © 1974, National League for Nursing.

Source: Guidelines for Continuing Education, Veterans Administration, 1977, #G-11, M2 Part V.

Table 34–2 Criteria for Evaluating Instructional Materials

☐ *Are the materials appropriate for the training objectives?* Materials selected must relate to the objectives. A trainer may use a set of existing materials to save development time, but learners may become confused and lose interest when there appears to be no relationship between the materials and the training objectives.

☐ *Are the materials relevant to the organization?* A commercially produced set of safety slides may show basic safety procedures, but if the equipment, products, and processes are not familiar to the learners, the effectiveness of the slides may be limited.

☐ *Are the materials compatible with existing media and media equipment?* If not, programs must be returned or modified, or new equipment must be purchased.

☐ *Is the format of the materials consistent with that of existing materials?* There are many sources of instructional materials appropriate for use in individualized training packets. The program designer may want to have all information sheets in the same format to ensure consistency.

☐ *Is the information contained within the instructional materials current?* Dated content, photographs, and references limit the effectiveness of materials.

☐ *Is the information contained within the instructional materials factual?* A subject matter expert should review the materials to ensure that the information presented is correct.

☐ *Is the information biased?* The program designer must review materials to ensure that there is no job denigration bias, sex-role stereotyping, ethnic bias, racial bias, age discrimination, or religious bias.

☐ *Is the quality of the materials consistent with that of existing materials?* Materials must be reviewed to ensure that the quality of sound, video, image, layout, and other factors meet the expectations of the organization.

☐ *Is the reading level of the materials appropriate for the learners?* A procedure sheet written at a 12th-grade reading level may be inappropriate for learners reading at a 9th-grade level. The program designer may need to determine the approximate reading level of the learners in order to consider reading level in the selection of materials. There are standardized tests for determining the reading level of instructional materials.

☐ *Is the cost of the materials reasonable?* A program designer may decide to use interactive video as part of an individualized training program. The final decision to use this medium may be a budgetary decision that takes into account the cost of developing and delivering interactive video.

Source: Richard L. Sullivan, Jerry L. Wircenski, Susan S. Arnold, and Michelle D. Sarkees, *The Trainer's Guide: A Practical Manual for the Design, Delivery, and Evaluation of Training*, Aspen Publishers, Inc., © 1990.

---

tional needs of professional nurse employees and the needs of the institution.

- Learning experiences of basic and higher degree programs in nursing should be monitored to determine the appropriateness of selected educational programs or learning activities for continuing education.

- The staff development program should be consistent with the overall goals and objectives of the institution.

- Objectives should be defined for each inservice education program and used as a basis for determining content, learning experiences, and evaluation. They should be

stated in terms of the terminal overt behaviors that indicate successful achievement of desired outcomes. Plans for continuous and terminal evaluation should be made at the time objectives are identified.

- An interdisciplinary approach to sponsoring, planning, and implementing educational activities is encouraged. Close working relationships should be developed between nursing service and staff development personnel.

- Inservice education programs for nurses should be developed under the direction of nurses who, as well as being competent nurse practitioners, are skilled in planning and implementing educational programs.

- Faculty expertise in the content to be taught is essential.
- A variety of formats and teaching methodologies should be used, with selection based on the objectives.
- The time allotted to any inservice education activity should be sufficient to ensure achievement of the objectives. Provision should be made for nurses to have time available to devote to these educational activities.
- Facilities and resources appropriate to the educational program should be provided, including instructional materials, libraries, learning laboratories, conference rooms, secretarial services, and consultants (if indicated).
- Adequate funds for planning, conducting, and evaluating the continuing education program should be included in the nursing services budget.
- Programs should be announced well in advance to enable all concerned to make personal and professional plans accordingly.
- Records of attendance should be maintained.
- Counseling and guidance should be offered so that staff will be informed about the range of continuing educational opportunities that may meet their intermediate and long-range career needs.
- Maximum opportunity should be provided for participants of continuing education programs to integrate new knowledge and skills into practice, share with others, and evaluate the effect on patient care.

CONTINUING EDUCATION— OUTSIDE THE HEALTH CARE FACILITY

Each nursing service should be constantly alert to available outside learning opportunities and the conceivable use that can be made of these in rounding out the program of development for its entire staff. Included in this category are the following types of experiences:

- institutes
- short courses
- conferences
- workshops
- clinical experiences in other facilities
- participation in a national professional meeting
- tuition support for part-time university study
- educational leave with or without tuition support for advanced study

Criteria for Selecting Individual Participants*

Planning *who* shall have *what* in terms of experiences outside the agency should be approached on a "first come, first served" basis. The selection of nurses for these experiences should depend to a large extent on the kinds of goals the nursing service has established for itself. The learning value to the individual and to the health care facility should be considered. The ability of the nurse to make functional adaptation of the experience to the local situation should be a criterion for selection of both the individual and the experience. Matching experience with the individual is not easy; however, one question that always has to be examined is how closely related the experience is to the nurse's regularly assigned duties. The nurse who is able to state clearly his or her objectives in requesting the educational experience is usually the one who can evaluate the experience in a way that has meaning for others. However, the position the nurse holds needs to be considered when projected plans include sharing this experience with many other persons. For example, a staff nurse may experience personal and professional development but is not in a position to readily implement new approaches or change existing think-

---

*Source: Guideline for Continuing Education, Department of Medicine and Surgery, Veterans Administration, 1977.

ing of other persons in his or her unit, as is the head nurse or clinical nurse manager.

Criteria for Funding*

In developing criteria for complete or partial defrayment of cost and/or authorizing absence and for an equitable allocation of time and funds for nursing personnel, consideration should be given to the following:

- benefit to patient care
- facility need for developing or updating staff skill and knowledge
- degree to which the individual can assume responsibility for sharing and applying learning
- preference for local continuing education activity over a distant equivalent offering
- frequency of facility support of the individual's participation in a continuing education activity

Evaluating Program Quality**

Curricula must be designed to foster the baseline tools of professional practice and to support the activities of the professional nurse. Continuing education classes must be performance centered, organized to promote problem-solving skills, analytic thinking, and critical decision making. Case scenarios and role play situations that teach conceptual content and provide multiple practical examples to demonstrate application of skills are necessary. Well-designed courses will use the nurse's expert clinical knowledge base as a foundational support and baseline for building principles of practice. For example, the nursing care needs of the ventilated patient are similar in the critical care unit and in the home; the application and implementation of the care plan, however, will vary and requires the use of the expanded skill set of the professional nurse.

The requirements of a practical, realistic continuing education program must include

- recognition of the skill set required for the nurse in the transformed work environment,
- acknowledgment of the effects of change on the learning environment,
- content necessary to build competence in standard care concepts,
- practical application and examples in multiple settings and situations,
- opportunities to role play or model the skill,
- mentoring or preceptorship when appropriate,
- sensitivity to the nurse's time constraints,
- accessibility and affordability, and
- availability on all days and shifts.

Continuing education is an integral component of the professional development of nurses in every diverse setting. Community and home care agencies, as well as acute care facilities, have invested in the development of their nursing staff and have acknowledged the need for such programs.

---

*Source: *Inservice Education Activities in Nursing Service*, Department of Medicine and Surgery, Veterans Administration, 1963.

**Source: Marjorie Heinzer et al., "The Challenge for Education in a Transformed Health Care System," *Nursing Administration Quarterly*, Vol. 20, No. 4, Aspen Publishers, Inc., © 1996.

Chapter 35

Evaluation: Performance Appraisal

CRITERIA FOR A PERFORMANCE APPRAISAL SYSTEM

The choice of a performance appraisal system (PAS) for a health care facility is a complex decision. Health care delivery systems are constantly being influenced by a variety of internal and external environmental factors. Consequently, the evaluation system that is selected must exhibit a number of characteristics. It must be flexible and capable of balancing the technical, social, and environmental aspects of the organization and their interactions with one another. By accomplishing this balance, the goals of the PAS will assist in the achievement of the goals of the organization. With respect to specific administrative goals, the appraisal system must accurately assess employee performance to ensure that the following interrelated goals are accomplished:

- All employees must be included in the system design and implementation process.
- The system must produce equitable compensation and career development decisions.
- The system must motivate employees to perform well and develop their capabilities.

- The system must be consistent with the rational planning of the human resource requirements of the organization.
- The system must promote constructive communication between managers and employees.
- The system must be in compliance with federal equal opportunity employment directives.*

The Legal Impact of Appraisal**

Performance appraisal presents a steadily growing number of potential legal traps for the unwary evaluator. Although employers have no legal obligation initially to establish a formal system for appraising performance, once an employer institutes a system, the employer may

---

*Source: Michael D. Wiatrowski and Dennis S. Palkon, "Performance Appraisal Systems in Health Care Administration," in Current Comments #108, Health Law Center, *Health Care Labor Manual*, Aspen Publishers, Inc., © November 1993.

**Source: Charles R. McConnell, *The Health Care Manager's Guide to Performance Appraisal*, Aspen Publishers, Inc., © 1993.

have inadvertently established a contract with its employees to use the system for the purpose for which it was established and in the manner in which it was described to employees.

Performance appraisal is used to provide a basis for making employment decisions, including promotions, transfers, layoffs, discharges, and pay raises. These decisions could be made fairly only if employee performance appraisals were consistent. A consistent performance appraisal system helps control arbitrary employment decisions based on likes, dislikes, biases, personalities, or whatever a particular decision maker might factor into a decision. In all probability, the legal entanglements arising from various employment decisions would be far more numerous and considerably more troublesome in the complete absence of performance appraisal.

The documentation of performance becomes evidence when legal discrimination charges are lodged by disgruntled employees with governmental agencies concerned with violations of rights based on race, religion, sex, age, disability, or pregnancy. The three most common forms of human resource actions giving rise to discrimination complaints are promotions, retirements or layoffs, and discharges. Honest, accurate, complete performance appraisals for all parties concerned can determine the outcomes of such complaints.

Complaints involving the issues of promotion and layoff or retirement usually do not turn on whether an individual was performing at a so-called satisfactory level or to some specific standard. Rather, in these actions the assessment of performance is relative; that is, performance documentation is used to show that one person was or was not performing at a higher or lower level than certain others.

Nurse executives must review the process and content of their current practices to measure them against the following elements of legally defensible performance appraisal systems.

The system is based on the job, with the appraisal criteria arising from an analysis of the legitimate requirements of the position. This is, again, the embodiment of the oft-repeated admonition to focus on the job itself and not on the person who does the job.

Performance is assessed using objective criteria as much as possible given the unique requirements of the job. That is, there must be reasons behind the assessments rendered, reasons that amount to more than simply the unsupported subjective opinion of the appraiser.

The appraisers have been trained in the use of the system and possess written instructions on how the appraisal is to be completed. This establishes that any appraiser is as reasonably capable of evaluating performance as any other appraiser using the same system, and that the system can be expected to be applied as intended.

The results of each appraisal are reviewed and discussed with the employee. This is a key area of concern. Documentation of performance problems and efforts to correct them are necessary if an employee fails to improve and must be let go, but it is also necessary to establish that the employee knew about the difficulties. Thus, the legally defensible appraisal system can be used to demonstrate that the employee knew of the problems and was given the opportunity to correct them.

OVERVIEW OF THE PROCESS

Work-Related Objectives of the Performance Appraisal System*

The work-related objectives of a performance appraisal system fall into three broad categories: identifying and remediating problem behaviors, enhancing professional growth and development, and strengthening team efforts toward meeting departmental goals cooperatively.

Monitoring Work-Related Behaviors

The first group of program objectives relates to monitoring, assessing, and remediating work performance. These are important as far as the "control" function of management is concerned. Without the ability and mechanisms to monitor

---

*Source: Therese G. Lawler, "The Objectives of Performance Appraisal—or 'Where Can We Go from Here?'" *Nursing Management*, Vol. 19, No. 3, March 1988. Reprinted with permission.

carefully each individual employee's performance, the manager can neither identify nor help solve work problems stemming from unacceptable job-related behaviors.

To achieve effective monitoring, managers should note the following requisite elements.

Assess individual performance in relation to practice/work standards. Managers should use specific work standards as criterion measures for performance evaluation. It should be remembered that evaluation is a comparison of present work-related behaviors of an individual with defined and delineated standards, which are related to that individual's particular role or job category. In assessing individual performance one looks for compliance with those standards or an acceptable level of competence.

Provide incentives for the improvement and maximization of work-related behaviors. Various types of behavior reinforcement can come into play in evaluation systems. These reinforcements, whether positive or negative, provide incentives toward improved behaviors. Positive incentives may include something as obvious as a merit pay increase, but incentives that also motivate include praise and recognition; employee awards for outstanding evaluations; and increased job responsibility, which acts as an enriching factor. Negative reinforcers or disincentives may be as simple as supervisory displeasure or docking of pay for habitual tardiness.

Establish a mechanism for the remediation of suboptimal performance. The manager builds into a performance evaluation system a "due process" system that can be used for dysfunctional staff problems. For instance, if a particular employee is habitually late for work, the established guidelines of the evaluation system or performance appraisal program would specify that after the second time the individual would be informally counseled. After the fourth incident, there would be a formal interview in which the discussion is noted and specific goals and objectives set. If the goals still are not realized in the specified time frame, the employee would be given an official warning and a final deadline for showing changes in behavior—that is, for being on time. Should additional infractions occur, due process would include, in sequential order, docking of pay, suspension, probation, and finally termination. The aim of the remedial mechanism always is to salvage the employee and to help direct him or her to an acceptable behavior pattern.

Maintain documentation of problem areas and remedial action. Documentation itself is different from the establishment of a remediation mechanism. The process of recording dysfunctional behavior of a problem employee is vital; however, not only are the interactions between nurse manager and subordinate noted but the mutually agreed upon solutions to the work-related problem are recorded and progress toward them is monitored. Documentation is not only important to ensure due process and equitable treatment of employee difficulty, but it also serves as an ongoing progress report to determine degrees and areas of improvement.

Document employee/manager interactions. Recordkeeping in this instance relates to keeping a log of what was said and what commitment to action was made. To accomplish this particular objective, as well as those previously mentioned, more than one conference yearly is necessary. Anecdotal records demand periodic dialogue and assessment, the foundations of any good appraisal program. Good behavior needs to be reinforced when it happens; likewise, suboptimal behavior needs to be confronted as soon as it occurs.

Stimulating Individual Growth and Development

The next group of expected outcomes or objectives of a performance appraisal system centers on contributions to individual growth and development. An essential underlying assumption about staff evaluation is that it should be approached as a learning experience. In this context, both the employee and the manager should be learning from the process. If an evaluation system is to achieve this, it must allow for the following elements.

Recognize and/or reward performance. There are many creative ways in which recognition, a major positive reinforcer of behavior, can be built into a standards-based system. For example, monetary recompense is an obvious and tangible reward that has both real and symbolic value to an employee.

Identify professional goals of the employee. An important function of the nurse manager's role is that of coach or director. A prime responsibility for anyone who supervises a group of employees is assisting with their personal and professional growth and development. To do this well, the manager helps each person identify (1) personal and career goals and (2) strategies that will aid in their achievement.

Enhance work performance through mutual goal setting. Goals can relate either to shoring up weak work behaviors or to increase skill and learning new competencies. Managers must remember how important it is that people who *want* to be better at what they do be given as much supervisory attention and backup as people who *need* to be better. Mutual goal setting between nurse manager and subordinate and periodic tracking through a well-delineated evaluation system will allow for growth.

Enhancing Team Development

The last group of objectives includes those that revolve around team development through the monitoring of *group* performance. Inherent in the definition of a manager as "one who gets things done through others" is a concept that individual employees band together under common direction to accomplish the unit's or agency's goals.

A performance evaluation system can assist the health care manager to do the following.

Stimulate constructive communication through a formalized feedback system. The evaluation process provides a formalized channel for two-way communication and it is to the manager's advantage to use this channel productively and wisely. The manager is able to collect data on common problem areas seen by staff members and to identify better the strengths and weaknesses in the group as a whole.

Identify training needs for both the individual and the group. If people are performing certain work behaviors poorly, there are many plausible explanations. One is that employees are not do-

ing well simply because they do not know that their shortcomings are a result of a deficit in knowledge or skills.

Evaluate the quality of aggregate practice and productivity within a unit or department. In the role of controller or monitor, the manager is responsible for overseeing the quality assurance program of his or her nursing unit or department. A valuable methodology to ensure quality of care is (1) to set up practice or performance standards and then (2) to compare work-related behaviors of both the individual and the group to the standards. A broader application of the principle of quality assurance through an evaluation system can be illustrated through identification of particular competencies related to patient care that are not being carried out by the majority of a particular staff.

Provide a means for participation and staff input into job practice standards and departmental planning. Input by staff is a key factor. Becoming involved in evaluations, which provides mutual benefits both to employees and to the nurse manager and ensures quality provision of care, can forestall many morale problems.

Benefits of Systematic Appraisal*

A formal evaluation system helps the manager consider these factors more carefully and reduces the chances that personal biases will distort the rating. It also forces the manager to observe and scrutinize the work of subordinates not only from the point of view of how well the employees are performing their jobs, but also from the standpoint of what can be done to improve performance. An employee's poor performance and failure to improve may be due in part to the manager's own inadequate supervision. A formal appraisal may serve to evaluate and improve the manager's own performance.

A formal appraisal system serves another important purpose. Every employee has the right to know how well he or she is doing and what

_____

Source: Copyright © 1977, Jonathan Rakich.

can be done to improve work performance. Most employees want to know what their managers think of their work. An employee's desire to know how he or she stands can be interpreted as a need for assurance that he or she has a future in the organization.

Regular appraisals are an important incentive, particularly to the employees of a large organization. Many workers have the feeling that because of the great amount of job specialization, the individual worker's contributions are lost and forgotten. Regular appraisals provide some assurance that the employee is not overlooked by his or her superior and the entire organization.

Regular appraisals of all subordinates should be made by the manager at least once a year, normally considered a sufficiently long period of time. If an employee has just started in a new and more responsible position, it is advisable to make an appraisal within three to six months. In some organizations, appraisals are made according to the dates each employee started; in others, all appraisals are made once or twice a year on fixed dates. As time goes on, periodic appraisals become an important influence on an employee's morale.

The Appraiser*

The ideal appraiser, one who observes and evaluates what is important and reports judgments without bias or error, probably does not exist. But since human judgments must be used, several criteria have been developed to aid in determining an appropriate appraiser.

Qualities of an Appraiser

An appraiser must have *sufficient opportunity to observe:* In other words, the appraiser must be in a position to collect relevant information about the person being evaluated. This can be

accomplished through personal observation, reviewing records, or talking with others who have direct knowledge of the person.

An appraiser's *ability to judge* depends on having a clear understanding of job requirements and standards of satisfactory performance. The objectives and procedures of the appraisal system must be understood as well. Research has shown that the most competent managers' appraisals are the most valid, while less effective managers tend to reward the conservative, co-operative employee who does not represent a threat to the manager's position.

An appraiser needs to possess an appropriate *point of view* for the purpose of the particular appraisal being prepared, because one's point of view usually influences which observed performance is considered desirable or undesirable. A clinical nurse manager and a head nurse might well have different perspectives on what constitutes excellence.

Position of Appraiser

The *position of an appraiser* helps determine opportunity to observe, ability to judge, and the appropriateness of point of view.

Nurse Managers. By virtue of their position, nurse managers have long been favored as appraisers. They have the necessary experience, knowledge, and ability, plus there is the fact that they represent the organization.

Peers. So far, peer appraisals have been used primarily for research purposes. It has not yet been determined how valid peer appraisals could be as a basis for administrative decisions.

Subordinates. Subordinate appraisals are considered to be deficient because the subordinate sees only a part of the manager's job. They have been successfully used, however, to gauge manager-subordinate relationships and in management development work where managers want feedback on how their subordinates experience them.

Self. Self-appraisals find their greatest use in performance discussions. When a person completes a self-appraisal prior to a performance

---

Source: Marion G. Haynes, "Developing an Appraisal Program, Part I," *Personnel Journal*, January 1978. Reprinted with the permission of *Personnel Journal*, Costa Mesa, California; all rights reserved.

discussion, the appraisal tends to be modest. Under most other circumstances, people tend to see themselves as better performers.

Reducing Individual Bias in Reviews

Appraisals by one individual can be influenced by personal bias. There are four ways to reduce this possibility.

Second-Level Review. By having appraisals reviewed by a nurse manager's superior, the chance of superficial or biased evaluations is reduced.

Group Appraisal. In a group appraisal, the judgment of a nurse manager is supplemented by others who have an appropriate relationship with the employee being appraised (e.g., the head nurse or team leader).

Multiple Appraisal. Here appropriate managers, in addition to an immediate superior, also appraise the subordinate. In selecting appropriate managers, the same criteria are used as in selecting appraisal groups.

Field Review Specialists. A field review specialist interviews a manager and prepares an appraisal form from the data obtained. With proper training, a specialist can contribute significantly to the quality of appraisals by maintaining consistency.

APPROACHES TO APPRAISAL

Subordinate Evaluation of the Boss*

In a 1988 study a number of managers were asked, "If your subordinates were to evaluate your performance, how valuable would you find such feedback for your personal development?" Three-quarters of those asked said they would find such feedback definitely or extremely valuable. One might wonder if in actual practice the proportion of managers favoring subordinate evaluation would remain as high as three-quar-

___

*Source: Charles R. McConnell, "The Supervisor's Performance Appraisal: Evaluating the Evaluation," *Health Care Supervisor,* Vol. 11, No. 1, Aspen Publishers, Inc., © 1992.

ters after they had all experienced subordinate evaluation. However, there are some definite advantages to having subordinate input in the evaluation of the supervisor. Specifically the rank-and-file employee is often sufficiently close to the supervisor to see the supervisor's true work performance. The employee is able to see aspects of the supervisor's conduct that higher management never gets to see, and is in the best position to judge whether the supervisor is appropriately visible to the department and available to the employees. Because of the rank-and-file employee's unique view of the supervisor, the employee is able to add perspective to supervisor development by helping to highlight management training needs that might not otherwise be readily uncovered.

But the disadvantages of subordinate evaluation can at times be significant. There are straightforward personality differences; like everyone else, the individual employee will like some people more or less than others and this will influence the assessment of any particular supervisor. There are often differences related to age—the older employee may resent the younger boss and rate accordingly; differences related to length of service or experience—the "older" resents the "newer" and rates accordingly; and differences founded in beliefs about capabilities—"I know that *I* could do that job better."

The supervisor who opts for subordinate evaluation needs to have developed a fairly thick skin. Overall the employees will be relatively kind in their assessments, and in many instances they will, on average, rate supervisors higher than the supervisors rate themselves. However, there will be some occasional surprises and some barbs from directions that never occurred to the supervisor. There will also be some predictable inconsistencies between supervisors' ratings and employees' rating of the supervisors; for example, the overwhelming majority of supervisors rate themselves higher in the communication skills than their employees rate them.

Because of the shortcomings described above, it is hazardous to use subordinate appraisal to provide specifics about supervisory behavior to the appraisal process. However, subordinate evaluations can be helpful in revealing trends and tendencies in a supervisor's behavior. In other words, if it is something said by just a person or two it is probably not valid, but if nearly everyone raises the same point, there is probably something to it of substance.

Another Approach: Upward Performance Appraisals*

While upward performance appraisal (UPA) is a measurement approach designed to let managers know how their skills, leadership, and behavior are being received and accepted by subordinates, others view UPA as a way to gauge whether or not managers fit the continuum between organizational purpose and staff expectations. Naturally, the organization cannot ask employees to appraise managers' performance unless there are clearly defined management practices that managers and employees understand and there are well-defined organizational values and goals.

If the UPA approach is taken, answers to preliminary questions must be established.

- Is the organization's mission clearly stated, evaluated, and articulated to staff?
- Does the organization want to hear from staff in a format that demands action and disclosure?
- Will action be taken to ensure that identified problematic performances are addressed?
- Do staff have experience and empowerment?
- How will upward performance appraisal fit into empowerment structures and processes?

It takes courage for managers to ask employees how they are doing; however, upward performance appraisals, if implemented properly,

can strengthen empowerment programs. Finally, if the organization solicits employee evaluations of managers, it must ensure that expected and necessary behavior modifications in manager practices will follow.

PERFORMANCE APPRAISAL INSTRUMENTS

Performance appraisal measurements are designed for a specific job or job classification. The PAS instrument developed for a nurse would be different from that for a medical record specialist, because the functions that the instrument is designed to measure are different. In the development of the instruments, two factors interplay: cost and effectiveness. The broader and less job specific the instrument becomes, the lower the developmental costs. This vagueness, however, lowers the usefulness of the instrument for improving the performance of an individual or specific jobs and almost forces the evaluator to return to the assessment of global personality dimensions that may not be related to job performance. Performance appraisal instruments are unique because they evaluate behaviors. Health care personnel can evaluate their performance with organizational expectations and know exactly what they have to do to improve the effectiveness of their work.*

Problems in the Use of Evaluation Measures**

A common problem encountered in performance evaluation is the "halo effect." This refers to the tendency of an evaluator to allow the rating assigned to one or more characteristics to influence excessively the rating on other performance characteristics. The rating scale meth-

---

Source: David G. Gyongyos, "Upward Performance Appraisals: Fad or Baldridge Criterion?" *Aspen's Advisor for Nurse Executives*, Vol. 9, No. 7, Aspen Publishers, Inc., © April 1994.

Source: Michael D. Wiatrowski and Dennis S. Palkon, "Performance Appraisal Systems in Health Care Administration," in Current Comments #108, Health Law Center, *Health Care Labor Manual*, Aspen Publishers, Inc., © November 1993.

**Source:* Charles R. McConnell, *The Effective Health Care Supervisor*, ed 2, Aspen Publishers, Inc., © 1988.

ods are particularly susceptible to the halo effect. For instance, if you have declared an employee to be excellent in terms of "initiative" and "dependability," so might you be inclined to rate high relative to "judgment" and "adaptability." Since it is extremely difficult to force oneself to separate completely the consideration of each performance factor from the others (many performance characteristics actually include shades of others), there is no guaranteed way of eliminating the halo effect.

Another common problem in most rating systems is the tendency of many managers to be liberal in their evaluations, that is, to give their employees consistently high ratings. Most approaches to rating are partially based on the assumption that the majority of the work force will be "average" performers. However, many people (managers included) do not like to be considered "only average."

Central tendency or clustering is another problem, one that some rating methods have attempted to overcome. Some managers are reluctant to evaluate people in terms of the outer ends of the scale. To many managers, it is "safest" to evaluate all employees consistently. This often leads to a situation in which everyone is average, contrary to the likelihood that in a work group of any considerable size there are, in fact, performers who are both better and worse than the so-called average.

Interpersonal relationships pose a considerable problem in performance evaluation. The manager cannot help but be influenced, even if only unconsciously, by personal likes and dislikes. Often, a significant part of an evaluation will be based on how well the manager likes the employee rather than how well the employee actually performs.

Types of Instruments*

Rating Scale Variations

Rating scales are the most numerous and popular appraisal mechanisms. All rating scales are

*Source: Adapted from Charles R. McConnell, *The Health Care Supervisor's Guide to Performance Appraisal*, Aspen Publishers, Inc., © 1993.

essentially of two kinds—continuous or discrete. In the *continuous scale* form, the evaluator simply places a mark somewhere along a continuous line to represent the value of the rating for a single performance criterion (see Figure 35–1).

A *discrete scale* contains a number of specific choices from which the evaluator must choose in describing performance against a particular criterion or characteristic. These choices are usually arrayed from poorest to best performance or vice versa.

Rating scales are easy to understand since they readily permit statistical analysis of scores. They facilitate ready comparison of scores among employees. However, there are drawbacks to rating scales. Unless a particular system is designed to highlight substandard scores on individual criteria, there is a chance of genuine performance problems being masked by scores that are satisfactory overall. This is complicated by the fact that, in practice, evaluations using rating scales tend to cluster on the high side. There are also frequent rating scale problems with words and their meanings, allowing for misunderstandings and disagreements.

Another variation of rating scales is the *behaviorally anchored rating scale* (BARS). Figure 35–2 is an example of such a scale for a single evaluation criterion. In the BARS system, a scale is created for each major component or task area of the position. Each scale ties sample kinds of behavior associated with a job description task to an overall description of task performance. This process steers the evaluator away from personality effect and focuses attention on behavior or actions.

Employee Comparison

There are two options in employee comparison. In *ranking*, the evaluator ranks his or her subordinates on an overall basis according to job performance and value to the organization. The evaluator designates the best and poorest performers first, then selects the best and poorest of the remainder, and so on until all in the group have been placed in order. *Employee ranking* may be a satisfactory method in a small group in which all members are known to the evaluator

Figure 35–1 Continuous-Type Rating Scale Excerpt

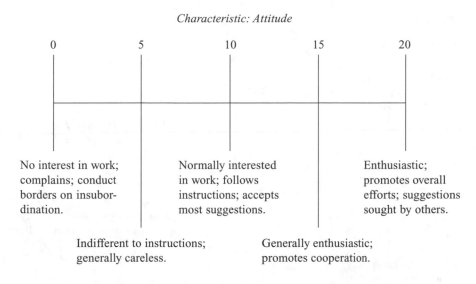

Characteristic: Attitude

0   5   10   15   20

No interest in work;   Normally interested   Enthusiastic;
complains; conduct   in work; follows   promotes overall
borders on insubor-   instructions; accepts   efforts; suggestions
dination.   most suggestions.   sought by others.

Indifferent to instructions;   Generally enthusiastic;
generally careless.   promotes cooperation.

equally well. However, this method is highly subject to personal bias.

In the *forced distribution method*, the evaluator must allocate rankings according to set percentages, for example, 10 percent to the top end of the ranking scale, 20 percent to the second highest group, 40 percent to the middle area, 20 percent to the next lowest group, and 10 percent to the lowest group (see Table 35–1).

Checklists

Checklist evaluation systems require a great deal of development effort.

The *weighted checklist* consists of a large number of statements describing types of behavior associated with a specific job or family of related jobs. The descriptions cover a number of variations in the appropriateness of the behavior in fulfilling the requirements of the job. There is a value or weight associated with every statement, and when rating an employee the evaluator checks all of the statements that most accurately describe the person's behavior. A total score is developed by averaging the weights of all of the statements selected by the appraiser. The actual weights of the statements are kept secret from the evaluator, supposedly so that it

is not possible to deliberately make a score come out as desired.

Critical Incident

Critical incidents are those events that occur during the evaluation period when the employee either makes an outstanding contribution or suffers a significant failure when trying to fulfill an important job responsibility. For each critical incident there should be no doubt that the event was the direct result of the employee's behavior. As the evaluation period proceeds, the evaluator simply records in a notebook or on a simple form all such important positive and negative instances of performance.

The primary advantage of this method is that a clear track of performance is being created while the information is current. The drawback is that many incidents get recorded incorrectly or not at all. There is also the danger of going too far in recording incidents and creating the impression with employees that everything they do is recorded.

Field Review

The most appealing feature of this approach, at least to the evaluators, is that the evaluators

Figure 35–2 Behaviorally Anchored Rating Scale Format

Position: Manager

Job Characteristic: Delegation

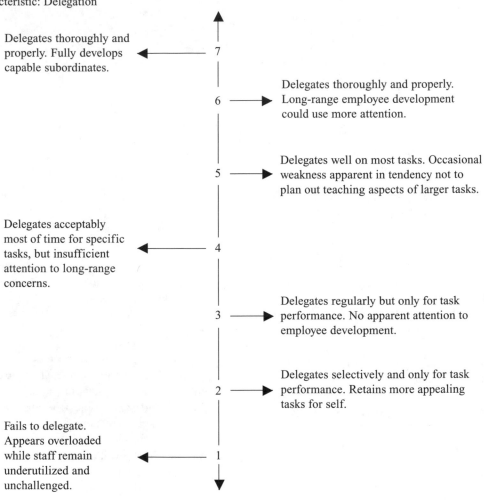

Delegates thoroughly and properly. Fully develops capable subordinates. ← 7

6 → Delegates thoroughly and properly. Long-range employee development could use more attention.

5 → Delegates well on most tasks. Occasional weakness apparent in tendency not to plan out teaching aspects of larger tasks.

Delegates acceptably most of time for specific tasks, but insufficient attention to long-range concerns. ← 4

3 → Delegates regularly but only for task performance. No apparent attention to employee development.

2 → Delegates selectively and only for task performance. Retains more appealing tasks for self.

Fails to delegate. Appears overloaded while staff remain underutilized and unchallenged. ← 1

fill out no forms and do very little paperwork at all. The nurse manager is interviewed by a human resource department interviewer to obtain all pertinent information on each employee. The human resource representative writes a detailed appraisal following whatever format the organization uses and submits this to the nurse manager for modifications or suggestions. Only overall ratings are used; there are no degrees, factors, or incremental scores, as such.

On the positive side, field review relieves the nurse manager of paperwork. On the negative side, the process consumes the time of two management representatives, the nurse manager and the human resource representative.

Essay

The essay method is essentially the same as the field review method but with all of the thinking, writing, correcting, and so on done by the evaluator. No specific form is used, although the evaluator is usually provided with some general questions to answer about the employee or an outline to follow.

Table 35–1 Illustrative Group of Statements: Forced Choice Appraisal

Circle the letter for the statement that is *the most* descriptive of the employee's performance or *the least* descriptive of the employee's performance.

Most	Least	
A	A	Makes mistakes only infrequently
B	B	Is respected by fellow employees
C	C	Fails to follow instructions completely
D	D	Feels own job is more important than other jobs
E	E	Does not exhibit self-reliance when expressing own views

The essay form of appraisal works best for relatively small groups of educated, self-governing professionals, especially if all such people report to a single manager.

Group Appraisal Methods

This approach is extremely valuable in revealing differences in group members' perceptions of each other. (It is best to use strict criteria-based appraisal when peer groups are involved.)

Although a peer group appraisal is done by all members of the group together, the appraisal interview should still be a traditional one-on-one conducted by the immediate superior. The manager, however, presents not just his or her own evaluation but a consensus rating developed by the group.

Properly done, peer group appraisal has some strong advantages and produces good, valuable appraisals. More often than not, an employee's peers are most knowledgeable about the work to be judged and about the employee's performance and behavior. (*Note:* This form of performance appraisal, encountered only occasionally in the past, may be more significant today with the growth of patient care teams.)

Developing Appraisal Forms

Essentially, the appraisal form stipulates various elements for appraisal in objective terms. Basic categories include criteria for measuring job performance, intelligence, and personality. The following are some of the factors most frequently included in performance rating forms for workers: supervision required, attitude, conduct, cooperation, job knowledge, safety, housekeeping, adaptability, absenteeism, tardiness, judgment, quantity of work, and quality of performance.

For each factor, the management may be provided with a number of choices or degrees of achievement. Some appraisal forms, as discussed previously, will use a series of descriptive sentences, phrases, or adjectives to assist the manager in understanding how to judge or evaluate the various rating factors. Many forms are of a "check the box" type and are relatively easy to complete.*

Language**

The language on appraisal forms must be precise, since appraisers tend to read each word very critically. The following thoughts will facilitate the design of forms that are clean, understandable, and relevant.

Express only one idea with each factor. If two thoughts are expressed, a person who is rated high on one and low on the other is difficult to appraise. For example, punctuality and attendance often appear together. Does a low rating indicate the person is often late to work or often absent?

Use words the appraiser will understand. Be particularly careful to design the form for the supervisory group who will be working with it.

---

*Source: Jonathan S. Rakich, Beaufort B. Longest, and Thomas R. O'Donovan, *Managing Health Care Organizations*, W.B. Saunders Company, © 1977. Reprinted by permission of CBS College Publishing.

***Source:* Marion G. Haynes, "Developing an Appraisal Program, Part II," *Personnel Journal*, February 1978. Reprinted with the permission of *Personnel Journal*, Costa Mesa, California; all rights reserved.

Have appraisers evaluate what they observe, not what is inferred. This is particularly appropriate in evaluating elements such as knowledge. Without extensive testing, it cannot really be said how much knowledge a person has on a given subject. However, one can observe the extent to which an understanding of the job is demonstrated.

Avoid double negatives. A positive, declarative approach is easier to understand and respond to.

Express thoughts clearly and simply. Qualifying clauses, ponderous words, and complex expressions serve only to confuse the appraiser. Avoid long, wordy introductions and definitions.

Keep statements internally consistent. Occasionally, direct contradictions may creep into the appraisal form.

Avoid universal statements. Words such as *all, always,* and *never* lead to ambiguity. When *never* appears, most people interpret it as meaning "hardly ever"; yet no two people have exactly the same understanding of *hardly ever*.

Concentrate on the present. Any attempt to go into the past for a rating will lead to distortion. Dramatic events in the past stand out in an appraiser's memory, while good daily work tends to be expected and therefore overlooked.

Avoid vague concepts. This is particularly apparent in attempts to appraise personality factors. The terms *honesty* and *integrity* frequently appear on forms; yet no one has a clear understanding of the two concepts.

EFFECTIVE PERFORMANCE APPRAISAL REVIEW

Processes of the Performance Evaluation Interview*

There are at least four managerial objectives for the interview: (1) to convey information,

*Source: Barbara Stevens Barnum and Karlene M. Kerfoot, *The Nurse as Executive,* Aspen Publishers, Inc., © 1995.

(2) to foster actual behavioral change, (3) to keep the interview situation comfortable and as free of tension as possible, and (4) to maintain control of the situation. These goals are facilitated if the manager goes into the interview with clear purposes in mind. The manager should know in detail what kinds of changes he or she wishes to bring about in the employee and how those suggested changes should be implemented.

To make the interview two-way, the employee should be advised to prepare for the evaluation just as adequately as does the manager. Another way to establish two-way communication is for the two individuals to discuss their mutual expectations of each other.

One of the best ways to maintain good communication during an evaluation interview is for the manager to avoid falling into common interview traps, such as

- conducting a one-way (telling) conversation
- interrupting the employee's thoughts, explanations, and questions
- criticizing the employee rather than the performance
- smoothing over real deficiencies and problems too fast
- failing to investigate facts before expressing opinions
- passing the buck by claiming that one's corrective measures originate higher up
- allowing the interview to fall into charge–countercharge cycles
- allowing the interview to fall into charge–denial cycles
- allowing the interview to fall into charge–excuse cycles
- allowing the interview to deteriorate into a social visit

During an interview, the manager continuously evaluates what is happening in the interaction, recognizing what he or she is doing as well as what the employee is doing.

Developing Improvement Plans*

The key objective of any appraisal system should be positive change on the part of the employee being evaluated.

Given that an appraisal system has presented an employee with valid and meaningful performance data, how does he or she proceed to develop an improvement plan?

The improvement plan is a simple document that allows an individual to determine and document areas in which he or she would like to change and how the change could be accomplished. It focuses on the priority of areas needing improvement as determined by the appraisers and employee and can serve as a commitment for improvement between those individuals. Once the priority areas for improvement have been determined, the following questions need to be answered by the employee.

1. Is it worth changing in this area? (What's in it for me?) This question is inserted because of a strong tendency for people to change behavior only when there is some tangible benefit for them to do so (e.g., career advancement, better boss-subordinate relationships, etc.).

2. How do I want to change? (What is the desired behavioral objective?) One can often change behaviors; however, productive change takes place only when a desired behavioral objective is well defined.

3. How will I change? It is important to be able to define the process to be used to reach the desired objective. Will the employee use outside courses, training, or consulting assistance? Will the employee meet with superiors more often or inform them more of his or her activities through written communications?

4. When will I do it? People have an innate tendency to procrastinate. Change is very often not an easy process and therefore tends to in-

crease this tendency. Therefore, the establishment of a timetable is extremely important.

5. How will I know it got done? There needs to be some means of allowing the employee to know that the commitment to change has been met. It can be feedback from others, the completion of specific activities, and so forth.

To ensure that appraisers continue to give timely and valuable performance data, the employee should be certain to share this plan with each of them and continue to solicit feedback on his or her progress.

Finally, within the time frame of six months to one year, the employee should begin the full appraisal process once again.

What the Employee Needs To Know

To make behavioral changes, the employee must understand which behaviors are desired and which must be corrected. During this final phase of the interview the employee must:[1]

- understand how he or she is going to change to the desired behavior and agree to do so
- understand the consequences of changing or not, identify desired behaviors, and participate in setting goals to change behavior
- develop an action plan on how the change will be accomplished, either at the interview or within one week of the interview
- establish a time frame in which the change will be accomplished
- ensure that the goal is measurable, achievable, and clear to the evaluator and to him- or herself
- understand that the nurse leader and other resource personnel are available to provide assistance as needed

Source: Len Schlesinger, "Performance Improvement: The Missing Element," *Personnel Journal*, June 1976. Reprinted with the permission of *Personnel Journal*, Costa Mesa, California; all rights reserved.

[1]Barbara A. Mark and Howard L. Smith, *Essentials of Finance in Nursing*, Aspen Publishers, Inc., © 1987.

- participate in setting ongoing checkpoints to receive feedback on how he or she is accomplishing specific goals

PREPARATION FOR THE PERFORMANCE EVALUATION INTERVIEW*

Supervisors should develop a method to track evaluation due dates to ensure their timely administration. Tag the anniversary date on the personnel file of each employee as one method of tracking. Mark the due date and the "begin to prepare" date on the annual calendar at the beginning of each year. Schedule the interview several weeks in advance of the annual review date. Inform the employee of the purpose of the interview and discuss any specific problems or administrative actions that may come up during the review; send him or her a copy of the standard evaluation form. Annual performance evaluations, conducted objectively, with clearly stated outcome goals and no surprises, should be constructive experiences for the employee and the nurse manager, not episodes of stress.

Ask the employee to prepare for the interview by doing the following:

- ranking performance on key functions of the job description
- completing a self-evaluation that includes strengths, limitations, current actions to correct deficiencies, type of assistance required from the evaluator, and annual goals for the new year
- obtaining written input from two peers, preferably someone who works on the same shift and someone who works on a different shift
- submitting any additional supportive data that will highlight performance, such as community performance and committee performance

---

*Source: Baillie et al., *Effective Nursing Leadership*, Aspen Publishers, Inc., © 1989.

PERFORMANCE EVALUATION INTERVIEW PROCESS

Take the following actions to ensure a positive interview process:

- Schedule the appointment to ensure there are no unavoidable interruptions. Allow adequate time for the interview, and state the time frame at the beginning of the interview.
- Provide a private, comfortable setting for the interview.
- Allow time for the employee to analyze the written evaluation. Give the employee a copy of the evaluation the day before the interview. The employee should submit a self-evaluation 24 hours in advance of the interview using the same form, performance criteria, and offering any additional documentation.
- Encourage a written response on the institutional evaluation form for the employee. Most evaluation forms have a "comments" section. Allowing the employee to write comments of agreement or disagreement reinforces the bidirectional nature of the evaluation process.
- Encourage free discussion in order to mutually identify problems and goals. Respect the employee's opinions and the right to express them.
- Identify processes by which goals can be achieved and problems solved.
- Assist and counsel with humanity and compassion, as indicated.
- Inform the employee of recognition, as indicated. Reward achievement with an appropriate salary adjustment, merit award, or promotion. State the consequences of unacceptable performance.
- Summarize the interview in a succinct note for the personnel record.
- Establish a mutually agreed-upon time for reassessment of progress.

PERFORMANCE APPRAISAL INTERVIEW GUIDE FOR THE EMPLOYEE*

Before the Interview

- Know your job description.
- Ask for a copy of the evaluation and perform your own appraisal.
- Expect that you will be allowed ample time to prepare.
- Be sure that the manager performing the evaluation is familiar with you and the quality of your work.
- Be prepared to discuss your performance.
- Be prepared to accept and to give constructive criticism professionally.
- Come to the meeting with potential solutions as well as opportunities for improvement.
- Think of ways in which management can help you to improve your performance and to decrease frustration.

During the Interview

- Engage in benign conversation with the rater.
- Listen to the agenda for the meeting.
- Share and discuss your self-appraisal with the appraiser.
- Listen to the rater's comments.
- Work with the appraiser toward mutual understanding and an honest and open dialogue.
- Share your feelings.
- Offer suggestions.
- Follow up on your commitment to improved performance.
- Ask for feedback at regular intervals.

After the Interview

- Expect coaching.
- Request feedback if it is not consistently offered.
- Continue to work with the rater toward better communication and mutual understanding.
- Strive to reach your potential.
- Explore career opportunities.

PERFORMANCE APPRAISAL INTERVIEW GUIDE FOR THE APPRAISER*

Before the Interview

- Know the employee and the job description.
- Give the employee notice that the appraisal will occur.
- Schedule the appointment at a mutually convenient time.
- Give the employee ample time to prepare.
- Gather information pertaining to the employee's performance.
- Refer to the rater training manuals for guidance in avoiding rater pitfalls.
- Choose a private place.
- Anticipate reactions, plan the course of the meeting, and try to prepare for any eventuality.
- Know the company policy regarding salary, merit pay, and appraisal.
- Give the employee a self-appraisal form.

During the Interview

- Do not allow interruptions.
- Do not rush the interview.

---

*Source: Jeanne Marcision, "The Appraisal Interview: Constructive Dialog in Action," *Health Care Supervisor,* Vol. 10, No. 1, pp. 41–50, Aspen Publishers, Inc., © 1991.

*Source: Jeanne Marcision, "The Appraisal Interview: Constructive Dialog in Action," *Health Care Supervisor,* Vol. 10, No. 1, pp. 41–50, Aspen Publishers, Inc., © 1991.

- Listen to the employee's self-appraisal.
- Create a comfortable atmosphere.
- Give the employee his or her evaluation.
- Invite discussion.
- Allow time for both parties to discuss views.
- Be calm, patient, and professional in the face of adversity.
- Encourage a 50/50 dialogue.
- Summarize discussion.
- Make an appointment for follow-up conference.
- Ask for input regarding your role in job enhancement.

After the Interview

- Critique your performance.
- Follow up on plans made for future meetings.
- Provide feedback all year round.
- Continue to work toward improving relations with the employee.

IMPLEMENTING AND MAINTAINING A NEW PERFORMANCE APPRAISAL SYSTEM*

Implementation

To implement a new performance appraisal system three steps should be taken.

Pilot Testing. A group should be selected that is large enough to provide a representative sampling. A measure of the effectiveness of that group's present appraisal program should be developed to serve as a basis against which to evaluate the test program. (Such a measure might be an attitude survey. A less elaborate measure

would be to identify problems with the present program.) After a reasonable time operating under the test program, an evaluation should be made to determine if it is better than the prior one and what changes, if any, should be made to improve it.

Announcing. When an acceptable program has been designed and tested, it needs to be announced to all involved by top facility management. The announcement should include communication with employees who will be covered by the new program as well as managers who will be applying it. This announcement should be made in such a way as to confirm top management interest and confidence in the program and to foster this interest and confidence in its use.

Training. For a program to meet its objectives, the managers involved need to be trained in its use. In general, training would cover the basic procedures material and should concentrate on the actual preparation of appraisals using the forms involved. Such training experience can greatly improve managers' confidence in a program by giving them an opportunity to see it in action and to discuss any reservations or misconceptions they may have.

Maintenance

Staff work is not complete with the implementation of a program. New concepts are continually being developed on appraisal methods, and departmental needs change. Therefore, to maintain a program that is current and that meets departmental needs, some staff unit must assume responsibility for its maintenance. An important part of this function will be to provide channels for feedback from managers on problems encountered in working with the program. From this information, modifications can be made that will result in a program that meets departmental needs and is understood by both the managers and the employees affected by it.

Source: Marion G. Haynes, "Developing an Appraisal Program, Part II," *Personnel Journal*, February 1978. Reprinted with the permission of *Personnel Journal*, Costa Mesa, California; all rights reserved.

Chapter 36

Promotions

CAREER LADDER MOBILITY

Multirole Promotional Ladder*

Most health care facilities have traditionally awarded promotional opportunities only to those professional nurses who assumed administrative or teaching roles. To overcome the inflexibilities of the traditional promotion systems, a new classification system was developed by one hospital. Its design was based on the four major elements of professional nursing practice—clinical practice, administration, research, and education.

In terms of the institution's needs and the skill level brought to the job by an individual nurse, it was possible to classify all nurses within this basic system regardless of the job to be performed. Since the system depended not on job titles but rather on graduated levels of skills, an infinite number of job classifications could exist. (See Table 36–1.)

To accommodate new nurses, all position specifications for professional nursing classifications contained entry qualifications for each

level above the beginning staff nurse position. These minimum qualifications were graduated on the basis of educational background and experience in the specialty field. (See Table 36–2.)

Dual Career Pathway*

A dual career pathway allows the professional nurse to pursue a career in either clinical or administrative nursing and receive equal recognition for whichever option chosen. The clinical ladder concept rewards nurses for their role in staff orientation, inservice, and patient education by providing an opportunity for clinical promotion instead of the traditional administrative promotion. A professional role model within the unit is an additional benefit inherent in the concept of the clinical ladder.

In the past, skilled practitioners who were often better suited for clinical nursing found the administrative track to be the only mode of promotion and the only method of professional advancement. Frustration often resulted because the clinical nurse may have wished to remain in clini-

---

*Source: Harold MacKinnon and Lillian Eriksen, "C.A.R.E.—A Four Track Professional Nurse Classification and Performance Evaluation System," *Journal of Nursing Administration*, April 1977. Reprinted with permission.

*Source: Julie A. Wine and Sara J. Mapstone, "Clinical Advancement," *Nursing Administration Quarterly*, Vol. 6, No. 1, Aspen Publishers, Inc., © 1981.

Table 36–1 Nurse Job Classifications

	NURSE I	NURSE II	NURSE III	NURSE IV	NURSE V
Clinical Practice	Assists in developing nursing care plans	Initiates, implements, and modifies nursing care plans	Develops care plans for complex patient problems	Makes innovative changes in care planning and practice	Analyzes clinical care problems and effects remedial modifications
Administration	Provides administrative support in the provision of nursing services in limited and specific areas of a nursing unit	Administers a nursing unit for part of a 24-hour period	Administers a nursing unit on a permanent round-the-clock basis	Administers several nursing units for either 8- or 24-hour periods	Provides administrative direction for a large nursing division on a 24-hour basis
Research	Assists in research that requires an unsophisticated approach to methodology	Does research that requires a moderate amount of sophistication in research methodology	Does research that requires sophisticated research methodology	Supervises research requiring complex and sophisticated research methodology	Plans and supervises research that requires highly sophisticated research methodology in a variety of areas of nursing and nursing administration
Education	Participates in nursing care conferences	Conducts pre- and post-patient care conferences	Provides learning opportunities through inservice programs, unit conferences, and individual conferences	Plans and coordinates learning conferences and projects	Demonstrates expertise in curriculum development and a thorough knowledge of educational principles

Table 36–2 Job Classifications by Educational Background

	Degree	Nondegree
Nurse I	New graduate	
Nurse II	Baccalaureate with three years' experience, one year in specialty, or master's in nursing with no experience	Three and a half years' experience, one year in specialty
Nurse III	Baccalaureate with four years' experience, two years in specialty, or master's in nursing with one and a half years' experience	Five years' experience, two years in specialty
Nurse IV	Baccalaureate with six years' experience and two years in specialty, or master's in nursing with two years' experience	Seven years' experience, two years in specialty

cal nursing or lacked the skills and motivation to be an effective administrator.

The lack of recognition for clinical expertise often leads to disillusionment with the nursing profession. Nurses may seek another career where they are better appreciated. Some nurses move into teaching or supervisory positions because of the traditional recognition these entail. Other nurses deal with their frustrations by maintaining the status quo and become passive and unmotivated. An increasingly large number of nurses pursue alternate career options or revert to an inactive status in the nursing profession.

Clinical Ladders

See Table 36–3 for factors to consider in implementing a clinical ladder.

Characteristics of Clinical Ladders*

1. Clinical ladders have various levels and titles. There may be multiple tracks that combine clinical and career ladder concepts, or there

_____
*Source: Reprinted with permission, *AORN Journal,* Vol. 37, May 1983, pp. 1209–1222. Copyright © AORN, Inc., 2170 S. Parker Rd., Suite 300, Denver, CO 80231.

may be a single track related to direct patient care. The tracks provide for lateral mobility within defined position descriptions that contain more than one level. From level to level, there are requirements for increasingly complex skills and increasing use of the nursing process (assessment, planning, implementation, and evaluation).

2. The nurse initiates the advancement process, requesting promotion and review and gathering documents to support the claim of being able to perform at the next level.

3. There must be a method of evaluation and periodic reviews and checkpoints to assess performance at that level based on established criteria. A mechanism must be included for advancing, staying at the same level, and being demoted.

4. There must be a reward system that offers incentives to enter the program and to remain in it. This may include titles, status, and benefits.

5. Each level must be defined by behaviors that are discrete, progressive, and stated as behavioral objectives. These behavioral objectives must be realistic and achievable. Performance is measured by established criteria rather than length of service or educational achievement. There may be formal or informal education requirements, however.

Table 36–3 Considerations in Developing a Clinical Ladder

The following aspects need consideration before implementing a clinical ladder program.

The Need for a Clinical Ladder Program

- Does the existing evaluation system provide for the advancement of the individual nurse in the practice setting?
- Does the health care facility recognize the need to reward the nurse who functions with advanced clinical expertise?
- Does the recognition provided for clinical expertise parallel the recognition provided to nurses for managerial or educational expertise?
- Do the nursing staff want a system that provides opportunities for advancement at a clinical level? Potential effects could be
  - pressure to compete for advanced clinical positions
  - perceived threat from change in the existing reward system
  - recognition based on performance rather than on length of service
  - changes in job security resulting in changes in status and potential changes in self-esteem (opportunity would be provided for increased accountability and responsibility and more comprehensive performance evaluations)

Impact on the Health Care Facility

- What are the economic implications of a clinical ladder program?
  - cost of developing and implementing program
  - salary and benefits related to clinical level
  - time and personnel to maintain the program

- time for individual to fulfill role responsibilities
- What are the organizational changes that must occur to implement a clinical ladder program?
  - determination of the number of personnel in levels based on facility needs
  - effect of clinical levels on staffing patterns
  - necessity of redesigning organization chart related to distribution of authority, responsibility, and accountability
  - timing of implementation of clinical ladders program appropriate to organizational climate
- What are the potential effects on personnel?
  - changes in personnel policies, benefits, and salary (benefit changes and salary adjustments should not adversely affect personnel)
  - current contractual agreements
  - effects on other categories of facility personnel
  - effects on retention of personnel
  - restrictiveness caused by penalizing interdepartmental transfers with possible demotion if proficiency at previous level cannot be demonstrated within an established time period
- What are the potential side effects on patient care?
  - greater patient satisfaction because care is provided by the most qualified professional nurse
  - improvement of consistency and efficiency of care throughout the health care facility because of appropriate matching of nursing expertise with patient care needs

---

6. Advance must be by choice and/or opportunity. A nurse must be allowed to remain at one level without penalty.

Benefits. Clinical ladders have a number of advantages.

- They have a positive or beneficial effect on patient care.

- They recognize the value of perioperative nursing practice.
- They provide a method for individual recognition of clinical expertise.
- They are a means of recognizing formal and informal educational achievement.
- They are a motivating force for individual growth and achievement.

- They provide advancement alternatives for nurses in direct patient care.
- They provide a reward system.
- They increase job satisfaction.
- They provide direction for increasing clinical expertise.
- They stimulate individual professional development.
- They aid in developing position descriptions.
- They provide criteria for developing performance evaluation tools.

Purposes of the Program. A clinical ladder program requires considerable deliberation and planning. A nursing unit cannot develop a clinical ladder program in isolation. The entire nursing department and facility administration must be involved and committed to its development and implementation.

Specific purposes of the clinical ladder program should be identified:

- Is this program for increased productivity?
- Is it a reward system?
- Is it a retention system?
- What goals are to be achieved through the program?
- Is this program to be a means of promotion on the individual clinical units, or is it to provide additional career opportunities in management and education?

Rules for Implementation of the Program*

Experience with clinical ladder programs indicates that there are some general rules that can facilitate successful implementation.

Minimize quotas. Limiting the number of nurses that can advance can sap motivation and discourage participation. Quotas limit the number of nurses who can be promoted, thus diminishing the impact of the clinical ladder system on nurse retention. The increasing acuity levels of patients and shortened patient stays indicate that an investment in the highly skilled nurse will produce its own reward by reducing complications that create significant losses over reimbursement. In addition, the highly skilled nurse can far more readily manage the increasingly complex patients who have become the norm on most of the inpatient units.

Maximize staff nurse participation. Clinical ladder programs developed by nursing administration and educators do not always reflect the complexities of the staff nurse role at the bedside. Staff nurses are more inclined to participate if the expectations are realistic and match their perceptions of the clinical environment. The involvement of staff nurses in the steering committee that develops the clinical ladder proposal will alleviate this problem.

Differentiate between the levels through monetary reward. In many clinical ladders the incremental increase in monetary reimbursement is so small that it appears to the staff nurse to belittle the effort involved for progression. The clinical ladder system is one meaningful way to address the very real problem of salary compression within the field of nursing.

Make monetary rewards directly proportional to the need for retention. The fact remains that administrative advancement is still more lucrative than clinical advancement. If nursing is to be perceived as valuable and as a career worth having, financial rewards will have to reflect that value more directly.

Design the program so that the criteria are consistent with program goals. Sometimes clinical ladder programs are too idealistic and heavily weighted toward professional outcomes that are unrealistic for the practice setting (e.g., programs that emphasize research with a predominately diploma education–based work force). In other cases, the criteria are clinically based and do not adequately take into account professional development, as in the case where years of experience are more heavily weighted than educational

---

**Source:* Abby M. Heydman and Nancy Madsen, "Career Ladders for Nurse Retention," in *Managing the Nursing Shortage: A Guide to Recruitment and Retention.* Terence F. Moore and Earl A. Simendinger, eds., Aspen Publishers, Inc., © 1989.

preparation. In either case, staff nurse participation will not be as meaningful and the desired outcomes will not be achieved.

A NURSE PRIVILEGING SYSTEM

Overview*

The use of a privileging process for nurses has the potential for both improving nurses' professional competency and self-esteem and increasing the quality of patient care. Through privileging, nurses are required to meet specific established criteria in order to practice particular nursing skills. Criteria typically distinguish nurses according to their education and experience. Thus, the privileged nurse is recognized for his or her level of professional expertise and experience.

Privileging can be defined as a system for authorizing the performance of selected advanced nursing tasks through peer review of nurses' clinical expertise and education. The purpose of privileging is both to acknowledge nurses' education and skill level and to protect nurses from receiving assignments for which they are not prepared. The process of providing documented evidence of the nurse's qualifications is called credentialing.

The privileging procedure often requires each nurse to complete an application and present credentials and documents supporting the request for privileges (such as performance reports signed by training managers) to the nursing committee. (See Figure 36–1.) At regular monthly meetings, the nursing committee reviews applications and verifies credentials from recognized licensing or certifying agencies such as the American Nurses' Association (ANA) , Nursing Registration and Licensure, or the state board of health. If approval is granted, the application is forwarded to the health care facility privileging committee and the facility's chief executive officer (CEO).

Rejection of an application or of certain privileges requested by an applicant can be challenged by the applicant during a meeting with the committee. If the applicant disagrees with the committee's decision following this meeting, the decision can be challenged through the facility's appeal process. A statement in the privileging application informs applicants that a nurse has 30 days in which to appeal an unfavorable decision.

Functions of the Nursing Service Clinical Privileging Board*

The nursing service clinical privileging board is composed of a variety of expanded role nurses representing areas such as rehabilitation, ambulatory care, medical/surgical psychiatry, and spinal cord injury. This cross section of clinical experts assures critical review of requested privileges and consistency of privileges across clinical specialties and within the nursing service.

The nurse requesting clinical privileges initiates the application process by submitting a packet of information that outlines the privileges requested (see the box entitled "List of Packet Contents"). The request describes educational preparation, relevant experience, certifications, and continuing education. The nurse applicant also secures supervisory and collaborating physician concurrence for the request.

The NSCPB reviews the application package and evaluates congruence between educational preparation, experience, and training with the requested privileges. If the request is unclear, the chairperson meets with the nurse applicant to clarify function and role. Ultimately the NSCPB recommends approval, disapproval, limitations of privileges, and time frames for review.

---

*Source: © Quality Review Bulletin, Oakbrook Terrace, IL: Joint Commission on Accreditation of Healthcare Organizations, 1987, pp. 382–386. Reprinted with permission.

*Source: Patricia Quigley, Andrea Kaye Hixon, and Sandra K. Janzen, "Promoting Autonomy and Professional Practice: A Program of Clinical Privileging," Journal of Nursing Quality Assurance, Vol. 5, No. 3, pp. 27–32, Aspen Publishers, Inc., © 1991.

Figure 36–1 Credentials Validation Chart

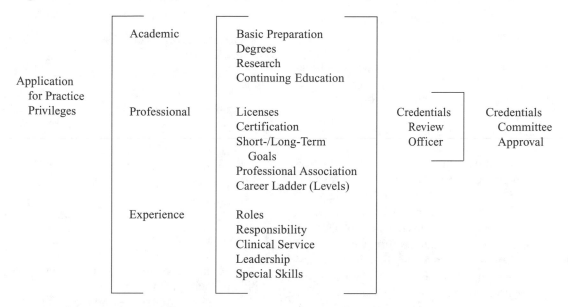

Mobility along the career ladder implies a structure for assessing standards, achievements, and the attainment of requisite credentials. The component items to be validated in a credential review process are outlined in the figure.

Source: Tim Porter O'Grady, "Credentialing, Privileging, and Nursing Bylaws: Assuring Accountability," *Journal of Nursing Administration*, Vol. 15, No. 12, December 1985.

(Occasionally, nurses have not needed privileges as functions were determined to be within the scope of nursing practice.) For initial privileges the review date may be 6 or 12 months; the review period for previously privileged nurses is 2 years.

Recommendations are routed for approval to the chief, nursing service. Upon approval, the packet is forwarded to the executive committee of the medical staff for review in accordance with medical staff bylaws. Signature of the chief of staff indicates final medical staff approval and the packet is forwarded to the hospital director, who is the final approving authority to grant privileges for expanded clinical practice. Results are communicated back to the board and to the applicant by the chief, nursing service.

The NSCPB maintains all records and expiration dates for staff nurses, clinical specialists, and nurse practitioners who apply and are granted privileges. Guidelines stipulate that it is the individual nurse's responsibility to initiate renewal of clinical privileges within a two-year time frame to assure that they do not expire.

DEVELOPING MANAGERS

Overview*

Managerial development for positions such as nurse managers, clinicians, and head nurses should be an integral part of the management process of any nursing department.

---

*Source: Addison C. Bennet, "Towards More Effective Management," *Hospital Topics*, July 1973. Reprinted with permission.

Management Personnel Planning

A logical first step is management personnel planning. To be consistently effective, planning should not be occasional or haphazard, but should be done on a regularly scheduled basis, perhaps once a year. It is a process that embraces three distinct phases—analysis, forecasting, and inventory.

The analysis calls for the administrator and members of administrative staff to review and discuss internal conditions relating to the objectives, structure, and policies. The task of forecasting estimates the number of managers who will be required in the next three to five years, not only for new positions to be established, but as replacements for normal turnover. The forecast should also indicate the functions and levels and when the managers will be needed.

The inventory phase identifies those individuals with a good potential for filling existing or projected managerial vacancies.

Identification and Selection

If the selection of managers is made from within the organization, the criteria must go beyond the candidate's technical skills and capabilities and tenure history.

Much of the problem of building management teams has been created by health care facilities themselves through their short-sighted pursuit of the best technicians at the first-hiring stage. It is the rare facility that shows the wisdom to choose for its management team the person with less-than-the-best technical skills but with a clear promise of administrative and managerial ability.

Currently, the primary criteria being used for the selection of management personnel appear to be technical and professional competence, the ability to deal successfully with interpersonal relationships, and personal stability and maturity. (See Table 36–4.)

Offhand, these would appear to be excellent attributes, but they are unreliable in predicting whether the individual will be a good manager.

A recent study identified the following far more reliable indicators of effective management:[1]

- viewing the organization as a part of a larger system
- perceiving the organization as a patient-oriented system
- establishing goals and objectives
- handling interpersonal relationships
- using personnel resources
- handling and imparting information
- implementing practices of financial administration

Promotions from Within

People are often the most visible yet overlooked resource within any health care organization. The heavy initial costs of recruiting, orienting, and training have already been borne, some degree of loyalty and stability has been demonstrated, and work appraisal, however informal, has at least begun. In short, you know much more about present employees and their potential than you will ever learn from a telephone call to an applicant's last employer. Further, bringing in an outsider at the same or higher pay level than that paid to existing employees who are performing what they believe to be work of equal value can do violence to all of your progressive employee relations. Overlooked workers would do you a favor if they complained. More often they remain silent and vent their frustration on patients, nurse managers, new employees, and the institution itself.*

*A Transfer/Promotion Program**

Opportunity for internal promotion and transfer should be an established and functioning

[1]United Hospital Fund of New York: *Toward More Effective Management*, A Special Study in Management Problems and Practices, 1973.

Source: Skoler, Abbott & Presser, *Health Care Labor Manual*, Aspen Publishers, Inc., © 1981.

Table 36–4 Competency Expectations of First-Level Nurse Manager

Unit Management

- Staffs the unit to meet patient care needs according to
  - classification system
  - staff level of responsibility/ability
  - contractual agreements
  - established patient care standards
- Determines priorities of unit activities based on
  - available resources
  - management principles
  - proven/commonly accepted practices
- Delegates responsibility/authority to those able to assume and implement them
- Proposes options for solving staffing problems that
  - are within legal parameters
  - use as few resources as possible
- Initiates methods for cost containment
- Submits timely written reports that communicate requested information accurately and succinctly
- Evaluates patient care given by staff for
  - achievement of intended outcomes
  - efficient use of resources
  - perceived satisfaction of patients/families
- Using facility guidelines and format, participates in the development of unit budget
- Initiates staff conferences for solving patient care problems
- Makes management decisions that are
  - consistent with delegated authority
  - based on management principles
  - effective in achieving intended results
- Follows established lines of communication for
  - suggestions/complaints
  - reporting unresolved unit problems
  - reporting results of independent decisions
- Uses communication strategies with other departments and individuals that result in
  - achievement of intended results
  - perception of satisfaction/acceptance

Staff Development

- Evaluates staff, using reliable and objective criteria
- Gives feedback to staff on both acceptable and unacceptable performance
- Implements disciplinary action consistent with organizational procedure and guidelines
- Sets goals with employees for improving/maintaining performance, including
  - measurable performance outcomes
  - action plan
  - time frame
  - consequences/rewards
- Holds staff accountable for achieving unit objectives
- Determines options for meeting identified learning needs of staff
- Using the established criteria and process, interviews prospective employees
- Participates in orientation plan for individual employees

Professional Development

- Participates in the development of departmental objectives
- With staff, determines patient care standards for the unit that are consistent with
  - organizational philosophy
  - resource constraints
  - current nursing theory and practice
- Participates in nursing research projects
- Participates in activities that meet own identified learning needs
- Evaluates own performance against competency expectations

Source: Donna R. Sheridan and Katherine Vivenzo, "Developing Prospective Managers: The Process," *Journal of Nursing Administration*, May 1984.

privilege. It is normally the human resource department's responsibility to exercise leadership in articulating the policy and making it work. Managers will not ordinarily oppose interdepartmental transfers and promotions—as long as they themselves do not feel injured in the process. But there is a pervasive natural instinct to use such a policy to "unload bad apples" (without the pain of discharge) while keeping good ones.

The ingredients of a sound transfer/promotion program include the following:

- an up-to-date skills inventory of the present work force
- a fair, easily understood policy along with forms and procedures to make it work
- a tuition assistant program together with on-site opportunities for skill improvement
- human resource department staff who can counsel employees who were considered for better things but were found unqualified
- good statistics on the number and kinds of people who were transferred or promoted during each quarter of the year

Encouraging Applications for Promotions*

The traditional method of promoting staff to managerial levels relies on the astuteness of the nursing service director in perceiving the "best" choice. Often, length of service and reliability determine the selection. Occasionally favoritism by an immediate superior plays a significant part. Some critics of nursing service personnel practices have observed that when such decisions are made only at the topmost level of administration, upward mobility is often stymied.

One method for overcoming such problems is through a system whereby employees can apply for promotion. This procedure allows the nurse

---

*Source: Sigmund G. Ginsburg, "The 'I' Test—Evaluating Executive Talent and Potential," *Personnel Journal*, April 1976. Reprinted with the permission of *Personnel Journal*, Costa Mesa, California; all rights reserved.

director to discover those employees who are interested in advancement and why they feel they are qualified. It also allows staff members to assess their own readiness for upper level positions.

To encourage applicants, notifications of job opportunities should be posted in a central location along with the specific qualifications for each position and the procedure for submitting the written application. A reasonable deadline should be set. A confirmation letter should be sent on receipt of the application, setting up an interview appointment. Interviews should commence promptly after the application deadline. The interview should avoid becoming a performance evaluation. The focus should be on the applicant's concept of management, personal aspirations, assessment of the available position, and view of potential challenges, changes, or obstructions.

After the interview process, the nursing director would most likely discuss tentative choices with the nurse manager under whom the successful applicant would work. The views of the immediate superior are of considerable importance, reflecting close experience with the demands of the job. Once the successful candidate has been selected, public announcement should be delayed till all nonappointees have received brief explanations of their shortcomings in terms of the position's requirements and have been offered guidance on developing needed strengths. This tone provides encouragement and gives direction for further preparation for promotion at a later date. These conferences should be scheduled within as short a period as possible, preferably within one day, to prevent harmful news leakage. The helpful conference softens disappointment, whereas whispered gossip might turn the rejected nurse into a resentful employee.

Do not overlook the selected candidate. Explain the exact requirements of the new position, indicate the associated salary and benefits, and set the date for transfer. Finally, provide recognition of the promotion through a formal announcement or notice to the staff.

Evaluating Subordinates for Management Positions*

In evaluating applicants for top- and middle-level positions, various types of structural formats are employed, including performance appraisals and potential assessment centers; merit systems; psychological, intelligence, and motivation tests; interviews; coworker evaluations; in-basket tests; managerial grid; transactional analysis; and so forth.

However, there are 10 traits, skills, or attributes that distinguish the very successful manager from those who do not quite reach that level of performance. Thus, whatever selection or evaluation devices are used, the goal should be to identify those candidates who have a proven track record and/or high potential in regard to the items listed below.

To use this list as a scoring device, place different weights on each of these factors. Some of the factors might have a weight of 1, others 1.25, and others 1.50. Thus, you could score individuals on a 1–10 scale, multiply by the weights involved, and then come up with a reasonably accurate differentiation among candidates.

The I-Factor Test: What To Look for in Managers

Intelligence. The individual demonstrates both broad and specific knowledge, understanding, and perception; quickly grasps the general as well as technical details; knows what information is needed and how to use it; demonstrates sharpness and clarity of thought and written and oral expression; comes up with creative solutions to difficult problems; shows flexibility in the face of changing times and needs; has ability to pose penetrating questions and deal with the main issues; has ability to learn from the past, deal with the present, and anticipate the future; has ability

---

Source: Sigmund G. Ginsburg, "The 'I' Test—Evaluating Executive Talent and Potential," *Personnel Journal*, April 1976. Reprinted with the permission of *Personnel Journal*, Costa Mesa, California; all rights reserved.

to plan, organize resources to meet the plan, supervise, and control.

Individual Confidence and Self-Knowledge. The individual has trust and confidence in own ability to handle the ordinary as well as new, future, or extraordinary demands of the position without ending up as an egotist; understands own strengths and weaknesses and has ability to build on the strengths, improve on the weaknesses, or to shore up the weaknesses; has ability to know when he or she does not know enough or even anything about a problem and to take steps to acquire the knowledge either personally or through staff assistance; has ability to handle defeats and bounce back with confidence.

Intestinal Fortitude. The individual has ability and courage to make tough decisions, to be decisive, to stick his or her neck out to take sides if needed, to do the unpopular but necessary before the crisis stage is reached—yet at the same time is willing to reverse time-honored practices, precedents, and policies and his or her previous decisions; has courage to be bold, to take a chance, to be unpopular, to be wrong.

Integrity. The individual's word and promises are good and he or she is fair, trustworthy, and unbiased in action; holds to high standards of truth, conduct, honesty, and ethics—and expects it of others.

Interpersonal Relations. The individual has ability to communicate and relate to people as well as problems; understands social and human dynamics, the effect of actions on individuals, and the various psychological, emotional, and ego needs of individuals at various levels; has ability to sympathize and empathize, to supervise and set high standards while earning respect and support.

Innovation. The individual has ability to think beyond the traditional or pedestrian, to see new opportunities and better approaches and ways of doing things, to "dream things that never were, and say, why not?"; possesses a healthy dissatisfaction with the status quo; is creative.

Intensity. The individual has ability to handle problems that vary widely in both scope and magnitude, and to bear up under pressure; possesses the physical, mental, and emotional stamina to meet the everyday as well as crisis pressures of management responsibility; has ability to see the tough, often long, grinding tasks accomplished.

Implementation. The individual demonstrates a concern for ensuring that plans, policies, and programs are carried through on a timely basis with modifications as necessary; demonstrates a concern for the details involved in bringing about successful implementation; has an ability to make things happen.

Identification. The individual has the willingness and ability to identify with the goals and aspirations of the department; to support and represent it with other departments; to identify with the hopes, aspirations, and needs of the staff of the organization; to be loyal to the organization and to superiors, subordinates, and peers commensurate with integrity.

Influence-Inspire. The individual is able—by word, action, interpersonal relations, achievements, standards of conduct, or how he or she carries out all the other factors—to influence all levels of the organization, inspire others to meet his or her high standards and expectations, and motivate others to develop their own potential fully.

Education of New Style Leaders

Leaders in a health care organization who are not provided with the opportunity to learn and practice new behaviors will not be able to contribute to the success of the organization. Without selected strategies for leadership development, the leaders will fail to build the necessary structures and processes that link the professional workers to the processes of care delivery. Instead, they will continue to use the command and control model of the past. Compliance may be achieved but not the commitment vital to surviving the stress of new configurations.

Regardless of whether shared governance, patient-focused care, or systems integration is the type of initiative, clear definitions of the organization's goals must be articulated in such a way that they are easy for managers to act on.

Without the managers' understanding of the revisions needed, they enter leadership development programs wary of broader accountability and unclear about just what their new role and skills should be. The rationale for change must be clearly and repeatedly articulated by the top leaders in the organization and by each manager's own superior. Although the managers may be aware of new leadership competencies, they will likely have little practical knowledge about how to actually perform in a new way.

To assist managers in the acquisition of practical knowledge, an organizationwide program encompassing *specific experiences* must be carefully designed and implemented.

The foundational work in planning a leadership program begins with a key set of questions that must be asked and answered by those charged with planning a leadership development program (see Table 36–5).*

Supporting a Management Development Program*

The development and implementation of a strong leadership development program must garner the same commitment as any other strategic initiative embraced by the organization.

The quality of personal management behavior is the result of a complex interaction between

---

Source: Adapted from Tim Porter O'Grady and Cathleen Krueger Wilson, *The Leadership Revolution in Health Care: Altering Systems, Changing Behavior*, Aspen Publishers, Inc., © 1995.

Table 36–5 Foundations of an Effective Leadership Development Program

- What is happening that demands that managers change their practices?
- How does the application of new leadership skills contribute to the organization's achievement of its goals?
- What specific actions are required from managers? Which practices should continue and which should stop?
- How will the rate of learning and progress in the application of new competencies be measured?
- What opportunities will there be for the development of new competencies?
- How will the application of new practices be rewarded?
- What will the consequences be of choosing not to develop new leadership competencies?

individual competencies, knowledge and experience, personal traits, and attitudes about work. Failure to recognize this complexity can result in the provision of management development programs that are irrelevant, poorly defined, and deficient in resources. The most common reasons why management development programs fail are indicated in Figure 36–2.

Content of a Leadership Program*

The leadership development program is designed to strengthen the overall management team by addressing team issues as they emerge in training, identifying the various strengths of individual members, surmounting obstacles to collaboration and leadership in the organization, and providing opportunities for managers from different departments to learn together. These high-level outcomes are pursued through the purposeful assignment of managers to "practice lab" groups, which will evolve new principles of management practice to be tested against the participants' experiences. The membership of each group consists of no more than eight people; they come from different departments and have different levels of experience in the managerial role. After the program has been completed, the practice labs commonly continue as support and continuous learning groups, extending the learning long past the end of the formal development program.

Instead of receiving a "canned program," each organization gets a customized package that takes into account where it is along the continuum of change. (See Table 36–6.)

Source: Tim Porter-O'Grady and Cathleen Krueger Wilson, *The Leadership Revolution in Health Care*, Aspen Publishers, Inc., © 1995.

Figure 36–2 Why Leadership Development Programs Fail

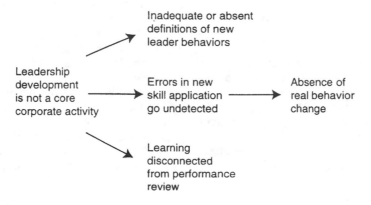

Table 36–6 A Course of Management Workshops

Month 1: The Manager as Facilitator

Objectives

At the end of the first workshop, participants will be able to:

- Critically analyze three key facilitation roles that can be assumed in a work group.
- Contrast the helping and hindering behaviors that people exhibit in the TQM process in a multidisciplinary work group or a team.
- Identify two alternatives for intervening in a problem behavior in empowered groups.
- Describe the construction, development, and maintenance needs of effective work groups.

Month 2: The Faultless Facilitation of Groups

Objectives

- Apply one method of tackling problems and making decisions in an empowered work group.
- Present a method for consensus decision making.
- Evaluate their personal strengths and weaknesses in communications and problem-solving skills in a group setting.
- Explain two methods for bringing forth a group's knowledge, candor, and trust.

Month 3: The Leader Manager as Coach

Objectives

At the end of the workshop, participants will be able to:

- Describe how coaching interactions contribute to employee commitment and sustained, superior performance.
- Define a process model for coaching and the requisite skills involved in each stage of the process.
- Practice the process model with feedback through videotape.

- Analyze the facilitators and the obstacles to coaching interactions in their workplace.
- Apply the coaching model to peer review, shared governance council work, CQI, and advanced nursing practice interventions (nursing groups only).

Month 4: Learning from Conflict

Objectives

At the end of the workshop participants will be able to:

- Distinguish between a supportive versus a defensive climate in conflict resolution situations.
- Anticipate potential areas of conflict in work groups of which they are currently members.
- Apply two strategies for resolving conflicts in work groups.
- Recognize when to create learning opportunities out of conflict situations.
- Evaluate a conflict situation that originates in the mismanagement of agreement.

Month 5: The Empowered Leader/Manager: The Personal Journey

Objectives

At the end of this workshop, participants will be able to:

- Recognize and define the five major characteristics of an empowered person.
- Assess how well they personally think that they exemplify empowering qualities.
- Identify how well the management/leadership team exemplifies empowering qualities.
- Recognize how they act and feel when they have responded in a confident and empowering manner.
- Identify how oppressed group behaviors interfere with the expression of empowering qualities (nursing groups only).

continues

Table 36–6 continued

Month 6: Developing Empowered Work Groups

Objectives

At the end of this workshop, participants will be able to:

- Create and communicate an empowering vision for their organization.
- Identify the actions needed to achieve that vision.
- Relate the concepts of commitment and contribution to vision and purpose.
- Analyze their own organizational structure for evidence of empowerment and determine an action plan for further development.

Month 7: Negotiating the Messy Terrain of Change

Objectives

At the end of the workshop, participants will be able to:

- Describe the characteristics of effective and ineffective strategies for leading a planned change.
- Identify the common roles assumed by individuals in professional groups during the implementation of change.
- Apply, through practice, the key communication, coaching, empowerment, and facilitation skills necessary to produce lasting change.
- Integrate and execute a planned change within a shared leadership group.

Month 8: Making Change Happen and Making It Work

Objectives

At the end of the workshop, participants will be able to:

- Describe how the human experience of change is expressed in health care organizations.

- List the steps and accompanying leadership activities in the project management cycle.
- Identify the characteristics of an effective project manager.
- Apply project management techniques to a planned or progressing change in their own organization.
- Describe the features of selected project management software (optional).

Month 9: Organizing Professional Work Systems

Objectives

At the end of the workshop, participants will be able to:

- Apply concepts of empowerment, teamwork, TQM, and change leadership into a whole systems approach to work redesign.
- Describe how structure, information flow, and reward systems impact output, quality, and job satisfaction.
- Apply facilitation skills to use teamwork in order to align the characteristics of work for maximum quality and dramatically improved results.
- Understand how employee knowledge of economic, social and technical traits of the system is the basis for work redesign in the continuous improvement environment.
- Recognize that there are many "right" ways to redesign work to improve results.

Month 10: Mastering Systems Thinking

Objectives

At the end of the workshop, participants will be able to:

- Describe the value of systems thinking to managerial work.
- Apply systems thinking principles to problem situations.
- Practice mindmapping techniques as a means of problem identification or resolution.
- Use casual looping to see connections to a larger system.

continues

Table 36–6 continued

Month 11: Developing Accountability in Health Care Organizations	Month 12: A New Day Is Dawning: Planning Your Career in the New Health Care Paradigm

Objectives

At the end of the workshop, participants will be able to:

- Identify accountability behaviors as they are expressed in the health care workplace.
- Recognize and modify at least two management practices that contribute to a lack of accountability.
- List characteristics of nonaccountable or "below the line" behaviors.
- Describe the results of a personal self-assessment regarding their own accountability behaviors.
- Lead a work group in the development of shared accountability.

Objectives

At the end of the workshop participants will be able to:

- Develop insight into their career competencies in order to manager career choices and moves.
- Apply a set of concepts and a framework for thinking about how careers develop and how people integrate careers into their personalities.
- Examine the future career choices possible in their own organization within the new health care policy environment.
- Apply concepts of career development in nursing in order to understand the Why and How of their present career path (nurses only).
- Develop a draft of a personal career plan.

Source: Tim Porter-O'Grady and Cathleen Krueger Wilson, *The Leadership Revolution in Health Care*, Aspen Publishers, Inc., © 1995.

Part VI

New Directions and Developments

Chapter 37

New Realities: New Structures, New Opportunities

TRANSITIONS IN HEALTH CARE SYSTEMS AND FACILITIES

No health care system in the world has undergone as much structural change as has that of the United States over the past three decades. Nowhere is this change more evident than in the transition to multiprovider systems. The previous cottage industry of individual, free-standing health care facilities has become a complex web of systems, alliances, and networks.

The development of hospital systems initially encompassed horizontal integration of facilities, with the creation of multihospital systems that provided similar acute care services in multiple locations. More recently, expansion of system capability has occurred by way of vertical integration and diversification into activities that may or may not be related to the hospital's inpatient acute care business. This system development reflects the transformation of linked multicare systems from multiple providers of acute care to various providers that, together, are capable of addressing a continuum of health care needs.*

Background of the Health Care System*

The growth and development of multifacility health care systems in the United States has been characterized by integration of services and economic concentration and consolidation of resources. The transition to multifacility systems reflected the horizontal integration of facilities that began with investor-owned acquisitions in the late 1960s. Investor-owned systems entered into multifacility system arrangements because they had access to capital markets and because federal reimbursement encouraged and rewarded growth. Not-for-profit organizations began to horizontally integrate in the mid-1970s in response to competition from investor-owned chains and the regulatory effects of state certificate of need legislation and rate review programs. Until the mid-1980s, the primary difference between investor-owned and not-for-profit systems was one of magnitude. Investor-owned systems concentrated on national markets and evolving into large national multifacility systems, whereas the not-for-profit systems focused on local and regional markcts.

*Source: Myron D. Fottler and Donna Malvey, "Multiprovider Systems," in Lawrence F. Wolper, *Health Care Administration: Principles, Practices, Structure, and Delivery*, ed 2, Aspen Publishers, Inc., © 1995.

*Source: Myron D. Fottler and Donna Malvey, "Multiprovider Systems," in Lawrence F. Wolper, *Health Care Administration: Principles, Practices, Structure, and Delivery*, ed 2, Aspen Publishers, Inc., © 1995.

Horizontal integration strategies dominated system development during the late 1960s through the mid-1980s and have diminished in significance with the implementation of the prospective payment system (PPS) and cost reduction programs of other payers. It is expected that there will be fewer systems purchasing hospitals because of the financial disincentives and increased risk. In addition, recent evidence suggests that there may actually be a saturation point for system horizontal integration and that hospital acquisition is selective.

Today's systems are characterized by trends toward vertical integration, regionalization, and related diversification. These new systems represent more than a collection of hospitals. Instead, they offer a continuum of health care services that extends beyond acute patient care.

Diversification and Vertical Integration

Diversification through integration of clinical services transforms a horizontally integrated system into a vertically integrated one. Vertical integration involves incorporating within the organization either stages of production (backward integration) or distribution channels (forward integration), that were formerly handled through arm's length transactions with other organizations.

A vertically integrated system is described as offering "a broad range of patient care and support services operated in a functionally unified manner. The range of services offered may include preacute, acute, and postacute care organized around an acute care hospital. Alternatively, a delivery system might specialize in offering a range of services related solely to long-term care, mental health care, or some other specialized area." The intended purpose of vertical integration is to increase the comprehensiveness and continuity of care while simultaneously controlling the channels or demand for health services. Thus, vertical integration emphasizes connecting patient services with different stages in the health services delivery process.

Vertical integration may be complicated by a number of legal problems (see Table 37–1). There

Table 37–1 Types of Arrangements for Vertical Integration

- Internal development of new services
- Acquisition of another organization or service
- Merger
- Lease or sale
- Franchise
- Joint venture
- Contractual agreements
- Informal agreements or affiliations
- Insurance programs

is also the difficulty of moving sick people through a dispersed system of care, since vertical integration does not mean that all services will be offered at one site.

Management implications for vertically integrated systems are as complex and diverse as the arrangements themselves.

- Initially, managers must ensure that the integration strategy is consistent with the mission of the system and its priorities, and that the communications structure supports the organizational changes.
- Capital requirements and financing must be examined for all system components with particular consideration given to financial incentives and economic benefits for these components.
- Managers must realistically determine whether expertise and other resources are available to establish and maintain vertically integrated arrangements.

If the system lacks the resources to achieve successful vertical integration, it may prove to be a better strategy for the system to collaborate with other organizations where risks and costs can be shared.

Diversification Trends

During the 1980s, diversification occurred primarily in nonacute care services and was intended to compensate hospitals that were losing revenues under PPS by generating revenue through new sources. In many instances, hospitals diversified into a wide range of businesses that were completely unrelated to health care, such as dude ranches and travel agencies. Many diversification efforts failed during this decade in part because management was unprepared to manage services unrelated to the hospital's core business of acute care. In the 1990s, the purpose of diversification shifted from generating revenues to offering health services that reduce hospital costs. What has become apparent is that diversification activities related to the hospital's care business tend to be more profitable than diversification activities that are partially or totally unrelated to acute care. (During both the 1980s and the 1990s, ambulatory care and physician joint ventures were the most profitable diversification strategies.)

The 1990s brought a period of reconfiguration, rebuilding, and redesign of systems. Chaos and creativity are the norms as traditional boundaries disappear and competition gives way to collaboration. The focus is now on the provision of comprehensive health services at regional and local levels.

The trend toward regionalization recognizes that 99 percent of health care services delivered in the United States will take place within the region where the patient resides. System strategies are shifting their focus to establish predominance in local and regional markets rather than national ones. The national companies learned that uniform corporate policies were not always sensitive to state and local market and reimbursement differences. Recent experience indicates that the role of larger investor-owned systems is declining and that system growth for the proprietary sector is occurring in small local and regional investor-owned systems, many of which are newly established systems. Vertical integration is consistent with the trend toward regionalization because it concentrates resources in local markets to establish a dominant presence in these markets.

As a result of all these factors, the industry, which was once moving toward rapid consolidation through national chain ownership, appears to be moving now toward regionally based operators with strong local ties. This is reflected in the acquisition activities of nonprofit organizations, health care facilities, and small regional operators. Many in the field now believe that vertically integrated regional delivery systems that emphasize primary care and preventive medicine will prove to be the best approach to providing health care services. The focus will be on development of a continuum of care that incorporates a range of services from preventive to long-term care (see Table 37–2).

OVERVIEW: MANAGED CARE PLANS AND SYSTEMS

Managed care is rapidly dominating the health care financing and delivery system in the United States. To illustrate, HMO enrollment reached 51 million in 1994. Although the estimates are less reliable, by all accounts the number of persons enrolled in PPOs and their variants rivals the number enrolled in HMOs. Even traditional plans are adopting principles of managed care; for example, hospital precertification and large case management, daring innovations as recently as a decade ago, have become the norm in indemnity insurance. Public sector, notably Medicare and Medicaid, reliance on managed care is growing rapidly.

When one thinks of managed care, one should distinguish between the techniques of managed care and the organization that performs the various functions. Managed care can embody a wide variety of techniques. These include various forms of financial incentives for providers, promotion of wellness, early identification of disease, patient education, self-care, and all aspects of utilization management.

A wide variety of organizations can implement managed care techniques, of which the HMO has the potential to align financing and delivery most closely by virtue of enrollees' being (with some

Table 37-2 Diversification and the Continuum of Care Services

Extended
Skilled nursing care
Intermediate care
Swing beds
Nursing home follow up
Respite care

Acute
Medical/surgical
Psychiatric
Rehabilitation
Comprehensive geriatric assessment
Geriatric consultation services

Ambulatory
Physician care
Outpatient clinics
Geriatric assessment clinics
Day hospitals
Adult day care
Mental health clinics
Satellite clinics
Psychosocial counseling
Alcohol and substance abuse services

Home Care
Home health—Medicare
Home health—private
Hospice

High-technology home therapy
Durable medical equipment
Home visitors
Home-delivered meals
Homemaker and personal care

Outreach
Screening
Information and referral
Telephone contact
Emergency response system
Transportation

Wellness
Educational programs
Exercise programs
Recreational and social groups
Senior volunteers
Congregate meals
Wellness clinics
Respite relief
Support groups

Housing
Retirement communities
Senior housing
Congregate care facilities
Adult family homes
Short-term housing/hotels

Source: Reprinted from Connie J. Evashwick, "Creating a Continuum," *Health Progress*, Vol. 70, No. 5, pp. 36–39, with permission of the Catholic Health Association of the United States, © 1989.

exceptions) required to use network providers. Managed care techniques can also be employed directly by employers, insurers, union–management (Taft-Hartley) trust funds, and the Medicare and Medicaid programs. They can also be implemented by PPOs, organizations that allow enrollees to be reimbursed for care delivered by nonnetwork providers, although the enrollees face higher out-of-pocket payments (i.e., cost sharing) if they do. Finally, a variety of hybrid arrangements have evolved, one example is the point-of-service (POS) program, which operates as a PPO except that, to receive the highest level of benefits, the enrollee must obtain a referral from a primary care physician who is part of the contracted network. Increasingly, the arrangements are difficult to characterize, let alone profile statistically, in a meaningful manner. (See Table 37–3).*

Source: Peter D. Fox, "An Overview of Managed Care," in *The Managed Health Care Handbook*, ed 3, Peter R. Kongstvedt, ed., Aspen Publishers, Inc., © 1996.

Table 37–3 Types of Managed Care Systems

Health Maintenance Organizations
- In HMO-type managed care plans, care providers agree to provide comprehensive care to enrollees for a fixed fee.
- Cost control occurs both through the limitations that are placed on enrollees' use of care providers and from financial disincentives for care providers to refer patients to specialists, to hospitalize patients, and to perform high-cost procedures.
- The primary feature of HMOs is the sharing of financial risk of health care delivery costs between the insurer and the care provider through fixed-fee schedules. Care providers shoulder the financial risk of overuse of health care services.
- Health services are delivered by the HMO through (1) group or staff model HMOs, which are designated groups of providers under control of the HMO and on a salary basis; (2) independent practice associations (IPAs) that contract directly with care providers in private practice; and (3) networks, which combine group and IPA models.

Preferred Provider Organizations and Point-of-Care Service Plans
- PPOs involve contracts between insurance companies and care providers who agree

to accept discounted usual and customary charges in exchange for patient volume.
- The plans involve financial incentives for patients to choose the preferred provider. That is, if an individual purchases health care outside of the designated list of preferred providers, the care will be more costly to him or her.
- Utilization review of inpatient services occurs in the majority of PPO contracts in the form of precertification, concurrent review, mandatory second optioning, and discharge planning.
- In point-of-service plans, patients can make their choice of provider at the time the service is needed rather than upon entry into the plan.

Relations with Hospitals
Note: Overall, insurers are most likely to use discounted usual customary and reasonable charges as their principal hospital reimbursement mechanism in both HMOs and PPOs. Diagnosis-related group (DRG) payments in PPOs and DRG and capitation payment by HMOs are more popular forms of payment for inpatient services because of the incentives to reduce the number of services as well as the length of stay.

Source: Nancy J. Packard, "The Price of Choice: Managed Care in America," *Nursing Administration Quarterly,* Vol. 17, No. 3, Aspen Publishers, Inc., © Spring 1993.

Managed Care Plans: The Efficiency Effect*

What effect will managed care plans have on health care organizations such as hospitals, clinics, and community health centers? Whatever managed care arrangement is in effect, the incentives for health care organizations are simi-

lar: to compete for patient volume or market share on the basis of efficiencies and willingness to accept a competitively low reimbursement rate.

Most important, health care organizations will compete on the basis of their efficiencies. The major challenge for managers will be to view traditional profit centers as cost centers. Specifically, organizational viability most likely will depend not on the alignment of organizations toward profit-making services, but on the ability of the organization to minimize utilization of

Source: Nancy J. Packard, "The Price of Choice: Managed Care in America," *Nursing Administration Quarterly,* Vol. 17, No. 3, Aspen Publishers, Inc., © Spring 1993.

high-cost services and maximize the value of their services.

Second, to achieve the kinds of efficiencies that are required within an organization providing managed care, the gaps in the cultures of health care practitioners and health care managers must be bridged. Specifically, managed care systems need to develop more innovative models of cooperation with practitioners.

Third, attaining increased efficiencies within organizations will mean maximizing the value of all human and technical resources within the organization. Developing cultural compatibility within an organization will require a shared sense of commitment to the organization and to the community.

Finally, health care organizations will have to demonstrate their efficiencies. For organizations to compete successfully with others, administrators will need good information systems for the collection and dissemination of data on organizational efficiencies and quality of patient care.

Impact on Nursing

Managed care will inevitably affect *nursing's agenda* to ensure the delivery of effective and efficient health care. Managed care integrates health care financing and care delivery in a way that places the financial burden of choice of resource use on the shoulders of patients and care providers. In doing so, it will profoundly affect all facets of care systems, including clinical encounters, access to health care, and the structure of health care delivery.

Nurses involved in the management of care systems within a managed care environment will require sophisticated skills in the areas of assessment of effectiveness and efficiency of services. Information systems will be a necessary tool for data processing related to these areas. Finally, nurse managers will need a range of administrative and leadership skills to advocate effectively for the creation of managed care systems that benefit all populations in their care.

Utilization Review Aspect*

Controlling the parameters of care through a well-detailed utilization review process is an important component of cost controls associated with managed care. Court cases have demonstrated that a plan's utilization review process is an operational exposure with the potential for considerable financial risk. A well-structured utilization review program is designed to limit the potential risks associated with attempts to structure care around predetermined criteria. The program should allow for retrospective, concurrent, and prospective review of care provided under the managed care plan. It should be remembered that underutilization presents real threats to quality and risk just as overutilization presents threats to cost control.

The one individual who is crucial to the success of a managed care program is the UM nurse. It is the UM nurse who will be the eyes and ears of the medical management department, who will generally coordinate the discharge planning, and who will facilitate all the activities of utilization control.

The scope of responsibilities of the UM nurse will vary depending on the plan and the personalities and skills of the other members of the medical management team. In some plans, the role simply involves telephone information gathering. In other plans, there will be a more proactive role, including frequent communication with attending physicians, the medical director, the hospitals, and the hospitalized members and their families; discharge planning and facilitation; and a host of other activities, including active hospital rounding.

The one fundamental function of the UM nurse is information gathering. Information about hospital cases must be obtained in an accurate and timely fashion. It falls to the UM nurse to be the focal point of this information and to ensure that

---

Source: Barbara J. Youngberg, "Risk Management in Managed Care," *The Managed Health Care Handbook*, ed 3, Peter R. Kongstvedt, ed., Aspen Publishers, Inc., © 1996.

it is obtained and communicated to the necessary individuals in medical management and the claims department.

Necessary information includes admission date and diagnosis, the type of hospital service to which the patient was admitted (e.g., medical, surgical, maternity, and so forth), the admitting physician, consultants, planned procedures (type and timing), expected discharge date, needed discharge planning, and any other pertinent information the plan managers may need.

MANAGING THE CONTINUUM OF CARE

Managing the continuum of care is not like any approach to management previously experienced. In an institutional model there is much greater control over the variables that affect the service, and supports are readily accessible on request. In a more decentralized service structure with many component parts, it is much more challenging to manage and integrate the service structures and activities.

The service manager will have to construct different relationships with workers and the system to be able to do his or her work. The challenge will be in keeping the system going and evaluating performance daily on some level of outcome measure so outcomes can be assessed and changes made as quickly as possible. Newer relationships with workers, which are not dependent or institutionally based, will challenge the role of the leader and create a whole new set of circumstances for providing leadership.*

Management Challenges*

• Workers will be spread over a broad network of service structures depending on service and consumer need. There will be expanded mobility in the health system, and therefore professional workers will increasingly be interdependent in their service relationship and independent in their functional activity. The number of manager roles used in an institutional setting will be substantially reduced in a continuum-of-care setting.

• The focus of the manager's work will be different from what it was in the past. As departmental structures collapse, the manager will serve a broader constituency than in the past. More often, managers will have workers from a wide range of disciplines and roles in an integrated environment, each with his or her own obligations and functions. The manager role will demand much flexibility and skill in consensus building, problem solving, and opportunity finding.

• The competence once necessary only at the executive level in the organization will now be required at the service level in the health system. The service leader will essentially be managing a strategic service unit and will be required to perform the full range of functions necessary to ensure that the service structure operates effectively and successfully. The leader must know how to make use of financial and service resources in a way that maximizes the efficiency and effectiveness of the service.

• Working across the continuum of care means a much broader frame of reference for work and a greater need for integration in the system and between the players. The service manager will play a larger role in smoothing the rough roads between workers and systems, ensuring that integration works in the best interest of the customer. Integrating service providers

Source: Tim Porter-O'Grady, "Managing along the Continuum: A New Paradigm for the Clinical Manager," *Nursing Administration Quarterly*, Vol. 19, No. 3, Aspen Publishers, Inc., © Spring 1995.

Source: Tim Porter-O'Grady, "Managing along the Continuum: A New Paradigm for the Clinical Manager," *Nursing Administration Quarterly*, Vol. 19, No. 3, Aspen Publishers, Inc., © Spring 1995.

means that care is well integrated too, so evaluating the service system will be an important corollary to the activity of building good provider relationships.

• Knowing a great deal about the market requirements and the quality indices for the service will tell the manager much about the quality of the services provided. Quality cannot be separated from cost in a capitated system. Therefore, the manager will need to be cognizant of the vagaries of the customers and the demands they make on the system in the form of service expectation and customer sensitivity. Failing in this area will ensure the loss of subscribers and compromise the future of the service.

• Management of information is perhaps the most critical role of the service manager. Information is the circulatory system of any organization. Knowing what information is needed, how it should be configured, and in what form it should be generated is an important job of the service manager. Since information will provide the database for the financial and service health of the system, carefully constructing it and using it will be the single most important activity of the leader.

Finally, since health is going to depend much more on what patients do or do not do, it will be necessary to ensure, at a much higher level of efficiency, that the outcomes of service are evidenced in healthier behavior of the consumer. Much more self-directed activity, education, and follow up will be a part of the service structure and will require careful and thorough preparation of the consumer with regard to his or her health.

It will, in fact, call for a different relationship with the patient. Different expectations between provider and patient will be essential to lower cost and will ensure better outcomes. Dependent relationships that take control away from the patient will no longer be acceptable, and a new partnership between patient and provider for health will be essential. The leader must create a context for this relationship and build a continuing set of expectations in the workers that these issues are at the center of their own performance expectation and evaluation criteria.

How the Continuum of Care Can Work: The Network Organization*

A continuum of care must be available. A continuum of care is a comprehensive array of health, mental health, and social services that span all levels of intensity and are coordinated and integrated into a system of care. Managing the broad continuum of care needed by the chronically ill is a complex undertaking.

It requires a shift from the current biomedical model to a biopsychological model.

It requires replacement of provider-centered care by patient-centered care, in which the ill person and family function as partners of health care professionals in specifying health care needs and assembling, producing, and delivering health care services.

It requires collaboration among service providers who are accustomed to functioning independently.

It requires the implementation of integrative mechanisms at the top management level of the organizations participating in the network and at the front lines, where the services are produced and delivered to the chronically ill and their families.

It requires health care professionals, across organizations, agreeing on critical pathways—on how the health and social service work is done, on the relative importance of functions, and on the sets of problem-solving processes and techniques to be employed.

Finally, it requires the development of financial arrangements that cover the continuum of care and allow participating providers to be paid in accordance with the value of the services they render to the chronically ill patients and their families.

---

*Source: Kenneth D. Bopp, Gordon D. Brown, and Robert H. Daugherty, "Continuum of Care," in *Manual of Health Services Management*, Robert J. Taylor, ed., Aspen Publishers, Inc., © 1994.

Although these are large managerial challenges, they are essential if the needs of chronically ill patients are to be adequately met. The network organization appears to be an effective organizational form for managing chronic illness. It uses existing community resources rather than building capabilities from the ground up. It offers the opportunity for each member entity to pursue its particular specialty or distinctive competence within the context of a unified framework and to jointly solve the problems of the chronically ill. However, the management of a network is radically different from management of a hierarchical organization. In the network model of resource allocation and control, transactions occur neither through discrete exchanges nor by administrative fiat but through participating organizations and individuals engaging in reciprocal, preferential, mutually supportive actions.

The "Broker" Manager

Many of the managerial functions in networks are performed by brokers, who assemble, locate, build relationships, and subcontract for specific services. The focus of the broker in network management is on developing among the members of the network a commitment to the goals of the network (e.g., better service to the chronically ill) and a mutual orientation. The key function of the broker is to establish, maintain, and enhance relationships. This involves

- bringing organizational members together and getting them to commit to an overall vision
- introducing members to each other and serving as a focal source of information about each other
- redirecting individual perspectives to encompass both the goals of the network and each organization's goals through joint planning and coordination of routines
- mutually reinforcing trust through social processes
- providing feedback to the members regarding the equity of payment to members for

their value-added contributions to the network

Although nurturing relationships between organizations is critical in network management, absolute harmony will not be obtained. Consequently, a very important broker role in network management is ongoing mediation and conflict resolution.

Management and Service Integration across the Continuum of Care

The shift in thinking about health care delivery requires a concomitant change in managerial strategies, methods, and techniques at the care coordination level. Health care traditionally has been a functionally organized service deliv-

---

The predominant focus in U.S. medical care has been on science-based diagnosis and treatment of disease—the so-called *medical model*. While the medical model has been reasonably efficacious in the treatment and elimination of infectious diseases and other acute illnesses, its application to chronic illness has been less than totally successful. The primary reason is that, historically, the treatment of chronic disease has focused mostly on the acute (and sometimes dying) phase, in which diseases are treated in the hospital, and the severe disability phase, in which the ill are cared for in a nursing home owing to the severity of their illness and/or their lack of support. The *biopsychosocial approach to chronic illness* treatment and management, however, will result in a shift away from this treatment of chronic illness in only the acute and severely disabled phases toward a proactive management of *all* phases of the illness.

Source: Kenneth D. Bopp, Gordon D. Brown, and Robert H. Daugherty, "Continuum of Care," in *Manual of Health Services Management*, Robert J. Taylor, ed., Aspen Publishers, Inc., © 1994.

ery system with strict divisions of labor among organizations as well as among departments and specialists within organizations. Although patients and families have been burdened with the responsibility of coordinating care services provided by diverse organizations within hierarchical organizations there is an obdurate belief that sufficient coordination occurs by virtue of management fiat.

Overcoming this and getting health care professionals to work as a team across organizations, functions, and specialties is one of the most difficult changes and challenges faced by the manager at the care coordination level. Of primary concern will be the development of knowledge and abilities to effectively manage a team of diverse professionals with their own distinct ideologies regarding how care should be rendered. Networking requires coordination with others. For the network to function effectively at the front lines, coordination must become a part of each provider's job rather than a responsibility of a few designated individuals. By making coordination everyone's responsibility, the network ensures that a lateral structure exists across all functions and specialties.

POTENTIAL HOSPITAL-RELATED SERVICES

While calls for hospital beds have diminished in the newly restructured and refocused health care environment, a number of health care organizations have found niches and needs between acute care and preventive care. There are patients who are not "sick enough" for the hospital but are too sick to go home without support, who need care for a while but not forever, who need a low level of care for an indeterminate amount of time, or who need a special type of care for a measured number of days.

Enterprising organizations have responded to these needs by developing facilities and agencies for subacute care, rehabilitative care, elder care, home health, and hospice care—all types of care that the hospital is eminently qualified to supervise and supply. These are briefly described in the following text.

Subacute Care

The International Subacute Healthcare Association (ISHA) defines subacute care as follows: Subacute care is a comprehensive and cost-effective inpatient program for patients who have had an acute event as a result of an illness, injury, or exacerbation of a disease process; have a determined course of treatment; and do not require intensive diagnostic and/or invasive procedures. The severity of the patient's condition requires physician direction, intensive nursing care and significant utilization of ancillaries, and an outcomes-focused interdisciplinary approach using a professional team to deliver complex clinical interventions (medical and/or rehabilitation).

The identification of need for postacute skilled health care and its potentially large market was based on six principle factors, which are listed in Table 37–4. The subsequent reduced occupancy of acute care hospital inpatient beds provided the economic incentive for developing an intermediary level of care.*

The Scope of Subacute Care*

Typically short term, the subacute level of care is used as an inpatient alternative to an acute care hospital admission or as an alternative to continued hospitalization.

Comprehensive Care. Subacute care programs are designed to provide the full range of necessary medical, rehabilitation, and professional services required to provide efficient and effective care for the specific medical conditions treated within a program.

Cost-effectiveness. Subacute programs are designed to maximize value to patients and payer sources through the delivery of necessary, appropriate care with optimal outcomes in the lowest cost setting.

Outcomes Orientation. Subacute programs are designed to achieve quantifiable, measurable

---

Source: Kathleen M. Griffin, "The Subacute Care Industry," in Kathleen M. Griffin, *Handbook of Subacute Health Care*, Aspen Publishers, Inc., © 1995.

Table 37-4 Factors Contributing to the Development of a Subacute Care Level

- Expanded outpatient services, growing day surgery, increased diagnostic capabilities, comprehensive home care services, and others
- The efforts of insurance companies, HMOs, and other managed care insurance plans to keep people out of the hospital
- The Health Care Financing Administration's implementation of DRGs
- The public's desire to remain at home and receive diagnosis, treatment, and care services as outpatients
- The clamor and rising need to curtail spiraling health care costs
- The recognition that certain hospital patients remain sick and weak upon completion of allowable DRG stay and require further stabilization, medication, monitoring, ongoing treatment, less than comprehensive inpatient rehabilitation therapy, and other therapy or specialized care without requiring the amenities of a full-service acute hospital

Source: Mary T. Knapp, "Introduction to the Hospital-Based Nursing Facility," in Mary T. Knapp, *Subacute Care: The Definitive Guide to Hospital-Based Nursing Facilities*, Aspen Publishers, Inc., © 1995.

---

outcomes such as, but not necessarily limited to, functional restoration, clinical stabilization, avoidance of medical complications or exacerbation of a disease process, and discharge to the patient's least restrictive living environment.

Professional Staffing. Subacute interventions, because of their duration, complexity, and intensity, are provided under the direction of a physician. An interdisciplinary team provides a coordinated program of care. The team may include a physician, nurses, therapists, social workers, psychologists, pharmacists, dietitians, case managers, discharge planners, and other professionals.

Program Description. Programs are organized around patient populations with related treatment or service needs that result in common goals, measures of outcomes, treatment plans, and resources delivered at similar levels of intensity. Subacute programs may include medical rehabilitation and respiratory nutrition, cardiac, oncologic, and wound care programs. Levels of intensity for specific disciplines will vary from program to program but will generally range from 3.5 to 8.0 nursing hours per patient day, up to 5 hours per patient day for therapy, as well as appropriate use of nutrition, laboratory, pharmacy, radiology, and other ancillary services.

Site of Care. The site of care is not a distinguishing characteristic of subacute care. Subacute programs can be delivered in a variety of settings, including acute hospitals, specialty hospitals, free-standing skilled nursing facilities, hospital-based skilled nursing units, outpatient ambulatory centers, residential living facilities, and home health settings.

Continuum of Care. Subacute care is essential to the development of a complete continuum of care. Subacute programs are necessary components of vertically integrated health care systems.

The Hospital-Based Nursing Facility*

The hospital-based nursing facility (HBNF) is the hospital industry's response to the demonstrated need for a specialized inpatient skilled care that allows a Medicare beneficiary to make a smooth transition from acute hospital care to a stepped-down, transitional level of care. HBNFs treat a greater proportion of patients with continuing medical problems that are beyond the capability of the free-standing or traditional skilled care nursing facility. Cost reimbursement is available for the first three to four years of operation, which enables the patient to remain in the hospital for continued care at a skilled care level and for the hospital to secure additional revenues.

---

*Source: Mary T. Knapp, "Introduction to the Hospital-Based Nursing Facility," in Mary T. Knapp, *Subacute Care: The Definitive Guide to Hospital-Based Nursing Facilities*, Aspen Publishers, Inc., © 1995.

By developing an HBNF, hospitals develop a better capacity to provide a continuum of care for their patients. Hospitals have also begun to identify and develop an array of health and social services for patients to use upon discharge. These services have been expanded and now include adult day care, home health care, respite care, transportation, and assistance with Medicare claims.

Categories of Care Delivered*

According to the ISHA, subacute programs may include medical rehabilitation and respiratory, nutritional, cardiac, oncological, and wound care. Other product lines in subacute care include ventilator dependent care, with or without weaning, tracheostomy, postoperative care, total parenteral nutrition, intravenous therapy, enterostomal therapy, total brain injury (TBI) or spinal cord injury, hospice, and continuing abdominal peritoneal dialysis (CAPD).

Transitional Subacute Care. Transitional subacute care can be described as a short stay (5 to 30 days) with high nursing acuity (5.5 to 8.0 hours per patient day). Transitional subacute facilities and units are used by payers, providers, and physicians for patients who require regular medical care and monitoring; highly skilled and intensive nursing care; an integrated program of therapies, both rehabilitative and respiratory; and heavy utilization of pharmaceutical and laboratory services. This type of subacute care unit or facility serves as a hospital step-down entity and results in a significant reduction of acute hospital days. A transitional subacute facility actually serves as a substitute for continued hospital stays, not as an alternative hospital discharge placement.

Hospital-based subacute units and staff model HMO-owned subacute units typically are in this category. Clinically, patients in traditional subacute units may require cardiac recovery from heart attacks or cardiac surgical procedures, pulmonary management for tracheostomies or ven-

tilator weaning programs, multiple stage III and IV decubiti or vascular or other surgeries, or oncology procedures, including chemotherapy and radiation therapy.

General Subacute Care. General subacute units are most often used for patients who require medical care and monitoring at least weekly, short-term nursing care at a level of approximately 3.5 to 5.0 hours per patient day, and rehabilitative therapies that may extend from 1 to 3 hours per patient day. Short stay in nature (10 to 40 days), general subacute care facilities see a significant number of Medicare patients who may require subacute rehabilitation or certain subacute nursing services, such as intravenous therapies for septic conditions, but have no other significant medical complications. (Younger patients at these acuity levels tend to be cared for by home health services.)

Chronic Subacute Care. Chronic subacute units manage patients with little hope of ultimate recovery and functional independence, such as ventilator-dependent patients, long-term comatose patients, and patients with progressive neurologic disease. Typically, these patients require nursing staffing at the level of the general subacute unit (3 to 5 hours per patient day), medical monitoring biweekly to monthly, and restorative therapies, usually provided by nursing staff with guidance from rehabilitation therapists. These patients either will eventually be stabilized so that they can be discharged home or be cared for in a long-term care facility or they may die. Their average length of stay is 60 to 90 days.

Long-Term Transitional Subacute Care. Long-term transitional subacute facilities most often are licensed as hospitals rather than as nursing facilities; they are PPS exempt as long-term care hospitals and have average lengths of stay of 25 days or more. Typically, these facilities provide care for acute ventilator-dependent or medically complex patients. Because the patients are hospitals, attending physicians may visit them daily. Nursing staff tend to be primarily registered nurses, and nursing hours per patient day may range between 6.5 and 9.0 depending on the types and acuity levels of patients.

Source: Kathleen M. Griffin, "The Subacute Care Industry," in Kathleen M. Griffin, *Handbook of Subacute Health Care,* Aspen Publishers, Inc., © 1995.

Provider Success and Profitability

See Tables 37–5 and 37–6 for keys to the success and profitability of subacute care providers.

Preparing To Care for Older Patients*

For hospitals to manage senior health needs effectively, they will need to take a number of steps that go beyond bringing long-term care

---

Table 37–5 Keys to Success for Subacute Providers

- *Attractive facility:* No one wants to go to a nursing home or a unit in the "old part of the hospital."
- *Programs of care:* The subacute programs should have specific protocols or care paths for the two to four programs in which the provider specializes. Admission criteria should be clear for each program.
- *Medical staff:* In addition to a medical director, a medical staff of credentialed and privileged physicians are attending or consulting.
- *Dedicated clinical staff:* Under the direction of a program director, nursing and social services staff, along with rehabilitation, dietary, and respiratory therapy staff, provide care in the subacute unit or facility.
- *Admissions:* Procedures are user friendly to all referral sources and allow for an expedited admissions process.
- *Outcomes:* Patient outcomes are measured and reported by means of a quantitative instrument.
- *Financial reports:* Management information systems are adequate to provide frequent and detailed reports on costs and profitability by patient.

Source: Kathleen M. Griffin, "The Subacute Care Industry," in Kathleen M. Griffin, *Handbook of Subacute Health Care*, Aspen Publishers, Inc., © 1995.

Source: "New Models and 'Best Practices' for Meeting Eldercare Needs," *Russ Coile's Health Trends*, Vol. 7, No. 6, Aspen Publishers, Inc., © April 1995.

Table 37–6 Keys to Profitability for Subacute Providers

- *Alternative to hospitals:* Patients, families, physicians, and referral sources must perceive that the subacute unit is a positive alternative to an admission or continued stay in an acute or rehabilitation hospital.
- *Payer mix:* The payer mix (Medicare and/or managed care) must be able to provide favorable profitability. Admission criteria must focus on the right payer mix.
- *Efficiency/quality:* Referral sources must believe that a high-quality integrated program is provided in a cost-effective way.

Source: Kathleen M. Griffin, "The Subacute Care Industry," in Kathleen M. Griffin, *Handbook of Subacute Health Care*, Aspen Publishers, Inc., © 1995.

---

services and facilities into the system. Some examples are as follows:

- Expand wellness and health promotion programs.
- Make prudent investments in high technology.
- Put case management systems into place.
- Link all providers with clinical information systems.
- Educate patients and families.
- Orient providers in care of an aging population.

Without a doubt, senior health care programs will expand in the future. Disease-specific case management programs will be needed for chronic conditions such as hypertension, diabetes, and emphysema. Special medical problems will grow, including in-home renal dialysis, sexual dysfunction treatment, stroke rehabilitation, obesity counseling, geriatric health assessment, and women's health services. The numbers of mental health, substance abuse, Alzheimer's disease, hospice, adult day care, and subacute and skilled nursing facilities are all predicted to grow in the next five years as hospitals increasingly shift their emphasis to the health needs of an aging population.

Best Practices Anticipate the Age Wave

At the leading edge of the age wave, new approaches can be found that will be models for restructuring the future health care delivery system. A fascinating study of California hospitals by Baxter Healthcare showed that only 5 percent were fully ready for the oncoming age wave and only half were "moderately" prepared. The Baxter age wave study then collected a series of "best practices" that identify new delivery modalities for care of older persons throughout the country.

Inpatient Programs. Special inpatient units are being designed for the care and coordination of older patients. These programs concentrate on extensive patient evaluation. The geriatric units provide a continuum of care, including acute, subacute, chronic, and rehabilitation services. Units like this are typically small—only 5 to 15 beds—and often serve patients who have not responded to treatment of their initial acute conditions. The emphasis of such geriatric units is on stabilizing medical conditions and optimizing the highest level of patient function before discharge. Features of inpatient geriatric units include the following:

- a comprehensive geriatric assessment on admission by a multidisciplinary team
- a cooperative care unit with facilities for a family member, who receives special training as a "care partner," to be accommodated in the same room
- a geriatric resource nurse (GRN) model, in which a minimum of two GRNs are assigned as care managers to every unit made up of more than 35 percent seniors
- greater emphasis on patient outcomes, functional improvements, after-care, and integration of treatment and management of acute conditions
- continuity of care facilitated by a postdischarge follow-up process, with outreach to the patient's primary care physician and family

Outpatient Programs. Ambulatory care clinics and programs designed for older adults focus on multidisciplinary assessment and coordination with other services in the community. Programs fill needs for seniors, from active to frail older adults. Ambulatory health programs for seniors can do the following:

- Locate a senior ambulatory center proximate to the hospital or on the hospital campus to facilitate the provision of after-care services after discharge.
- Decentralize the network of senior multiservice health centers across the community to encourage access to health care, mental health, and social service needs.
- Experiment with locations close to senior populations, such as residential hotels, continuing care retirement centers, and senior activity centers.
- Broaden the spectrum of ambulatory services to include dentistry, optometry, podiatry, nutrition, and audiology.
- Develop extended care pathways that anticipate the chronic and acute care needs of patients with chronic diseases.
- Computerize medical records systems to link all senior services and sites.
- Develop brokerage models to contract for services with other community-based organizations and arrange for support activities such as transportation, housekeeping, medical equipment, and personal care.
- Use case managers to coordinate care for 30 to 45 clients, providing individualized care plans and continuous monitoring.

Specialty Care and Treatment Facility. An expanding number of specialized health facilities provide an array of disease- and patient-specific services. Such specialized facilities can concentrate resources on a single focus. The best of these specialty care programs can reach "center of excellence" status to manage and treat high-cost, complex conditions, such as Alzheimer's disease and stroke, and offer rehabilitation and oncology services.

Specialty Treatment Facilities. Chronic care facilities are often large, multidimensional, and located on a multiacre campus, and they provide "single-door" access to a comprehensive range of services for patients. Some institutional services may be provided in a licensed hospital facility with other levels of licensed care such as skilled nursing, psychiatric care, or rehabilitation. Other beds are DRG exempt, providing postdischarge care for patients needing another two to three weeks of treatment.

Home Care Services*

Home care before the late 1890s consisted primarily of house calls by physicians for the affluent and nursing care by charity organizations for the poor. Initially, communicable diseases and child health and nutrition (with an emphasis on prevention) were the focus of home care visits. The Visiting Nurses' Association was the first formally organized home care network, funded and designed by the community and charitable funds to service the needs of the community. The enactment of Medicare legislation in 1966 provided for federal insurance reimbursement for home care services. The beneficiary of home care services paid no out-of-pocket fees for covered services. Providers of home care services were paid based on cost reimbursement. It was not until the early 1980s that hospitals rapidly expanded into home care programs to help offset the newly instituted cost-containment measures of the Medicare DRG guidelines. Private insurance carriers and HMOs only recently have offered covered for home care services in order to reduce hospital utilization.

Independently owed home health agencies proliferated during this time as intermittent home care was viewed as a lucrative area of health care. Other home health providers altruistically saw home health as a way to improve the quality of care and the quality of life for clients who were being discharged from hospitals earlier due to DRG regulations. This rapid growth in home care, however, meant that many home care providers were without adequate experience or even state licenses. This led to the closure of many Medicare-certificate agencies. The current trend for home care companies is to provide profitable ancillary services such as pharmacy services, durable medical equipment services, and private duty nursing and to decrease dependency on traditional Medicare services.

The most traditional as well as most common service provided in the home is nursing. The purpose of intermittent nursing care is to augment or complete the nursing care program required by the client and to ease the transition from clinic or hospital to home. Nursing services include wound, intravenous, catheter, ostomy, drainage tube, and tracheostomy care and management. Nurses also assess patients' physical status and psychosocial environment, as well as monitor new disease processes and response to new medications. Education of clients and their families regarding medications, disease processes, nutrition, skilled nursing care procedures, skin care, and bowel regimes is an important part of the medical team effort. All nursing services are under the direction and guidance of the patient's personal physician. Intermittent services are those performed at the patient's home over a period of time. The duration and frequency of visits is dependent on the patient's needs and the physician's orders.

Specialty nursing services are becoming more available to the patient in the home setting. Enterostomal therapists, for example, are available to provide management of clients who have undergone an ostomy or have skin problems. Some home health agencies also offer the services of pediatric nurse specialists to deal with the specific and complex needs of pediatric patients and their parents. Perinatal and neonatal services are being offered as an alternative to extended hospital stays and as an adjunct to early postpartum discharge. These services include instructions on neonatal care, postpartum checks, and management of equipment such as bili-lites and apnea monitors in the home. Rehabilitative nursing services focus on bowel, bladder, and

Source: Helga Bonfils, Denise E. Stanton, and Sharon Guller, "Home Care Services," *Ambulatory Care Management and Practice*, Barnett and Mayer, eds., Aspen Publishers, Inc., © 1992.

skin problems and the regaining of maximum function by the neurologically impaired.

Hospice services emphasize the emotional and physical comfort of the terminally ill patient. They focus on pain control, body function control, and support of the client and family so as to maximize the quality of life remaining.

Private duty nursing or shift care provides round-the-clock care for patients who require or desire continuous nursing care. These services are generally available to patients who are unable to care for themselves, have no caregiver available, or have chronic conditions that require skilled nursing care.

Among the most popular home care services are those provided by home health aides. These services include bathing, nail and hair care, meal preparation, bedmaking, and some light housekeeping to ensure a clean and safe environment. Home health aides can also assist with a range of motion exercises, ambulation, and transfer activities and are available on an intermittent or shift basis.

The Hospice Alternative*

The word *hospice* was used first in Europe during the Middle Ages to identify a place that provided shelter to travelers or crusaders on their journeys. The word came into its current usage in the 1960s when Dr. Cecily Saunders, a British physician, sought a way to care for dying patients different from the acute care setting of British hospitals. She popularized the word *hospice* to mean an approach to caring for dying patients and their families that focuses on palliation of symptoms and emphasizes the quality of life, rather than attempts to treat the disease aggressively. In addition to physical symptoms, this approach addresses emotional, spiritual, and social symptoms common to terminally ill patients and their families.

Hospice programs developed rapidly during the late 1970s and early 1980s, with the hospice concept of care quickly spreading from the Northeast throughout the United States. Landmark legislation in the early 1980s provided Medicare coverage for terminally ill beneficiaries electing to receive care from a participating hospice. It also required that an interdisciplinary team be used.

The Structure of Care. The composition of the team must include at least the following individuals as employees of the hospice: a doctor of medicine or osteopathy, a registered nurse, a social worker, and a pastoral or other counselor. Trained volunteers in defined roles must be available working under the supervision of a designated hospice employee. The role of the team is to participate in the plan of care, provide or supervise hospice care or services, periodically review and update the individual plan of care, and establish policies governing the day-to-day provision of hospice care and services. The interdisciplinary team in hospice is not a suggested organizational structure to deliver care services, it is a required element of care.

The hospice team, composed of core members and other consulting members, meets on a weekly basis to discuss, review, and revise the plans of care for patients and families. All disciplines are in attendance; they discuss the needs and goals of the patient and family and share their past assessments and plans for ongoing intervention.

A record of these meetings and plans of each team member are recorded in the team plan of care. During these meetings, insights are also shared so that other team members may benefit from information that has been learned. It is also a time when team members may ask for assistance with a particular problem from other disciplines or from members of the same discipline.

Working together from different perspectives to improve the care delivered reflects the synergistic aspect of the hospice team. When this happens, the sum of the parts is truly greater than the whole.

---

*Source: Maureen A. Eng, "The Hospice Interdisciplinary Team: A Synergistic Approach to the Care of Dying Patients and Their Families," *Holistic Nursing Practices*, Vol. 7, No. 4, Aspen Publishers, Inc., © July 1993.

Chapter 38

Management of Opportunities
for the Nursing Service

RESPONDING TO CHANGING NEEDS

Nurses must anticipate and prepare for the considerable threats and *substantial opportunities* that will evolve if a relatively pure form of managed competition emerges as the economic strategy guiding health care reform.

—Peter I. Buerhaus
Harvard Nursing Research Institute, 1994

Requirements for Nurse Leaders*

Nurses must remember that nursing work is a part of a continuum that moves toward a future that is ever in transition. Both the nurse executive and staff nurse must be willing to take advantage of opportunities to create new frameworks for nursing service and be ready to accept challenges from others related to providing health care services in a broad variety of settings.

The nurse executive will always have to be alert to the impact of major social change on the management of the practice of nursing. The nurse

---

Source: Tim Porter O'Grady, *Reorganization of Nursing Practice: Creating the Corporate Venture*, Aspen Publishers, Inc., © 1990.

executive will often be the front person on the road to assessing and evaluating both the nature and impact of change on the way health care services are provided and the nurse's role in their provision. As a leader, the nurse executive will have to be the visionary, conceiving as well as creating and facilitating the opportunity for nurses to assume roles that effectively move the nursing service into newer areas of opportunity. Reading the signposts of change and reflecting on their meaning will be the first steps in creating models within which nursing services will be provided.

In his or her role as leader, the nurse executive will always be challenged to provide the milieu in which nurses will seek new ways of rendering services and new settings within which to offer nursing care. Often it will be the staff who have the best perspective on how nursing work is offered and the way in which it can unfold to best suit the community or constituency nurses seek to serve. Staff spend their professional lives on the front lines of services and are often positioned to identify opportunities for new services or different ways to provide existing services. The challenge for staff is to explore these options for service and undertake creative efforts to deliver health care services.

What is expected of the nurse executive is sensitivity not only to the opportunities that can be suggested by the nurse in practice but also to the changing milieu that provides the framework that will permit the practicing nurse to explore his or her options and opportunities and provide a plan and a strategy for making it live. Indeed, it is a part of the emerging role of the nurse executive to create and maintain an internal working environment that provides the expectation that newer staff roles will emerge as the new service opportunities are created.

The Limits of Diversification in Nursing*

Diversification is a major direction for health care organizations today. Diversification generally means moving into nonrelated businesses. The critical aspect of diversification that therefore needs examination is the relation of the new business to the mission. The critical questions are: What is our business? What should our business be?

Diversification in nursing is carefully weighed by considering the mission of the nursing department. First, it is unlikely that the nursing department will be creating a spinoff, non–health-related business. Second, if the diversification is not in line with the mission, it is likely to create an additional workload, driving up nursing costs and reducing profit margins.

The emphasis now is on the consumer as a purchaser and user of the product: *health care*. Consequently, management efforts are shifting from decision making based on institutional needs to decision making based on customer research and careful matching of customer needs with the capabilities of the organization. In market-based management, customer wants and needs are best identified by those closest to the customer. This requires a participative process, with the manager being the knowledgeable facilitator. The management style, therefore, is participative.

Nursing, more than any other department, is for a longer period closer to the primary cus-

tomers of the hospital: the patients, physicians, and registered nurses. Therefore, nursing is in a position to design, develop, implement, and market service programs effectively. In addition, because of the competitive environment, the marketing model is an appropriate nursing management tool in developing and implementing objectives designed to meet customer needs.

Nursing Intrapreneurship*

Nursing programs are now being asked to do more than just control costs. They are also encountering requests to enhance health facility revenues. This new mission is generally captured by the term *intrapreneurship*—the creation and implementation of new, creative, vibrant, and profit-oriented ideas that will instill renewed vigor in service delivery.

Intrapreneurship in nursing settings is commonly characterized by the following attributes:

- emphasis on creative efforts to control costs or to enhance profit generation
- reinforcement of innovative ideas through intrinsic and extrinsic rewards
- search for methods to generate revenues for nursing services and for the total organization
- enhanced financial viability of nursing programs, with expanded support (e.g., seed money) for new program efforts
- promotion of a supportive culture that retains nursing personnel and facilitates personal growth
- expansion of nursing business lines or products

In addition, intrapreneurship is a mechanism for increasing the power of nursing services. Instead of taking a traditional stance as a support service, nursing is allowed more freedom through intrapreneurship. Nurses can redefine what it

---

*Source: Vi Kunkle, *Marketing Strategies for Nurse Managers: A Guide for Developing and Implementing a Nurse Marketing Plan*, Aspen Publishers, Inc., © 1990.

*Source: Judith F. Garner, Howard L. Smith, and Neill F. Piland, *Strategic Nursing Management: Power and Responsibility in a New Era*, Aspen Publishers, Inc., © 1990.

means to offer nursing care. Intrapreneurship fosters a new way of looking at service delivery. It is an optimistic and constructive approach for improving nursing services and the return from the delivery process.

The way to think of intrapreneurship in nursing is in terms of the products or services delivered in nursing care. In many respects, nurse managers need to think in terms of marketing their product or service line. Once a nursing program has delineated its product or service line, it is in the position of being able to promote excellence in the services or products and to expand the services or products offered. At the heart of this issue is marketing nursing care as a profitable, cost-controlling, and valuable service.

Entrepreneurship: Decision-Making Process for Developing a New or Modified Service*

Current emerging trends of new service development, as well as new applications of delivery systems, accentuate the critical need for managerial resourcefulness and responsiveness to the swiftly evolving environment. Entrepreneurship exploits opportunities, optimizes what already exists, and obtains desired results. An entrepreneur continually searches for plausible and effective methods to respond to the market (the people served) and its shifts in preference.

Developing new services or significantly modifying existing services is an essential management pursuit in the process of adapting to a changing environment. However, the development of a new service must stand the test of appropriateness and risk evaluation.

Developing new or modified services also requires considerable planning and cost analysis—including revenue projections and interfunctional cooperation and coordination. The more complex the information, the better the decision and the greater the ultimate level of success.

---

*Source: Kenneth R. Emery, "Developing a New or Modified Service: Analysis for Decision Making," *The Health Care Supervisor*, Vol. 4, No. 2, Aspen Publishers, Inc., © 1986.

The format presented in Table 38–1 and discussed below addresses critical management issues for making effective and timely decisions. It is the responsibility of the new or modified service sponsor (manager or supervisory manager) to respond thoroughly to each question or to request information from appropriate resource personnel.

Part I attempts to provide the reviewer of the proposal with a complete description of the service, the purpose of the service, and who is to benefit by the service and to identify duplicate or similar services that have already been established in the service area. This information lays an important foundation. Defining the need and the rationale supporting that need secures the underpinnings of the proposal. All service efforts should be market oriented, responding to a special need for a defined market.

Part II provides important pieces of environmental information that will help in assembling the complex overall market puzzle. Every service should be associated with a specific market to be served. Each market consists of distinguishable segments that can be identified either geographically or demographically. If the employer conducts formal marketing surveys, the proposal could be augmented with information about consumer behavior, attitudes, and patronage.

With the use of the information contained in this section, promotional strategies can be developed and implemented once the program is approved. Therefore, all the effort expended to obtain the most complete information possible will lead to rewards not only in the decision-making process but also in the promotion process. Promotion strategies will be vital to the success of the service. The responses to items 10 through 15 supply the reviewer of the proposal with important supportive information and serve as a basis for the action that will be requested in item 30.

The operational information gathered in *Part III* is, in effect, the nuts and bolts of the proposal. Can the proposed service be successful given the realities of the internal and external environment? Health care organization managers are increasingly concerned with having the

Table 38–1 Developing a New or Modified Service Analysis

Part I: Service Description and Need

1. Describe the proposed new or modified service.
2. Describe the extent to which the service is compatible with the organization's philosophy and mission.
3. Identify the benefits of the service to the patients (community).
4. Describe how the need for the service was determined.
5. Fully explain the need for the service.
6. Identify the alternatives that exist to serve the need.

Part II: Market Information

7. Identify the segment of the community to be served: market (geographic) area, age group, sex, diagnosis, and other patient-origin information.
8. Describe how patients will be directed to the service.
9. Determine whether the location of the service will be convenient for patients: accessibility, parking, directions, and reception.
10. Identify who will provide the service.
11. Identify the hours of operation of the service and waiting time.
12. Describe the price structure for the service and how it was determined.
13. List the prices charged by primary competitors for the same or comparable services.
14. Describe the full scope of competition (name, location, range of service, and the strengths and weaknesses of the competitors).
15. Explain how the new or modified service would be better than each competitor's service.

Part III: Operational Information

16. Identify the persons who will be responsible for the management of the service.
17. Identify the persons who will be responsible for the medical direction of the service.

18. Attach job descriptions of any new positions to be created.
19. If there is a need for a medical director's contract, describe the suggested provisions of that contract.
20. If there is a need for malpractice insurance, explain why.
21. Indicate whether all necessary coordination with other functions has been completed.
22. Fully define and explain all legal ramifications (liability, contracts, regulatory restrictions, etc.).
23. If a certificate of need (CON) is required, explain why and provide details.
24. Identify any support resources required (personnel, material, space, facilities, equipment, etc.).

Part IV: Success Indicators

25. Describe the strengths of the service.
26. Describe the weaknesses of the service.
27. Identify all major areas of concern.
28. Describe all medical staff support that may be needed.
29. Describe how the necessary acceptance of the medical staff will be achieved.
30. Describe how the service will be promoted.
31. Outline the proposed buildup and implementation schedule (activities and dates).
32. Estimate the probability of success (rank success on a scale of 1 to 10, with 10 being high).

Part V: Financial Plan and Information Verification

33. Attach a complete three-year financial plan. Consider revenue, expense, labor and nonlabor costs, capital equipment, billing, collection, bad debts, indirect expenses, and renovation costs.
34. Calculate a three-year projected return on investment.
35. Ensure that all information is reviewed and verified: interdepartment, intradepartment, and fiscal services.

proper resources and the capabilities to capitalize on growth opportunities.

The success part of the analysis in *Part IV* provides the program reviewer with supportive information so that the reviewer is able to gain a clear perspective on the possibilities for success. The service viability factor becomes more evident with the answers to these questions. Knowing constraints as well as opportunities provides decision makers with information vital in the decision-making process. Every service goes through a product cycle consisting of the introduction phase, the growth period, the maturity period, and the eventual decline of the product or service. An objective assessment of the product's strengths and weaknesses provides a reasonable means of assessing success during the initial and growth phases of a new or modified service.

Part IV also examines the proposed strategy for promoting the service. The approach for communicating the service to various groups of potential consumers begins to unify the entire proposal.

Once all the information in the analysis is reviewed, item 32 (the success scale) must be considered. This places the entire package in a nutshell—a simple and straightforward subjective assessment. Considering today's environment, if the answer is not 8, 9, or 10, then it is suggested that the person who is making the proposal return to the drawing board and strengthen all supporting information.

Part V helps establish priorities based on reasonable risks and available resources. For an organization to remain financially viable, prudent decisions must be made. Therefore, a proposal should have complete financial data, including forecasts based on projected business volume and expenses. Without a thorough financial analysis and a clearly projected return on investment, it may be virtually impossible to obtain an informed decision. The final question of the analysis should not be overlooked. The information contained in the analysis should be accurate; therefore it is advisable to receive verification from all individuals who either contributed to the analysis by submitting information or who have reviewed the information for accuracy. This effort not only supports the validity of the information but also expedites the decision process because there is no need for the final decision makers to request verification of the information.

PRODUCT LINE MANAGEMENT

Overview*

A pure product line structure is developed by organizing under customer services, not health care facility departments. Traditional lines of authority are used, but the scope of responsibility includes cost centers for services identified by the facility as major strength areas. The major areas of strength are the facility's product mix. For example, in the box below each product item has a business plan identifying budgetary income and expense included in a cost center under rehabilitation services.

Source: Vi Kunkle, *Marketing Strategies for Nurse Managers: A Guide for Developing and Implementing a Nurse Marketing Plan*, Aspen Publishers, Inc., © 1990.

Sample Rehabilitation Services Product Line

Rheumatology Center	Vocational Rehabilitation Center
Spinal Cord Injury Center	Developmental Pediatric Rehabilitation Center
Stroke Rehabilitation Center	Rehabilitation Inpatient Care
Head Trauma Center	Rehabilitation Outpatient Care

Each product item is a separate business within the facility. In addition, each product item has a product manager who develops a product team and reports to the vice president of rehabilitation services. Under this organizational structure, the vice president of nursing also manages a product line.

The emphasis in this organizational structure is service to customers, not operations or traditional departmental issues. The entire organization, staff to management, is brought into the product lines through participation in product teams. Administration and marketing are represented on the product teams, with the marketing representative being a facilitator and educator. The cost and revenue of nursing services, professional services, ancillary services, and support services are allocated appropriately to each product item cost center. This structure provides

- increased unity in implementing facility objectives
- increased focus on customer service
- increased creativity in developing programs
- increased specialization and enhancement of expertise
- increased efficiency in defining the target market
- increased market attractiveness and competitiveness because of specialization

The disadvantages include the lack of attention to operations, policies, procedures, and detail as well as loss of some time-honored values of the organization. The matrix organizational structure addresses the disadvantages with the retention of traditional lines of authority but in the process creates confusing dual authority relationships.

Implications for Nurse Managers*

Product line management (PLM) has been successful in industries based on discrete and tangible products that can be mass produced. When the product is a clinical service that is provided by a team of health care professionals and does not lead to a discrete outcome, PLM faces inherent difficulties.

The basic premise of PLM is that one decision maker is responsible for all aspects of the product: design, development, production, marketing, sales, service evaluation, and profitability. This decision maker has the ultimate authority over the product. In the health care setting, the product is patient care and services. This product is created by interdependent departmental systems. It is difficult to separate clinical departments like nursing, laboratory, radiology, and special diagnostics and essential support departments such as food service, housekeeping, and materials management into distinct product lines.

If PLM addresses only those departments involved in the product of patient care, fewer departments are affected. The nursing department may become the primary focus for restructuring, as the nursing units are the essence and, in some product lines, the only component of the product. In this scheme, each nursing unit or service is responsible to a product manager or administrator who holds the ultimate decision-making authority. Consequently, this shift in the table of organization eradicates unified reporting to a central nursing department and fragments nursing with multiple reporting relationships to various product managers.

Fragmentation of nursing could mean a loss of power and influence, division of impact, and the eventual erosion of standards of patient care and nursing practice across an institution. Alliance to a product line as opposed to patient care stimulates interunit competition, rivalry, and dissonance.

The PLM structure does not usually view nursing as the primary product for health care facilities; rather, nursing is defined as a means to provide products such as cardiovascular services, oncology services, and so forth.

Questions To Ask about PLM

The following questions may be helpful in projecting the consequences of PLM:

---

*Source: Nancy Higgerson, "Product Line Management for Nurse Executives," *Aspen's Advisor for Nurse Executives*, Vol. 4, No. 7, Aspen Publishers, Inc., © 1989.

- Given that nursing care is the primary product in a health care facility, how does PLM support and enable the "nursing product"?
- How will PLM affect the facility's reputation for nursing excellence, which, as studies demonstrate, affects physicians' and patients' selection of facilities (market share)?
- What message does PLM convey about the position, influence, and importance of nursing?
- How will professional standards and quality assurance be established, maintained, and coordinated under PLM?
- How will PLM affect the recruitment and retention of professional nurses?
- How does PLM address the issues nurses identify as major contributors to nursing burnout and the growing shortage, such as participation in decision making and position within the institution?
- Will PLM increase or diminish nurses' participation in the organization's decision-making process?
- How does PLM affect the design and evolution of care delivery systems that are patient focused, satisfying to professional practitioners, and cost-efficient?
- Under PLM, how will the health care facility satisfy Joint Commission on Accreditation of Healthcare Organizations (Joint Commission) standards requiring a professionally qualified person to be accountable for nursing practice?
- What efficiencies will be gained or lost with PLM?
- How will nursing activities and systems among product lines and across the department be coordinated and integrated?
- How will nursing be represented on the board of trustees and at the executive level?
- How will the nursing department accomplish functions that are more efficient if centralized, such as core orientation and nurse recruitment?
- Where do nursing units that do not relate to a specific product fit in the organizational structure?

Structure for Product Line Management*

In a health care facility setting, the ways in which product lines are differentiated are as many and as varied as the accompanying organizational structures. Traditionally, each product line has its own product manager, and the product line is treated as a business within the business.

Product Lines Defined

A *product line* is a group of products within a product mix that are closely related, either because they function in a similar manner, are made available to the same consumers, or are marketed through the same types of outlets. A product mix (width of consumer offerings) is defined, then each product line in the product mix is lengthened by the product items. The product line can be organized in several ways. Tables 38–2 and 38–3 show two options for presenting product lines in a university school of nursing. Table 38–2 shows product lines developed by product items that are similar in function. Table 38–3 shows a variation that defines product lines more progressively, and is organized by the similarities of consumers using the programs. Whereas the product lines in Table 38–2 are organized by similarities of the products, the product lines in Table 38–3 are organized by similarities of the consumers who use the product lines. The product lines in Table 38–2 are oriented toward the organization, and the product lines in Table 38–3 are oriented toward the consumer.

A change in the way products or services are differentiated has major implications for the organization, one of which is a change in structure to facilitate the success of the product line. The other major implication is that product lines require product managers. For example, a product manager will cross departmental lines in developing and implementing the product items in the product line. That is, the product items in the health education product line will be developed from the offerings of other departments, such as

*Source: Vi Kunkle, *Marketing Strategies for Nurse Managers: A Guide for Developing and Implementing a Nurse Marketing Plan*, Aspen Publishers, Inc., © 1990.

Table 38–2 Functional Product Mix and Product Lines

Science	Psychiatry	Humanities	Business	Practicum	Curriculum Development
SC 101	PSY 101	SOC 110	BUS 110	MS 110	Revision
SC 300	PSY 102	ENG 110	BUS 210	PED 110	New Courses
SC 310	PSY 200	SPN 110	COM 110	OB 110	Textbooks
SC 312	PSY 310	REL 110		RHB 110	Sequencing

Table 38–3 Consumer-Oriented Product Mix and Product Lines

Generic	Degree Completion	Master's	Health Ed	Continuing Ed	Marketing
Course A	Course A	Courses	Mental Hlth	Course A	Recruitment
Course B	Course B	Clinical	Child Dev	Course B	Planning
Course C	Course C	Thesis	Nutrition	Course C	Curriculum
Course D	Course D		Family	Course D	Advertisement
			Planning		Promotions

psychiatry, pediatrics, sociology, nutrition, and so forth.

Selecting Product Lines

Various methods are used by health care facilities to define appropriate product lines. Certainly, the driving force is the market-based planning process itself. Criteria, then, are

- recognized strength in the marketplace (includes clinical, educational, and research expertise)
- marketability in the area of strength (includes high profitability, high demand, and positive exchange relationships)
- capability for expanding the area of strength
- compatibility with the mission
- consistency with the interest of the program experts

The market-based planning process identifies the five or six major areas that need development, and these can be used in defining the product lines. During the annual market-based planning process, the product mix is widened, the product lines are lengthened, and existing product lines are continued, dropped, or expanded.

Nursing uses the market-based planning model to identify product items and product lines. If product lines determine the organizational structure, only the most significant product lines are developed, product line managers are named, and separate cost centers are allocated.

Modified Approach

In the absence of a product line–oriented organizational model, integrating nursing product lines into cost centers is difficult. Matrix and project organizational structures are innovative approaches designed to change the organizational focus from departmental operations to services. This customer-oriented approach recognizes that services and programs are both more important and marketable than operations.

However, even if traditional lines of authority are retained, product lines and product items can be integrated under the already established structure. Table 38–4 shows an example of product lines and product items organized under traditional organizational structures. The nurse manager of pediatrics manages the inpatient and same-day surgery units as well as the various other programs. In this example, the unit staff nurses become the project managers for the various product items. Cost centers include only the

Table 38–4 Product Items or Product Lines Organized under Traditional Lines of Authority

Title: Nurse Manager   **Service:** Pediatrics   **Product Line:** Children's Center

Inpatient Pediatrics
  Routine Care
  Intensive Care
  Orthopaedics
  Juvenile Diabetes
  Rehabilitation
  Leukemia

Same-Day Surgery
  Unit Tours
  Preadmission Screening

Parental Education
  Child Development
  Pediatric Toxicology
  Pediatric Nutrition

Support Groups
  Death and Dying
  Diabetes Support
  Pediatric Emergencies
  Pediatric Newsletter

Outreach Education
  Intensive Care Course
  Annual Seminar

Physician Relations
  Office Nurse Seminar
  Physician/Nurse Mini-Grand Rounds
  Primary Nurse Program

Nurse Retention/Recruitment Program

inpatient units of routine care and intensive care. The same-day surgery income and expense are included in the routine care unit cost center. The costs of the various programs are written in a business plan format but are a part of the units' budget.

MARKETING PROCESS

The Role of the Nurse*

The product of health care facilities and health care providers is health care. Nursing produces and delivers this health care. The outcome and purpose of patient care are patient compliance with the health care regimen and a resulting physical and mental state called *health*, restored at least to the previous level. In the process of producing and delivering health care, nursing is simultaneously selling an image of both nursing and the health care provider to the patient.

Nursing, by definition, is the primary interface between the health care facility and its custom-

ers. Because patients in some facilities (e.g., hospitals) are too ill to coordinate their own plan of care, nurses also act on behalf of patients, representing patients to physicians and other professional disciplines. Although nursing at the organizational level works in close collaboration with the planning, marketing, and communications departments of the health care facility, bedside nurses are key figures in microlevel nursing.

The Marketing Concept

- The process of listening to consumers and the marketplace
- The philosophy of organizing to satisfy needs of a group or groups of consumers
- The satisfaction of these needs in a profitable fashion

The nurse does marketing for the health care facility in three ways. First, in the provision of excellence in patient care, nurses sell the facility to physicians. Second, by their manner and approach to care delivery, nurses sell the facility to patients. Third, by their positive attitudes and job satisfaction, nurses influence the retention of other nurses.

---
*Source: Vi Kunkle, *Marketing Strategies for Nurse Managers: A Guide for Developing and Implementing a Nurse Marketing Plan*, Aspen Publishers, Inc., © 1990.

Planning versus Marketing*

There is a great deal of confusion regarding the relationship of planning to marketing. Some believe a corporate plan should be established before a marketing plan is developed. For example, the organization establishes its mission and then develops its marketing plan within the context of its mission and goals. Although this is an interactive process, marketing can play a key first-step role by helping to determine which direction to go. However, most health care organizations that develop plans do not incorporate a market-based approach. The typical process begins with the wants and needs of people who work in the facility or own the clinic and their views of the marketplace. The market-based approach starts with customer wants and needs, and these become the basis for a program or service to address those needs.

An Overview of the Process*

A marketing plan begins with an analysis of the market. Most health care organizations think of their internal needs first and the marketplace second. This is a nonmarket-based approach. A market-oriented manager, however, begins with a determination of external needs and focuses internal actions on these external needs. This is a market-based approach. The two approaches vary in just a few instances (see Figure 38–1), but the difference in the results obtained with these two planning approaches can be dramatic.

A market-based approach is not "right" and the nonmarket-based approach is not "wrong." Yet, as financial resources became more restricted, mistakes (in terms of programs that do not meet expectations) are more costly for the organization. A market-based approach helps improve the odds of success. It is easier to listen

*Source: Steven G. Hillstead and Eric N. Berkowitz, *Health Care Marketing Plans: From Strategy to Action*, ed 2, Aspen Publishers, Inc., © 1991.

to buyers and provide the necessary programs than to attempt to divine what buyers may need.

Marketing Planning Sequence

The sequence of the market-based approach is relatively simple. It incorporates six steps:

1. setting the mission
2. performing an external/internal analysis
3. determining the strategy action match and marketing objectives
4. developing action strategies
5. integrating the plan and making revisions
6. providing appropriate control procedures, feedback, and integration of all plans into a unified effort

At each step, three types of activities are necessary for success:

- the process of doing the staff work necessary to support decision making
- the process of actually making decisions
- the process of integrating the activities of all units or services to enhance coordination between the functional units, such as operations and finance

The collection of the details and data needed in the decision-making process constitutes the staff work. Here, marketing plans differ substantially from other planning approaches, because they require not only internal data but also information on the attitudes, the opinions, and the environment of those outside the organization.

In the decision process, the actual steps of a marketing plan are charted. As health care facilities or nurse executives assess the external market data, they must decide how to react to external conditions in light of its internal capabilities.

The integration process involves the coordination of marketing plans with finance, human relations, operations, and resource allocation.

Figure 38–1 Diagram of Internal Planning versus Marketing Planning

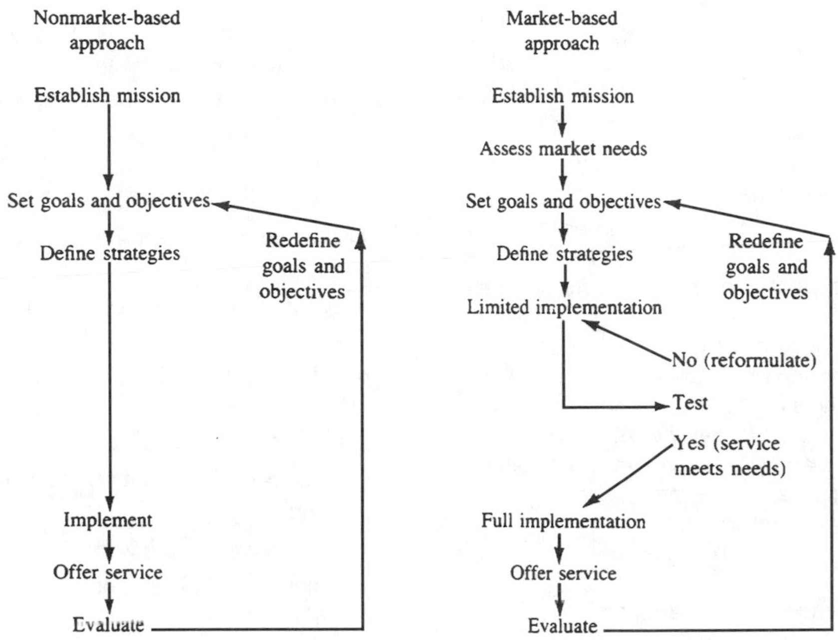

Nonmarket-based
approach

Establish mission

Set goals and objectives

Define strategies

Redefine
goals and
objectives

Implement

Offer service

Evaluate

Market-based
approach

Establish mission

Assess market needs

Set goals and objectives

Define strategies

Redefine
goals and
objectives

Limited implementation

No (reformulate)

Test

Yes (service
meets needs)

Full implementation

Offer service

Evaluate

Also included are the development of the organization's entire product or service portfolio and the sharing and coordination of plans with the other services within the health care organization.

The Marketing Plan

To establish an effective marketing plan, it is necessary to understand the first premise of marketing. Marketing is the process of determining customer wants and needs and then, to whatever extent possible, designing appropriate programs and services to meet those wants and needs in a timely, cost-effective, competitive fashion. It is the process of molding the organization to the customers rather than convincing customers that the organization provides what they need.

When completed, a marketing plan contains answers to the questions in Table 38–5. Answering these questions in sequence is the foundation for most marketing strategy sessions.

Table 38–6 summarizes what a marketing plan must do.

Key Questions for Conducting an Internal/External Analysis*

The internal/external analysis is a key component in developing the marketing plan, as it is the foundation from which the strategy action match is determined. It is also important in determining which specific action-oriented marketing tactics are appropriate. The following list is a reminder of which questions should be asked as part of the analysis.

---

*Source: Steven G. Hillstead and Eric N. Berkowitz, *Health Care Marketing Plans: From Strategy to Action,* ed 2, Aspen Publishers, Inc., © 1991.

Table 38–5 Marketing Planning Questions

Who is the market?
Where is the market?
What are the needs and demands?
Where are you now?
- as an institution
- as a department
- as an individual
- with respect to the environment and competition
- with respect to capabilities and opportunities

Where do you want to go?
- assumptions/potentials
- objectives and goals

How do you want to get there?
- policies and procedures/levels of initiative
- strategies and programs

When do you want to arrive?
- priorities and schedules

Who is responsible?
- organization and delegation

How much will it cost?
- budgets and resource allocations

How will you know if you did it?
- feedback and review sessions
- continuous monitoring

Table 38–6 Marketing Plan Summary

- Describe characteristics, trends, market share, and competitive factors.
- Describe business mission and goals.
- Describe key customers (segment) and key needs as they relate to your service area.
- Describe the product and key advantages.
- Describe four key strategies, tactics, and strategy action match.
- Describe economic profile.

The Environment and the Market

- What kinds of external controls affect the organization?
  - local
  - state
  - federal
  - self-regulatory
- What are the trends in recent regulatory rulings?
- What are the main developments with respect to demography, economy, technology, government, and culture that will affect the organization's situation?
- What are the organization's major markets and publics?
- How large is the service area covered by the market?
- What are the major segments in each market?
- What are the present and expected future profits and characteristics of each market or market segment?
- What is the expected rate of growth of each segment?
- How fast and far have markets expanded?
- Where do the patients come from geographically?
- What are the benefits that customers in different segments derive from the product (e.g., economics, better performance, displaceable cost)?
- What are the reasons for buying the product in different segments (e.g., product features, awareness, price, advertising, promotion, packaging, display, sales assistance)?
- What is the market standing with established customers in each segment (e.g., market share, pattern of repeat business, expansion of customers' product use)?
- What are the requirements for success in each market?
- What are the customer attitudes in different segments (e.g., brand awareness, brand image mapping)?
- What is the overall reputation of the product in each segment?
- What reinforces the customer's faith in the organization and product?
- What reasons force customers to turn elsewhere for help in using the product?
- What is the life cycle status of the product?
- What product research and improvements are planned?

- Are there deficiencies in servicing or assisting customers in using the product?

The Competitive Environment

- How many competitors are in the industry?
  - How are competitors defined?
  - Has the number increased or decreased in the last four years?
- What is the organization's position in the market (size and strength) relative to competitors?
- Who are the organization's major competitors?
- What trends can be foreseen in competition?
- Are there other companies that may be enticed to serve the organization's customers or markets? This should include conglomerates or diversified companies that may be attracted by the growth, size, or profitability of these markets.
- Are these facilities on the periphery—that serve the same customers with different but related products? This may include related pieces of equipment. It is impossible to list all related items, but those closest should be included.
- What other products or services provide the same or similar function? What percentage of total market sales does each substitute product have?
- What product innovations could replace or reduce the sales of the organization's products? When will these products be commercially feasible? (*Note:* Information about potentially competitive products can be found by searching the U.S. Patent Office or foreign patent offices.)
- What are the choices afforded patients in services and in payment?
- Is competition on a price or nonprice basis?
- How do competitors (segment/price) advertise?
- Are there competitors in other geographic regions or other segments who do not currently compete in the organization's markets or segments, but may decide to?

- Who are the customers served by the industry? Are there any who may want to move backward?
- Who are the suppliers to the industry? Are they moving? Why?

The Internal Assessment

- What has been the historical purpose of the facility?
- How has the facility changed over the past decade?
- When and how was it organized?
- What has been the nature of its growth?
- What is the basic policy of the organization? Is it health care or profit?
- What has been the financial history of the organization?
- How has it been capitalized?
- Have there been any accounts receivable problems?
- What is the inventory investment?
- How successful has the organization been with the various services promoted?
- Is the total volume (gross revenue, utilization) increasing or decreasing?
- Have there been any fluctuations in revenue? If so, what caused them?
- What are the organization's present strengths and weaknesses in the following?
  - management capabilities
  - medical staff
  - technical facilities
  - reputation
  - financial capabilities
  - image
  - medical facilities

The Marketing Function and Programs

- Are there specialized training programs for key personnel that emphasize the marketing concept?
- Do the administrator and other key personnel have marketing experience?
- Does the marketing department have a key role in the planning activities of the organization?

- Does the person with marketing responsibility report directly to the chief executive officer or top administrator?
- Is marketing research appreciated as an ongoing task necessary for the development of effective marketing plans?
- Are policies and procedures in place to coordinate the marketing activities with the other ongoing activities of the organization?
- Does the organization have a high-level marketing officer to analyze, plan, and implement its marketing work?
- Are the other persons who are directly involved in marketing activities competent people? Do they need more training, incentives, or supervision?
- Are the marketing responsibilities optimally structured to serve the needs of different activities, products, markets, and territories?
- What is the organization's core strategy for achieving its objectives, and is it likely to succeed?
- Is the organization allocating enough resources (or too many) to accomplish its marketing tasks?
- Are the marketing resources allocated optimally to the various markets, territories, and products of the organization?
- Are the marketing resources allocated optimally to the major elements of the marketing mix (i.e., product quality, personal contact, promotion, and distribution)?
- Does the organization develop an annual marketing plan? Is the planning procedure effective?
- Does the organization implement control procedures (e.g., monthly, quarterly) to ensure that its annual plan objectives are being achieved?
- Does the organization carry out periodic studies to determine the contribution and effectiveness of various marketing activities?
- Does the organization have an adequate marketing information system to service the needs of managers in planning and controlling various markets?

Products/Services

- What are the organization's products and services, both present and proposed?
- What are the general outstanding characteristics of each product or service?
- How are the organization's products or services superior to or distinct from those of competing organizations?
  - What are the weaknesses?
  - Should any product be phased out?
  - Should any product be added?
- What is the total cost per service (in use)? Is service over- or underutilized?
- Which services are most heavily used? Why?
  - Are there distinct groups of users?
  - What is the profile of patients/physicians who use the services?
- What are the organization's policies regarding the following?
  - number and types of services to offer
  - needs assessment for service addition/deletion
- What is the history of the organization's major products and services?
  - How many did the organization originally have?
  - How many have been added or dropped?
  - What important changes have taken place in services during the last 10 years?
  - Has demand for the services increased or decreased?
  - What are the most common complaints against the services?
  - What services could be added to make the organization more attractive to patients, medical staff, and nonmedical personnel?
  - What are the strongest points of services to patients, medical staff, and nonmedical personnel?
- Does the organization have any other features that individualize its services or give it an advantage over competitors?

Pricing Strategy

- What is the pricing strategy of the organization?
  - cost plus
  - return on investment
  - stabilization
  - demand
- How are prices for services determined?
  - How often are prices reviewed?
  - What factors contribute to a price increase/decrease?
- What have been the price trends for the past five years?
- How are the organization's policies viewed by the following?
  - patients
  - physicians
  - third-party payers
  - competitors
  - regulators
- How are price promotions used?
- What would be the impact of demand on a higher or lower price?

Promotional Strategy

- Is the sales force large enough to accomplish the organization's objectives?
- Is the sales force organized along the proper principles of specialization (e.g., territory, market, product)?
- Does the sales force show high morale, ability, and effort? Is it sufficiently trained and motivated?
- Are the procedures adequate for setting quotas and evaluating performance?
- What is the purpose of the organization's present promotional activities (including advertising)?
  - protection
  - education
  - search for new markets
  - development of all markets
  - establishment of a new service
- Has this purpose undergone any change in recent years?

- To whom has advertising been largely directed?
  - donors
  - patients (former, current, or prospective)
  - physicians (staff or potential)
- Is the cost per thousand still favorable?
- Is it delivering the desired audience?
- What media have been used?
- Are the media still effective in reaching the intended audience?
- Are the objectives being met?
- What copy appeals have had the most favorable response?
- What methods have been used for measuring advertising effectiveness?

Public Relations Strategy

- What is the role of public relations?
  - Is it a separate function/department?
  - What is its scope of responsibilities?
- Has the public relations effort led to regular coverage?
- Are the public relations objectives integrated with the overall promotional plan?
- Are procedures established and used to measure the results from the public relations program?

Distribution Strategies

- What are the distribution trends in the industry?
  - What services are being performed on an outpatient basis?
  - What services are being performed on an at-home basis?
  - Are satellite facilities being used?
- What factors are considered in location decisions?
- How important is distribution in establishing a competitive advantage for a particular service?
- Where does the organization stand on this component?

SELLING THE NURSING SERVICE

Monitoring the Pulse of Nursing's Customers*

The concept of monitoring the pulse of the customer is a strategy requiring continuous feedback concerning the perceptions of nursing care in the mind of its customers. Responsive nurse managers devise and implement ongoing systems for continuous feedback.

Patients' Perceptions

Patients are the primary customers of the nursing department, and as such, their satisfaction with care is of paramount value to the providers. With so many classifications of personnel coming in contact with patients, it is difficult to control and standardize approaches to patient care. One of the best methods of obtaining immediate feedback concerning patient perceptions of care is to simply ask patients about the care received. (See Chapter 15 on patient-centered care.)

A positive and high-visibility program to determine the efficiency of the admission process is the *administrative welcome rounds*. The nurse administrator, accompanied by the manager or staff nurse, chats briefly with each patient admitted the night before, giving a welcome and leaving a business card for future use by the patient in contacting the nurse administrator. This program sets a positive tone for the admission and leaves the patient with an accessible person's name if problems should occur later.

A *postdischarge follow-up* call program continues to set this positive tone. Primary nurses call the discharged patient within three days postdischarge to reinforce patient compliance with the treatment regimen, express concern about the patient's condition and health status after discharge, and inquire about satisfaction with care. The telephone call, in and of itself, is a powerful marketing strategy for nursing. It shows that the nursing organization cares about the customers.

Physicians' Perceptions

The responsive nurse manager keeps a constant pulse on the perceptions and attitudes of physicians. A physician questionnaire is developed and administered to physicians monthly to monitor perceptions. Discussions on patient-physician problems can be initiated. Using a patient-oriented questionnaire as supportive evidence avoids the evaluation of nursing based on subjective criteria such as likes and dislikes of a particular unit, nurse manager, or nurse. A more informal method is face-to-face discussions with physicians about items on the questionnaire. The feedback is used to assess physicians' satisfaction level, and immediate action is taken where appropriate.

Nurses' Perceptions

Responsive nurse managers continuously monitor not only the supply of nurses but nurse vacancy rates and the reasons for the vacancies. Analyzing the reasons for resignations requires an accurate monitoring system of the attitudes and beliefs of the resigning nurses and those who are still employed. Continuous feedback strategies for nurses include exit interviews, staff attitude questionnaires, and a nurse ombudsman program.

Ideas for Patient Promotional Programs*

Promotional programs designed to attract or retain patients are based on programs or services that are already developed but that need special promotions to be competitive. These strategies are primarily based on augmented services rather than on price, although, occasionally, price competition is one of the strategies. Highly competitive areas or services design special promotional services to link current patients and potential patients to the institution. This is especially common in obstetrics and pediatrics but can also occur when there is more than one of any spe-

Source: Vi Kunkle, *Marketing Strategies for Nurse Managers: A Guide for Developing and Implementing a Nurse Marketing Plan*, Aspen Publishers, Inc., © 1990.

Source: Vi Kunkle, *Marketing Strategies for Nurse Managers: A Guide for Developing and Implementing a Nurse Marketing Plan*, Aspen Publishers, Inc., © 1990.

cialized program in the community such as oncology, rehabilitation, home, emergency, and ambulatory care. Although these promotions are often designed by the marketing and promotions departments, staff at the unit level are indeed creative in generating ideas for the promotion of their specific services. Examples include

- birthday cards for newborn nursery infants
- free pictures for newborns at birth and ages one and two
- exercise classes for obstetric patients (designed with physician input)
- child development classes for parents of young children
- quarterly health update newsletters for cardiac patients
- reunions for rehabilitation patients
- support groups for relatives who have lost loved ones
- hot lines for obstetric, emergency, and psychiatric patients with qualified response staff
- follow-up telephone calls to the patient from the primary nurse

Promotions such as these are topics of controversy in health care and are often labeled *gimmicks* by critics. Actually, they are augmentations of already developed services and programs. Although they are designed to attract patients, these augmentations also improve services to the customer. Additionally, such promotions provide increased top-of-mind name awareness of the health care facility among customers.

Physician Bonding*

The changing environment of health care requires nurse executives to examine more closely the *physician as customer*. Faced with declining admissions and reimbursements, health care fa-

cilities are competing to attract and retain physicians. Nurse executives know the significant contributions physicians make to patient care revenues. Health care facilities are in fierce competition to attract and retain physicians.

The nurse executive must include physician relations and satisfaction with the organization and services provided in the long-range planning for service excellence. The development of a program to "bond" physicians to the nursing department will greatly assist in meeting the organization's overall objective of long-term survival through enhanced revenues and the delivery of quality care.

The nurse executive plays a key role in developing a successful physician bonding program. Physicians are most attentive to patient care and the quality of services offered to produce favorable outcomes. Because nurses are the administrators of patient care, the nurse executive can facilitate successful bonding strategies to enhance the quality of patient care as well as foster loyalty and bonding of physicians to the nursing department and ultimately the health care institution. For the variety of strategies available, see Table 38–7.

Perhaps the greatest challenge to the nurse executive is selling the concept of the bonding program to the chief executive officer and governing body. When selling the program, the nurse executive should focus on the overall benefits to the organization. Two major benefits are as follows:

- Physician bonding programs lead to increased physician commitment to the facility and thus increased utilization of services and patient admissions. The end result is a real increase in patient-generated revenues and stronger, more secure operating margins.
- Bonding programs have a positive effect on the entire morale of the institution: Staff members and physicians gain a better understanding of each other's priorities and agendas; communication and cooperation increase, thus providing a more professional and satisfying work environment; and nurse and physician retention and recruitment are

*Source: Dominick L. Flarey, "Physician Bonding: The Role of the Nurse Executive," *Journal of Nursing Administration*, Vol. 20, No. 12, December 1990.

Table 38–7 Strategies To Promote Physician Bonding

- *Nurse-physician liaison committees* promote collaborative problem solving and program planning.
- *Joint nurse-physician question and answer programs* enhance professional working relationships and ensure mutual goal setting and direction.
- *Physician lecture series* allow participation of physicians in the continuing education of nurses.
- *Patient teaching programs* position nursing as a primary deliverer of preventive and restorative care and assist physicians in overall patient management.
- *Patient screening programs* assist physicians in overall patient care and preventive health care (e.g., breast exams, cholesterol screening).

- *Nurse-physician team conferences* bridge the gap between medical practice and professional nursing practice, foster collaboration, increase communications, and facilitate quality care planning.
- *Collaborative practice models* enhance mutual goal setting for quality care, enhance communications, increase bonding and physician commitment to the nursing department and the delivery of nursing care, and position nursing as an integral and primary component of patient care.
- *Physician office training programs* assist physicians in the continuing education of their office staffs and position nursing as an important resource for medical practices.

enhanced. This results in considerable cost savings and increased profit margins for the institution.

Follow-up interviews after implementation of the bonding program will ascertain physicians' perceptions and feelings about the program as well as verifiable evidence of increasing satisfaction with care services offered, the nursing department, and the institution. The degree of customer satisfaction by the physician is an important indicator of program success or failure.

Chapter 39

Grant Proposals and Research

PLANNING FOR GRANTS*

Literally millions of dollars are available through grants and contracts from government agencies, private foundations, and individuals. Although religious and related charities are the most popular recipients of such donations, health-related programs usually receive the second largest sum.

The dollar amounts fluctuate from year to year, but large sums of money are available each year and often go unclaimed. Grant writers must start with the assumption that the dollars are there and continue to be optimistic and enthusiastic.

Agencies and institutions usually have mission statements, goals and objectives, and long-term plans to implement the goals and objectives and fulfill the mission statement. Possible grants should be reviewed and discussed in this context. Most important, grant applications should be prepared only for tasks that an agency would like to undertake, even if external money were not available.

Rational planning is also essential in development of the proposal. Grant reviewers look for a proposal that is stated clearly and convincingly. They look for documentation that a problem exists and for a plan that will help alleviate the problem. They look for measurable objectives that are feasible. They look at the credibility of the agency and the credentials of the staff. They look for the probability of success and how such a project will be evaluated.

Stated differently, agency personnel that review and act on grant applications are concerned that their money is spent wisely and that full value will be received. Rational planning and sound administrative practices are therefore essential parts of the grant preparation process and the program that is proposed.

The committee approach is recommended for grant development, although one person usually needs to do the actual writing for the proposal to be coherent. The value of having several people involved in generating ideas and in reviewing drafts cannot be overstated. If a proposal represents the best thinking of several people, it will be better than if it represents the good thinking of only one person.

*Source: Adapted from Donald J. Breckon, John R. Harvey, and R. Brick Lancaster, *Community Health Education: Settings, Roles, and Skills for the 21st Century,* ed 3, Aspen Publishers, Inc., © 1994.

Guide to Nursing Research Grants

Those in search of research and project grants in nursing can find funding sources quickly in a comprehensive directory edited by the American Association of Colleges of Nursing (AACN). The guide, *The Complete Grants Sourcebook for Nursing and Health*, is a single-source reference designed specifically to help nursing and other health professionals develop effective grant-seeking strategies and find the best sources of funding for a variety of research, practice, and educational programs.

The AACN *Sourcebook* provides information on corporate, foundation, and federal sources that have funded nursing- and health-related research and projects or whose interests match those of the nursing and health professions. Listings include details on eligibility and application requirements, deadlines, financial data, contact persons, and the funds each has contributed to nursing and health activities.

Source: Holly A. De Groot, "Patient Classification System Evaluation, Part I: Essential System Elements," *Journal of Nursing Administration*, Vol. 19, No. 6, June 1989.

THE GRANT PROPOSAL

The Steps in Development of Grant Proposals*

Grant writing is no longer limited to securing funds for research purposes. Major changes in the allocation of health care funds require that administrators develop and seek more funds. Unfortunately, the amount of grant funds available is often limited and competition for the funds intense. Therefore, the ability to develop a successful grant proposal is crucial.

*Source: Deidre Richards, "Ten Steps to Successful Grant Writing," *Journal of Nursing Administration*, Vol. 20, No. 1, January 1990. © 1990 J.B. Lippincott Company.

Step 1: Identify a Funding Source. Funding sources include government agencies (at the federal, state, and city or county levels), private foundations, corporations, and associations, and academic institutions. Each funding source has different policies, missions, and application forms. To determine the best funding source, familiarize yourself with each funding source's history, dollar limitations, objectives, and areas of interest. A guide like *The Complete Grants Sourcebook for Nursing and Health*, which contains in-depth profiles of corporation, foundation, and government sources, could be of great help.

Grant applications should be tailored to meet the priorities of the funding source. One of the most inefficient methods of developing a grant application is to write the proposal and then look for a funding source. A thorough library search to analyze funding sources before developing the proposal will save countless hours of revising the proposal to fit the funding source.

Step 2: Obtain Application Materials from the Funding Source. Thoroughly read the application materials before you begin to write the proposal. This is very important and often ignored. These materials provide instructions on content and format of the application and are often developed by the same individuals who will review the application. The instructions will assist you in preparing a complete application that meets all requirements of the funding source.

Step 3: Identify Content Essential to Developing the Proposal and Note Areas in Which You Need Clarification. Underline the content essential to the actual writing of the proposal, for example, application format, required signatures, number of copies. Take special note of proposal deadlines. Missing a deadline in all likelihood will disqualify your proposal. Contact the funding source to clarify points of confusion such as questions relating to the forms, budget, or instructions.

Step 4: Follow the Application Instructions Precisely. It is very important to adhere strictly to proposal page limits. Do not include information that is not requested. If you think additional information is essential to the reviewers' understanding of how the project will operate, then place the information in an appendix and reference it in the proposal narrative. Reviewers appreciate a proposal that is easy to read and includes only what must be known.

However, do not omit requested information because it is not readily available to you. Keep in mind, the grant reviewers will definitely notice if requested information is omitted or unrelated information is added. These practices will jeopardize the success of your proposal.

Step 5: Clearly Describe Project Goals, Objectives, Implementation Strategies, and Evaluation Criteria. Identifying the need for grant funds, explicitly describing what will be done with the grant funds, and evaluating the project are extremely important parts of the grant proposal. Most funding agencies adhere to a general grant format.

Step 6: Proofread the Proposal. Carefully proofread the final draft of the typed proposal. Proof for typographical errors and to determine that all of the required information is included, the application forms provided by the funding source are completed correctly and signed when necessary, and the application is arranged in the order requested by the funding source.

Step 7: Complete a Presubmission Review of the Finished Proposal. Give a copy of the application instructions and the completed proposal to a colleague who is knowledgeable about the project but not directly associated with developing the proposal. Your colleague should read the proposal for required content and critique each section for clarity, specificity, and overall "flow" of the proposal from assessment of need to evaluation.

Step 8: Review the Proposal Based on the Presubmission Review. Frequently, grant writers do not allow sufficient preparation time to permit the presubmission review and subsequent revision. "The uninitiated seldom appreciate the number of revisions and the amount of time consumed in preparing a sound proposal."

Step 9: Avoid Common Mistakes. These mistakes reflect a rushed and disorganized grant writer. Common mistakes to avoid include submitting the proposal after the deadline; omitting literature citations that support the needs assessment or implementation strategies; incorrectly completing the application forms; omitting required signatures; mathematical errors in the budget; inconsistent budget figures throughout the application; goals, objectives, or implementation strategies that do not pertain to the identified need; evaluation criteria that do not include project outcomes; padding the application with unnecessary information; and using a format that does not conform to the application instructions. For the grant reviewer's convenience, include a table of contents and number all the pages.

Step 10: Submit the Proposal to the Funding Source. The application should be sent by certified mail, return receipt requested. Occasionally, applications have been lost in the mail or delivered to the wrong person. If the application is sent by certified mail, you have documentation of when you sent it and who received it. This documentation may mean the difference between a review or a disqualification.

ELEMENTS IN A GRANT PROPOSAL

Letter of Transmittal*

The letter of transmittal, or cover sheet, is the fist page of a grant but may, in fact, be the last part of the application to be prepared. It provides, at a minimum, the name and address of the organization submitting the proposal, a concise summary of the problem, and the proposed program. In an initial attempt to establish credibility, it often includes a statement of the organization's interest, capability, and experience in the area. It must contain the contact person's

Source: Donald J. Breckon, John R. Harvey, and R. Brick Lancaster, *Community Health Education: Settings, Roles, and Skills for the 21st Century*, ed 3, Aspen Publishers, Inc., © 1994.

name, address, and telephone number and an authorized signature from a chief administrative officer. The authorized signature is necessary because the proposal is offering to use agency space, equipment, and staff to do specific tasks. Grant reviewers want to know that the agency is committed to such tasks. When funded, such a project has the effect of a contract.

Table of Contents

If the application is large, a table of contents usually follows the letter of transmittal. Use of headings in the body of the proposal facilitates development of a table of contents. Headings also make it easier for reviewers to follow the organization of the project and should be used even if a table of contents is not needed.

Introduction

An introductory statement that puts the proposal in context is appropriate. The statement may or may not include a description of the problem; the description can be a separate section. In either case, it is important to establish that there is a problem and that it has serious consequences to the citizenry. Documentation is usually necessary at this point and, even if not necessary, is helpful.

Applicant Agency Description

Funding agencies need to know if the organization is able to carry out the proposed project. Items to describe include organizational structure, past experience, qualifications of the staff, and budget.

Target Group

The target group should be described in detail and put in the context of the geographical area in which the program will take place. The number and kind of clients is valuable information. A description of the client group's involvement in the project planning process is also important.

Objectives

The specific objectives should be included in measurable form. Although behavioral objectives are not necessarily required, they lend themselves well to grant application specifications. A timetable for accomplishing the objectives should also be included.

Procedures

The procedures that will be used should be detailed. A logical, sequential timetable for the work plan is helpful. Specific methods and materials should be identified, with emphasis given to the innovative features of the program.

Evaluation

A plan for evaluation should also be included and is often a key part of the proposal. The tools and methodology to be used should be described in enough detail to ensure funding agencies that the results of the program will be summarized accurately.

Budget

A budget sheet is usually included in the application form. Because this varies from agency to agency, the forms of the grant agency should be used when possible. However, grant budgets do have some commonality. Usually they list salaries, by position. Salary schedules of the applicant agency should be used in calculations. Fringe benefits are ordinarily figured on a percentage of salary. They include employer contributions to Social Security, health insurance, unemployment compensation, workers' compensation, and so on. The figures vary from agency to agency and from year to year but are usually about 25 percent of the total salary costs.

If consultants are needed on technical projects, a realistic per diem fee should be used in a separate section of the budget. Consultants are not entitled to fringe benefits.

Supplies and materials should also be described in a separate section. They should be itemized by major types, such as office supplies, mail, telephone, duplication costs, and printing.

Equipment is usually itemized in a separate category, giving such specifics as model number and vendor.

Travel should be categorized as in country/out of country, in state/out of state; it can be divided by personnel or by program function. Reviewers usually want to know how travel allowances are going to be used.

Indirect costs include such items as utilities, space procurement, and accounting staffs. Governmental funding agencies usually have a maximum allowable indirect rate. The rate is often negotiated; it may approach 50 percent of salaries and wages for the project.

Matching Funds

If matching funds are being used, they should be described. They represent the portion of the project cost that the institution is providing. In some instances, in-kind contributions have been used for this purpose. Institutions may agree to provide space, office furniture, and so on, and place a monetary value on that. In other instances, matching funds are required. In any case the larger the amount of matching funds or in-kind contributions, the more attractive the application will be.

Assurances

When applying to government agencies it is also necessary to provide assurance compliances. There are a number of such assurances and they change from time to time. They might include such items as treatment of human subjects, following affirmative action procedures when hiring, handicapped accessibility, and accounting practices. Again, funding agencies can readily provide copies of such required assurances.

Appendices

As in other written documents, the appendices are used to include material that, if included in the body of the proposal, would interrupt the flow. Vitae of key personnel in the project and supporting letters of other agencies are usually appended. Brochures, flow charts, diagrams, and other supporting material may be included.

RESEARCH IN THE NURSING SERVICE SETTING

Scope*

To establish a successful research section within a practice setting requires a commitment to the value of research in terms of guiding decision making as well as allocating and generating resources. The consistent pressure in practice settings for accurate information to guide administrative and clinical decisions and long-term policies stimulates the endeavors for integrating research. However, the integration process is not without its challenges. For example, not all problems confronting nurse administrators and clinicians are researchable. Some are more amenable to immediate problem-solving techniques than to research strategies. Experience, however, suggests that clinical and administrative problems with the following characteristics are researchable:

- The problems or issues are repetitive.
- The problems or issues occur across multiple clinical settings.
- The problems or issues are testable empirically and are not philosophical stances representing values such as "should" or "ought."
- The problems or issues represent long-term practices and/or policies for which accurate

---

Source: Ada Sue Hinshaw and Carolyn H. Smeltzer, "Research Challenges and Programs for Practice Settings," *Journal of Nursing Administration*, Vol. 17, Nos. 7 and 8, July-August 1987.

information or data will be necessary for decision making.

Defining researchable problems in this manner requires that the department of nursing's long-term strategic plans outline the type of information that will be needed for policy decisions.

Setting Limits and Guidelines

It is important when research is integrated in the clinical setting that realistic guidelines are set for each individual investigation, either clinical or administrative, in terms of the time frame that the project can be expected to require. Establishing such a time frame in the early stages of the research process allows personnel in the practice setting to understand what can be expected in terms of feedback about the results or involvement in different stages of the research project. Ongoing team meetings about the project allow for all parties to remain involved with the research decisions and to be realistic about the time frame in which the project is progressing.

Where information is available at several key points in the research process, data can be reported as long as they do not bias further data collected within the project. This strategy allows the practice personnel, as well as the researcher, to be aware of the progress of the research findings and to be involved in their interpretation at appropriate points. Finally, it is useful for administrators/clinicians and researchers in the service setting to have negotiated together a set of explicit guidelines for when investigative results will be considered appropriate for use in the practice arena. This strategy curbs the researcher's natural inclination to hedge as well as the practitioner's premature push for the use of inappropriate findings.

Conducting Research

One of the major research programs in a clinical agency, just as in an academic setting, is the actual conduct of scientific investigations. In a clinical setting, purposes for these investigations are usually twofold: the provision of information for long-term practice decisions and policies as well as the generation of knowledge for the discipline.

The investigations are generally multiphased in nature; that is, they consist of a number of phases in the same content area. Two types of substantive research investigations tend to be prominent in clinical settings: health services research and clinical nursing research. Health services or nursing administration research consists of investigations targeted at providing information for administrative decisions and policies. These investigations are often initiated by nurse administrators or head nurses with the intent to study structural or system type variables that impact heavily on the delivery of nursing care.

Investigations that focus on the study of clinical nursing phenomena often reflect questions about the efficacy of nursing interventions and are cost-efficient in terms of producing certain kinds of desired patient outcomes. Nurse managers and staff nurses generally initiate these types of investigations because of recurring clinical issues on their particular units for which there do not seem to be a standardized set of interventions or a well-understood set of alternatives.

The various types of research projects cited are conducted within a collaborative model. A collaborative model involves merging the expertise of the clinician or nurse administrator with the research expertise of the nurse scientist. Staff nurses and nurse administrators are not expected to conduct independent research, but neither is the nurse scientist expected to have the detailed clinical knowledge, although they need to be sensitive to the clinical issues of the project. Integrating the expertise of these various types of people, however, provides a very strong base from which to conduct nursing research.

Using Research

Research findings may be generated by investigations that have been conducted by the organization itself or may be gathered from the research literature of the discipline. The primary focus of research utilization programs is to put into practice, in terms of nursing activities and polices, findings that meet the following criteria: They have been replicated and have been substantiated.

Because of the tailoring that must occur with research findings in order for them to be fully effective within any given clinical agency, the nurse scientist can carry the application of research findings only so far and does have responsibility for making research findings available, understandable, and generalizable across numerous settings. It then becomes the responsibility of nurse administrators and clinicians in practice settings to actually use the results within specific agencies.

Research-Based Practice

Nurse executives must be committed to providing the best care based on the latest in research-based outcomes and on the latest information available for developing financially sound practices.

Using the latest research in practice is often easier said than done. The nurse executive must develop a research surveillance system so that new data are continually assessed and, when valid, implemented in practice. The staff in charge of the various specialty units within the division must be aware of the latest findings presented at national meetings and published in nursing journals. The practice of these units must incorporate the implications drawn from this research.

Research-based staff development programs reinforce this pattern. A departmental newsletter that describes new research, references pertinent articles, and reports on news presented at meetings throughout the nation, encourages a research-based practice.

Source: Barbara Stevens Barnum and Karlene M. Kerfoot, *The Nurse as Executive*, ed 4, Aspen Publishers, Inc., © 1995.

Role of the Nurse Administrator: Initiator, Facilitator, and Implementer of Nursing Research*

As an *initiator*, the nurse administrator participates in or may originate research. As a *facilitator*, the nurse administrator is responsible for supplying resources and encouraging research to take place. As an *implementer*, the nurse administrator operationalizes research findings.

The role in each of these areas of nursing research may vary depending on the setting, contextual management, organizational control, extent of collegial relationships, and preparation and expectation of nurse administrators. The nurse administrator is expected to maximize research to the greatest extent possible regardless of the setting and situation.

Associated Activities

As an initiator, the nurse administrator generates research proposals in nursing practice and nursing administration, including the following activities:

- writing grants
- preserving data for research
- organizing studies of both experimental and nonexperimental nature
- initiating interdisciplinary and intradisciplinary proposals and studies

As a facilitator, the nurse administrator develops an organizational design, including philosophy and structure, in which scientific inquiry is the norm rather than the exception. This includes the following activities:

- providing support for personnel for research, including the generation of grant proposals
- ensuring control in the case of both inter and intradisciplinary efforts and intervening as necessary

---

Source: Copyright © 1982, B.J. Brown and P.J. Chin.

- ensuring nursing's access to and share of technological resources such as computers
- providing time for nursing staff to explore problems needing research as well as for application discussions
- promoting placement of graduate students on human subject review committees
- promoting or creating new coalitions of individuals in practice and education to facilitate research and research application

As an implementer, the nurse administrator evaluates and applies research findings to the practice of nursing. Activities may include the following:

- keeping up-to-date with published research
- evaluating research findings
- functioning as part of a network to identify research in process as well as forming coalitions of nurses to promote research utilization
- promoting research colloquia to explore research findings and their application
- modifying administrative and organizational systems to promote utilization of findings
- applying change theories in the promotion of research findings

Nursing Administration Research Issues*

Nursing administration research includes inquiries into factors that influence the effective and efficient organization and delivery of high-quality nursing service, factors that are particularly important given the harshness of the contemporary health care environment. More specifically, nursing administration research is concerned with establishing the costs of nursing care, with examining the relationships between nursing services and quality patient care, and with viewing problems of nursing service delivery within the broader context of policy analysis

and delivery of health care services. Therefore, nursing administration research can be used to influence health care policy and examine how the organization of care affects patients, the care delivery process, and both patient and organizational outcomes. (See Table 39–1 for an excerpt of the research priorities formulated by the Association of Nurse Executives [AONE].)

Redirecting nursing research to embrace nursing administration research will facilitate comparing the process of care delivery across settings, assist in identifying differences in outcomes in response to changes in the environment, and support a more sophisticated assessment of the care process and the results of care.

PREPARATION FOR NURSING RESEARCH

The Nursing Research Committee*

Through the establishment and support of a nursing research committee, the nurse executive creates an important vehicle to assist staff in developing an appreciation for the merits of nursing research while providing a climate conducive to fostering nursing research.

Specifically, the development of a nursing research committee (NRC) within a clinical agency serves several important purposes for nurse executives. First, research findings generated from well-developed projects can be instrumental in formulating new solutions and approaches in practice to unsolved or persistent problematic situations. Instituting ideas that have been grounded in research can offer new and validated ways for handling difficult and time-consuming problems. Second, the establishment of an NRC dictates the implementation of a systematic process of inquiry to test hypotheses and questions using a logical, analytic, and clearly defined method of investigation. Therefore, results generated through this approach have greater validity and application across clinical disciplines.

*Source: Bonnie Mowinski Jennings, "Nursing Research: A Time for Redirection," *Journal of Nursing Administration*, Vol. 25, No. 4, April 1995, J.B. Lippincott.

*Source: Helene J. Krouse and Suzanne Diffley Holloran, "The Nursing Research Committee," *Journal of Nursing Administration*, Vol. 18, No. 12, December 1988. © 1988 J.B. Lippincott Company.

Table 39–1 AONE Research Priorities for Nursing Administration (Excerpt, 1993–1994)

- What is the impact of significant organizational change (i.e., new reimbursement models, downsizing, acquisitions, or mergers) on clinical and administrative nursing practice?
- What is the cost/quality impact of differing systems of nursing care delivery (primary, modular, team, functional, nursing diagnosis based, case management, etc.)?
- What is the relationship of specific nursing interventions to specific patient outcomes (length of stay, readmission rates, etc.)? What are the cost and quality implications of these interventions?

- What is the cost/quality impact of clinical and nonclinical support services on the professional nursing staff and care delivery systems?
- What is the impact of technology (clinical, managerial, informational) on administrative and clinical nursing practice?
- What factors and data elements contribute to the creation of an effective decision support system for nurse managers?
- What elements are required for the successful redesign of the nurse manager role in contemporary health care environments?

Last and most important, the formation of a functioning NRC acts as a device that enables nurse administrators and executives to present information and make administrative decisions based on facts and clinical findings. Decisions made on the basis of well-substantiated information are more likely to be accepted by clinicians, because they have a history of success as demonstrated in clinical trials. This allows administrators to

- become increasingly comfortable with decisions that they make
- decrease judgments primarily grounded in tradition or ritualistic behaviors
- generate facts that support ideas as demonstrated on smaller projects and pilot studies before general implementation
- use facts together with intuition to guide the development and modification of policies and procedures used within the nursing department

Specific Functions

The NRC within the health care facility functions to strengthen and facilitate clinical nursing research. The NRC can support nursing research in three major ways:

- It establishes a mechanism to assist the researcher and reviewers in preparing and critiquing proposals.

- It contributes to the positive climate of nursing research within the department and throughout the facility by encouraging and soliciting proposals.
- It reviews nursing research proposals for scientific merit and protection of human subjects' rights as well as for feasibility in the organization.

An NRC review should occur in relation to the facility's mandated institutional review process. Once reviewed and changed as recommended, the proposal is approved. An approved proposal receives the support of nursing administration within the agency and is then sent to the institutional review board (IRB). The major thrust of the IRB review is the evaluation of scientific merit and protection of human subjects. Once the proposal is approved by the IRB, steps are taken to implement the study.

A nursing review process serves to complement the IRB process. The researcher contacts the nursing and protocol or research offices at the agency and obtains information and guidelines for preparing the research proposal. The researcher has the responsibility of initiating contact with health care facilities and agencies being considered as data collection sites early in the process. Because time is a critical factor, speaking to nursing administration can be helpful before contacting the IRB. Carefully following the guidelines as an initial step facilitates review and passage of the proposal.

If a facility has an NRC, researchers can request information, preferably written, about the necessary process and forms that must be submitted to institute review boards. In preparing the proposal for review, the researcher should consider (1) professionally preparing the proposal; (2) what reviewers will be looking for in terms of study design and procedure, subjects' time involved, use of staff, and information to be obtained; (3) solicitation of subjects; (4) weaknesses in study design; (5) procedures and implementation of the study; and (6) how the study will enhance nursing's current or future practice and professional development.

The principal role of the reviewer is to give careful and thoughtful review to the researcher's proposal. The reviewer should be allowed approximately three weeks to read the proposal before the scheduled meeting. In reviewing the proposal, the committee member should pay close attention to guidelines or review criteria established by the NRC.

In general, the points and concerns raised by reviewers and nursing administration often help to clarify and strengthen the proposal. Issues raised at the initial review will frequently be brought up later at the IRB if not properly resolved by the researcher. Used properly, members of the NRC can be catalysts for initiation and maintenance of research in the clinical area. The concept of peer review by other clinicians, administrators, educators, and researchers will permit the profession to influence its own destiny regarding research and theory development.

The Institutional Review Board and Human Subjects Review*

Human subjects review refers to the required review process for any research proposal involving the use of human subjects. Over the years the United States Public Health Service (USPHS), the Department of Health, Education,

and Welfare (DHEW), the National Research Act and its Commission for the Protection of Human Subjects of Biomedical and Behavioral Research, and the Department of Health and Human Services (DHHS) have issued reports and guidelines for protecting the rights of human subjects in research. Federal guidelines requiring review of funded studies came in 1966. This development spurred research-conducting institutions to acknowledge their ethical responsibility to protect the rights of human research subjects.

Current Federal Guidelines

Since most nursing studies involve human subjects, nurse researchers need to know that there are federal regulations protecting the rights of human subjects in research. Further, nurses must anticipate that any proposed study will be reviewed according to federal guidelines to ensure that subjects are respected as persons and will have the freedom to participate or not participate, to receive no harm if at all possible, and to be treated fairly. (See Table 39–2.)

How To Prepare for the Human Subjects Review

- Obtain from your local departmental review committee (DRC) or IRB a copy of its procedures or guidelines for human subjects review.
- If possible, obtain a copy of the federal guidelines for protection of human subjects.
- To ensure that you have included all essential elements or requirements, consult local and federal guidelines as you write the methodology section and develop the consent form of your proposal.
- If you intend to apply to an organization other than your own for funding of the project, or if you plan to collect data at multiple sites, each of which requires its own DRC or IRB review, contact those agencies and ask for their procedures and guidelines for human subjects review. Use these guidelines in developing your proposal.

---

*Source: Daniel W. Tetting, "Preparing for the Human Subjects Review," *Critical Care Nursing Quarterly*, Vol. 12, No. 4, Aspen Publishers, Inc., © 1990.

Table 39–2 Basic Requirements for Studies Involving Human Subjects

For local IRBs to approve research involving human subjects, a proposal must ensure that seven major requirements are met.

- The study will minimize risks to subjects by using procedures that are consistent with established research designs.
- The risks to subjects will be reasonably outweighed by the anticipated benefits and the importance of the knowledge that may reasonably be expected to result.
- Selection of subjects will be equitable, taking into consideration the purpose and setting of the research.

- Informed consent will be documented according to requirements, and records will be maintained.
- Informed consent will be obtained from each potential subject or the subject's legally authorized representative.
- The research plan will include provisions for monitoring the data collected to ensure the safety of subjects.
- There should be plans to protect the privacy of subjects, to maintain confidentiality of information given by subjects and obtained during the course of the study.

Source: Protection of Human Subjects (45 CFR 46) *Code of Federal Regulations.* Washington, DC: U.S. Department of Health and Human Services publication 0-406-756, 1983.

- Find out specifically if your proposed project must undergo a total or an expedited review. Obtain a list of research categories that are exempted. This information should be included in your institution's procedures or guidelines. If it is not, ask for it from the chairperson of the DRC or IRB that will be reviewing your proposal.
- Obtain copies of previously approved projects and look at their sections on human subjects and consent forms. Use these as examples or models to follow.
- Locate other successful researchers; seek their advice.
- Ask local DRC or IRB committee members for assistance or advice.
- Prepare your materials according to federal guidelines. If you do, you can be reasonably confident that you have included everything, and local approval should therefore be easily obtained.
- If total review (nonexempt) is anticipated, offer or request to attend the DRC or IRB committee meeting at which your proposal will be discussed so that you can provide clarifying information.
- When you have successfully negotiated the human subjects review, offer to share your work and experiences with others.

- Last, offer to serve on a DRC or IRB as a member; it will be an excellent learning experience.

Misconduct and Fraud*

The potential for misconduct and fraud is always present during research activities. Data may be fabricated (a practice known as "drylabbing"), or manipulated ("trimming"), or interpreted so that one hypothesis is favored over others (a process called "cooking"). If the researcher enrolls ineligible subjects in a study, false data may result. If research data are misappropriated, their ownership misrepresented, or interpretations improperly reported and acknowledged, charges of plagiarism may be leveled. All of these activities are considered scientific misconduct or fraud because they are deviations from accepted practices in proposing, carrying out, or reporting results from research.

To ensure the integrity of nursing research, the community of nurse researchers must do the following:

Source: Sara T. Fry, "Outlook on Ethics—Ethical Issues in Research: Scientific Misconduct and Fraud," *Nursing Outlook,* November-December 1990.

- Carry out funded studies with accuracy and with an adequate "audit trail."
- Closely supervise graduate students, postdoctoral students, and other faculty associated with funded studies.
- Remain knowledgeable about misconduct policies in their schools and institutions.
- Teach the ethical requirements of research activities to the next generation of nurse researchers through course content and by example.

Data fabrication, plagiarism, falsification of data, and deviation from accepted research practices are clear indications of scientific misconduct. However, sloppy recordkeeping, duplicate or selective reporting of research results, honorary authorship of publications, and the underreporting of research results are equally serious and may qualify as scientific misconduct in some instances. Nurse researchers will need to conduct research activities very carefully in order to meet their moral obligation to contribute to patient well-being. They also need to carefully consider their obligations to report reliable research results and to conduct research according to acceptable standards recognized by the community of nurse researchers.

Appendix A

Management Tools for Scheduling Activities

GANTT CHART

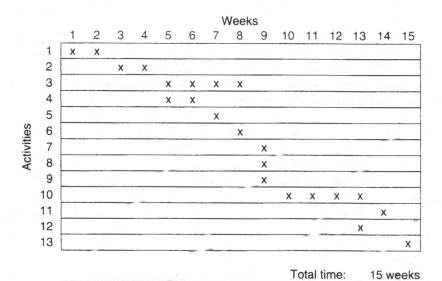

The Gantt chart is a graph with activities listed on the vertical axis and time units on the horizontal axis. It is used to determine the shortest total time required to reach a goal by showing how much time each activity requires and which activities can and cannot be performed simultaneously. In the chart note the overlapping of several of the activities.

PERT CHART

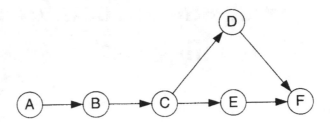

PERT (program evaluation and review technique) charts were developed to minimize and control the time required for large projects. The PERT chart is composed of activities and events. Events are represented by circles. Arrows show the time necessary to complete events. When there are steps that are carried out simultaneously, different times are needed for each of these parallel steps. In the PERT chart above, the lines could represent the following steps:

A–B	=	time for request to reach a work station
B–C	=	time for blood collection and delivery to laboratory
C–D	=	time for serological testing
D–E	=	time for immunohematological testing
E–F	=	time for delivery of blood product to patient

The critical path represents the sum of the times for individual steps in the path that require the most time. In the chart, the critical path is A–B–C–D–F because it takes longer to perform the serological tests than to do the routine compatibility tests.

Source: William Umiker, *Management Skills for the New Health Care Supervisor*, ed 2, Aspen Publishers, Inc., © 1994.

Appendix B

Management Tools for Planning

The main purpose of these planning tools is to help the members of a quality improvement team work together toward a quality goal and to help focus their activities. The set of seven management planning tools aids groups in generating and organizing verbal (non-numerical) information, ideas, concepts, intuition, attributes, descriptions of tasks, and so forth.

The tools are pictorial in nature—a key feature—and therefore the set of seven management planning tools makes the methods of systematic planning accessible to all members. Although they are shown as individual entities, the tools are most powerful when used as an integrated set. They can help planning groups move forward together based on verbal knowledge, and they therefore complement the traditional statistical tools of quality management. Decisions made using this set of tools can help a team or committee analyze ideas and verbal information and compile them into coherent pictures that all members can understand. These idea-based pictures may help define areas where the committee can collect and analyze new data to verify its thinking.

Source: Paul E. Plsek, "Tutorial: Management and Planning Tools of TQM," *Quality Management in Health Care,* Vol. 1, No. 3, Aspen Publishers, Inc., © Spring 1993.

TOOL 1: AFFINITY DIAGRAM

☐ *Description.* An affinity diagram is a group brainstorming and organizing technique that results in a picture displaying ideas that were randomly generated and written on individual pieces of paper and then sorted into categories based on natural relationships among the ideas.

☐ *Application.* The affinity diagram is most useful when facts or thoughts are voluminous and seemingly chaotic—a typical situation at the beginning of most planning tasks. The brainstorming allows everyone to participate freely, while the silent grouping allows new patterns of information to emerge by postponing the critical thinking that tends to mold information into preconceived patterns. Finally, the process of naming the groups establishes a common understanding among team members of the central themes reflected in the collection of their ideas.

**Affinity diagram showing brainstormed ideas
grouped under headers that capture the central themes**

TOOL 2: RELATIONS DIAGRAM

☐ *Description.* A relations diagram (also known as an interrelationship digraph or ID) documents the complex cause-and-effect relationships among items to lead to better understanding. The items under discussion might be the result of an earlier affinity diagram exercise or some other brainstorming technique.

☐ *Application.* The relations diagram is useful when causal relationships are complex and not well quantified or when priorities and starting points for action are unclear. Again, these two conditions often apply in the early phases of planning and leadership tasks. The result of the planning team's work is a common understanding of the factors that seem to drive the causal system and insight into ways to measure the overall performance of that system.

**Relations diagram showing relationships within a
complex system of causes and effects**

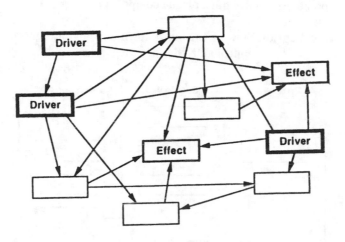

TOOL 3: TREE DIAGRAM

☐ *Description.* A tree diagram (also known as a systematic diagram) starts with an end result to be attained and then describes in increasing detail the full range of tasks that contribute to that result. Graphically, it resembles an organization chart or family tree.

☐ *Application.* The tool is best used when the team feels the need to "really get down to details" following the free flow of broad ideas that occurs in constructing an affinity or relations diagram. It is important to note that the tree diagram simply maps out activities and categories; it does not evaluate the relative importance of these, nor indicate how to allocate resources. (The matrix diagram tool—Tool 4—can help address this need.) The group effort needed to construct the tree diagram ensures that there are no major gaps in the planning team's thinking about what needs to be done and that, in the end, the people working on individual tasks will be able to see how what they are doing fits into the bigger picture. Seasoned organizational leaders might recognize from past experience that gaps in thinking and lack of a broad perspective often plague complex planning efforts.

Tree diagram showing the breakdown of a goal into more detailed activities or categories

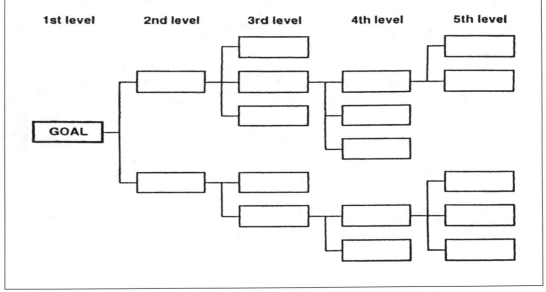

TOOL 4: MATRIX DIAGRAM

☐ *Description.* The term *matrix diagram* is a generic name for any of a broad class of tables that use rows and columns to hold information about relationships between items in lists. Planning teams can use matrix diagrams employing symbols (rather than numbers) to indicate subjective relationships. These planning matrices can take forms that go beyond the simple two-by-two table columns. There are five generic matrix formats—the L, T, Y, X, and C matrix shapes—that can be used to show relationships among two to four lists of items.

☐ *Application.* Like tree diagrams, matrix diagrams are most useful in the middle phases of a planning effort, when it is necessary to get down to specifics following the freewheeling, high-level discussions that often accompany the construction of affinity and relations diagrams. The key benefit of using a matrix diagram is that it allows a planning team to work simultaneously at the level of the detailed tasks and the level of the overall system of tasks.

T-shaped matrix diagram showing relationships among tasks, project success criteria, and involved departments

Dept 1	Dept 2	Dept 3	Dept 4		Criteria 1	Criteria 2	Criteria 3	Criteria 4	Criteria 5
	◎	△		Task 1					
	◎			Task 2			◎		△
	◎	△	△	Task 3	△	◎		◎	
△		△	◎	Task 4	◎			△	
△	◎			Task 5		◎	◎	◎	
	◎	△		Task 6	◎		◎	◎	

Key: ◎ Strongly related.   △ Somewhat related.

TOOL 5: MATRIX DATA ANALYSIS

☐ *Description.* Matrix data analysis is a way of summarizing and identifying key factors in a large array of data. The technique relies on a multivariate statistical method known as principle-component analysis. Calculations often require the use of a computer. Matrices depend on the data fed to the computer.

☐ *Application.* A planning committee could use matrix data analysis to help it analyze patterns in complex market, competitor, and patient demographic data. But the committee would likely require the services of an in-house analytical market researcher, statistician, or consultant to lead it through the analysis.

TOOL 6: PROCESS DECISION PROGRAM CHART

☐ *Description.* The process decision program chart (PDPC) maps out conceivable but undesirable events in a plan and indicates appropriate responses. The completed chart resembles a tree diagram.

☐ *Application.* The PDPC is typically used near the end of a planning effort as a final check of potentially problematic elements of an implementation plan.

Process decision program chart used to develop contingency plans

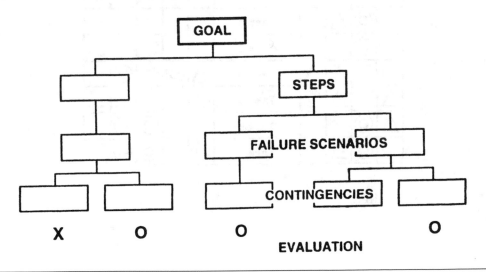

TOOL 7: ACTIVITY NETWORK DIAGRAM

☐ *Description.* The activity network diagram is a flowchart with an additional twist. The diagram shows the sequence of tasks required to accomplish some objective (like a flowchart), but it adds time estimates for each task. By adding the time estimates, a planning team can define start and completion dates, identify the critical path of activities that dictate the minimum total time required to accomplish the objective, manage the slack time resulting from tasks done in parallel, and monitor progress toward the objective.

☐ *Application.* The activity network diagram is one of the last planning tools that a team might use. The activity network diagram is most helpful when an implementation objective is clear, the set of tasks needed to accomplish the objective is easily identified, the time needed to complete each task can be estimated, and schedules are critical.

Activity network diagram showing the critical path of the series of activities that dictate the minimum total time needed to accomplish the objective

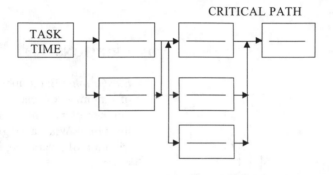

Note: It is important to understand that, while the seven tools provide a way to make use of verbal information and intuition, they should not be taken as license to ignore the need for data and facts. These tools are intended to comple- ment, not replace, the traditional data analysis tools of quality management. Wherever practical, planning teams should seek to gather data to confirm the subjective relationships documented in the various management and planning tools.

Appendix C

Tools for All Stages of Data Gathering

DIAGRAMS

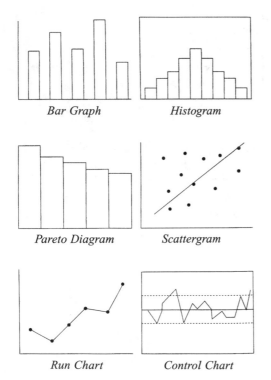

Bar Graph   Histogram

Pareto Diagram   Scattergram

Run Chart   Control Chart

DESCRIPTIONS

- *Bar Graphs:* Bar graphs display the values of a number of related items, such as the number of patient visits on each day of the month. When a bar graph shows the distribution of a variance, it is called a histogram.
- *Pareto Diagrams:* Pareto charts display the frequency of occurrences listed in order of importance or frequency.
- *Scattergrams:* A scattergram shows the correlation between two variables.
- *Run Charts:* Run charts plot data over periods of time. They exhibit trends, cycles, or other patterns in a process (e.g., attendance records, turnover, or customer complaints).
- *Control Charts:* Control charts illustrate values that are either in control or out of control. In the chart, the solid horizontal line represents an average or normal value. The spaces between the solid line and the dotted lines are acceptable values, usually plus or minus two or three standard deviations. Any value outside the dotted lines is an out of control value.

Source: William Umiker, *Management Skills for the New Health Care Supervisor*, ed 2, Aspen Publishers, Inc., © 1994.

Appendix D

Tools for Analytical Stages

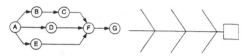

Flowchart *Cause-and-Effect Diagram*

Pie Chart *Gaussian Curve Chart*

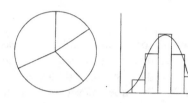

Force Field of Lewin

Test/Procedure	May Perform	Date/ Supervisor
Ova and parasites	✔	5/31/9_ SH
Clotting time	✔	5/30/9_ SH
Lee White clotting time	✔	5/30/9_ SH
Hema, QC	✔	5/30/9_ SH
Hema, PM	✔	5/30/9_ SH
Sed rate	✔	5/31/9_ SH
Sperm count	✔	5/31/9_ SH
Urinalysis	✔	5/30/9_ SH
Pregnancy test	✔	5/30/9_ SH
Urinalysis QC	✔	5/31/9_ SH
PT	✔	5/31/9_ SH
RPR	✔	5/31/9_ SH

Checklist

DESCRIPTIONS

- *Flowcharts:* A flowchart represents a series of steps or events arranged chronologically.

- *Cause-and-Effect Diagrams:* Also known as fishbone charts, these devices are useful in an early stage of problem solving or when one is considering potential problems. A cause-and-effect diagram forces a focus on potential causes. On each leg (fishbone), possible factors are recorded and grouped according to different categories (e.g., process, human, equipment, or policies).

- *Pie Charts:* Pie charts illustrate relative numbers or percentages.

- *Gaussian Curve Charts:* The bell-shaped curves show frequency distributions. These are among the most common quality control charts.

- *Force Field Charts:* When one is considering the advantages and disadvantages of a new service, process, procedure, or piece of equipment, the opposing considerations can be illustrated and quantified by a force field chart.

- *Checklists:* Checklists are used as reminders or for documentation of activities. Shopping lists, daily "to do" schedules, and validation of records are just a few uses for this ubiquitous tool. Shown here is a partial list of tests that a new laboratory technician must be qualified to perform.

Source: William Umiker, *Management Skills for the New Health Care Supervisor*, ed 2, Aspen Publishers, Inc., © 1994.

Statistics: Descriptive Measures of Distribution Parameters

PART I—MEASURES OF CENTRAL TENDENCY

Measures of central tendency are useful in reporting the results of quality improvement (QI) studies. Data points often cluster around a central value that is between two extreme values of the variable under study. A measure of central tendency describes this center of a distribution of data points. The measures of central tendency are the mean, median, and mode.

Mean

The mean is a reliable and stable measure of central tendency. The mean is the sum of all scores divided by the number of scores.

Median

The median is the preferred method of locating the center of skewed distributions.

The median is the middle-most score in a distribution, or the score above and below which one half of all scores fall.

The median for an odd number of measurements is the middle measurement when the values are arranged in ascending or descending order. If the total number of scores is even, the median is the sum of the two middle values divided by two.

Mode

The mode is the score that occurs with the greatest frequency. It is the most easily determined measure of central tendency because it can be obtained by inspection rather than computation. For example, if nine units reported blood transfusion errors in one year as 5, 9, 3, 5, 7, 2, and 5, then the mode is 5. In a frequency histogram, the mode is the class with the highest frequency.

PART II—MEASURES OF VARIABILITY

In reporting QI data, there is a need not only to describe the center of the distribution, but also its spread. Two distributions can have the same means, but have different variabilities. Although

Source: Divina Grossman and Janice Neubauer, "Basic Statistical Concepts in Quality Improvement," *Journal of Nursing Care Quality*, Vol. 6, No. 1, Aspen Publishers, Inc., © July 1992.

a mean falls within an acceptable standard, the range of variability may show that a problem exists.

Range

The range is the simplest and most straight-forward measure of variability. It is the difference between the highest and the lowest scores in a distribution. If there is one extreme score in the distribution, the range will appear large. Hence, the range is a highly unstable index and cannot provide a precise measure of variability. At best, it can only be used as a crude or preliminary index of dispersion.

Standard Deviation

Standard deviation measures the average variability in a distribution. The following formula is used in computing the standard deviation:

$$S = \sqrt{\frac{\Sigma(X-\overline{X})^2}{N-1}}$$

The standard deviation measures the average deviation from the mean. The greater the variability around the mean of a distribution, the larger the standard deviation. Thus, the standard deviation indicates how variable the scores in a data set are.

Statistical Terms and Formulas

Terms	Formulas

ADMISSION

Hospital patient
An individual receiving, in person, hospital-based or coordinated medical services for which the hospital is responsible.

Inpatient admission
The formal acceptance by a hospital of a patient who is to be provided with room, board, and continuous nursing service in an area of the hospital where patients generally stay at least overnight.

Number of patients in the hospital
at midnight April 29 535
Plus ...... Number of patients admitted
April 30 .... +30
565

Hospital inpatient
A hospital patient who is provided with room, board, and continuous general nursing service in an area of the hospital where patients generally stay at least overnight.

Minus ..... Patients discharged (including
deaths) April 30 .... −18
Patients in hospital at 12 AM
(midnight) April 30 547

Inpatient census
The number of inpatients present at any one time.

Plus ...... Patients both admitted and discharged (including deaths) on
April 30 .... +3

Daily inpatient census
The number of inpatients present at the census-taking time each day, plus any inpatients who were both admitted and discharged after the census-taking time the previous day.

Inpatient census (inpatient service
days) April 30 550

Source: Kathleen A. Waters and Gretchen F. Murphy, *Medical Records in Health Information,* Aspen Publishers, Inc., 1979. The information has been adapted from Edna K. Huffman, *Medical Records Management,* Physicians Record Company Publisher, 1972; *Glossary of Medical Terms,* American Medical Record Association, 1974; and Candace Dillman, RRA, who designed the section on "Psychiatric Survival Rates" for use in the Alaska Psychiatric Institute.

Terms	Formulas

Inpatient service day (also called census day)
A unit of measure denoting the services received by one inpatient in one 24-hour period.

Example of Care Unit Breakdown: — Intensive Care Unit Inpatient Service Days

Census .... Patients remaining midnight April 29 8
Plus ...... Patients admitted April 30 ...... +1
Plus ...... Patients transferred on unit from another unit in hospital .... +1
Minus .... Patients discharged .... −0
Minus .... Patients died .... −2
Minus .... Patients transferred off unit to another unit in hospital .... −1
Midnight census April 30 7
Plus ...... Patients both admitted and discharged on April 30 .... +1
(These patients have already been counted as admission and discharges or deaths. However, since their patient days have been canceled out by adding them as admissions and subtracting them as discharges, they must be added again to determine the inpatient service days on this unit.)

Total inpatient service days (also called census days)
The sum of all inpatient service days for each of the days in the period under consideration. Notice it is the numerator in the formula.

The formula to obtain the average daily inpatient census for a whole hospital is:

$$\frac{\text{Total inpatient service days for a period}}{\text{Total number of days in the period}}$$

Average daily inpatient census
Average number of inpatients present each day for a given period of time. This is always calculated by a formula such as indicated in the example.

The average daily inpatient census (average daily census) for newborn inpatients is generally reported separately. When it is, the following formula is used to determine the average daily inpatient census excluding newborns:

$$\frac{\text{Total inpatient service days (excluding newborns) for a period}}{\text{Total number of days in the period}}$$

Inpatient bed occupancy ratio
The proportion of inpatient beds occupied, defined as the ratio of inpatient service days to inpatient bed count days in the period under consideration.

Synonymous terms: percent occupancy, occupancy percent, percentage of occupancy, occupancy ratio

$$\frac{\text{Total inpatient service days for a period} \times 100}{\text{Total inpatient bed count days} \times \text{number of days in the period}}$$

Example: A hospital has an inpatient bed count (bed complement) of 150 (excluding the newborn bassinet count of 15). During April, the hospital rendered 3,650 inpatient service days to adults and children. April has 30 days. According to the formula, this is $(3,650 \times 100) \div (150 \times 30) = 365,000 \div 4,500 = 81.11\%$. Therefore, the inpatient bed occupancy percentage for April was 81.1%, or 81%.

Terms	Formulas

EVENTS DURING HOSPITAL STAY

Transfer (intrahospital)
A change in medical care unit, medical staff unit, or responsible physician of an inpatient during hospitalization.

Not applicable

Adjunct diagnostic or therapeutic unit
  (ancillary unit)
An organized unit of a hospital, other than an operating room, delivery room, or medical care unit, with facilities and personnel to aid physicians in the diagnosis and treatment of patients through the performance of diagnostic or therapeutic procedures.

Not applicable

Medical consultation
The response by one member of the medical staff to a request for consultation by another member of the medical staff, characterized by review of the patient's history, examination of the patient, and completion of a consultation report giving recommendations and/or opinions.

Consultations may be viewed from two perspectives.

1. Total consultations rendered. This may be used to show specialty activity, such as the total number of psychiatric consultations rendered by the psychiatric service.

2. The percentage of consultations rendered per patients treated in the hospital. The formula for this would be:

$$\frac{\text{Total number of patients receiving consultations} \times 100}{\text{Total number of patients discharged and died for the period}}$$

Surgical operation
One or more surgical procedures performed at one time for one patient via a common approach or for a common purpose.

The formula approved by the Joint Commission on Accreditation of Healthcare Organizations for computing the postoperative infection rate is:

$$\frac{\text{Number of infections in clean surgical cases for a period} \times 100}{\text{Number of surgical operations for the period}}$$

Complication
An additional diagnosis that describes a condition arising after the beginning of hospital observation and treatment and modifying the course of the patient's illness or the medical care required.

Usually calculated in a rate only in infection cases, since the formula above clearly assigns the source of the complication.

Hospital live birth
The complete expulsion or extraction from the mother, in a hospital facility, of a product of conception, irrespective of the duration of pregnancy, which after such separation breathes or shows any other evidence of life such as beating of the heart, pulsation of the umbilical cord, or definite movement of voluntary muscles, whether or not the umbilical cord has been cut or the placenta is attached; each product of such a birth is considered live born.

Live births may be classified according to the birth weight:
  1,000 grams (2 pounds, 3 ounces) or less
  1,001 grams to 2,500 grams (5 pounds, 8 ounces)
  over 2,500 grams.

Hospital Caesarean section rate
Hospital Caesarean section rate is the ratio of Caesarean sections performed to deliveries. For statistical purposes, when a delivery results in a multiple birth, it is counted as one delivery.

Formula:

$$\frac{\text{Total number of Caesarean sections performed in a period} \times 100}{\text{Total number of deliveries in the period}}$$

Terms	Formulas

Inpatient discharge
The termination of a period of inpatient hospitalization through the formal release of the inpatient by the hospital.

Discharge transfer
The disposition of an inpatient to another health care institution at the time of discharge.

Length of stay (for one inpatient)
The number of calendar days from admission to discharge.

Admit Jan 20
Disch Jan 24

Calculation:

$$\begin{array}{r} 24 \\ -20 \\ \hline \text{Disch days} = 4 \end{array}$$

or

Admit Jan 20
Disch Feb 14

$$\begin{array}{rl} \text{Total days in} & \\ \text{Jan} & 31 \\ & -20 \\ \hline \text{days in Jan} & = 11 \\ \text{days in Feb} & +14 \\ \hline \text{Disch days} & =25 \end{array}$$

The length of an inpatient's hospitalization is considered to be one day if he or she is admitted and discharged the same day and also if he or she is admitted one day and discharged the next day.

Total length of stay (for all inpatients)
The sum-of-the-days stay of any group of inpatients discharged during a specified period of time.

Total duration (discharge days) of inpatient hospitalization (including deaths; excluding newborns)

Average length of stay
The average length of hospitalization of inpatients discharged during the period under consideration.

$$\frac{\text{Total duration (discharge days) of inpatient hospitalization (including deaths; excluding newborns)}}{\text{Total discharges (including deaths; excluding newborns)}}$$

Gross death rate

$$\frac{\text{Total number of deaths (including newborns) for a period} \times 100}{\text{Total number of discharges (including deaths and newborn deaths) for the period}}$$

Net death rate (also called institutional death rate)

$$\frac{\text{Total number of deaths (including newborns) minus those under 48 hours for a period} \times 100}{\text{Total number of discharges (including deaths and newborns) minus deaths under 48 hours for the period}}$$

Postoperative death rate

$$\frac{\text{Total number of deaths within 10 days postoperative for a period} \times 100}{\text{Total number of patients operated on for the period}}$$

Maternal death rate

$$\frac{\text{Total number of maternal deaths for a period} \times 100}{\text{Total number of maternal (obstetrical) discharges (including deaths) for the period}}$$

Anesthesia death rate

$$\frac{\text{Total number of deaths caused by anesthetic agents for a period} \times 100}{\text{Total number of anesthetics administered for the period}}$$

Hospital fetal death
Death prior to the complete expulsion or extraction from its mother, in a hospital facility, of a product of conception, irrespective of the duration of pregnancy; death is indicated by the fact that after such separation, the fetus does not breathe or show any other evidence of life such as beating of the heart, pulsation of the umbilical cord, or definite movement of voluntary muscles.

Early: Less than 20 complete weeks of gestation (500 grams or less)

Intermediate: 20 completed weeks of gestation, but less than 28 (501 to 1,000 grams)

Late: 28 completed weeks of gestation and over (1,001 grams and over)

Usually only intermediate and late fetal deaths are included.

Terms	Formulas
Abortion Abortion is the expulsion or extraction of all (complete) or any part (incomplete) of the placenta or membranes, without an identifiable fetus or with a live-born infant or a stillborn infant weighing less than 500 grams. In the absence of known weight, an estimated length of gestation of less than 20 completed weeks (139 days) is calculated from the first day of the last normal menstrual period.	$$\frac{\text{Total number of intermediate and/or late fetal deaths for a period} \times 100}{\text{Total number of births (including intermediate and late fetal deaths) for the period}}$$
Gross autopsy rate ────── The ratio during any given period of time of all inpatient autopsies of all inpatient deaths.	$$\frac{\text{Total inpatient autopsies for a given period} \times 100}{\text{Total inpatient deaths for the period}}$$
Net autopsy rate ────── The ratio during any given period of time of all inpatient autopsies to all inpatient deaths minus unautopsied coroner's or medical examiner's cases.	$$\frac{\text{Total inpatient autopsies for a given period} \times 100}{\text{Total inpatient deaths minus unautopsied coroner's or medical examiner's cases}}$$
Hospital autopsy rate (adjusted) ────── The proportion of deaths of hospital patients following which the bodies of the deceased persons are available for autopsy and hospital autopsies are performed.	$$\frac{\text{Total hospital autopsies} \times 100}{\text{Number of deaths of hospital patients whose bodies are available for hospital autopsy}}$$

SPECIAL NEEDS

Psychiatric survival rates
The monthly statistics provided to staff gave no information as to how long a patient was able to function independently.

This formula was created when it became evident that staff were being discouraged by the high reported readmission rate, in spite of additions to staff and improved therapy programs.

The use of survival time statistics demonstrated two factors to administration that were then used to revise procedures:

- The survival time for which patients were functioning without support was increased with each discharge.
- There was no evidence that outpatient visits increased the survival time between hospitalizations. (Patients were returning due to attachments to staff.)

A program was developed to introduce outpatient clinic staff to patients and create attachments to the appropriate staff prior to discharge to reduce dependency on the patient facility.

Admission date
− discharge date of last visit = Survival time

$$\frac{\text{Cumulative survival time for all patients for the period using outpatient clinics}}{\text{Total number of admissions for the period}} = \begin{array}{l}\text{Average survival}\\\text{rate of patients}\\\text{using clinics}\end{array}$$

$$\frac{\text{Cumulative survival time for all patients for the period not using outpatient clinics}}{\text{Total number of admissions for the period}} = \begin{array}{l}\text{Average survival}\\\text{rate of patients}\\\textit{not}\text{ using clinics}\end{array}$$

Index